THE OBSTETRICIAN'S ARMAMENTARIUM

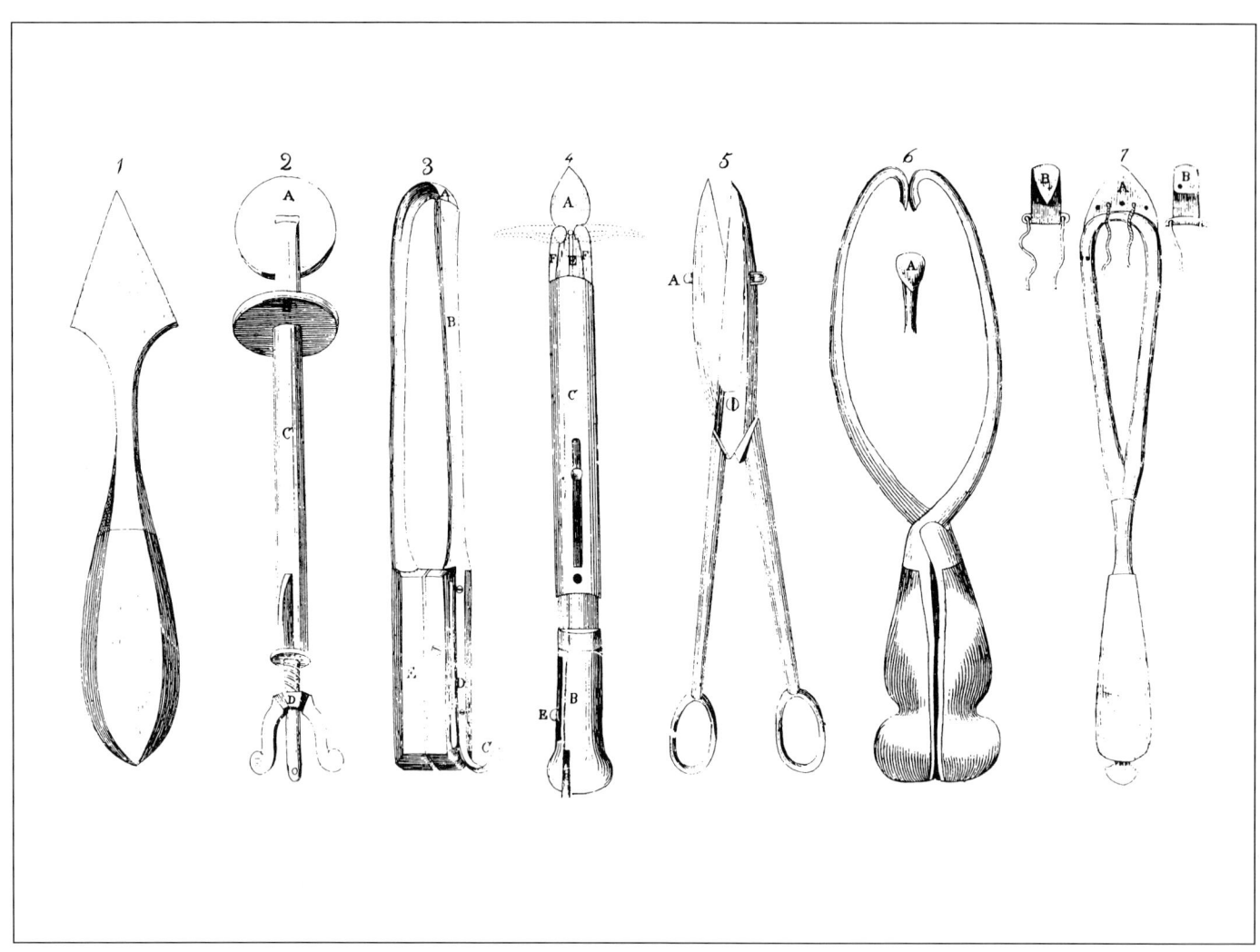

An assortment of instruments from Aitken, *Principles of Midwifery, or Puerperal Medicine*. For details, see figure 18.20 on page 226.

THE OBSTETRICIAN'S ARMAMENTARIUM

Historical Obstetric Instruments and Their Inventors

BRYAN HIBBARD

MD (London), PhD (Liverpool), FRCOG, FRANZCOG (Hon)

Best wishes to Don from Bryan Hibbard

San Anselmo, California   Norman Publishing   2000

Copyright ©2000 by Bryan Hibbard

All rights reserved. No part of this publication may be reproduced, stored in a retrieval system, or transmitted, in any form or by any means, electronic, mechanical, photocopying, recording, or otherwise, without the prior written approval of the publishers, except in the case of brief quotations embodied in critical articles and reviews.

Library of Congress Cataloging-in-Publication Data

Hibbard, Bryan M.

    The obstetrician's armamentarium : historical obstetric instruments and their inventors / by Bryan Hibbard.

    p.   cm.

    Includes bibliographical references and index.

    ISBN 0-930405-80-3 (alk. paper)

    1. Obstetrics—Instruments—History. 2. Medical instruments and apparatus—History. 3. Surgical instruments and apparatus—History.

    I. Title

    [DNLM: 1. Obstetric Surgical Procedures—instrumentation. 2. Surgical Instruments—history. WQ 11.1 H6240 1999]

    RG103.H53 1999

    618.2' .0028—dc21

    DNLM/DLC

    for Library of Congress   99-36288

                                          CIP

This book is printed on acid-free paper and its binding materials have been chosen for strength and durability.

Norman Obstetrics and Gynecology Series, No. 4

Manufactured in the United States of America.

Copies may be ordered from:
NORMAN PUBLISHING
normanpublishing.com
e-mail: orders@jnorman.com
1-800-544-9359
343 San Anselmo Avenue
San Anselmo, California 94960
Mailing address:
P. O. Box 2566
San Anselmo, California 94979

CONTENTS

Preface viii

Introduction   The Sixteenth Century and Before: Decoctions, Destruction, and Divine Intervention   1

1. The Chamberlens and the Origins of Obstetric Forceps   9
2. The Secret Emerges: The Early Eighteenth Century   22
3. Smellie and Levret: Trend Setters for the Late Eighteenth Century   33
4. British Man-Midwives and Their Conservatism: Late Eighteenth-Century, Early Nineteenth-Century Practice   45
5. The Evolution of European Forceps from the Late Eighteenth to the Mid Nineteenth Century   59
6. The British Renaissance of the Nineteenth Century   79
7. American Forceps of the Nineteenth Century   98
8. Hinged and Detachable Handles and Blades and Other Articulations   109
9. Antero-Posterior and Asymmetric Forceps   126
10. Noncrossed, or Parallel, Forceps   136
11. Aids to Traction (*Tractions mécaniques*) and Dynamometers   150
12. Early Axis-Traction Forceps and Their Precursors   160
13. Tarnier Axis-Traction Forceps and Their Modifications   170
14. Other Axis-Traction Forceps and Attachments   185
15. Vacuum Extractors   195
16. Fillets, Levers, and Other Nondestructive Extractors   199
17. Metreurynters and Cervical Dilators: Induction and Augmentation of Labor   213
18. Perforators and Extractors   219
19. Comminutors and Comminutor-Extractors   234
20. Embryotomy   254
21. Symphysiotomy and Pubiotomy   260
22. Pelvimetry   265

Appendix: Measurements of 17th-Early 20th Century Forceps in the RCOG Collection   275

Bibliography   283

Illustration Credits and Sources/Acknowledgments   303

Index   305

PREFACE

*"If no use is to be made of the labours of
past ages, the world must remain always
in the infancy of knowledge."*
JOHNSON

There are many well-known collections of obstetric instruments but perhaps the greatest excitement and pleasure comes from discovering the unknown or forgotten. Such was the case when in 1960 I retrieved from storage the Briggs Collection that is housed in the Department of Obstetrics and Gynaecology at the University of Liverpool and catalogued and restored them, stimulated by an old friend and expert in the field from Melbourne, the late Dr. Frank Forster. Many years later my latent interest was reawakened when the opportunity came to undertake the same task at the Royal College of Obstetricians and Gynaecologists, where the museum had been dismantled several years previously. As soon as the museum reopened new donations came from many sources, notably the Radford collection from the Department of Obstetrics and Gynaecology, St. Mary's Hospital, Manchester, which had disappeared when the hospital had been rebuilt; it was found subsequently in a cellar. Here was a real treasure trove including, unexpectedly, a set of David Davis's instruments as depicted in his *Elements of Operative Midwifery* of 1825. This led to the unearthing of a neglected collection at University College London, where Davis had been the first professor of midwifery and diseases of women and children and included two pairs of experimental forceps that had never been described in the literature, designed by Davis and bearing his name. Such are examples of the serendipity and of the interest of many colleagues that resulted in the stimulus to write this book.

After outlining events prior to the sixteenth century I have attempted to trace the gradual evolution and development of obstetric instruments up to the end of the nineteenth century, highlighting seminal contributions at different phases. Each section centers on representative developments of the period and the men primarily responsible for innovations, setting these in the medicosocial context of the time.

The twentieth century has brought so many developments, particularly in the broader aspects of operative obstetrics and in the involvement of other disciplines, that a different approach would be needed to chronicle these matters and would be more appropriately dealt with separately, as would the history of Caesarian section. It is for these reasons that I have drawn the line at the end of the nineteenth century.

I have tried to cover the field fully without being too exhaustive. For a comprehensive cataloguing of obstetric forceps I would not attempt to compete with Das whose classical work *Obstetric Forceps: Its History and Evolution*, published in 1929, contained details of about six hundred different designs. One of the other major sources derives from a *conversazione* organized by the Obstetrical Society of London and held at the Royal College of Physicians in 1866, at which there was an extensive exhibition of mainly nineteenth-century British and European obstetrical instruments. The material was well catalogued by A. Meadows, with illustrations, in the 1867 publication, *Catalogue and Report of Obstetrical and Other Instruments Exhibited at the Conversazione of the Obstetrical Society of London*. This work has become a key reference source for mid mid-nineteenth-century instruments. Many of these instruments became incorporated into the collection of the museum of the Obstetrical Society of London, the contents of which became the property of the Royal Society of Medicine, who in turn presented it as a loan collection to the Royal College of Surgeons of England in 1912. Alban Doran recatalogued the collection and the other obstetric instruments in the Royal College of Surgeons in considerable detail. His descriptive catalogue was not illustrated but several pairs of forceps were illustrated in the guide to the museum published in 1929 and Doran also published a number of illustrated articles on various of the instruments. Regrettably this outstanding collection was almost totally destroyed by bombing during the Second World War. I acknowledge my debt to these writers in particular and to all the other great chroniclers of the past referred to in the text.

Wherever possible I have referred back to the original material and the great majority of the references cited are accessible in one or more of three major collections in London. For help in tracing the literature I am particularly indebted to Miss Pat Want, Librarian at the Royal College of Obstetricians and Gynaecologists, whose extensive knowledge of and dedication to the historical literature of obstetrics and gynecology is unique. Her willing help and guidance has greatly eased my task.

The other major sources have been the libraries of the Royal Society of Medicine and of the Wellcome Institute for the History of Medicine. I am greatly indebted to the librarians and staff of these institutions. The Thackray Medical Museum in Leeds holds a unique collection of surgical instrument catalogues and Alan Humphries has given me considerable help. Other sources of significant material have been the Ryland collection in the University of Manchester and the libraries of the British Medical Association, the Royal College of Surgeons of England, and the Royal College of Physicians of London.

The illustrations are taken mainly from the original publications of the authors; from the photographic collection of the instruments at the Royal College of Obstetricians and Gynaecologists, which I have assembled over the years and which includes, *inter alia,* two hundred pairs of obstetric forceps; and from The Wellcome Collection now held by the National Museum of Science and Industry, another extensive and unique collection on which I have had the privilege and opportunity to draw extensively. I am particularly grateful for the assistance of Dr. Ghislaine Lawrence, Senior Curator, and Mr. Neil Irvine, Assistant Curator, at the Science Museum. I am also indebted to those institutions where I have been allowed to catalogue and photograph material, including the Rotunda Hospital and the Trinity Centre for Health Sciences, Dublin; the obstetric departments of the Universities of Edinburgh, Liverpool, University College and Middlesex School of Medicine, London, Charles University, Prague; the York Medical Society. These sources and others are acknowledged later and in the text.

For a publisher to take on a new work of this nature is something of an act of faith. I am grateful to Jeremy Norman for his ready acceptance of my manuscript. Since then Martha Steele, Managing Editor, has pandered to my idiosyncrasies while firmly guiding me in smoothing the edges and making the text more readable as well as, with her astute eye, meticulously checking the text, bibliography, and cross references.

Throughout this venture I have been encouraged and assisted by my wife, Elizabeth, who has been critic, proofreader, photographic assistant, and sustainer. Without her support this book might never have been completed. Likewise, without the long hours of my writing many of her tapestries might not have been completed.

"Even old roads may be sometimes profitably trodden."
THOREAU

Bryan Hibbard
Cardiff, 1999

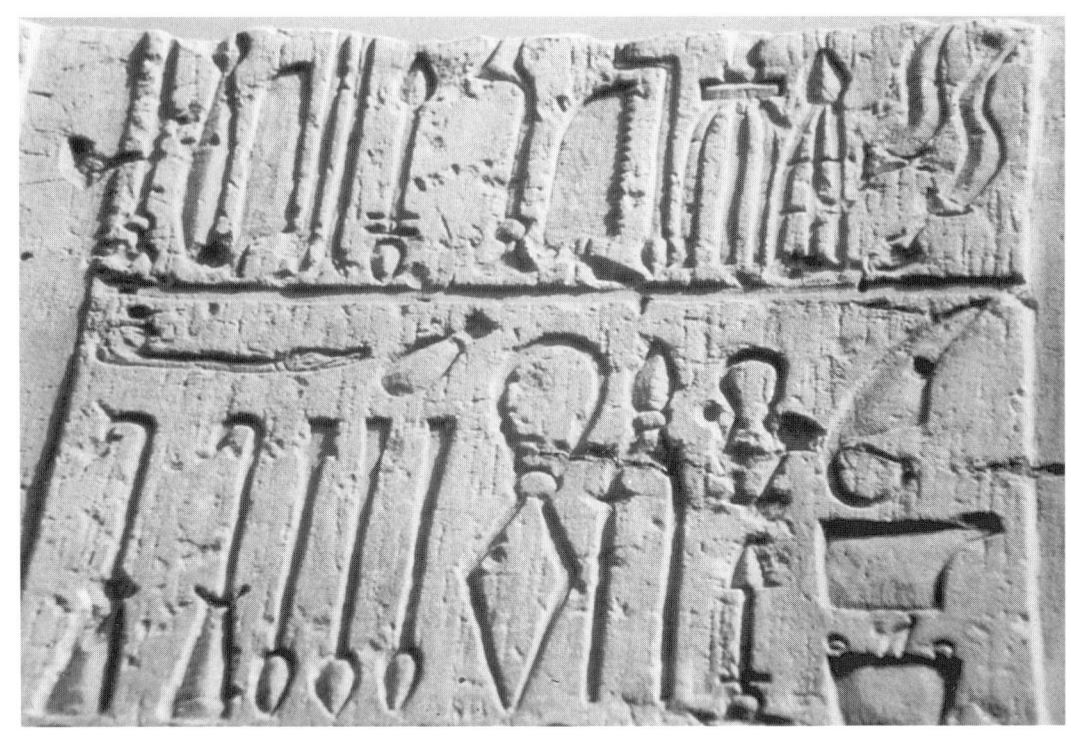

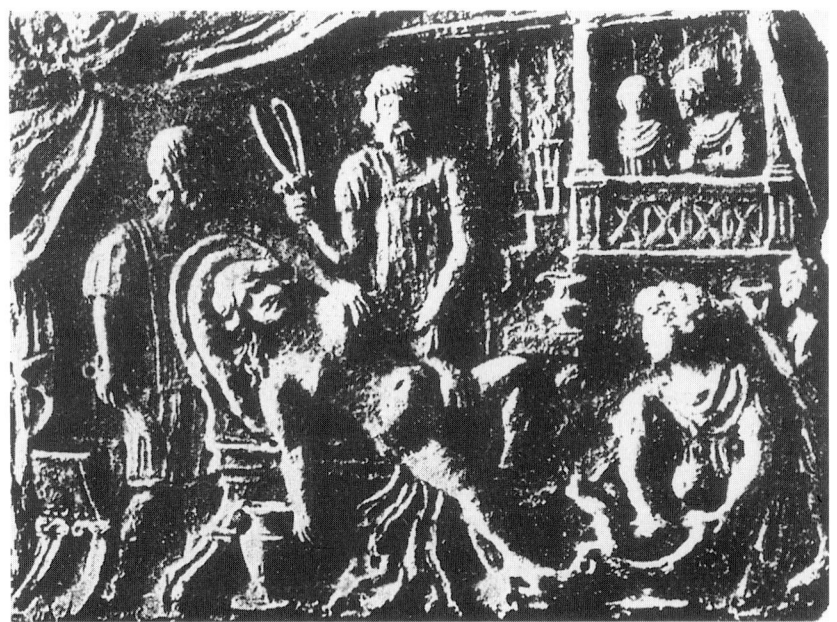

FIGURE I-1.
Kom Ombo temple carvings. The instruments depicted are probably for sacrificial rites although an obstetric function has been suggested.

FIGURE I-2.
Bas-relief, purported second century A.D. It was subsequently revealed as a hoax.

INTRODUCTION:
THE SIXTEENTH CENTURY AND BEFORE:
DECOCTIONS, DESTRUCTION, AND DIVINE INTERVENTION

In ancient times all manner of devices were used for bringing forth the child, but not the living child. Apart from podalic version delivery was assisted mechanically, usually with destructive intent, using a variety of instruments commonly selected from the surgeons' armamentarium and sometimes even from the kitchen, such as pot ladles. Many instruments depicted in illustrations were interpreted as being specifically for obstetric use, but after discussion with experts in the field, those seen in the Ptolomeic temple carvings of ancient Egypt were more likely instruments used in sacrificial rites (Figure I.1).

John Stewart Milne, in *Surgical Instruments in Greek and Roman Times* (1907, reprint 1970), gave a detailed account of Greco-Roman surgical instruments, including many unearthed at Pompeii. He also discussed a number of specific obstetric instruments, such as traction hooks and a sharp decapitation hook recommended by Celsus (27 B.C.–A.D. 50), and a traction hook for removal of a dead fetus:

> Then if the head present there ought to be inserted a hook, smooth all round, with a short point that is properly fixed in the eye or the ear or the mouth, sometimes even in the forehead, which being drawn on extracts the child. Nor is it to be drawn on without regard to circumstance. For if the attempt is made with an undilated cervix, not getting exit the foetus broken up, and the point of the hook catches on the cervix and inflammation follows and much danger of death.

A modification of the traction hook was used for decapitation in cases of transverse lie that in essence continued to be used into the twentieth century:

> The treatment is to divide the neck so that each part may be extracted separately. This is done with a hook which, though similar to the last, is sharpened on its inside only along its whole border. Then we must endeavour to bring away the head first, and then the rest of the body.

Milne could find no evidence of instruments designed to extract a living fetus in this Greco-Roman period. He also concluded that loose translation resulted in a sometimes unjustified use of the term *forceps*, which was subsequently misconstrued by later authors. The belief arose that in the first and second centuries A.D. the Romans had obstetric forceps of a pattern similar to modern forceps and this belief was reinforced by the purported discovery of a bas-relief of that period (Baglioni, 1937). Its authenticity was challenged by Crainz in 1941, however. It was subsequently revealed as a hoax and destroyed by Baglioni's family after his death. In spite of this information, the bas-relief continues to be widely reproduced (Figure I.2).

The decline of the Roman Empire was associated with the ascendancy of Arabian medicine in the second half of the first millennium. Arabian teaching was founded on Greco-Roman principles and translations of Greco-Roman manuscripts. Two of the most influential Arabian physicians at the end of the millennium were Avicenna and Albucasis.

In the *Liber canonis* Avicenna (circa A.D. 980–1037), a physician in Baghdad, recommended the use of a fillet to extract the impacted head, failing which the forceps should be applied. This has been interpreted by some as a description of the obstetric forceps as we understand them. It more likely refers to craniotomy forceps as depicted by many subsequent writers, such as Albucasis. The first Latin translation of

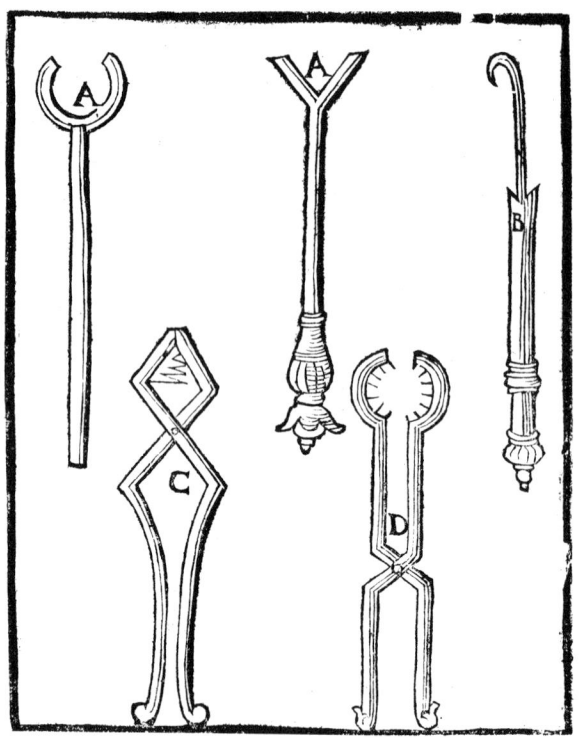

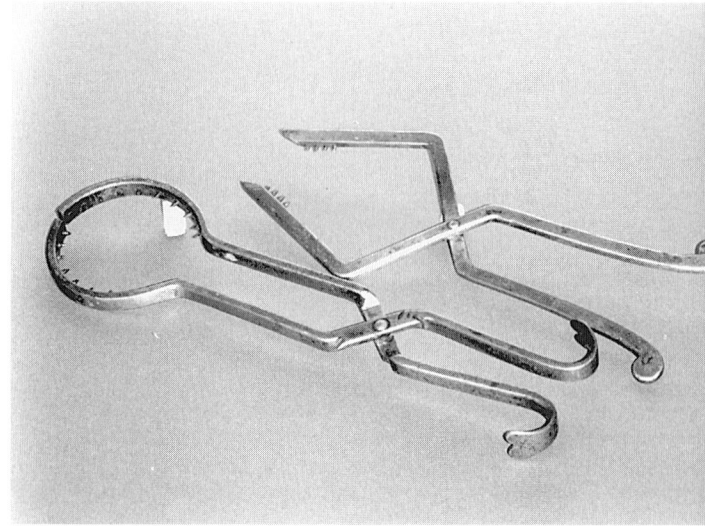

FIGURE I.5.
Mercurio's instruments. Facsimiles of his crushing forceps in the Department of Obstetrics, University of Edinburgh.

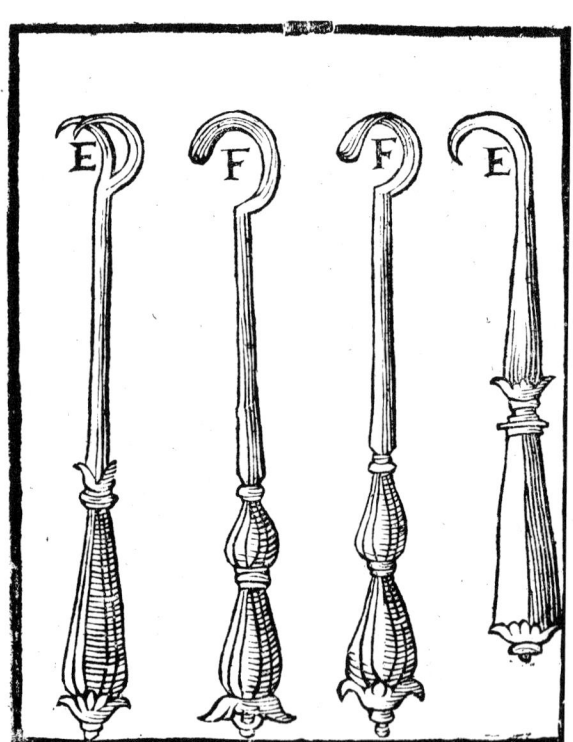

FIGURES I.3, I.4.
Mercurio's instruments for extraction of a dead fetus. The crushing forceps in particular are clearly copied from Albucasis. (Mercurio, 1601) (The Wellcome Institute Library, London)

Avicenna appeared in the twelfth century and throughout the Middle Ages remained one of the essential texts for the study of medicine. It was still in use in some Continental centers, including Louvain and Montpelier, as late as 1650 (see also Grunner, 1970).

The eleventh-century Arabian physician Albucasis (1013–1106) gave detailed instructions in his *Chirurgica* on the use of hooks to extract a dead fetus with, if necessary, up to three hooks fixed in the eyes, neck, mouth, collar bone, or ribs. If the fetus did not come out entire the hooks were reapplied to the remaining parts. M. S. Spink and G. L. Lewis translated the original and wrote extensive commentaries on the work (1937). Chapter 77 is devoted to descriptions of instruments for extracting the fetus. Among these are strong forceps with curved jaws and teeth for crushing, another pair of forceps for extracting, and various hooks and crotchets. Aveling concluded that

> [i]t is beyond doubt a fact that Arabian surgeons used forceps to deliver the foetal head in difficult labours. Avicenna mentions them and Albucasis gives drawings of barbarous instruments which were invented to be used as cranioclasts. It is not however proposed to consider these or any other evidences of the existence of midwifery forceps in remote times, for to whatever state of perfection they might have been brought, all knowledge of them had for centuries been lost and reinvention had become a necessity. (1882)

2 INTRODUCTION

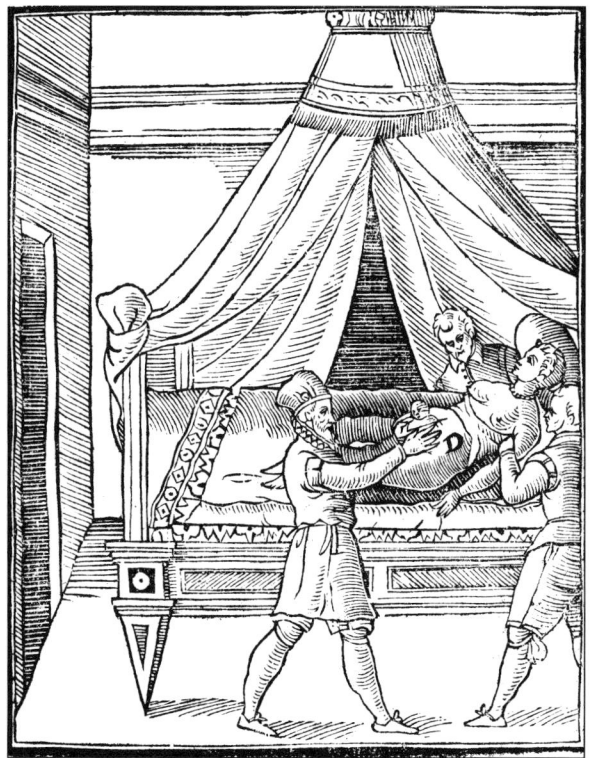

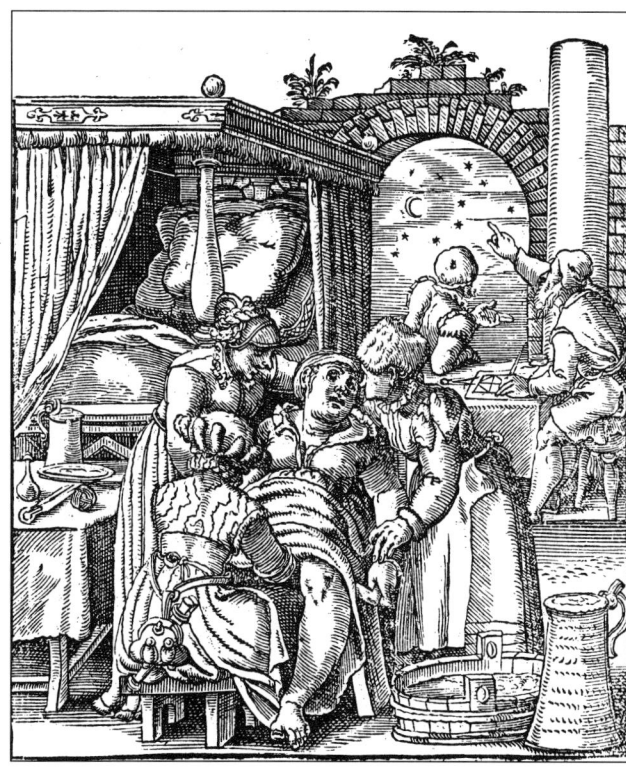

FIGURE I.8.
Sixteenth-century birth scene as depicted by Rueff. Note the use of a birth stool, the midwife's flask and table with sustenance, and the presence of astrologers at the window. (Rueff, 1580)

Later writers, such as Scipione Mercurio (circa 1540–1615) in *La Commare o riccoglitrice...* (1601) illustrated instruments clearly copied from Albucasis (Figures I.3, I.4). Facsimiles of the crushing forceps are in the Department of Obstetrics, University of Edinburgh (Figure I.5). Mercurio also gave a very detailed account of how to perform Caesarian section through a paramedian incision (Figures I.6, I.7).

The Middle Ages

In the Middle Ages midwifery was primitive and dominated by midwives whose practice was steeped in folklore and superstition. These women relied on astrologers, herbal potions, fumigations, and the occasional flask of wine to perform their duties (Figure I.8).

The Hippocratic teachings, dating from the third and fourth centuries B.C. persisted into the Middle Ages and were analyzed by R. W. Johnson in *A New System of Midwifery* (1769). Most importantly there was a persistent belief that

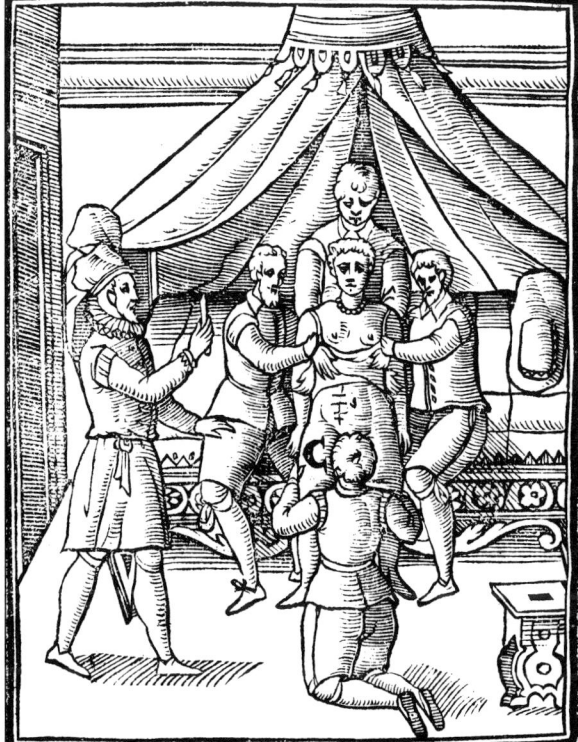

FIGURES I.6, I.7.
Caesarian section as depicted by Mercurio. (The Wellcome Institute Library, London)

the living fetus was solely responsible for his/her escape from the uterus. Thus there was no indication for the mother to actively assist during labor so long as the fetus was alive. By the same reasoning the dead fetus was incapable of delivering itself; assistance would be required in this situation. Hippocrates recommended that the head be opened with a small knife, the bones of the head broken, and the extraction performed with forceps. For shoulder obstruction the arms were to be divided at the articulations; for trunk obstruction the ribs were to be divided, the scapula removed, and the belly perforated if necessary.

Although physicians wrote tracts on the management of difficult labor, until the seventeenth century the actual procedures were largely assisted by women without the benefit of learning from these texts. However in the eleventh century a work dealing with the sicknesses of woman, *De passionibus mulierum curandarum,* was written by Trotula, purported to be a midwife from Salerno. Whether or not this work was a compilation of the experience of Trotula or one or more other midwives and whether or not the author was a Salernican doctor using a penname is a matter of conjecture (Tuttle, 1976; Rowland, 1981). Whatever the case, the work certainly had enduring appeal in various versions. According to Tuttle (1976) at least sixty manuscript versions still exist and there were eleven printed editions in the second half of the sixteenth century, the first printed version appearing in 1544. The *Trotula* comprised a set of precepts, mainly practical in nature, even if not very efficacious. However there was little advice on mechanical assistance as we understand it, as is illustrated in the following: "When there is a difficult labour with a dead child place the patient in a sheet held at the corners by four strong men, with her head somewhat elevated. Have them shake the sheet vigorously by pulling on the opposite corners, and with God's will she will give birth."

From the fourteenth century onward in parts of Europe there had been an awareness of the need for midwifery teaching. The Hôtel Dieu in Paris had a Mistress of Midwives in the fourteenth century and in Regensburg, Germany, a Midwifery Code was instituted in 1452. In Zurich Jacob Rueff (1500–1558) was responsible for the instruction and examination of midwives. He published a popular guide for midwives and pregnant women in 1554 entitled *Ein schön lustig Trostbüchle*, an improved version of the *Rosengarten* (see below). The information contained in this work eventually became the basis of their examinations. Gradually examination of midwives by the medical profession became an established practice and by the seventeenth century midwives in Bohemia were required to take examinations in the medical faculty of the university.

By the beginning of the sixteenth century little had changed: though the influence of the Catholic church had become dominant, with only the most cloistered male celibate considered pure enough to discuss midwifery. (No males were allowed to attend confinements, so these discussions were from borrowed knowledge.) Intrusion of a man into the birth chamber was unthinkable, as is illustrated by the fate of Dr. Wertt of Hamburg in 1522. Being anxious to study the process of birth first hand, he disguised himself as a woman and attended a confinement. During the course of labor a midwife recognized this subterfuge and raised a storm of protest. Wertt was promptly burned at the stake, observed by other physicians who quickly realized the hazards of trying to usurp the authority of the midwives.

Toward the end of the sixteenth century and into the seventeenth century midwifery practice began to emerge from its stagnation to become a more scientific discipline based on sounder anatomical knowledge. These changes were implemented in particular by an abundant talent in France, including Ambroise Paré (circa 1510–1590) and, later, François Mauriceau (1637–1709) and André Levret (1703–1780). In the Hôtel Dieu in Paris training was given for physicians, surgeons, and midwives, and some of the surgeons trained as man-midwives.

The common procedures of the time were the use of the crotchet, the blunt hook, and the lever. However, Paré, who worked at the Hôtel Dieu but was principally a very successful army surgeon, in 1549 reintroduced podalic version for the management of malpresentations and antepartum hemorrhage. The concept was not new, having been first advocated by the Arabs and Soranus as a substitute for craniotomy, but it was Paré who brought it to common knowledge and usage. Here was a practical alternative to Caesarian section, which at the time meant a death sentence for the mother, in order to try to obtain a living child in cases of severe dystocia. Instruction in podalic version became the keystone of Paré's teaching in the field of obstetrics and was widely adopted throughout Europe and Britain. Another example of Paré's advanced thinking was the induction of labor, followed by version when feasible, in cases of antepartum hemorrhage in order to minimize blood loss. An example of the clarity of his teaching is found in the English translation of his works:

> . . . and then let him [the man-midwife] put his hand gently into the mouth of the womb, having first made it gentle and slippery with much oil; and when his hand is in let him find out the form and situation of the child . . . and so turn him that his feet may come forwards. And when he hath them

both out, let him join them both together, and so little by little let him draw the whole body from the womb. (Johnson, 1665)

Paré devised a number of instruments to assist delivery but alternative methods of dealing with the head seem to have come from lithotomists, whose armamentarium included spoon-like forceps and a three-bladed calculus extractor commended by Pierre Franco, a cutter for stone, in 1556. This extractor probably provided the idea for Levret's *tire-tête*, which is described in Chapter 3. While Paré was the innovator who established and organized midwifery training in the Hôtel Dieu, his pupil and successor Jacques Guillemeau (1520–1613) was the recorder. As well as carrying on the Paré traditions and becoming surgeon to the Hôtel Dieu, he saved the life of Paré's daughter, using the techniques learned from his mentor. The incident was described by Guillemeau and appears in the English translation of his book *Childbirth, or the Happie Deliverie of Women* (1612).

> Madame Simon . . . being near to term was surprised by a great haemorrhage. Finding her nearly pulseless, with feeble voice and blanched lips, I made the prognosis to her mother and her husband that her life was in great danger. The only way to save here was to deliver her immediately, the which I had seen practised by Monsieur Paré, her father, who caused me to do the like unto a gentlewoman of Madame de Senneterre. The mother and husband entreated me to save her and put the case in our hands. Thus promptly, following the advice of Messieurs the Physicians, she was happily delivered of a lively infant.

In England in the sixteenth century midwives were still for the most part ignorant and illiterate, yet they were regarded as important people and were licensed by the bishops. They were often called upon to baptize the baby and were versed in this, a practice that was officially banned in 1576 but in fact continued until the time of James I (1603–1625). They were also forbidden to use any witchcraft, sorcery, or charms, except those allowed by the Catholic Church. Aveling, in his treatise *English Midwives, Their History and Prospects* (1872), concludes that by the mid-sixteenth century women were becoming dissatisfied with the midwives and were "alive to their ignorance and impressed with the necessity to educate them." They also wanted some guarantee of their skill. Unfortunately there were no female midwifery practitioners equal to the task and so male influence began to take hold. *De partu hominis,* referred to below, was translated into English in 1540 by Richard Jonas "at the request of diverse honest and sad matrons, being of his acquaintance. . . ." This was part of a major awakening in medical practice, for also at this time the medical profession in Britain was making strenuous efforts to put its house in order. The College of Physicians was established in 1518 and soon afterward the surgeons joined with the barbers who practiced surgery to form the United Company of Barber-Surgeons, which organized lectures and examinations in addition to the established apprenticeship training. Textbooks in English began to replace those in Latin, making information more accessible to the masses. However, knowledge of anatomy and the processes of childbirth were still rudimentary and practice was largely still that of the ancients, with the use of fumigations, fomentations, suppositories, bathings, and manipulations, even in normal labor.

Major Early Midwifery Texts

The earliest English work on midwifery is a fifteenth-century illuminated manuscript in the Sloane Collection (MS 2463) in the British Library. Although it has sometimes been referred to as the English *Trotula* and shares some of the remedies with this Italian work, it should not be thought of as a translation of the original *Trotula*. There is no evidence that it was ever printed (Aveling, 1874; Rowland, 1981), but a transcript by Rowland of the complete text from Middle English is readily available. The work is remarkable for its practical advice on dealing with "unnatural births," of which some sixteen manners in which "the chyld comyth forth unkyndely" are illustrated (Figure I.9). For the most part the advice was for the midwife to liberally anoint the birth canal, to push the baby back into the uterus and to manipulate it into the "natural" position.

The last desperate advice if the child could not be brought out was to kill it by giving the mother a complex herbal decoction, anointing the stomach and back with oil and gall, and inserting a vaginal pessary of oil, ox gall, and iris juice.

The first printed midwifery text was that of Eucharius Rösslin (or Rhodion) of Worms (d. ?1526), *Die swangern Frawen und hebammen Rosengarten,* which was dedicated to Princess Katherine of Saxony and was granted a copyright by Emperor Maximilian in 1513. The original German version was reprinted at least thirteen times in the next fifty years (Power, 1927; Ballantyne 1906, 1907). There were also six editions in Dutch (1540–1730), four in French (1536–1577), and at least one in Czech. However, the medical lingua franca of the day was Latin and the Latin version, *De partu hominis,* had at least nine editions between 1532 and 1563.

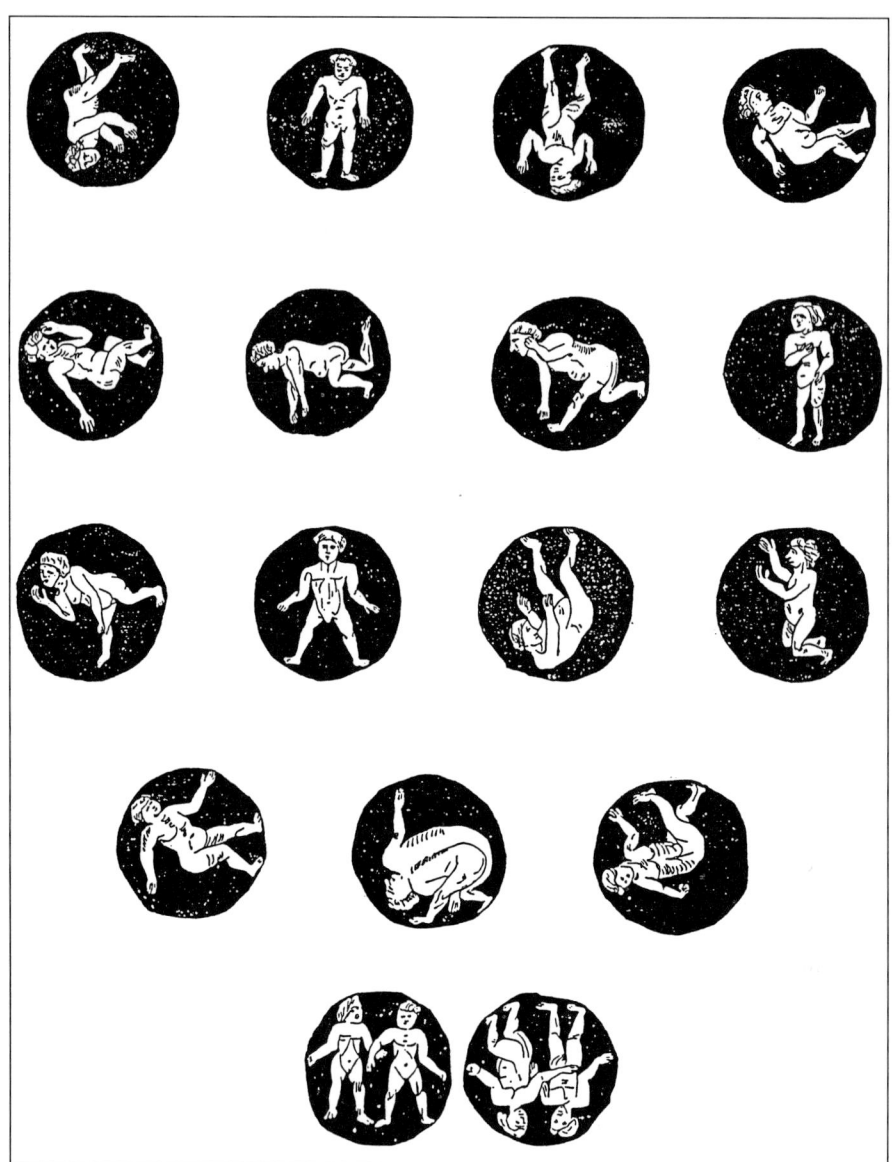

FIGURE I.9.
Malpresentations in Sloane Manuscript 2463. (Aveling, 1874) (By permission of the British Library)

The emergence of the first English version of *De partu hominis* has been the subject of much uncertainty and debate but the most plausible history is derived from the considerable researches of Aveling (1874), Ballantyne (1906), and Power (1927). A translation by Richard Jonas was printed by Thomas Raynolde and published in 1540. It was dedicated to Queen Katherine of England (Katherine Howard), who became queen in July 1540, and was addressed to "all honest and noble matrons." Thomas Raynolde, a physician unrelated to the printer with the same name, edited and enlarged the next edition, published in 1545 as *The Byrthe of Mankynde or the Woman's Book*. His name appears on all the subsequent editions (at least eight extending over the next hundred years) and he was probably actively involved in those published in 1545, 1552, and 1560. According to Power, "The book had a large sale for many years and was read extensively by doctors, midwives and ladies bountiful." The illustrations in this work come from two different sources. The birth figures can be traced back to Soranus's *Gynecology* (first century A.D.) and the anatomical plates that appeared for the first time in the 1545 edition can be traced to Thomas Geminus's (circa 1510–1562) copperplate illustrations for his work *Compendiosa totius anatomie delineatios...*, which had been taken from Andreas Vesalius's (1514–1564) works

6 INTRODUCTION

(Crummer, 1926). The text accompanying the anatomical illustrations is largely a straight translation from the Latin of Vesalius's *De humani corporis fabrica libri septem* (1543).

Raynolde entreated midwives who read the book to pay special attention to the anatomical descriptions and illustrations. Although it was addressed primarily to women readers he felt that if, by any chance a husband should read the book, he may, if of a gentle and loving nature, do his wife good: "[I]t shall be no displeasure to any honest and loving woman, that her husband should read such things: for many men there be of gentle and loving nature towards their wives, that they will be more diligent and careful to read and seek out anything that should do their wives good being in that case, then the women themselves."

For the conduct of labor he recommended the woman's stool (Figure I.10), then in use in France and Germany, with the midwife diligently observing and waiting, meanwhile instructing and comforting the mother and refreshing her with good meat, drink, and sweet words. For malpresentations cephalic version was advocated whenever possible. However, there was a paucity of instruction on how this was to be achieved. Ointments, plasters, and fumigations, as well as perfumes and potions, were used commonly, both in preparation for labor and when difficulties ensued. To encourage delivery of a retained placenta a "fume" (fumigation) of brimstone, ivy leaves, and cresses was advised, although the alternative of encouraging sneezing with white hellebore or pepper might have been more effective! When the fetus died in utero fumigations and plasters were advocated, not only those made from the herbal remedies commonly used but also those made of items savoring more of the occult, such as the skin of an adder or the hoof or dung of an ass. Only when these remedies had failed were "more severe and hard remedies" using instruments such as hooks and tongues (lever or vectis?) recommended. The arms and legs were to be cut off if necessary and the head opened with a sharp penknife. Piecemeal extraction could be undertaken with "such instrumentes as the Chirurgions have readye and necessarye for suche purposes." Should the mother die in labor the mouth and nether places should be opened so that the child might continue to breathe prior to carrying out a Caesarian section through the left flank. No details of this operative procedure were given. Subsequent twentieth-century commentators have viewed the book differently. "An illustrated manual of midwifery compiled from somewhat ancient sources for it contains little that is original" (Power, 1927), and "[This work is] the head and source of English obstetric literature, and has profoundly influenced the practice and art of midwifery in these Islands for more than three centuries" (Ballantyne, 1906). In 1554, Rueff published *Ein schön*

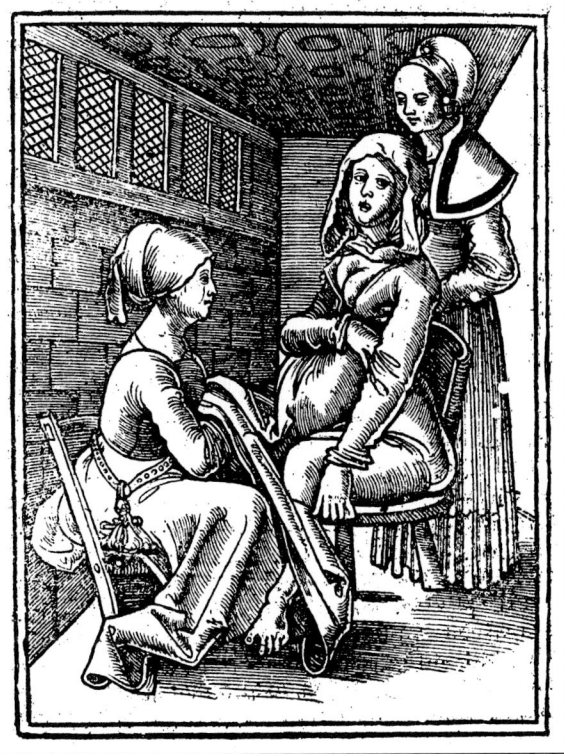

FIGURE I.10.
Illustrated title page from Eucharius Rösslin's *Rosengarten*. (Rösslin, 1513).

lustig Trostbüchle, an improved version of the *Rosengarten*, referred to previously, which appeared in Latin the same year as *De conceptu et generatione hominis* and then in English as *The Expert Midwife, or An Excellent and Most Necessary Treatise of the Generation and Birth of Man*. It was addressed "To all grave and modest matrons, especially such as have to do with women in that great danger of childbirth." Rueff described with illustrations instruments to extract both living and dead babies (Figures I.11, I.12). When the child was alive cervical dilatation was recommended. The *apertorium*, or opening instrument, was first lubricated and then the blades closed and inserted through the neck of the matrix [cervix]. The handles were then closed using both hands "to enlarge the mouth of the matrix as much as sufficeth." The mother was then refreshed and comforted with "sweet spices and convenient meat and drink." The *speculum matricis*, or looking-glass of the matrix, was similarly used to dilate the cervix. With its screw mechanism it clearly had the greater me-

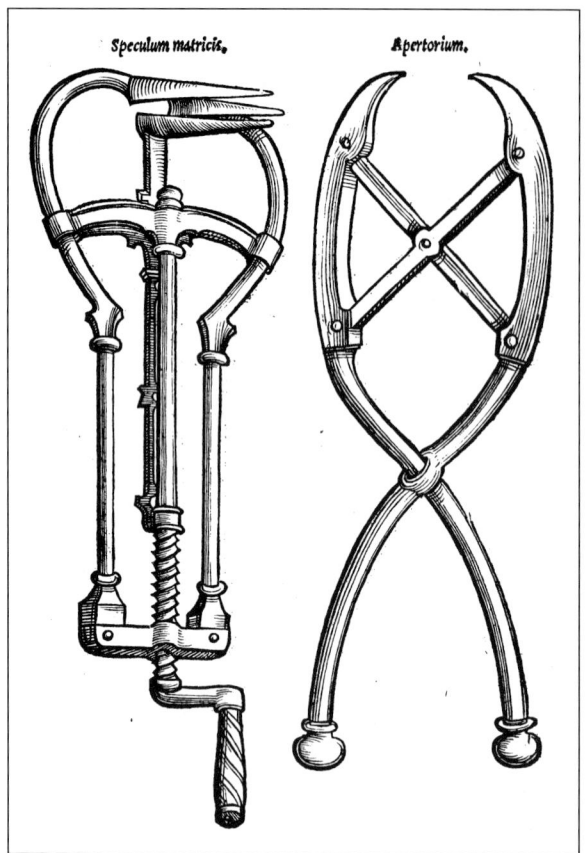
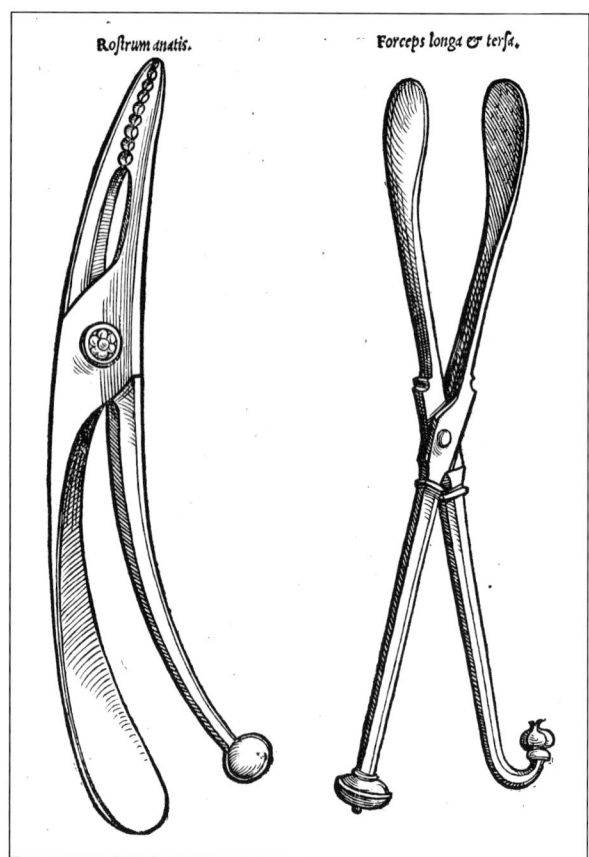

FIGURES I.11, I.12.
Sixteenth-century instruments illustrated by Rueff. Left to right: *speculum matricis, apertorium, rostrum anatis, forceps longa et tersa* (Rueff, 1554). (The Wellcome Institute Library, London)

chanical advantage. In the case of a dead fetus, dilatation of the cervix was also recommended. However, if the fetus was too big it was to be grasped with instruments "without hurt of the mother and be pulled forth with a discreet and prudent care." The operator then applied the *rostrum anatis*, or duck's or drake's bill, taking care to protect the maternal parts with the other hand. If necessary the operator could employ pincers used for tooth extraction or the *forceps longa et tersa*, the long and smooth fingers of tongs.

Although some suggestions were made that the concept of the obstetric forceps as we know them originated with Rueff it is clear from his illustrations that this was not so. Rueff laid no claim to the invention and Aveling summarily dismissed any claims to Rueff as primogenitor for the forceps saying that his book. "bears no evidence of his being an obstetrician of exceptional talent. The book was inferior to that of Rhodion which preceded it, and contained a large amount of useless and mischievous matter." (1875)

It was not until the early seventeenth century that the progressive teachings of Paré and Guillemeau appeared in textbooks for midwives. What was most likely the first of these appeared in 1609 and was entitled *Observations diverses sur la sterilité, perte de fruict, foecondité, accouchements, et maladies des femmes, et enfants nouveaux naiz*. The author was a well-educated Parisian midwife, Louise Bourgeois (1563–1636). Part of the book is devoted to midwifery and is a condensate of the teachings of Paré and Guillemeau. It was clearly written in the vernacular and therefore readily accessible to the Parisians of the day. Louise Bourgeois was married to a barber-surgeon, Martin Boursier, one of Paré's former pupils (Gebbie, 1981).

. . .

Thus, by the middle of the sixteenth century, midwifery was at last beginning to emerge from the stagnation of past centuries. Men-midwives increasingly attended difficult cases and new writings appeared, based not on the mythology of the past but on the personal, practical experience of managing childbirth.

THE CHAMBERLENS AND THE ORIGINS OF OBSTETRIC FORCEPS

The Chamberlen Family

Many British triumphs and inventions have been consequent on our ready acceptance of refugees. The obstetric forceps as we know them today are no exception, for the concept and original designs are generally attributed to an immigrant family of Huguenot refugees. William and Genevieve Chamberlen arrived in England with their family in 1569 after the Battle of Jarnac in which the Huguenots suffered a huge defeat (Figure 1.1). The Chamberlens settled in Southampton initially, in company with many other Huguenot refugees. After the St. Bartholomew's Day Massacre in 1572, it was obvious that they could never return to France and thus the family moved to London, except for the elder son Peter who stayed in Southampton until his father's death in 1596. He was probably the originator of the forceps at about the end of the sixteenth century, with other members of the family making subsequent modifications.

The story of the family and their invention of the forceps is well told by Walter Radcliffe in *The Secret Instrument* (1947; reprint 1989). The family were natural entrepreneurs and opportunists, undaunted by opposition. Their strong personalities and successful practice resulted in antagonism from the physicians, midwives, and the Church, but gained them the favor of the people and the court. They served through three generations as surgeons to the royal household and were successful obstetricians on the Continent as well as in England, consequent on their ability to achieve delivery in even the most difficult of cases using their "secret instruments." By present-day public and professional standards they might be judged as unethical rogues because of their scheming, their retention of the family secret to favor their own interests, their self-aggrandizement, and their flamboyancy, but such behavior was more or less in keeping with the times. However, many of their schemes were ostensibly for the public good as well as for their own benefit. For example the attempts of the brothers Peter to form a guild of midwives might be regarded as a forward-looking project forestalled by the Bishop of London who was at that time responsible for licensing midwives. The concept only came to fruition 250 years later with the passing of the Midwives Act in 1902.

The Chamberlen Family Tree (Figure 1.2)
Understanding the Chamberlen family tree is complicated by a rather unimaginative choice of Christian names. William named two of his children Peter and they came to be known as "Peter the Elder" (d. 1631) and "Peter the Younger" (1572–1620). Peter the Younger had eight children, the eldest of whom was also called Peter (1601–1683) who, because of his formal medical training and qualifications, came to be known as "Dr. Peter."

The brothers Peter both became members of the Barber Surgeons Company and set up their striped poles in London. However they were both fined for nonattendance at the Company's lectures and were arraigned by the College of Physicians for the prescribing of medicines, which, as nonphysicians, they were not entitled to do. Indeed, in 1612 Peter the Elder was committed to Newgate Prison for malpractice but was released following the intercession of his royal patron, Queen Anne (wife of James I), and the Archbishop of Canterbury. This episode did not appear to mar his relationship with the court. He remained as Court Surgeon, attending Henrietta Maria, wife of Charles I, for the delivery of her son and heir to the throne, Charles, who was to become King Charles II. Peter the Younger also had a very

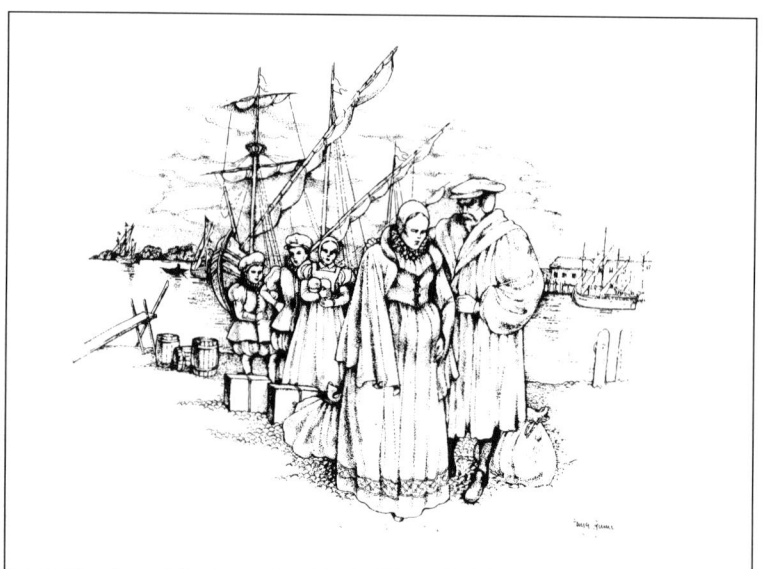

FIGURE 1.1.
The arrival of the Chamberlen family at Southampton. The two boys are Peter the Elder and Peter the Younger. (Original by Fenja Gunn)

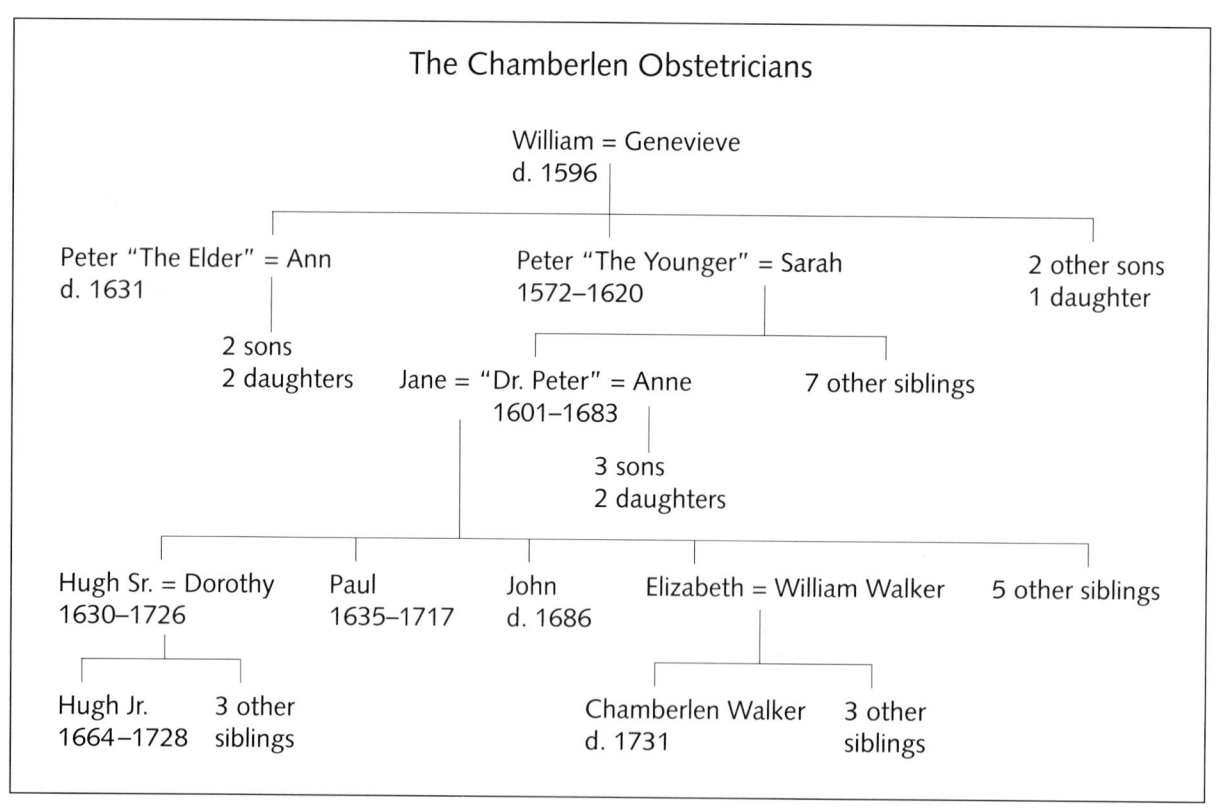

FIGURE 1.2.
The Chamberlen family tree.

10　CHAPTER 1

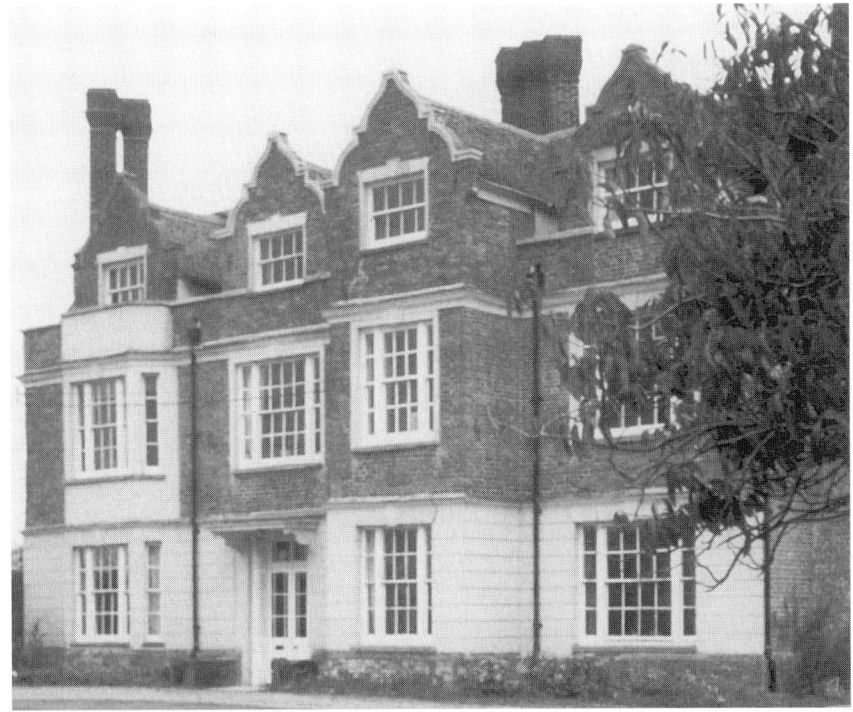
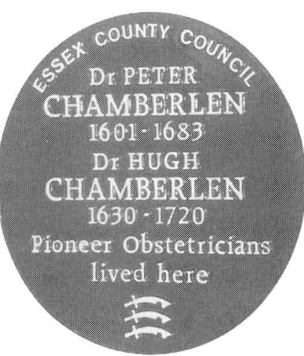

successful practice, but did not achieve the same recognition as his brother.

Dr. Peter, of the third generation, studied at the Universities of Cambridge, Heidelberg, and Padua, and achieved an M.D. in 1619 at the age of eighteen. In 1621, as soon as he was established in practice, he applied for fellowship to the College of Physicians but was rebuked by the president because of his frivolous dress style; he was not admitted until 1628. During the Commonwealth Dr. Peter ceased attending meetings of the College of Physicians and as a consequence was dismissed from the College in 1649 and moved outside their jurisdiction to Woodham Mortimer Hall in Essex (Figures 1.3, 1.4). It was here that the original Chamberlen instruments were discovered in 1813.

According to J. H. Thirtle (1910), Dr. Peter was initially in Cromwell's favor but was subsequently passed by and neglected. During this period he became increasingly puritanical and wrote numerous religious and sociological tracts. On the restoration of the monarchy in 1660 he was brought back into Court circles and appointed Physician in Ordinary to King Charles II. In his later years he became increasingly involved in politics and religion and was for some years a Baptist minister. He died and was buried at Woodham Mortimer, where his tomb gives details of his extensive family (fourteen children by his two wives [Figure 1.5]). Dr. Peter

FIGURES 1.3, 1.4.
Woodham Mortimer Hall, Essex, the home of Doctors Peter and Hugh Chamberlen. The trapdoor under which the box of keepsakes was found, including the original Chamberlen instruments, is in the attic in the bay to the right of the front door. The heritage plaque (Figure 1.4) was mounted in 1990.

also promoted various projects that are discussed in some detail by Thirtle and by J. H. Aveling (1882), including plans for a public bank, labor houses for thieves, and an attempt to obtain a monopoly on the manufacture of baths and bathstoves. Also, and in the family tradition, he attempted to organize a Sisterhood of Midwives of London, a scheme which he promoted with wine and a promise of various benefactions. His proposal required that midwives be licensed by him, that he be paid a fee for each delivery, and that he be called to all difficult cases. However the opposition was strong and the conflict prolonged. The scheme failed to materialize after complaints from midwives and their supporters had been upheld by the College of Physicians and lodged with the Archbishop of Canterbury and the Bishop of London. The protestors claimed that his proposals were an intrusion on ecclesiastical jurisdiction. His response and defense were contained in a document *A Voice in Rhama; or*

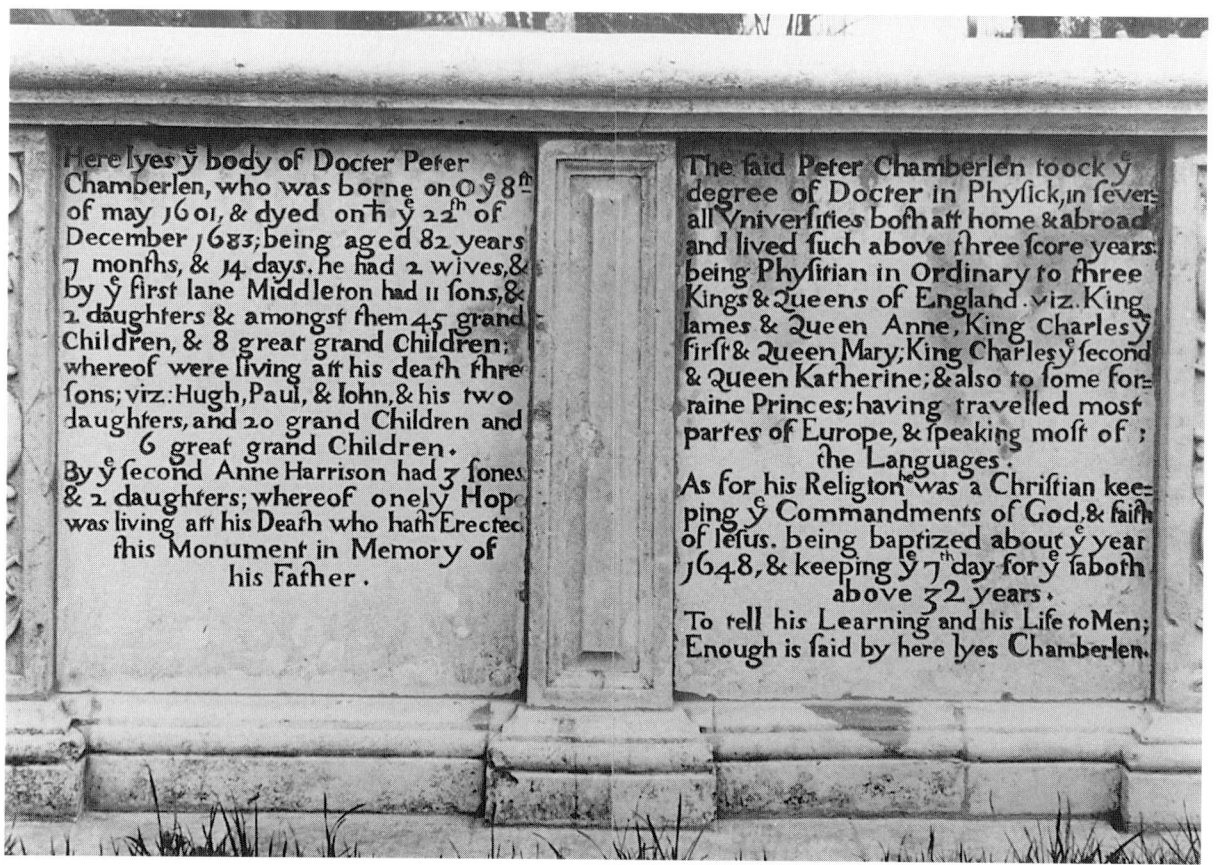

FIGURE 1.5.
Dr. Peter Chamberlen's tomb in the churchyard adjoining Woodham Mortimer Hall.

the Crie of Women and Children (1647) in which, having given an autobiography and details of his qualifications and experience in somewhat expansive terms, he claimed, "Fame begot me envie and secret enemies which mightily increased when my father added to me the knowledge of deliveries." According to Radcliffe Dr. Peter's wild and impractical schemes led people to believe that he was not a little out of his mind. However he was sane enough to get his son Hugh appointed as Physician in Ordinary at the Court in 1673, although by his death in 1683 he is said to have been quite mad.

Hugh Chamberlen, Senior (1630–1726), was the eldest son of Dr. Peter and, following family traditions, he also promoted various schemes for the public good, including public health insurance and a land bank, and was also prosecuted for practicing without proper qualifications. However, in his favor, he was one of the few practitioners to remain and practice in London during the plague of 1665. He was a man of considerable intellectual standing and in 1681 was elected a Fellow of the Royal Society of London for the Promotion of Natural Knowledge (commonly known as the Royal Society), where he was in the company of such outstanding contemporaries as Sir Christopher Wren, Sir Isaac Newton, and Samuel Pepys.

Hugh Senior became physician to Charles II and to James II. In 1688 he was due to attend on the wife of James II. The labor was premature, however, and he did not arrive in time for the birth of James Edward Stuart, who became known as "the Old Pretender" because it was alleged that the baby had been stillborn and that a substitute male child had been smuggled into the birth chamber in a warming pan. An investigation was instituted by the king to prove that the alleged substitution was without foundation. Hugh testified, "I am certain that no such thing as bringing a strange child in a warming pan could be practised without my seeing it." Since he was not present at the birth, Hugh's evidence did not carry much weight. Hugh Senior developed a bank scheme based on the successful Bank of Amsterdam, but this had rather shaky foundations and crashed. Because of this and suspected Jacobite sympathies he fell out of favor with society and he left England under a cloud. He eventually settled in Amsterdam; the date of his death is unknown. An anonymous contemporary critic, quoted by Aveling, wrote of him:

> He's a little old man very pale of complexion
> Into many deep things makes a narrow inspection
> His head's very long and his hand's very small
> Fit to fathom a gentle Tuquoque withall.
> To give you his character truly compleat
> He's Doctor, Projector, Man-midwife and Cheat.

Paul (1635–1717) and John Chamberlen (d. 1686) were Dr. Peter's second and third sons and both practiced as man-midwives. Although they were known to use the forceps, there is no evidence that they disclosed or attempted to sell the secret. Very little other information about their practice exists, though Paul was reputedly a quack who sold charm necklaces.

Hugh Chamberlen, Junior (1664–1728), the eldest son of Hugh Senior, was regarded as a trustworthy and popular physician in court circles. Although he made no notable contribution to medicine he achieved lasting notice by way of his court and ecclesiastical connections in the form of a magnificent cenotaph in the north aisle of Westminster Abbey (described in detail by Aveling).

Dr. (later Sir) Chamberlen Walker of Southwark (d. 1731), grandson of Dr. Peter and nephew of Hugh Senior, was the last obstetrician in the family dynasty. Little is known of Sir Chamberlen, except that he made important modifications to the forceps, which will be described in Chapter 2.

The Chamberlen Practice

Stories of how the Chamberlens went about their business abound and have been embellished over the years, but no doubt there was an element of showmanship as well as secrecy to their dealings. It is recorded that the Chamberlens traveled to confinements in a closed carriage with their secret device contained in a huge gilded box that required two men to lift it. It was only opened after the birth chamber had been cleared and the patient had been blindfolded. As was standard practice, in the interests of modesty, the man-midwife worked only by touch under cover of a blanket, thus providing yet another way for concealing the instrument (Speert, 1973).

It was Hugh Senior, possibly supported by the rest of the family, who endeavored to capitalize on the family secret by selling it abroad; interestingly, there is no record of any similar attempt at disclosure in Britain. In 1670 he went to Paris where Louis XIV had made man-midwives fashionable by utilizing their services in his mistresses' deliveries. Hugh Senior offered the family secret to the royal accoucheur, Jules Clement, for the sum of ten thousand crowns. He and his secret were put to the test by the celebrated physician and teacher, François Mauriceau, who set him the task of delivering a grossly deformed rachitic dwarf who had already been in labor for eight days. (Mauriceau detailed the case as Observation Number 26 in his *Des maladies des femmes grosses*.) Hugh struggled to deliver the woman but, after being locked in the room with her for three hours, he admitted defeat; the mother died from a ruptured uterus. Mauriceau claimed that it was this episode that induced him to invent his *tire-tête* (page 22).

Thus Hugh Senior returned to England with the family secret still unrevealed. However his journey was not without profit because he acquired a copy of Mauriceau's very successful textbook and published an extremely successful English translation, *The Accomplisht Midwife*, in 1673. (Mauriceau rather peevishly claimed that it netted Chamberlen thirty thousand pounds.) It was in the preface to this translation that the existence of the family secret was first mentioned, apart from Dr. Peter's vague hint in *A Voice in Rhama*.

> My father, brothers and myself (tho' none else in
> Europe as I know) have by God's blessing and our
> own industry, attained to and long practised a way to
> deliver women in this case without any prejudice to
> them or their infants; tho all others (being obliged,
> for want of such an expedient, to use the common
> way) do and must endanger, if not destroy one or
> both with hooks. By this manual operation, a labour

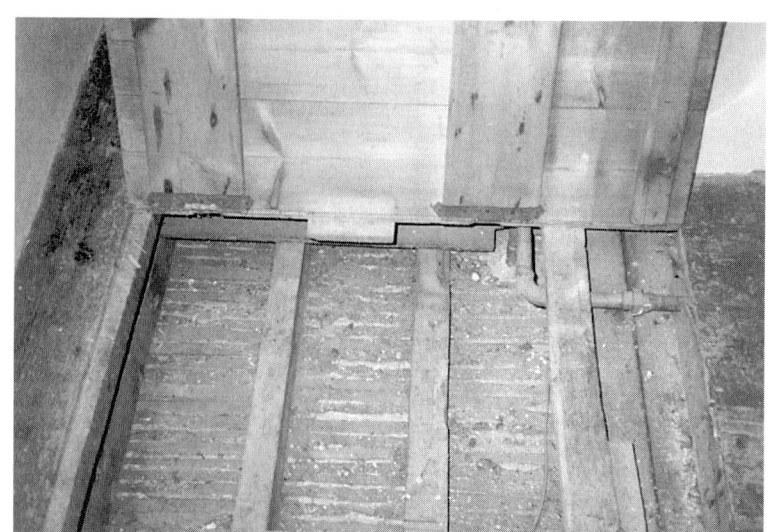

FIGURE 1.6.
The trapdoor in the attic.

may be dispatched (on the least difficulty) with fewer pains and sooner, to the great advantage and without danger both of woman and child.

I will now take leave to offer an apology for not publishing the secret I mention we have to extract children without hooks, where other artists use them, viz., there being my Father and two Brothers living, that practise this art, I cannot esteem it my own to dispose of nor publish it without injury to them; and think I have not been unserviceable to my country, altho I do but inform them that the forementioned three persons of our family and myself, can serve in these extremities, with greater safety than others.

The Discovery of the Original Instruments at Woodham Mortimer

The Chamberlen family sold Woodham Mortimer Hall in about 1715 and at the beginning of the nineteenth century it was occupied by the family of William Codd, Coroner to the County of Essex. In 1813 Dr. Codd's mother-in-law, while visiting the family, found in an attic a trap door, well constructed and concealed (Figure 1.6).

In the space beneath several boxes were discovered, the contents of which were described to Dr. May, a local practitioner, by Mrs. Codd and later recorded in R. Lee's work *Observations on the Discovery of the Original Obstetric Instruments of the Chamberlens* (1862).

> This [space] contained some boxes in which were two or three pairs of midwifery forceps, several coins, a medallion of Charles I, or II, a miniature of the Doctor [Dr. Peter], damaged by time, a tooth wrapped in paper, written on, "My husband's last tooth"; some little antique plate; a pair of ladys [sic] long yellow kid gloves, in excellent preservation; a small testament date 1645.

In fact there were four pairs of forceps, three levers, three crotchets, and three fillets (Figure 1.7).

Das concluded, without any supporting evidence, that the "rational and inevitable explanation, therefore, of this remarkable coincidence must be that the instruments found were those not only of Dr. Peter Chamberlen, but of his father and uncle. . . ."

The instruments were presented to a surgeon and friend of the family, Mr. H. H. Carwardine, who deposited them with the Royal Medical and Chirurgical Society of London in 1818, from where they passed to the Royal Society of Medicine and eventually to the Royal College of Obstetricians and Gynaecologists.

The Chamberlen Instruments

There is no written record of the development of the instruments; their conception and gestation are uncertain and surrounded by mystery, myth, and conjecture. While the broadest history of the instruments is given by Radcliffe in *The Secret Instrument*, the earlier account by Aveling (1882) deals in much more detail with the family members and their place in society, with frequent recourse to original documents. Kedarnath Das (1929; reprint 1993) claimed that there was evidence (which he did not substantiate) that the Chamberlens were sworn enemies of sharp hooks and that their first idea was to use two blunt hooks, which they after-

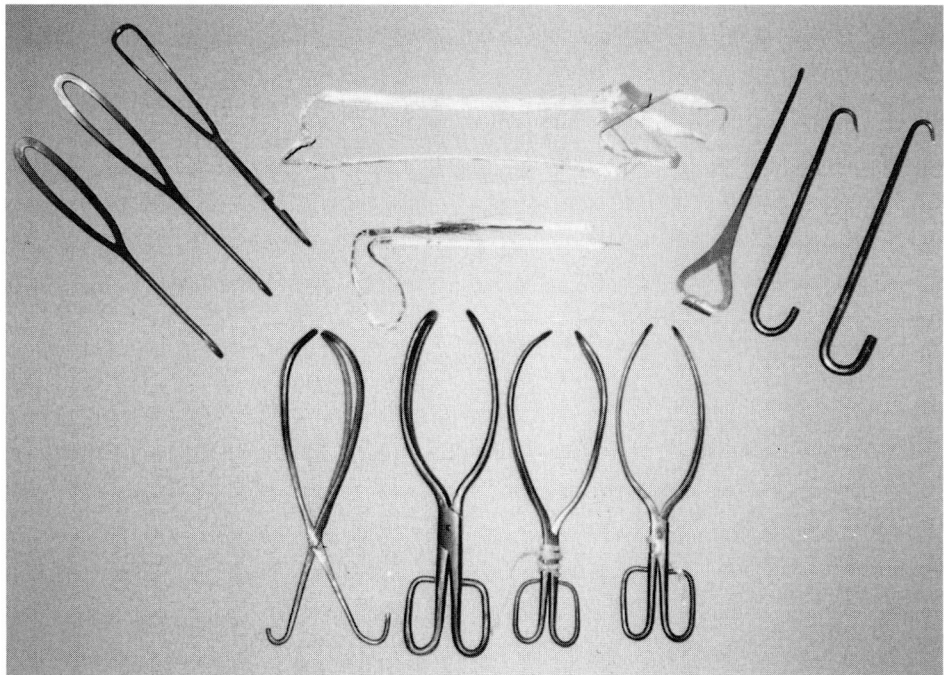

FIGURE 1.7.
The Chamberlen instruments discovered at Woodham Mortimer Hall in 1813. Top: Levers, fillets, and blunt hooks. Bottom: The four pairs of forceps showing progressive development in design. (RCOG)

ward modified. Almost certainly the original instrument was devised by Peter the Elder but whether it was based on the fenestrated lever or whether the lever was a later development, as suggested by M. Thiery (1992), is uncertain. The conventional tools of the time, blunt hooks, fillets, and—contrary to Das's assertion—sharp hooks (crotchets), were also included in the Chamberlen armamentarium.

The four pairs of forceps from Woodham Mortimer, now in the collection of the Royal College of Obstetricians and Gynaecologists, show progressive refinement in design and manufacture. The blades are curved to embrace the head and are fenestrated to give a better grip and to avoid undue compression. Devising an effective and functional articulation was clearly a problem and remained so for subsequent practitioners even into the eighteenth century. The first pair of forceps was of crude construction and had a riveted joint that made it almost impossible to introduce the blades. The second pair had a pin on one blade to act as a pivot and a hole to receive it on the other blade. However, this required accurate application of the blades to achieve alignment and locking of the joint. Subsequently this design was abandoned and both blades had a hole at the crossover. The blades were united by a tape that passed through the holes and was wound around the joint, thus allowing a degree of flexibility.

Did the Chamberlens Sell the Secret?
While Hugh Chamberlen's journey to Paris in 1670 and his failure to sell the family secret is well documented, subsequent events and developments in the Low Countries have remained a matter of dispute, encompassing rival claims with nationalistic undertones relating to the true inventor of the forceps. There are no contemporary descriptions by the purported inventors and subsequent chroniclers are often vague in regard to design detail and chronology. The waters are further muddied by perpetuated romanticizing, myths, and misinterpretations. It must be remembered that the eighteenth-century writers, referred to in Chapter 2, were unaware of the existence of the original Chamberlen instruments, which were concealed at Woodham Mortimer until 1813, and would probably not have had any details of the final form of the developed forceps. Thiery, in his scholarly dissertation *Obstetric Forceps and Vectis: The Roots,* proposed a triple lineage for the origins of the obstetric forceps. Hav-

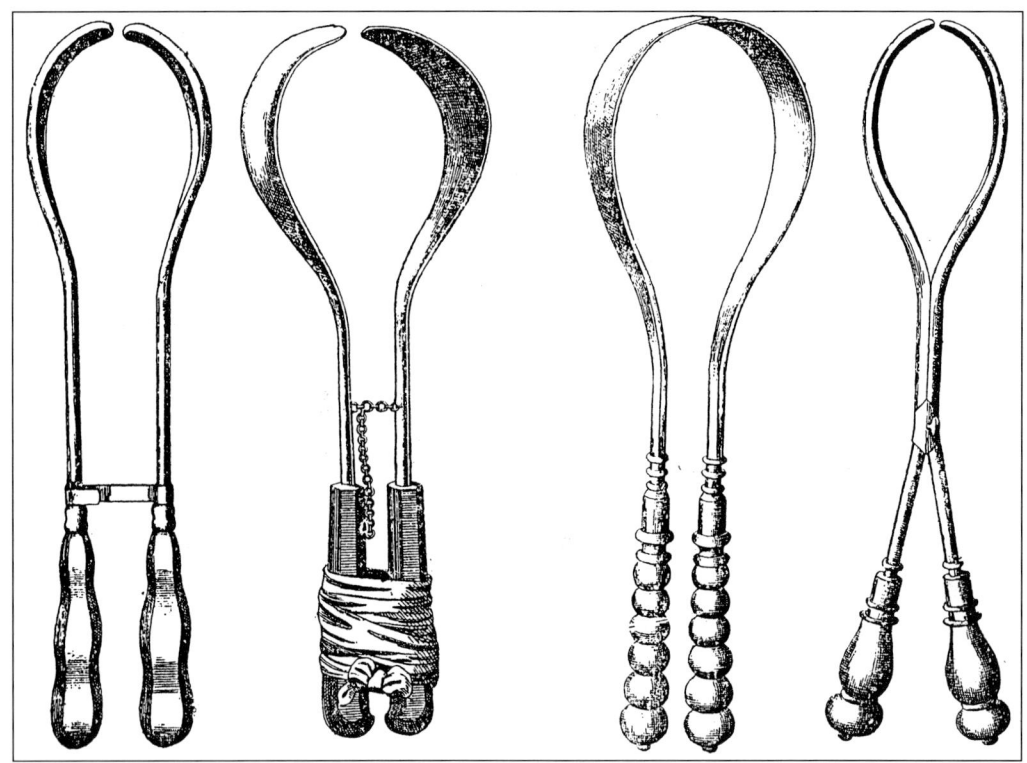

FIGURE 1.8.
Palfyn's *mains de fer* and modifications as illustrated by Kilian, 1835.

ing justifiably discarded earlier claims (pages 18, 20, 21), he argued that they were invented independently, and more or less contemporaneously, in England by the Chamberlen family, in Ghent by Johannes Palfyn, and in Amsterdam by Hendrik van Roonhuysen or his son Rogier. However it is safe to conclude that the Chamberlens and their neighboring successors were the first to develop and refine, through a number of models, instruments that were clearly functional.

Johannes Palfyn

Johannes Palfyn (1650–1730), who practiced in Ghent, devised his *mains de fer* in about 1716. Radcliffe claimed that Palfyn had visited London early in the eighteenth century and suggested that he there heard an account of an instrument used by the Chamberlen family; this account gave him the germ of an idea that developed into his own instrument. Thiery challenged the veracity of this account and there is certainly no documentary evidence to support Radcliffe's proposition that Palfyn had contact with the Chamberlen family. In addition, Palfyn's design was clearly inferior and lacked the essential features of the Chamberlen instruments.

The spoonlike Palfyn instruments were intended to be used in pairs to grasp the sides of the fetal head like human hands, hence the name *mains de fer*. Radcliffe suggested that the spoon-shaped blades were derived from the large curettes used since the time of Paré for piecemeal removal of fetal parts. Palfyn never published a description of the instruments but alluded to them in a letter to the University of Ghent in 1717 and exhibited them at the Royal Academy of Science in Paris in 1720. They received official approval three years later but did not achieve popularity. Guillaume La Motte (1722) confirmed that Palfyn had exhibited his instruments in Paris but he condemned their use.

> One of the master surgeons of Paris, who had been directed to examine this instrument with reference to the practicability of its use, did me the honor of asking me what I thought of the matter, without describing the instrument, for he had been requested to keep that a secret. I did not hesitate to assure my friend that whatever the design of the instrument, its use would be as impossible as to pass a cable through the eye of a needle. (Thiery, 1992)

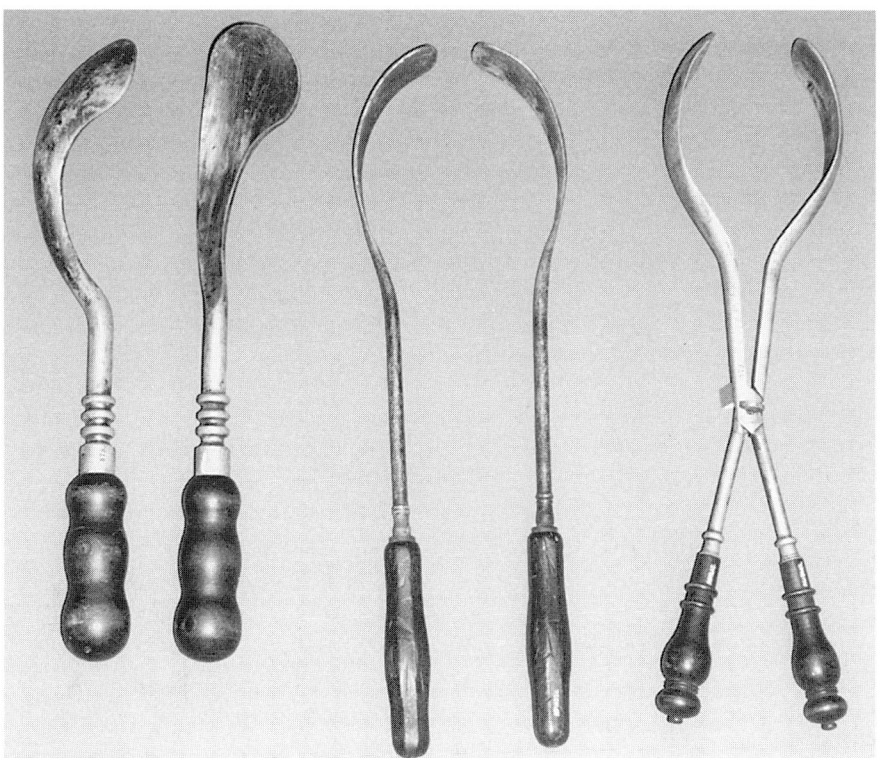

FIGURE 1.9.
Palfyn's *mains de fer* in the Wellcome Collection. They have been attributed as, from left to right, Types I, II, and III respectively. (Science Museum, London)

The credit for tying the two blades together with a ribbon was attributed by Levret (1747) to Gilles le Doux of Ypres.

There are numerous illustrations purporting to show Palfyn's *mains de fer* (Figures 1.8, 1.9). The first was in Lorenz Heister's textbook of surgery (1724, 1739, 1743), where he depicted a single blade with a pelvic curve. Heister is believed to be the originator of the more secure union of the blades using a chain or hook. However, in the 1763 edition of his book he concluded that the instruments were ineffective because they failed to achieve satisfactory compression of the head and also because they slipped off. Mulder, who produced the first atlas of obstetric forceps in 1794, showed a pair of blades with a pelvic curve, as in Heister's plate (Table XXXIII), held together with a tape or napkin that he called "Palfyn Type I" (Figure 1.9, left), and a longer pair without a pelvic curve held together with a metal clip ("Palfyn Type II") (Figures 1.8 left, 1.9 center). Kilian (1835) also showed a "Palfyn Type II" forceps but united by a chain (Figure 1.8, second from left) and another pair with a crossover joint and screw (Figures 1.8 right, 1.9 right), which Mulder had designated as "unknown" but which Kilian also attributed to Palfyn. There were other modifications of Palfyn's forceps but they were all unstable and the basic design only became functional with Dusée's modifications, particularly the addition of the screw lock (Chapter 2.)

Although there is little written on the acceptance or otherwise of Palfyn's forceps, Paulus de Wind's comments on the situation in Paris are of interest. He described how he went to Paris in 1734 to study under Grégoire. In his time with Grégoire he only saw him use the crotchet. Grégoire demonstrated the Palfyn instrument with the crosshook joining the blades but de Wind noticed that it was very rusty and concluded that Grégoire did not make use of it, having found it unfavorable. He subsequently stayed with Dusée (Chapter 2).

The Van Roonhuysian Accoucheurs

The third contenders for the invention of the obstetric forceps are the Van Roonhuysen family. The cunning and deception of the Van Roonhuysens and their disciples exceeded the bounds of even their liberal times. Thiery, in a fascinating description of ploy and counter-ploy in this saga, still leaves doubt as to when the Van Roonhuysen forceps did appear. Thiery's thesis is that the Van Roonhuysen instru-

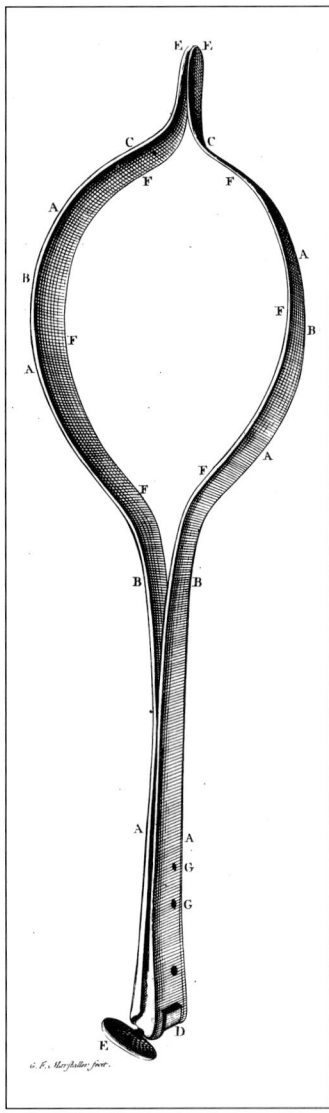
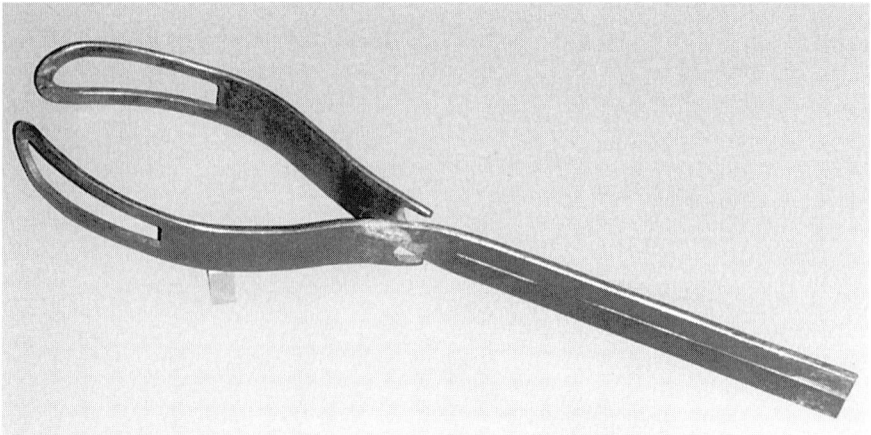

FIGURE 1.10 (ABOVE LEFT).
Rathlauw's original forceps. (Rathlauw, 1747)
(The Wellcome Institute Library, London)

FIGURE 1.11 (ABOVE RIGHT).
Rathlauw's improved fenestrated forceps.
(Science Museum, London)

FIGURE 1.12 (OPPOSITE LEFT).
Schlichting's forceps. Note the leather covering.
(Science Museum, London)

FIGURES 1.13, 1.14 (OPPOSITE RIGHT).
Schlichting's forceps. Figure 1.13 shows the construction. Figure 1.14 shows their purported use in a twin delivery. (Schlichting, 1747) (The Wellcome Institute Library, London)

ments owe nothing to the Chamberlens, which is likely to be correct when one considers the detail of design and the impracticability of the Van Roonhuysen flexible blades. Likewise the Van Roonhuysen lever was of an inferior design to that of the Chamberlens. It is hardly likely that the Van Roonhuysens would have devised inferior instruments if they had possessed knowledge of the Chamberlen designs.

The widely held belief, propounded by Aveling, is that when Hugh Chamberlen, Senior, left England for personal reasons in 1699, he settled in Amsterdam. In need of money, he sold what he claimed was the secret (but possibly only one blade or even a lever) to a surgeon, possibly Hendrik van Roonhuysen (1625–1672) or more likely his son, Rogier (circa 1650–1709). This account was questioned by Radcliffe, who pointed out that Hugh was already a very old man when or if he settled in that city. Hugh first went to Scotland before going to Amsterdam in about 1702, by which time he was in his seventies; there is no evidence that he set up a practice in Amsterdam.

Thiery referred to the researches of A. Geijl (1905) in archives that were subsequently destroyed in the First World War. He supported Geijl's argument that the chronology of possible visits of members of the Chamberlen family to the Low Countries makes it unlikely that there were opportunities for interchange of information between members of the two families. For example, there is the suggestion that Hendrik might have had contact with Dr. Peter Chamberlen when he visited London in 1646. However, Dr. Peter was at that time living in The Hague. Geijl concluded that Hugh Senior had not resided in Amsterdam, based on the lack of documentary evidence in contemporary records. It is possible that Aveling confused father and son, since Hugh Junior's name appears in the Amsterdam records of inhabitants in 1685.

Whatever the initial secret and its origin, it was alleged that the Van Roonhuysens shared it with close associates and

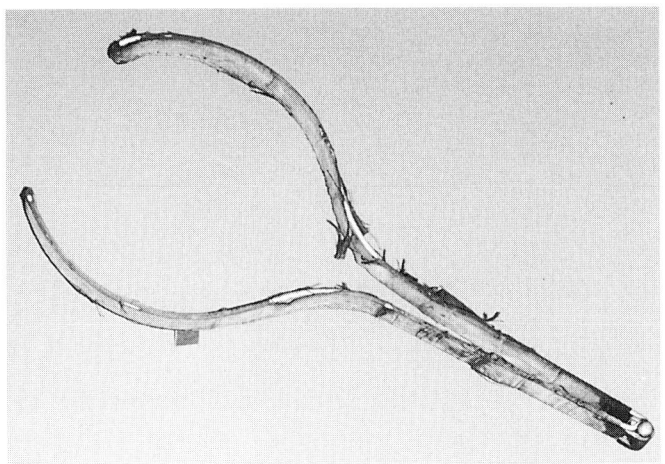

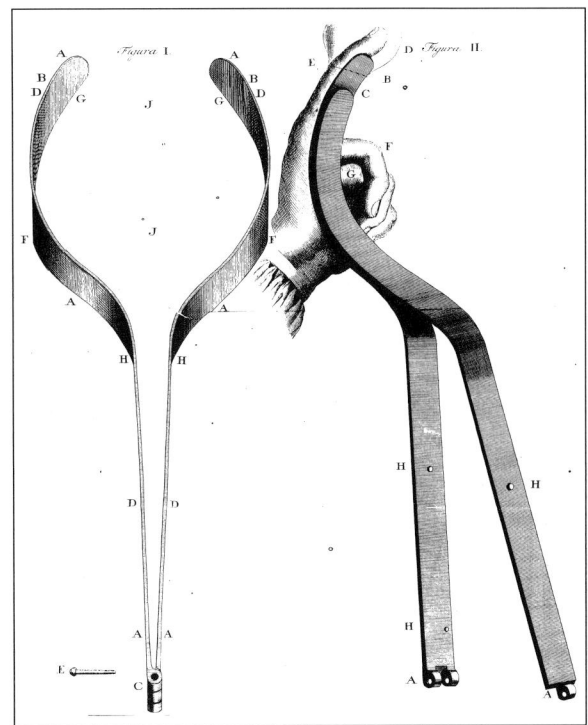

pupils, including Johannes de Bruin and Regner Bloom of Amsterdam and Paulus de Wind of Middleburg. These "Van Roonhuysians" retained the secret long after the death of both Hendrik and Rogier and continued to sell it to licentiate candidates.

The manner of disclosure of the Van Roonhuysian secret has been chronicled in several different versions. The first written account came from Jan Rathlauw (or Rathlaw). Rathlauw passed the examination of the Surgeons Guild in Amsterdam in about 1745, but from 1746 onward practitioners had to pass a special examination in order to be able to perform obstetric operations. The Van Roonhuysians were still in a strong position in the Amsterdam College and a license was only likely to be granted if the candidate had purchased the Van Roonhuysen secret, which Rathlauw apparently had not done. Rathlauw sought revenge and was put in touch with a Dr. Velsen of The Hague who claimed to have a sketch that had been made by a Van der Swam (or Suam), a former pupil of Rogier van Roonhuysen, behind his master's back. Rathlauw was granted his license to practice and was encouraged to publish the secret, which he did in 1747. He asserted that the instrument (Figure 1.10) was that which Hugh Senior had supposedly sold to Rogier van Roonhuysen.

When the Van Roonhuysian secret eventually leaked out in the middle of the eighteenth century, the instruments described were a pair of forceps and a lever. Rathlauw devised improved versions of the instrument by fenestrating the blades; increasing the cephalic curve, thereby providing a better grip; and adding a pin lock at the end of the handle, a version of which is in the Wellcome Collection (Figure 1.11).

In 1747, another surgeon from Amsterdam, Daniel Schlichting (1703–1765) also published a description of a pair of forceps, similar in design to Rathlauw's, that he claimed were of Van Roonhuysian origin (Figures 1.12–1.14). Schlichting claimed that he had found them in the house of

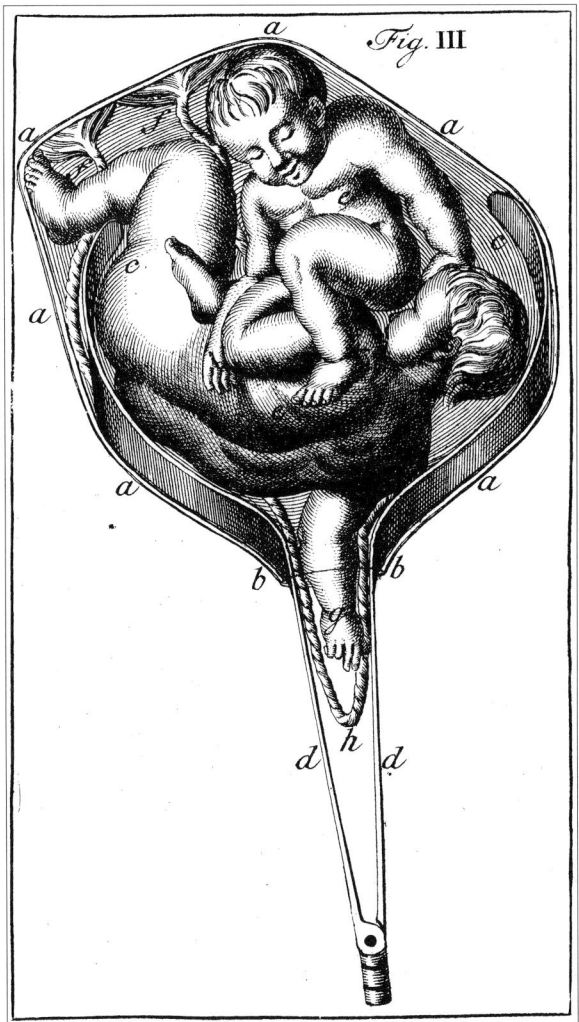

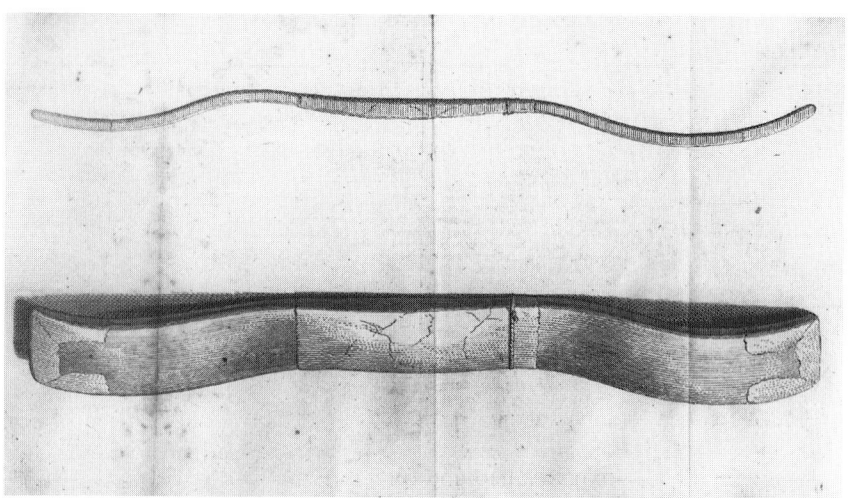

FIGURES 1.15, 1.16 (OPPOSITE). Levers of van Roonhuysen and De Vischer and Van de Poll.(De Wind, 1751; De Vischer and Van de Poll, 1753) (The Wellcome Institute Library, London)

a surgeon who had obtained them from a colleague who in turn had inherited them from a third generation Van Roonhuysian—rather a tenuous connection! (see also Thiery, 1992) However both Rathlauw and Schlichting agreed that the elastic nature of the blades still meant that they were unsatisfactory, though they could be used as cervical dilators.

The privileged group of Van Roonhuysians denied Rathlauw's and Schlichting's claims and declared that the secret was still inviolate. Indeed the "true" secret was not disclosed until 1753. On his deathbed Johannes de Bruin (1681–1753), who had been an assistant of Rogier van Roonhuysen, handed over a package of his instruments and instructions for their use to his family with a request that the contents should be published by two friends, J. de Vischer and H. van de Poll. This occurred promptly as *The Obstetric Secret of the Roonhuysians Discovered*. An expanded edition appeared in 1754. The instrument described was a flat steel lever slightly curved at the ends and covered with dog leather. The later publication also depicted some modified versions. Any other instruments that may have been in de Bruin's package were not disclosed (Figures 1.15, 1.16).

Robert Bland, who practiced in London at the end of the eighteenth century, wrote in 1790 that at the time the knowledge of the lever seemed to be almost exclusively confined to the Netherlands, the rest of Europe being preoccupied with rival instruments. He extolled the virtues of the Van Roonhuysen-type lever, particularly for those with limited obstetric practice who lacked expertise with the forceps. Use of the lever instead led to minimal use of destructive instruments. Bland gave an English translation of the detailed instructions for its use, based on the original paper by Vischer and Van de Poll.

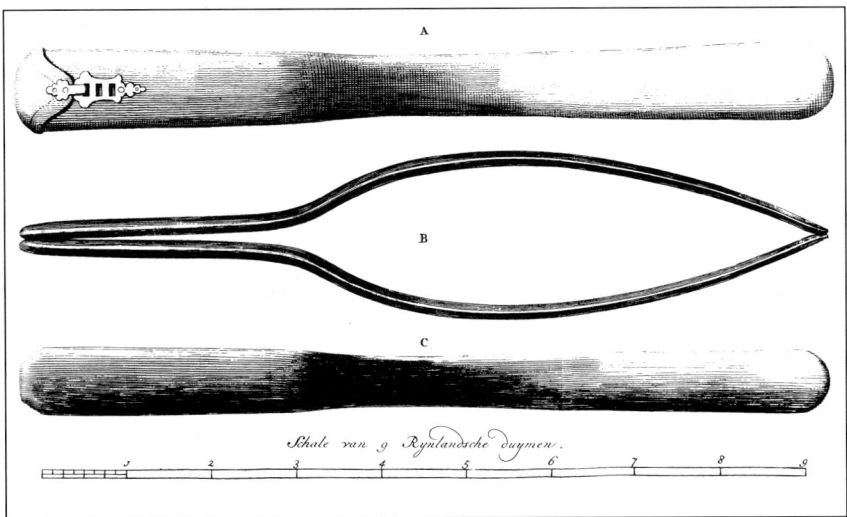

Thiery concluded that the Van Roonhuysians had two secrets, a forceps devised by either Hendrik or Rogier van Roonhuysen and subsequently modified by their followers but eventually discarded in favor of the lever. He concluded that levers were the preferred instrument on the Continent until the end of the nineteenth century. This may be so as far as the Low Countries are concerned but elsewhere on the Continent, as well as in Britain, the forceps were undoubtedly in the ascendancy, as will be seen in the following chapters.

· · ·

However, although knowledge of the forceps was widespread by the middle of the eighteenth century they were in use by only a limited number of enthusiastic practitioners and even they were conservative in their indications. Progress was also slowed by professional, religious, and lay opposition, as well as by constraints imposed by factors such as deficiencies in the available wrought irons, which was only fully remedied with the advent of crucible steel of consistent quality in the latter part of the eighteenth century.

Even by the beginning of the nineteenth century the use of forceps was still very limited. For example, at the Dublin Lying-in Hospital, which was regarded as being in the forefront of obstetrics, forceps were hardly ever used, reliance was still placed on the lever and crotchet. By the second quarter of the nineteenth century the factors that had militated against progress were lessening and more rational policies with scientific bases were emerging, as will be evident in subsequent chapters.

2 THE SECRET EMERGES: THE EARLY EIGHTEENTH CENTURY

In the late seventeenth and early eighteenth centuries attitudes toward operative delivery were changing and new instruments for assisting delivery of the fetus were emerging, but these were mainly destructive in nature. There was also still a substantial body of noninterventionists and advocates of herbal remedies. The Chamberlen instruments remained a secret and it was not until the second quarter of the eighteenth century that there was more than a hint of really functional and potentially lifesaving forceps, replacing the cruder devices discussed in the previous chapter.

The teachings of the influential Ambroise Paré (Introduction) were continued into the late seventeenth and early eighteenth centuries by his worthy successor, François Mauriceau (1637–1709). As did Paré before him, Mauriceau gave details of the options of the use of the crotchet and of perforation of the head to reduce its size when all else had failed, including his *perce-crâne* and *tire-tête* (1675) (Figure 2.1).

For abnormal presentations, podalic version and, if necessary, decapitation and/or perforation were performed, thus allowing piecemeal extraction with large lithotomy forceps. The severed head would be removed manually or with hooks, although other safer contrivances were emerging, such as the *tire-tête* (Figure 2.2) of Pierre Amand (1715)—a sort of net bag. It should be noted that the term *tire-tête* was use by various accoucheurs to describe a variety of devices for holding the head, decapitated or intact. The two described above are indicative of the range of devices used but the term was even used by some to describe conventional forceps, with which a linguistic purist might well agree. Linen bandages, precursors of the fillet, were also used for this purpose. Heister (1724) recommended stone (lithotomy) forceps for extracting a dead fetus as being better than hooks or any other instruments (Figure 2.3).

William Sermon (1629–1679), in his *Ladies Companion* of 1671, still concentrated on the use of herbals and a noninterventionist approach. However, he did state that "when it falleth out that none of these medicines shall take effect there are several other ways . . . as the crotchet, hooks, tongs and other instruments." It has been suggested that Sermon was alluding to the obstetric forceps but in the context of the book this statement related to the extraction of the dead fetus; the "other instruments" remain unidentified.

John Maubray (d. 1732), who was the first teacher of practical midwifery in London, published *The Female Physician* in 1724 (second edition 1730), addressed to both male and female practitioners as well as to women in general. He claimed that at that time in France only men practiced midwifery, while in Italy and Germany there were both men and women practitioners. In England, Scotland, and Holland men were styled "Extraordinary Midwives, being seldom or never called but in extraordinary cases of difficult or preternatural births."

Maubray, in spite of subtitling his book *The Whole Art of New Improv'd Midwifery,* added nothing to the traditional body of knowledge and believed that most difficulties could be overcome by tender care and herbal remedies with, if necessary, internal manipulation of the head position and stretching of the birth passages. He also described the procedure for internal version in detail. In a somewhat self-righteous dissertation (not uncommon for the times), he took the view that those who use instruments

kill many more INFANTS than they *save,* and *ruin* many more WOMEN than they *deliver* fairly: . . . .when they have perhaps wounded the

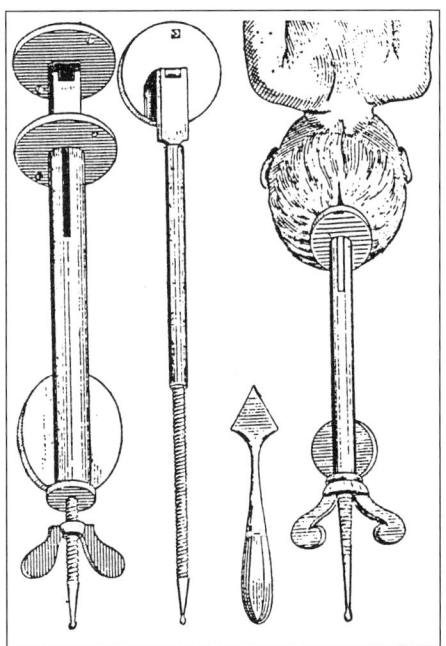

FIGURE 2.1.
Mauriceau's *perce-crâne* and *tire-tête*.
(Mauriceau, 1675; Witkowski, 1887)

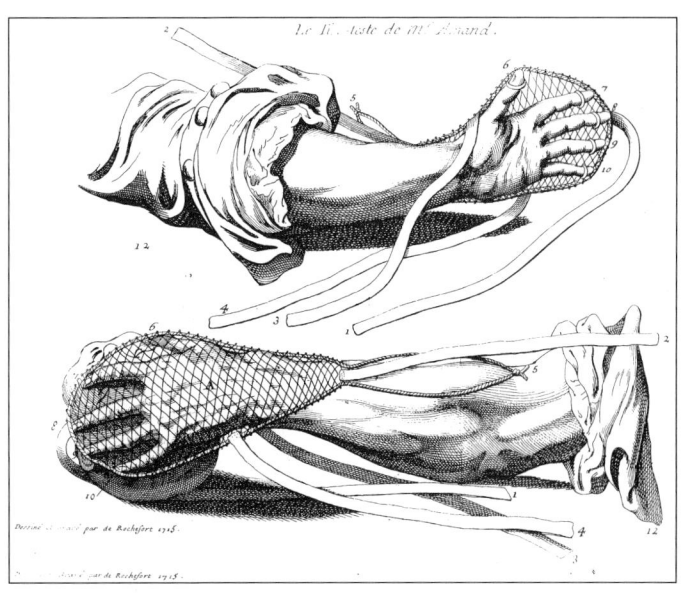

FIGURE 2.2.
Amand's *tire-tête* for extraction of the head after decapitation. (Amand, 1715)

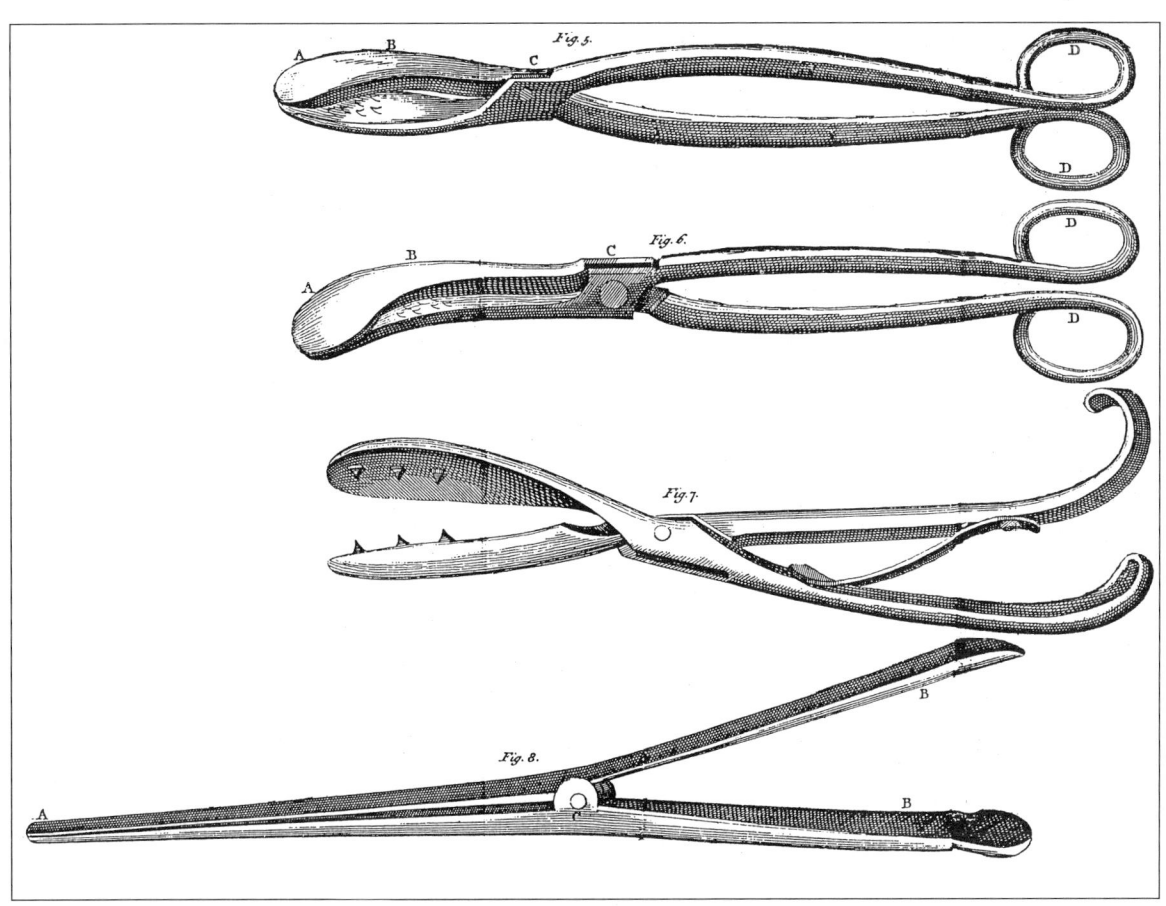

FIGURE 2.3.
Heister's lithotomy forceps. (Heister, 1724)

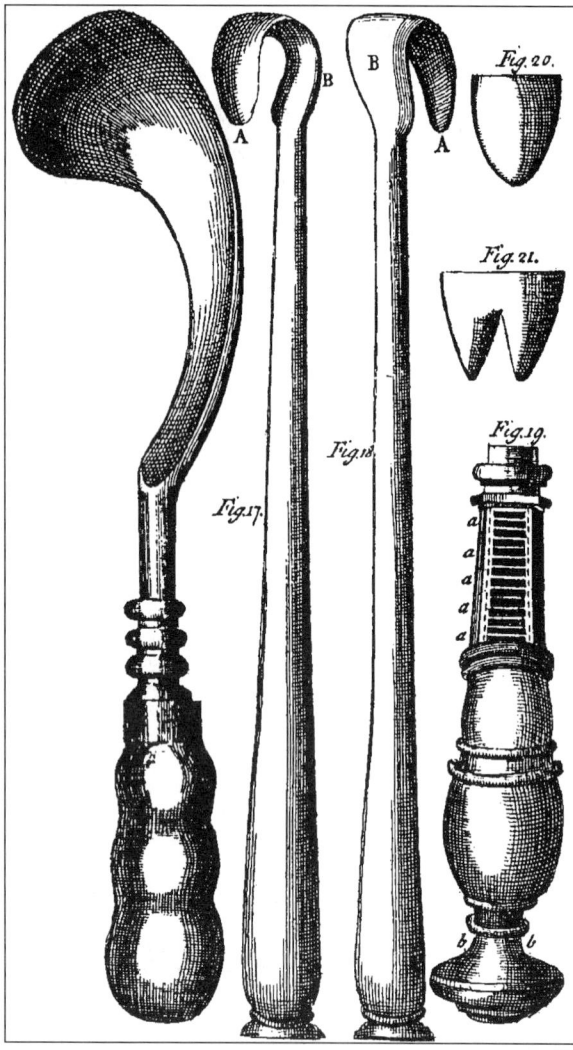

FIGURE 2.4.
Some of Heister's instruments for extraction of a dead fetus. (Heister, 1724)

complet des accouchements (1722).

So it was that in the first quarter at least of the eighteenth century the forceps were still largely unknown. John Douglas, a well-known physician in London, wrote in 1736 that "the operation necessary for the safety of women in labour, and their children seems to have been left entirely to a parcel of ignorant women, or to men little better than they, who, upon any extraordinary difficulty took hooks and knives and carved the children to pieces, and often also destroyed the mother."

There are few detailed descriptions of operative procedures at the beginning of the eighteenth century. A notable exception is *A General System of Surgery* by Lorenz Heister, Professor of Physic and Surgery at the University of Helmstadt, and based on thirty-years' experience. The English translation from the Latin edition was published in 1743 and gave considerable practical detail of methods for extracting a dead fetus, which could also be used on a living fetus when the mother's life was in the utmost danger. After clysters (enemas) and catheterization a broad ligature could be passed round the neck, failing which well-polished hooks could be "prudently fastened into some convenient Part of the Infant's Head, as the Eye, Ear, Mouth, and sometimes the Forehead and Occiput together... and, if those Instruments are not at hand, a large Nail may be bent into a Hook." He did not favor the *tire-tête* of Mauriceau but made passing mention of Palfyn's hooks and stated that a pair might be required. He illustrated many of his instruments (Figure 2.4) but obstetric forceps received no mention at all.

The First British Records of Obstetric Forceps

In the second quarter of the eighteenth century there were several publications describing forceps designs based on the Chamberlen concepts. However, prior to this an instrument belonging to a Dr. Drinkwater (d. 1728) of Brentford, Middlesex, was later described by R. W. Johnson (1769) as being similar to both Chapman's and Giffard's forceps (see below). Johnson did not say that they were Drinkwater's invention, merely that he reputedly had owned them. They were also mentioned later by Mulder (1794) and he dated them as 1668. However, this seems unlikely since 1668 was, according to Johnson, the year that Drinkwater began practice. Considering the lack of a contemporaneous description, the doubt as to whether Drinkwater designed or merely owned the instrument, and the interval of about a century before any written record emerged, claims for a "first" by Drinkwater have little substance.

MOTHER, kill'd the INFANT, and with violent *torture* and inexpressible *pain*, drawn it out by *Piecemeal*, they think no *Reward* sufficient for such an extraordinary Piece of mangled work. BUT, in short, I would advise such to practise *Butchery* rather than MIDWIFERY; for in *that Case*, they could *sell* what they *slay*....

Likewise, on the Continent there remained a cautious attitude to intervention with instruments. Guillaume La Motte (1665–1737), who trained at the Hôtel Dieu, favored manual manipulation. He disapproved of the crotchet, saying "I have not used it twice these thirty years" and supported this statement with some graphically described horror stories of trauma created by other practitioners in his work *Traité*

By the second quarter of the eighteenth century in London and elsewhere forceps based on the Chamberlen principles had, according to Edmund Chapman (1680–1756) in his 1735 *Treatise* (see below), become an open secret and were being used by many obstetricians. However it remains unclear as to how the secret leaked out; who were the first practitioners, other than the Chamberlens, to use forceps; and who first publicized the secret. The practitioners of the day were not driven by any academic desire to be first in print with details of a new invention and publication was expensive. Rather they were driven more by self-interest, as the Chamberlens had been, to enhance their practice. Publications consisted mainly of case reports and how difficulties had been overcome, rather than details of the instruments used. Indeed, written details usually came at a later date and frequently from the pens of other practitioners. Often there were inaccuracies in the artists representations of the instruments and possibly they were making depictions from descriptions or modifications of the originals.

The many designs of forceps in use in England by the second quarter of the century had features in common with the Chamberlen instruments. The fenestrated blade was almost universal but the pelvic curve had not yet emerged. The handles were hooked and could be used as extraction hooks. It was also common to modify one handle for use as a crotchet. There appeared to be two common practical difficulties, one of design and one of manufacture. The nature of the articulation, a problem with which the Chamberlens had wrestled, was still not resolved, and the iron used was so soft and malleable that distortion occurred.

Many historians consider that the strongest contender for the earliest use of forceps based on the Chamberlen concept was Edmund Chapman. Certainly he gave fuller discussion of their use but it is not clear to what degree his designs were original and how much he owed to his contemporaries (Figure 2.5). Starting in about 1708, Edmund Chapman practiced in Halstead, Essex, less than twenty miles from the Chamberlen's home at Woodham Mortimer. Later, he moved to London and, following the success of his book, he became the Public Teacher in Midwifery.

Chapman's knowledge of forceps may well have come from a member of the Chamberlen family or other associates in the neighborhood and he publicized through his works and teaching as much as he could discover of Hugh Chamberlen's methods of forceps delivery. He published the first written account of the use of obstetric forceps in English in 1733 in his *Essay on the Improvement of Midwifery*. This work was enlarged and revised and reappeared as a *Treatise* in 1735, with a further edition in 1753.

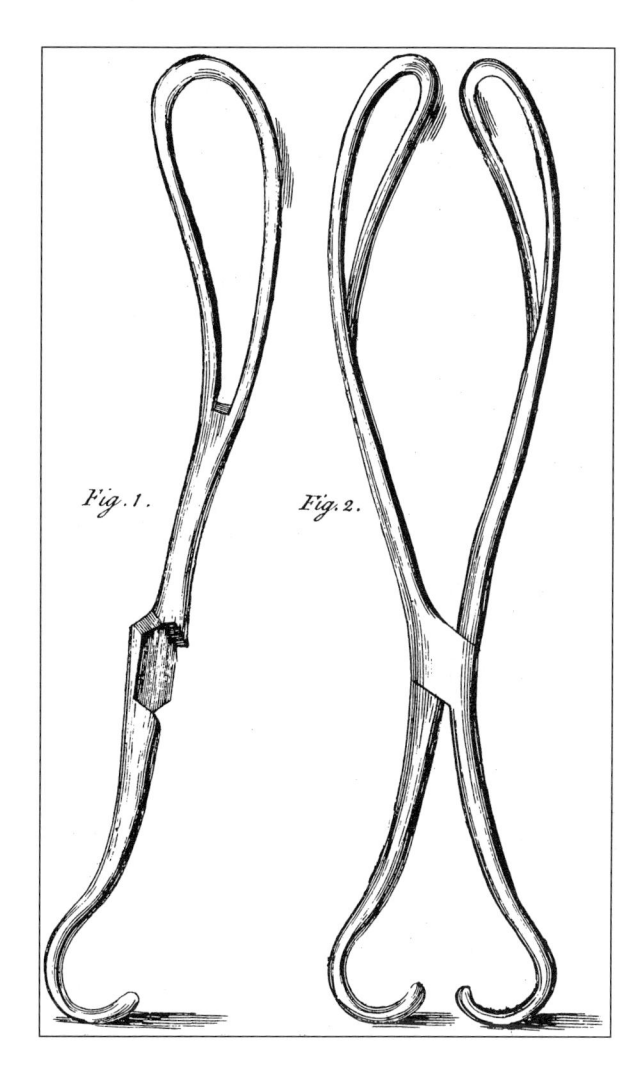

FIGURE 2.5.
Chapman's forceps, as illustrated in his *Treatise*.
(1735)

Chapman did not agree with some of his brethren who thought that (operative) midwifery should be a male prerogative and thus wrote his *Essay* primarily for midwives. He considered that they should know how to turn the child, at that time the preferred maneuver adopted for obstructed labor. He condemned the practice of "braining the child" and the use of crotchets and other instruments that resulted in the destruction of living children. "Some . . . being ignorant of the Method of Turning a Child, made frequent use of the Hook and Knife and several other shocking and barbarous Instruments, even while the Child was living."

Chapman recommended the use of a fillet or the forceps when the head presented and was low. He claimed the fillet to be an invention of his own and followed the Chamberlen precedent of not revealing the details of its design and use.

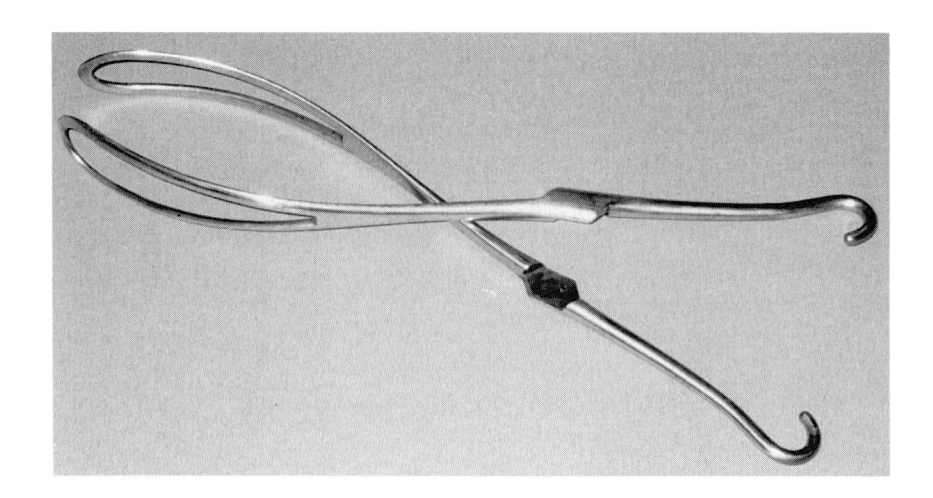

FIGURE 2.6.
Chapman's forceps, showing the articulation. (RCOG)

He was taken to task about this claim, which appeared in his *Essay* and in the 1735 edition of his *Treatise*. He admitted that the fillet was in common use for turning the child by securing one foot with it but that passing it over the head to use as a tractor was not so universally known and practiced. He described the forceps as "a noble instrument to which many now living owe their lives as I can assert from my own knowledge and practice" but gave no detailed description or measurements.

He had apparently been using forceps for some years prior to publishing his *Essay*, and almost certainly before 1725. He referred to "several different Sorts of Forceps . . . far from being all equally proper" and claimed that the use of the forceps "is now well known to all principal men of the profession both in town and country." His early forceps had a screw joint and, in common with other practitioners, he recounts difficulties with bending because of the soft metal. In consequence his "opinion of the instrument was so much lessened, that for many years after, [he] used it but seldom, and even not once for the space of ten years." He subsequently used a pair with a removable screw but recounts how he lost the screw during the course of a delivery and, having need for the forceps again soon after, had to use them without the screw. He found "that the instrument did its office much better without the screw or the two parts being fixt." He therefore abandoned the screw in favor of a simple mortise crossover joint (Figures 2.5, 2.6), and it is this instrument that he described in the 1735 edition of his *Treatise* (with the addition of "2nd edition" in the title but in fact the first appearance of the *Treatise*, an expanded version of his *Essay* of 1733). By 1736 he had adopted a design with deep grooves that were reputedly nearly as firm as a pivot joint and it was probably from this model that Smellie added the lugs that became the classic "English lock." (see Mulder, 1794)

Alexander Butter of Edinburgh took Chapman to task for not giving details of his own instrument.

> The Forceps for taking hold of a Child's Head, when it is fallen so far down among the Bones of the Pelvis, that it cannot be pushed back again into the Uterus, to be extracted by the Feet, and when it seems to make no Advances to the Birth by the Throws of the Mother, is scarce known in this country, though Mr. Chapman tells us, it was long made use of by Dr. Chamberlane [sic] who kept the form of it a secret, as Mr. Chapman also does. I believed therefore that the Sight of such an Instrument which I had from Mr. Dusè [sic], who practises Midwifery at Paris, and who believes it to be his own Invention, would not be acceptable to you, and the Publication of a Picture of it may be of Use to some of your Readers. (1735)

To which Chapman promptly responded in the 1735 edition of his *Treatise*:

> I must acknowledge myself short, in not giving the Figure of my Forceps in the former edition. I was not indeed so thoroughly sensible of this Defect, till I found my Essay honourably mentioned by a Learned Society established at *Edinburgh* for the improvement of *Physic* and *Surgery*, in the *Medical Essay* and *Observations, &c.* Vol. III. Art. XXXI. As these Gentlemen, by saying I have not given a Description of that Instrument as I used it seem to insinuate that something is wanting to render this Work more complete and satisfactory; I have now subjoined an exact Draught of my *Forceps* which is very little different from That used by the late Mr. William Giffard. . .

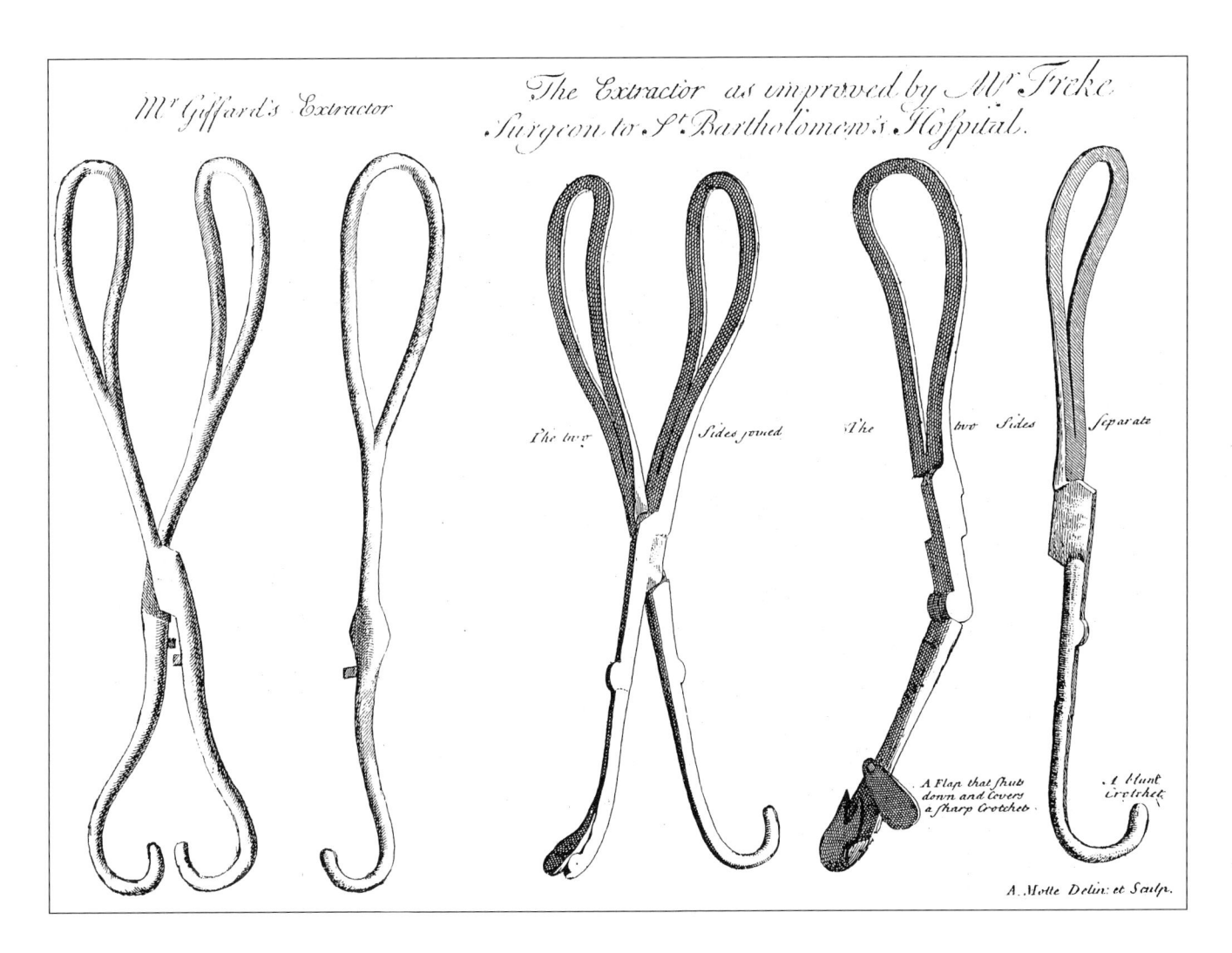

FIGURE 2.7.
Giffard's and Freke's forceps. Illustrated by Hody in his edition of Giffard's *Cases in Midwifery* (1734).

Chapman illustrated his version of the forceps with fenestrated blades similar to those of Giffard, and without a screw joint. William Giffard (d. 1731), claimed to have first used an "extractor" of his own design in a delivery on April 8, 1726. He continued to use the extractor with varying success until his death in 1731. However, the instrument was not described in detail and it was left to Edward Hody to give a full description and illustration when he revised and published Giffard's *Cases in Midwifery* in 1734, although the plates had been made in 1733. The forceps had a simple crossover articulation with the addition of small locating lugs but no screw (Figure 2.7). Other forceps with a screw joint have also been ascribed to Giffard but are not well authenticated.

Hody also referred to and illustrated an improved extractor (Figure 2.7) designed by John Freke (or Freake) (b. 1688). Freke was a surgeon at St. Bartholomew's Hospital, a Fellow of the Royal Society, and a contemporary of Hody (see also Moore, 1918). Radcliffe suggests that Freke persuaded Hody to include his forceps in the Giffard publication but there is no supporting evidence. Johnson said that Freke was a mechanical genius but was never distinguished in midwifery. Freke incorporated a folding sharp crotchet at the end of one handle and the other handle was shaped as a blunt hook. Freke was also the first to add a hinge to one handle, a feature not used again until much later in the century by the French obstetricians (Chapter 5).

An analysis of Giffard's cases is of interest and importance in that it gives some insight into the practice of the time. In Giffard's 225 cases he mentioned the use of his extractor on 60 occasions. In most of these the head was "locked in the pelvis" but he also used the extractor in cases of prolapsed cord and eclampsia; for the high head he favored turning. He would apply the extractor through an incompletely dilated cervix if necessary but always tried to get a proper cephalic application when using both blades. In 41 cases he initially applied one blade only and attempted to improve the position of the head or to lever it out; this was attended with success in 27 cases and loss of only 3 babies. In 33 cases he used both blades; on 14 occasions this was after failing with a single blade. Twelve of these 33 babies were lost. In 3 cases he failed to deliver with the forceps, resulting in podalic version in 1 case and craniotomy and hooks in 2 cases.

Thus it remains uncertain which practitioner first used forceps of the Chamberlen pattern but Hody's 1734 revised edition of Giffard's *Case Reports* illustrating both Giffard's and Freke's forceps just antedates Chapman's 1735 illustrated description of his forceps but not his written description of 1733.

None of these authors in their descriptions mentioned any derivation from the Chamberlen instruments but Chapman, in his 1735 *Treatise*, reproduced a letter dated October 30, 1734, which he had received from Dr. John Page of Lutterworth, a former pupil whom he had instructed in the use of the forceps, in which Page expressed his gratitude to Chapman for his "candid and ingenious Directions during the time I had the pleasure to be your pupil" and said "I do not wonder that Dr Chamberlen became so eminent in midwifery, when he had so safe an instrument to practice with." This appears to be the first written reference acknowledging the Chamberlen instruments.

The Beginnings of New Features in British Design

Soon after these instruments came to the public notice in Britain some novel ideas began to emerge that were of seminal importance and resulted in changes that endured in British design. Of particular note are two features, which subsequently were generally ascribed to Smellie but which might have had their genesis elsewhere. The first was a new articulation described by Chamberlen Walker and the second was the introduction of a second curve to the blades, the pelvic curve, described by Benjamin Pugh.

About the same time as Chapman, Chamberlen Walker (Chapter 1) introduced a forceps of similar overall style and with a general resemblance to the Chapman instrument but shorter, the important difference being a novel articulation (Figure 2.8). The forceps first came to public knowledge sometime between 1735 and 1740 and thus are contemporaneous with those of Chapman. The joint was a male/female hinge comprising a notch on one blade into which the flattened surface of the other blade fit. The description given by A. R. Simpson (1900) accords with an unnamed pair of forceps described by J. Mulder (1794). It seems that Walker was close to resolving the problem of the articulation that had troubled so many for so long and his description antedates the Smellie articulation, usually known as the English lock, which was a further development of it. Indeed, some would claim that Walker, rather than Smellie, was the inventor of the English lock.

Benjamin Pugh (circa 1710–1775) practiced in Chelmsford, not far from the Chamberlen household at Woodham Mortimer. In his *Treatise of Midwifery* (1754) he described three pairs of forceps, two long (355 millimeters/14 inches) and one short (280 millimeters/11 inches), all with a pelvic curve and with an articulation not unlike Smellie's (Figure 2.9). He emphasized the benefit over the straight forceps both in introduction and extraction. He claimed to have been using these instruments for "fourteen years past" (that is, 1740 or before because publication of his book was delayed for four years from lack of funds), thus making him a contender for originating the pelvic curve. In addition one of the long pairs had a small crotchet at the top of the bow, which he said he would prefer to the common crotchets though he had never used them.

Early European Forceps

The Grégoires, *père et fils*, had an extensive practice in Paris in the early eighteenth century. The Grégoires published no papers and the first written description of their forceps was from a pupil, A. Böehmer of Halle, in 1746, who is said to be the first person to introduce obstetric forceps into Germany (Doran, 1913a).

Numerous versions of the Grégoire forceps have been described and have been documented by Doran (1913a) (Figures 2.10–2.12). Mulder (1794), a generally reliable source, illustrated in detail a more complicated version of the locking mechanism than is generally described (Figure 2.13). Hellier (1912) described a pair that matched earlier descriptions detailed by Doran, but was of light construction and lacked the crotchet. The pair described by Doran (now destroyed) was much heavier and had a hinged crotchet. Their straight forceps, probably the design of the son, bore a resemblance to the English forceps of the time but were distinguished by a unique lock comprising a pivot on one shank that passed through a hole in the other shank and was secured by a sliding bolt that engaged in a groove on the pivot. This was a feature subsequently taken up by Levret. Also, in some versions, a sharp-hinged crotchet was incorporated in one handle, similar to Freke's forceps.

Dusée (d. 1734), was a pupil of the Grégoires but his forceps were developed from Palfyn's *mains de fer*. Like so many practitioners of the time he unfortunately left no written description of his instruments. His instruments, or modifications of them (Figures 2.14, 2.15), were first described by

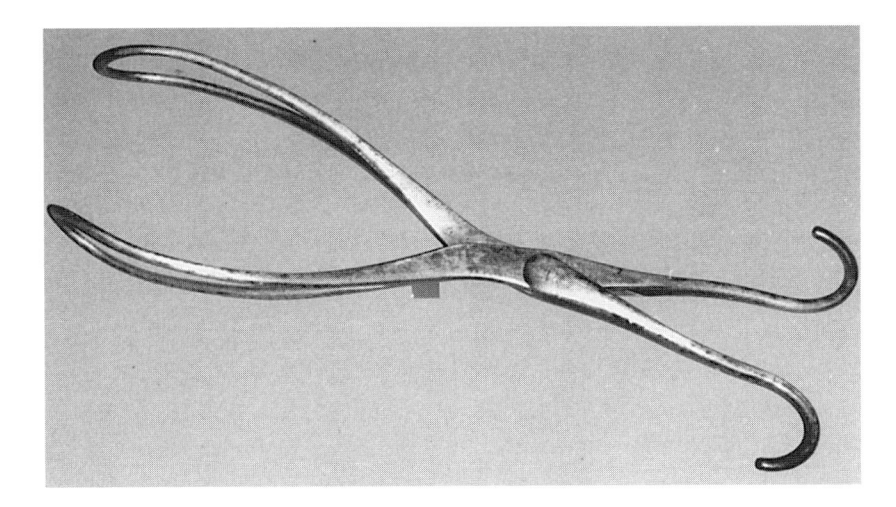

FIGURE 2.8.
Chamberlen Walker's forceps. Note the articulation. Although the date of the construction of these forceps is uncertain they probably antedate the Smellie forceps and could thus be considered the forerunner of the English lock. (The Science Museum, London)

Alexander Butter in Edinburgh in 1733 in the article in which he criticized Chapman (see above). Dusée is also believed to be the first person to teach the practice of fundal massage to control uterine hemorrhage. Butter gave a detailed description of Dusée's forceps. Dusée's main contribution was the addition of a mortise joint, or hinge, fixed by a removable screw pivot. He increased the versatility of the instrument by adding a second position for the lock for use in delivery of the head from high in the pelvic cavity—a procedure that had not been contemplated in British practice before this. This construction also enabled the instrument to be used as an asymmetric forceps. The solid blades had a marked cephalic curve in the Palfyn style but no pelvic curve. The exaggerated cephalic curve was intended to avoid compression of the temporal arteries. A notch at the end of the blade was supposed to avoid the risk of compressing the carotid arteries. In some illustrations only a single articulation is shown and there is no notch at the end of the blade. Butter agreed with Chapman that a screw was difficult to insert and remove and was unnecessary, so he discarded it. E. von Siebold suggested that Butter exhibited the Dusée forceps "to stir up his countrymen, not wishing that they should keep their instruments secret" (1839). Certainly it had the desired effect on Chapman.

Although Dusée's forceps are important historically, particularly because they were the first European forceps with a crossed articulation and could, at least in theory, be used for high forceps delivery, they were unsatisfactory in use, as is recorded by his own pupil, Paulus de Wind, and by Levret, Smellie (Chapter 3), and others.

When De Wind (Chapter 1) left Grégoire *fils* he and J. Boswell of Edinburgh went to live with Dusée in Paris in 1734. Dusée showed them his own forceps but they never saw the instrument in use because he died soon afterward. Boswell purchased the forceps from Dusée's heirs before re-

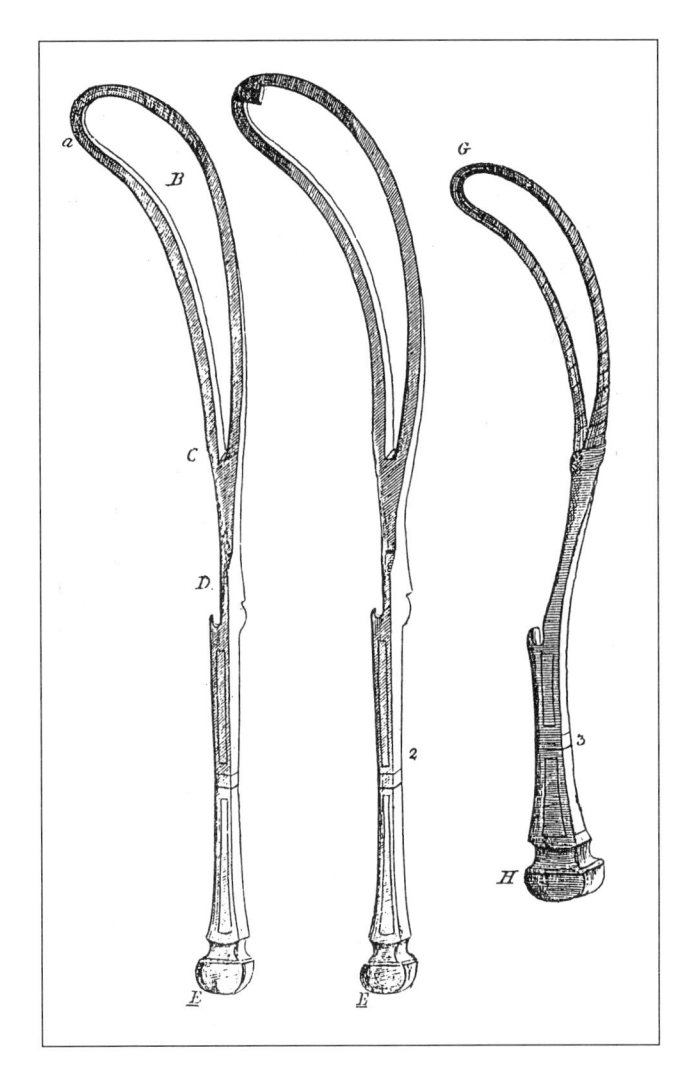

FIGURE 2.9.
Pugh's forceps. Pugh illustrated three pairs, two long (355mm/14ins) and one short (280mm/11ins). Note the introduction of the pelvic curve, the sharp hook on the tip of the middle blade, and the leather thonging on the short blade. (Pugh, 1754)

THE SECRET EMERGES 29

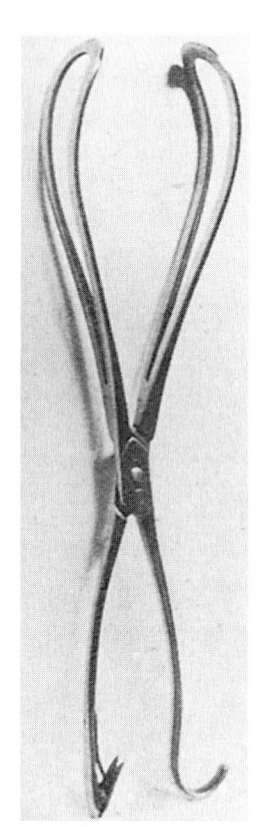

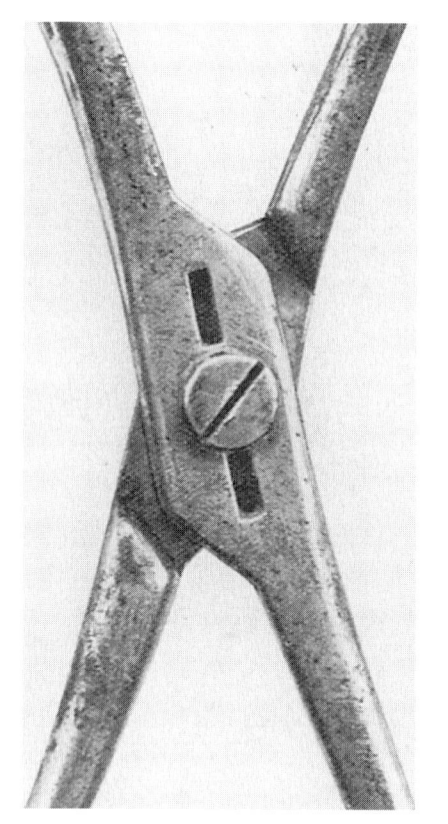

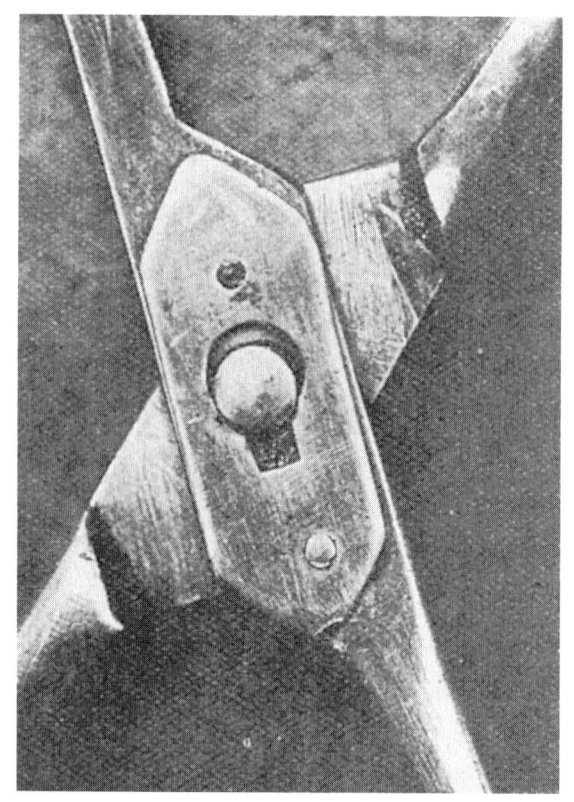

FIGURES 2.10–2.12.
Grégoire's forceps as described by Doran (1913a), showing different versions of the locking mechanism.

FIGURE 2.13.
Grégoire's forceps as illustrated by Mulder (1794). The design was more complicated than those shown by Doran (1913a).

turning to Edinburgh, where Butter had demonstrated his version of the Dusée forceps in the previous year. However, there is no mention that Boswell was aware of Butter's demonstration. De Wind had another pair made but found it "unsuited for its purpose. It was far too large and I could not introduce it into the body of my patient."

The translation concludes:

> It too often happens that teachers, after they have found that instruments which they have designed on theoretical principles are of no use in practice, cannot desist from demonstrating and expressing approval of them to their pupils. Thus we see the useless instrument of Dussé [*sic*] described in full in the Scottish transactions above quoted, and that of Palfyn in Heister's excellent work. I think that a good book might be written on bad surgical instruments; it is with such contrivances as with bad books, men who have laid out money on them are not inclined to throw them away and people buy them so as to give themselves a name be saying that they possess them.

30 CHAPTER 2

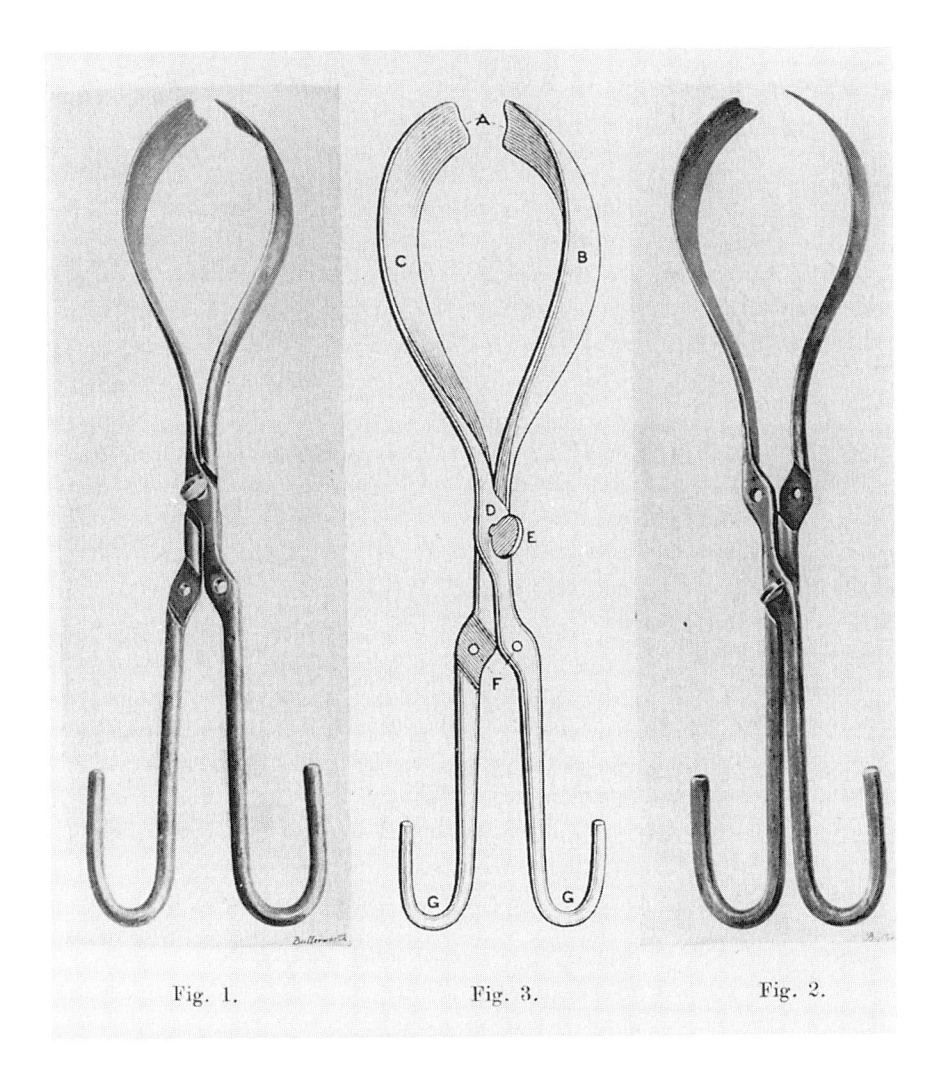

FIGURE 2.14.
Dusée's forceps. The center pair of forceps are those depicted by Butter of Edinburgh (see text). The others were in the museum of the Royal College of Surgeons of England but were destroyed during World War II. (Doran, 1912a)

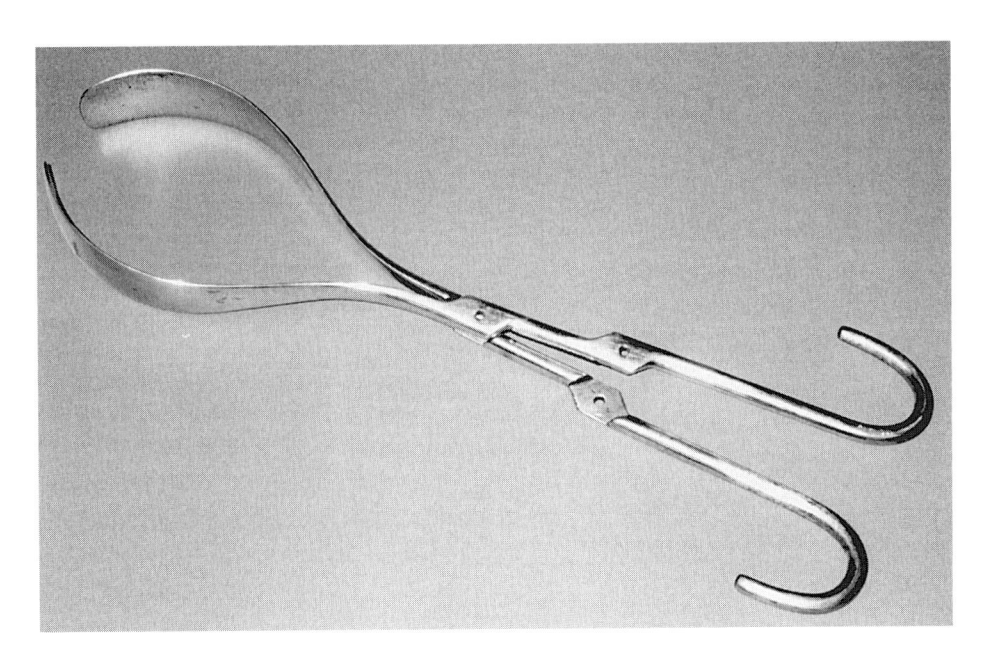

FIGURE 2.15.
Dusée's forceps. A pair in the RCOG collection, made by Still of Edinburgh and probably the Butter version of the original Dusée forceps.

In Paris in 1774, Antoine Petit, a professor of anatomy and surgery at the University of Paris, added to the confusion. He taught that there were only three kinds of forceps: Palfyn's, Smellie's, and Levret's (Petit, 1798–1799). He claimed that Palfyn brought the forceps to Paris between 1730 and 1734 and passed them off as his own invention, but that they had really been invented by a Dr. Douglas of London many years previously. He also claimed that a forceps of similar design originated from Gilles le Doux of Ypres, which he showed to Palfyn. Strangely, he made no mention of Dusée's instruments, though Mulder claimed that Petit described an instrument similar to Dusée's.

The Dusée type of forceps was also used in Ireland, and was probably introduced by Fielding Ould (1710–1789). Ould was born in Galway but after studying in Paris with Grégoire he practiced in Dublin from about 1736 and became the second master of the Rotunda Hospital in 1759. In his *Treatise* (1742) he stated that "[t]he best adapted instrument is the large forceps, which is in general use all over Europe." He described the essential features of the blade shape and gave details of how they should be applied. He mentioned a screw joint and handles that could be used as hooks for delivering the shoulders. Although Ould ascribed no name to the instrument the description fits with the Dusée type of forceps described above as Levret (Chapter 3) had not yet published details of his design.

. . .

The early eighteenth century saw the beginning of moving from herbalism and, as a last resort, traumatic operative procedures to more rational and practical obstetrics. Also, a small number of man-midwives in England who had previously relied on crude destructive instruments for dealing with obstructed labor had become acquainted with the concept of obstetric forceps. From where they had acquired this knowledge remains uncertain, but the Chamberlen secret was almost certainly leaking out by this time. It is notable that the earlier written descriptions of forceps design came from practitioners living in the same part of the country as the Chamberlen family and common features of their design were fenestrated blades and crossover articulation. Probably their acquired knowledge was fragmentary and they each made their own interpretation of the instruments.

In France attempts were being made to improve and articulate the Palfyn *mains de fer*. The Dusée design became the dominant pattern and his style of forceps became known and used in Scotland and Ireland, although they found little place in England.

These prototypes were relatively crude and had significant weaknesses in practice but they set the scene for a more scientific approach that was soon to follow.

SMELLIE AND LEVRET: TREND SETTERS FOR THE LATE EIGHTEENTH CENTURY[1]

Toward the middle of the eighteenth century a new breed of men-midwives was emerging who wanted to acquire knowledge of the new instruments and methods of delivery, and especially of the forceps, which would give them a skill denied to the midwives. R. W. Johnstone (1952) ascribes these developments to three factors: progress in medical science; fashion—in France Louis XIV had started the trend by employing a man-midwife, or *physician accoucheur,* for the delivery of at least one of his mistresses; and the spreading knowledge of the benefits of the obstetric forceps.

In the mid-eighteenth century there was increasing dissatisfaction with the old-fashioned teachings of such people as Maubray. Chapman had started as a teacher in London but apparently was not a great success, one of his pupils describing him as self-opinionated and too fond of the forceps.

The stage was set for the emergence of two of the most outstanding and influential British teachers of obstetrics, William Smellie and William Hunter. They began the evolution of obstetrics as a science, discarding medieval concepts and basing their teaching on a careful study of anatomy and practical observation, with operative procedures based on anatomical principles. Meanwhile, on the Continent the development of the design and use of forceps was dominated by André Levret.

The introduction of the pelvic curve in the 1740s was a major advance, especially for the high forceps operation that was favored by some, and pride of place for this has been claimed on behalf of both Smellie and Levret. Certainly as influential teachers with wide followings they popularized this innovation but in a carefully analyzed and well-reasoned paper McClintock (1876) concluded that the modification was first made and used by Benjamin Pugh in about 1740 (Chapter 2).

William Smellie

William Smellie (1697–1763), whose career has been well documented by J. Glaister (1894) and by Johnstone, practiced in his native Lanark, Scotland, for nineteen years, from 1720 to 1739. For the first thirteen his only instruments to assist delivery were crotchets and hooks, as had been used for centuries, and the perforator and lever. When the head was presenting and labor was obstructed the generally favored method of delivery, which was also used by Smellie, was to perform internal podalic version and to extract the baby by traction on a leg or with a breech hook.

Smellie's interest in forceps arose from a desire "to avoid this loss of children which gave me great uneasiness." His first experience with forceps was in 1737, using a pair of French forceps recommended by Alexander Butter of Edinburgh, which were in fact Dusée's forceps and were 432 millimeters (17 inches) long (Chapter 2). He later stated in his *Treatise* (see below) that he found them "so long and ill-formed that I could not introduce them safely to take a proper hold."

In 1739 Smellie went to London (where Chapman was still teaching) but soon left for Paris and attended the lectures of Grégoire from whom he learned the use of the "machine," or manikin, on which to practice operative procedures, which stood him in such good stead subsequently. On his return to London, somewhere between 1740 and 1741, Smellie's clinical practice was predominantly among the

---

[1] The material relating to Smellie and Hunter is derived from a lecture to the Hunterian Society on November 16, 1992.

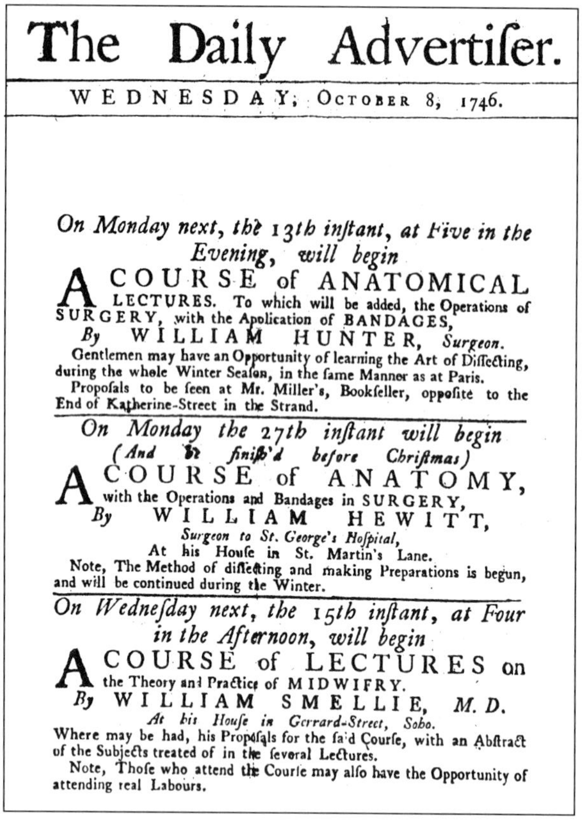

The Daily Advertiſer.

WEDNESDAY, OCTOBER 8, 1746.

On Monday next, the 13th inſtant, at Five in the Evening, will begin

A COURSE of ANATOMICAL LECTURES. To which will be added, the Operations of SURGERY, with the Application of BANDAGES,

By WILLIAM HUNTER, *Surgeon.*

Gentlemen may have an Opportunity of learning the Art of Diſſecting, during the whole Winter Seaſon, in the ſame Manner as at Paris.

Propoſals to be ſeen at Mr. Miller's, Bookſeller, oppoſite to the End of Katherine-Street in the Strand.

On Monday the 27th inſtant will begin (And be finiſh'd before Chriſtmas)

A COURSE of ANATOMY, with the Operations and Bandages in SURGERY,

By WILLIAM HEWITT,

Surgeon to St. George's Hoſpital,

At his Houſe in St. Martin's Lane.

Note, The Method of diſſecting and making Preparations is begun, and will be continued during the Winter.

On Wedneſday next, the 15th inſtant, at Four in the Afternoon, will begin

A COURSE of LECTURES on the Theory and Practice of MIDWIFRY.

By WILLIAM SMELLIE, *M. D.*

At his Houſe in Gerrard-Street, Soho.

Where may be had, his Propoſals for the ſaid Courſe, with an Abſtract of the Subjects treated of in the ſeveral Lectures.

Note, Thoſe who attend the Courſe may alſo have the Opportunity of attending real Labours.

FIGURE 3.1.
The Daily Advertiser of October 8, 1746. A broadsheet of news and advertisements, showing the advertisements of William Smellie and William Hunter.

poor. He was never on the staff of a lying-in hospital nor did he ever attend nobility. In 1741, he began teaching from his own house, offering instruction to midwives in the mornings and to men in the afternoons. As was the custom of the day he advertised his courses in broadsheets such as the *Daily Advertiser* (Figure 3.1). He charged two pounds, two shillings for twelve lectures, including demonstrations on "machines"; one pound, one shilling to witness a labor; and five pounds, five shillings for two lecture courses, four labors, and the supervision of one delivery by the student. In 1751 he published his *Treatise on the Theory and Practice of Midwifery*, which embodied the essence and application of the subject. The *Treatise* was illustrated with simple drawings of great clarity and contained the first accurate description of the mechanism of parturition. It was written with some elegance, unlike much of his correspondence, and thus it is likely that this work and his other publications were ghostwritten by his fellow doctor, friend, and essayist from Lanarkshire, Tobias Smollett.

Smellie's own assessment of his work, echoed by Johnstone, was that he showed a combination of uncommon industry and independent thinking, having a great ability to see things for what they were. According to A. H. McClintock in his annotation to the *Treatise* Smellie "cleared away an immensity of the rubbish and superstition which enveloped the whole theory and practice of midwifery."

Smellie probably used forceps of the Chapman type initially, having rejected Dusée's pattern, but soon set about designing his own instruments. His first pair were short, had small blades, and were made of wood (Figure 3.2). These were a failure, however, as their wooden construction necessitated undue thickness of the blades, which made insertion difficult. Also, the blades were of inappropriate shape and did not afford an adequate grip on the head. Smellie himself apparently only used them on four occasions. His first pair of steel forceps came into use in 1748. In his *Treatise* he described his new forceps, with features that have endured to this day, including the "English lock" and the pelvic curve (Figures 3.5, 3.7), although the latter was also being introduced at about the same time by Pugh in England (Chapter 2) and by Levret in France (see below).

Smellie's articulation, or lock, was a natural progression from the grooves in the later designs of Chapman (Chapter 2). He claimed that the design of the crossover lock had all the advantages of earlier articulations without the inconveniences. It was simple, with no screws or loose parts, and achieved a firm and stable union, while the lugs and grooves had sufficient tolerance to allow articulation when the fit on the head was less than perfect. Smellie also introduced into British practice the wooden-faced handle, which thereafter became a standard feature of British forceps designs. He may have got the idea from Mesnard's *Le Guide des accoucheurs* (Chapter 10), although wooden handles were not commonly used in Europe until much later.

Smellie recommended that the forceps "should be so short in the handles that they cannot be used with such violence as will endanger the woman's life," a sentiment reiterated by J. Wrigley almost two hundred years later when he was concerned with the excessive use and abuse of the forceps operation (1935). If the head was low in the pelvis Smellie regarded forceps delivery as justifiable to save the infant, even though the mother's life was not in danger—a novel philosophy for the time, since operative intervention had up to this point only been employed to save the life of the mother when the fetus was already dead. However, when the head was high in the pelvis he taught that "the Forceps ought not to be used except in the most urgent necessity," since their use increased the risk to the mother. The blades of Smellie's early forceps, which were slender and broadest near their

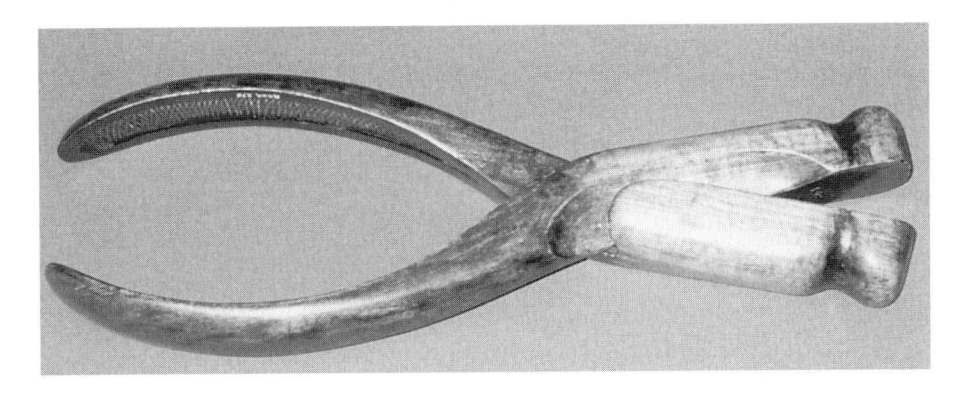

FIGURE 3.2.
Smellie's wooden forceps. Facsimile in the RCOG museum.

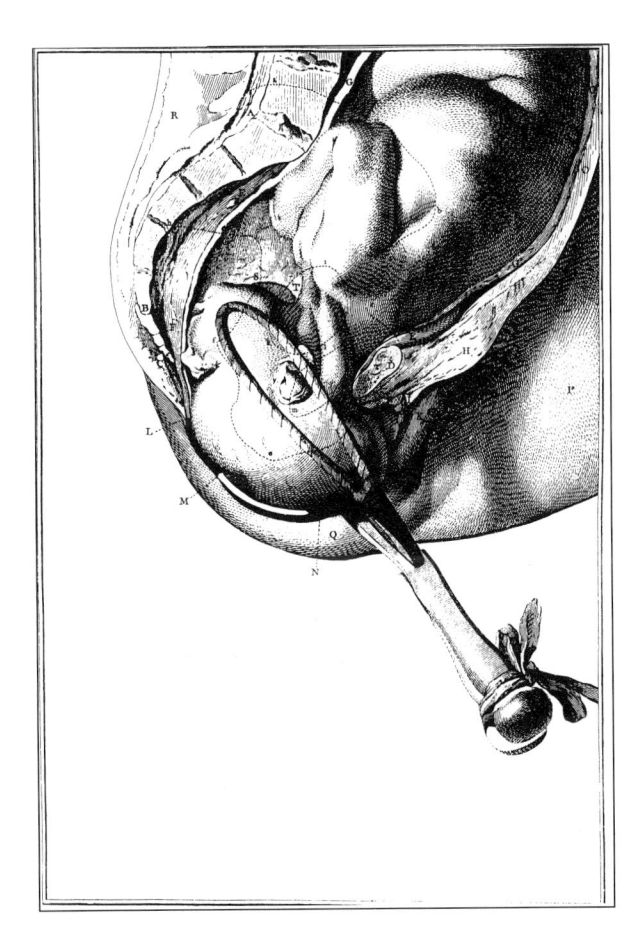

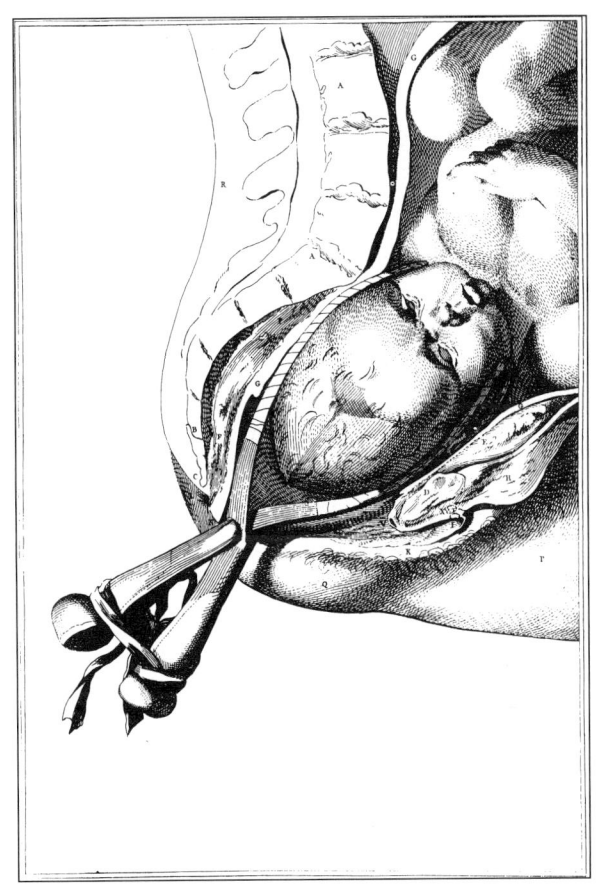

tips, were made of iron, covered with leather, and lubricated with hog's lard. Later the blades were wrapped in a ribbon of thinner material that was changed between deliveries (though not every time!) to reduce the risk of transmitting venereal infection (Figures 3.3, 3.4). When closed the tips of the blades touched but the maximum distance between the blades (averaging 64 millimeters [2.5 inches] in the examples at the Royal College of Obstetricians and Gynaecologists) meant that when applied to the head the handles would not approximate. However because of the shortness of the

FIGURE 3.3 (LEFT).
Smellie's straight forceps. Table XVIII from his *Atlas*. Occipito-anterior outlet delivery. Note the changeable leather thonging covering the blades.

FIGURE 3.4 (RIGHT).
Smellie's straight forceps. Table XVI from his *Atlas*. Delivery from the occipito-lateral position. Note the correct cephalic application.

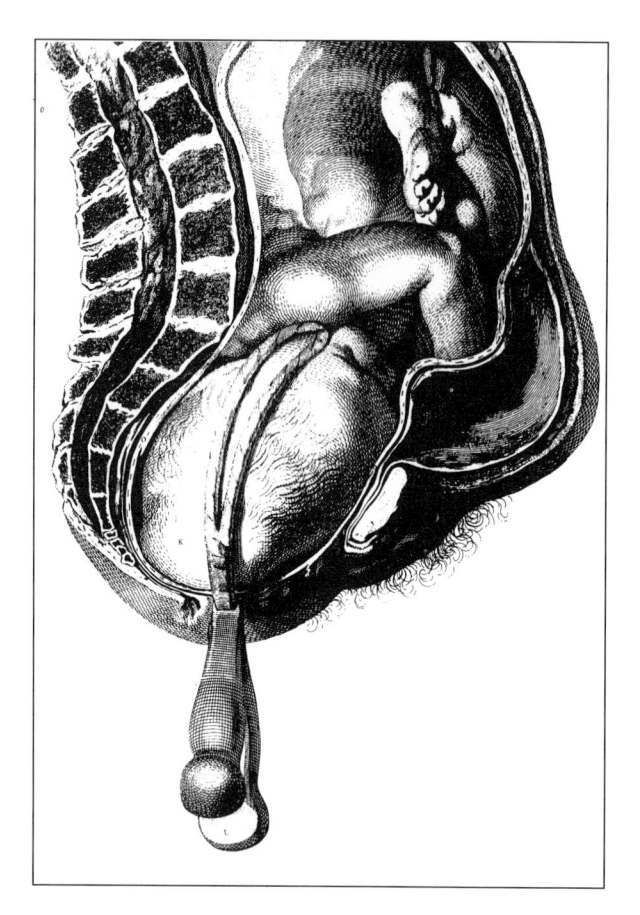

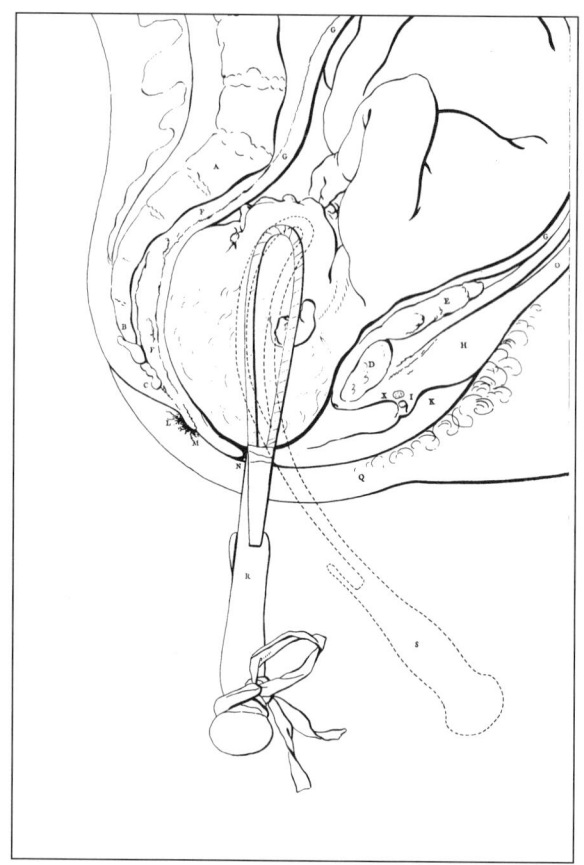

handles excessive compressive force could not be applied to the head, thus decreasing the danger to the infant. Smellie made many modifications to the shape and measurements over the years until he found those that suited him best, but he conceded that his choices should not restrict others who might want to alter the forceps further.

The introduction of the pelvic curve resulted in a better application and less risk of damage to the perineum. Figure 3.5 shows the curved forceps applied to a grossly molded occipito-posterior head. If traction was unsuccessful Smellie recommended rotation of the head to a favorable position with the forceps, historically the first mention of this procedure. In Case 258 from his *Treatise* Smellie recorded the following:

> While I paused a little, considering what method I should take, I luckily thought of trying to raise the head with forceps, and turn the forehead to the left side of the brim of the pelvis, where it was widest, an expedient which I immediately executed with greater ease than I expected. I then brought down the vertex to the right ischium, turned it to below the pubes, and the forehead into the hollow of the sacrum; and safely delivered the head by pulling it up from the perineum and over the pubes. This method succeeding so well gave me great joy.

Smellie subsequently lengthened his curved forceps from 280 millimeters (11 inches) to 318 millimeters (12.5 inches). These longer forceps are compared with the short straight forceps in Figure 3.6 and one can see that the lock is now well away from the perineum. The long forceps were also advocated in breech delivery for application to the aftercoming head if it was arrested.

It is difficult to identify or ascribe forceps of this period with certainty because no two pairs were identical, being made and copied approximately by local blacksmiths or cutlers, who sometimes worked only from a rough description or hearsay, with variations to suit the individual obstetrician. However, there are several pairs of the Smellie type in the museum at the Royal College of Obstetricians and Gynaecologists for which there are no obvious claims from other designers (Figure 3.7).

Smellie was not without his opponents. Midwives, as ever, were feeling threatened by the men-midwives because of

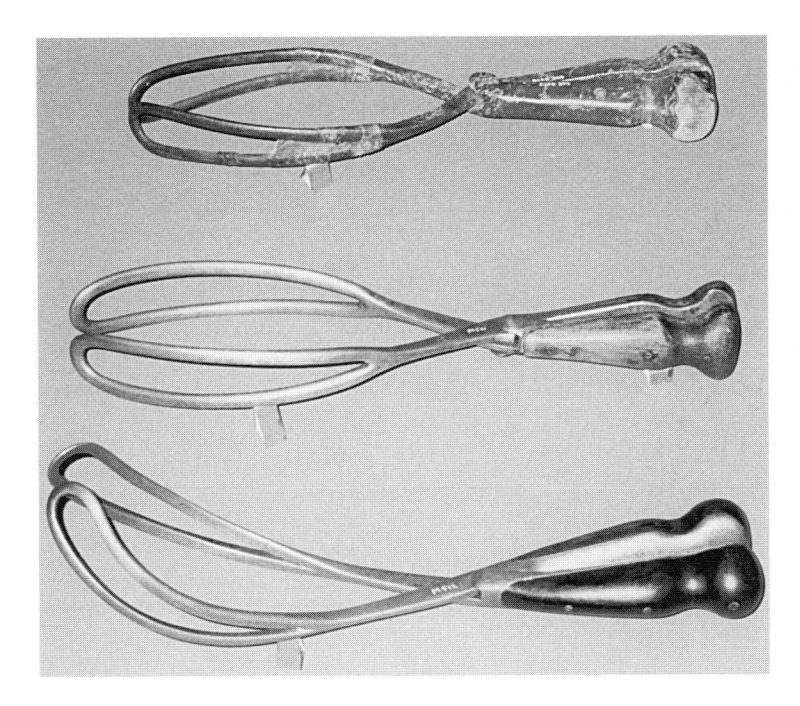

FIGURE 3.5 (OPPOSITE LEFT).
Smellie's curved forceps. Table XXI from his *Atlas*. Delivery from the occipito-posterior position.

FIGURE 3.6 (OPPOSITE RIGHT).
Smellie's long curved forceps and short forceps compared. Table XVII from his *Atlas* showing the advantage of the pelvic curve.

FIGURE 3.7.
Smellie forceps. Examples of his short, long, and curved forceps from the RCOG collection.

their instruments and operative skills. J. H. Aveling, in his *English Midwives* (1872), recounts some of the antagonisms that arose from the time of the Chamberlens onward. In the late seventeenth century prominent characters included Elizabeth Cellier, a colorful and deceitful midwife and political activist who petitioned King James II to establish a corporation of licensed midwives (with considerable financial benefit to herself). One doctor who questioned her received the reply "I hope, Doctor, these considerations will deter any of you from pretending to teach us midwifery, which ought to be kept a secret amongst women as much as possible." Sarah Stone, who established herself as a midwife in London in 1736, was prominent in continuing the campaign of Mrs. Cellier, expressing alarm about men-midwives and their instruments. Later in the century, Elizabeth Nihell was one of the most prominent campaigners and in 1760 published *A Treatise on the Art of Midwifery*, a somewhat venomous attack on the new breed of man-midwives and on Smellie in particular, whom she identified as the leader of this dangerous new profession. She also attacked Smellie's use of the forceps as a means of entry into midwifery practice. His *Treatise* she dismissed as being "just as insignificant and foolish a gimcrack as any of the rest."

It was not uncommon for practitioners to openly publish attacks on the skill and integrity of their competitors in books, essays, and pamphlets that they published themselves, never hampered by modesty nor fear of libel, nor peer reviewers. One such was William Douglas, (no relation to John Douglas [Chapter 2] or James Douglas [see below]) who, in an open letter to Smellie in 1748, first criticized Chamberlen Walker for pretending to improve the Chamberlen forceps by making them male and female (referring to the articulation), which had, in his opinion, spoiled them. He then attacked Smellie's wooden forceps and embarked on a diatribe against Smellie, attacking his motives, money grabbing, teaching, skills, even his hands: "Such *monstrous Hands* are like *Wooden Forceps*, fit only to hold horses by the Nose, whilst they are shod by the *Farrier*." Douglas claimed he knew of eight deaths in a few months caused by wooden forceps, to which Smellie replied that he had only used them twice, both times successfully, before Douglas's letter was published, and then twice subsequently. Douglas was correct at least in criticizing the materials from which many forceps were made at the time, particularly French instruments, which were too malleable and bent easily. He emphasized the need for properly tempered steel.

One of Smellie's fiercest critics was John Burton of York (1710–1771). Burton is credited with introducing the practice of delivering women lying on their sides rather than on their backs, referred to by the French as the *pruderie britannique*, and with devising his own complex forceps, which worked in the manner of a lobster claw (Figure 3.8). These he described in his *Essay towards a Complete New System of Midwifry*, published in 1751, claiming that his forceps

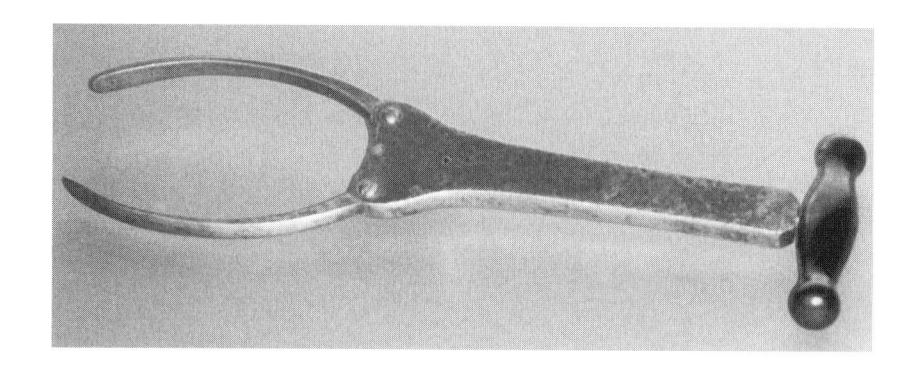

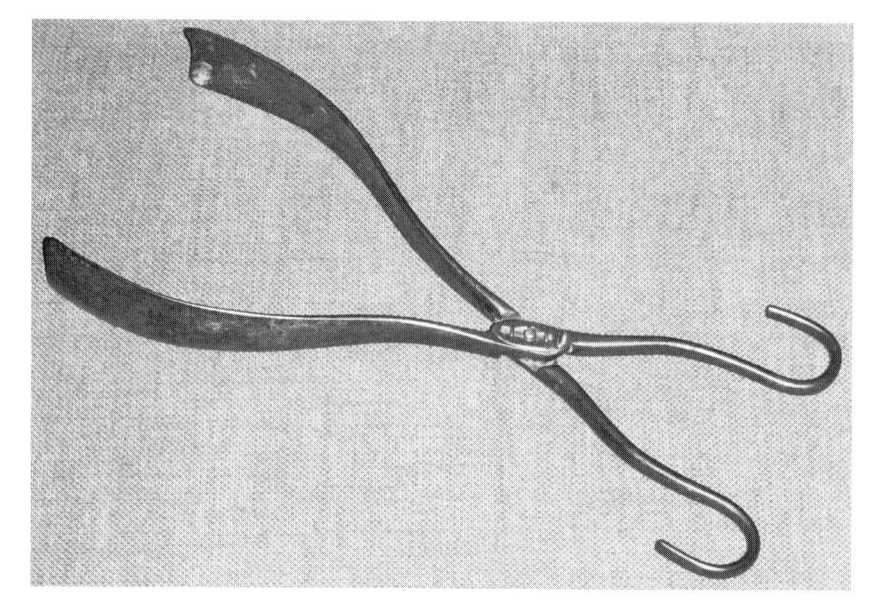

FIGURES 3.8, 3.9.
Burton's forceps. 3.8: The "lobster claw"
forceps described by Burton (University of
Edinburgh). 3.9: The forceps in his instrument
set at the York Medical Society. They are of the
Dusée type but with a single articulation.

were "better than any yet contrived" and that he delivered cases where Smellie had failed. In fact it is uncertain to what extent he ever used this device as it was well known that his standard armamentarium included a long forceps of the Dusée pattern, but with a single joint (Figure 3.9).

Burton was not a popular man and antagonized many people, including the Archdeacon of York, Laurence Sterne, who rewarded him with immortality in the thin disguise of Doctor Slop in *Tristram Shandy*. Slop, having damaged Uncle Toby's hand during a demonstration of his forceps, has an argument as to whether the head or breech was presenting (the midwife being right) and eventually delivers Tristram with forceps. He then goes missing and on inquiry it is reported that "in bringing him into the world with his vile instrument he has crushed his nose, Susannah says, as flat as a pancake to his face—and he is making a false bridge with a piece of cotton and a thin piece of whalebone from Susannah's stays. . . ."

Long after his death Smellie continued to be a target for criticism and the 1793 cartoon *Man Midwifery Dissected* is believed to depict Smellie (Chapter 4). The background and details of the fascinating Burton-Slop story were well reviewed and analyzed by A. Doran (1913b).

William Hunter

William Hunter (1718–1783), famous as an anatomist, teacher, and polymath, practiced as an obstetrician in London and, like Smellie, ran courses of lectures that were very popular and that influenced British obstetric practice, through his pupils and successors, for the rest of the eighteenth century and into the nineteenth. Twenty-one years younger than Smellie, Hunter moved to London from Lanark in 1740 with various letters of introduction. He used a letter from his mentor Cullen, a professor of medicine in Edinburgh, to introduce himself to Smellie, with whom he lodged for his first few months in the capital. Although from similar backgrounds, Smellie and Hunter possessed very different personalities and were described respectively by Johnstone as "a rough diamond and a cut and polished diamond of the first water." Smellie retained his humble and provincial lifestyle and did not pursue the social circuit. This way of life was not to Hunter's liking and he soon moved to live in the household of James Douglas, brother of John Douglas (Chapter 2) and a fashionable obstetrician and well-known anatomy teacher. It was from this point, around 1740, that his career in both anatomy and obstetrics blossomed. Apart from his brilliance as a teacher of anatomy and maintaining his anatomy school he soon had an ultrafashionable medical practice and was appointed as physician to Queen Charlotte in 1762. He made full use of the social and cultural opportunities that came his way in the flourishing era of Handel, Hogarth, Fielding, Smollett, Garrick, Reynolds, and Gainsborough.

Although Hunter's professional life was developing quite differently than that of Smellie he frequently alluded to Smellie's teaching during his lectures, often favorably but sometimes critically, particularly suggesting that Smellie was too interventionist. He was reputed to carry with him a pair of rusty forceps, which he would show to his students to emphasize how little they were used—not surprising when one compares his society practice of potentially normal cases with Smellie's clientele among the poor, who usually summoned Smellie only when problems had already developed. Nevertheless Hunter was not as anti-interventionist as many would believe and in his lecture notes devotes fifteen pages to the details of forceps application (Wilson, 1985). The guidelines for the use of forceps as designated by Smellie and Hunter can be summarized as follows:

(1) use only on the most urgent occasions;

(2) head on the perineum for six hours;

(3) if the head advances, no matter how slowly, no interference unless the child be dead;

(4) use the forceps sparingly—"Where they save one they murder many." (Hunter)

André Levret and Mid Eighteenth-Century European Developments

While William Smellie was instrumental in setting the scene in Britain for obstetrics and forceps design, parallel developments were occurring in France, the seminal character being André Levret (1703–1780) of Paris. Born and educated in Paris, Levret was able to pursue his obstetric interests following a bequest and rapidly gained a reputation that drew students from all over Europe. He was a member of the Royal Academy of Surgery of Paris and was also favored in court circles. His patients included the dauphiness, mother of Louis XVI.

Levret's monumental text *L'Art des accouchemens demontré par les principes de physique et de méchanique* (1753) earned him the title of founder of rational obstetrics. This work included his observations on the facility of delivery depending on the concordance of the diameters of the fetal head with the diameters of the pelvis and explained that retention of the placenta was due to poor uterine action rather than uterine abnormality.

Levret devised various instruments for assisting delivery, including a crotchet with a guarded hook (Chapter 16) and a three-bladed *tire-tête* for extracting the retained decapitated head. The mechanics of the latter instrument were rather complex although the principles were simple. The curved blades were made of spring steel and fit inside each other concentrically. After introduction they were fanned out to encompass the fetal head. Levret's original design (1747) is illustrated in Figures 3.10 and 3.11, while Figure 3.12 shows a modified and simpler version in the museum of the Royal College of Obstetricians and Gynaecologists.

Levret wrote extensively about this instrument but his greatest contributions were his modifications of Palfyn's *mains de fer* and of Grégoire's forceps, based on experiences with the practical difficulties in their use that were similar to those Smellie had experienced. Levret's contributions were achieved by a gradual process of experimentation and evolution, as is evident from his various designs that followed. The modifications were mainly in the blade shape and length and in the articulation, which appeared in various forms (Figures 3.13–3.15)

Because Levret made many modifications to his forceps over the years and some earlier references to them were vague there are variations in the descriptions and chronology given by different authors. For example, the description of a pelvic curve is usually dated at 1747, but Levret's own contemporary description does not mention a pelvic curve and the Mulder illustration of "Type I" forceps shows no pelvic curve (Figure 3.16, left).

Levret described his three-position joint but no pelvic curve (designated Type I by Mulder) to the Academy of Sciences in Paris in 1747 (Figure 3.16, left). Although this was, in his own words, a "novel instrument," his most important development was the introduction of a pelvic curve, the *forceps courbé*, in 1751 (Mulder Type II, Figure 3.16, center). This

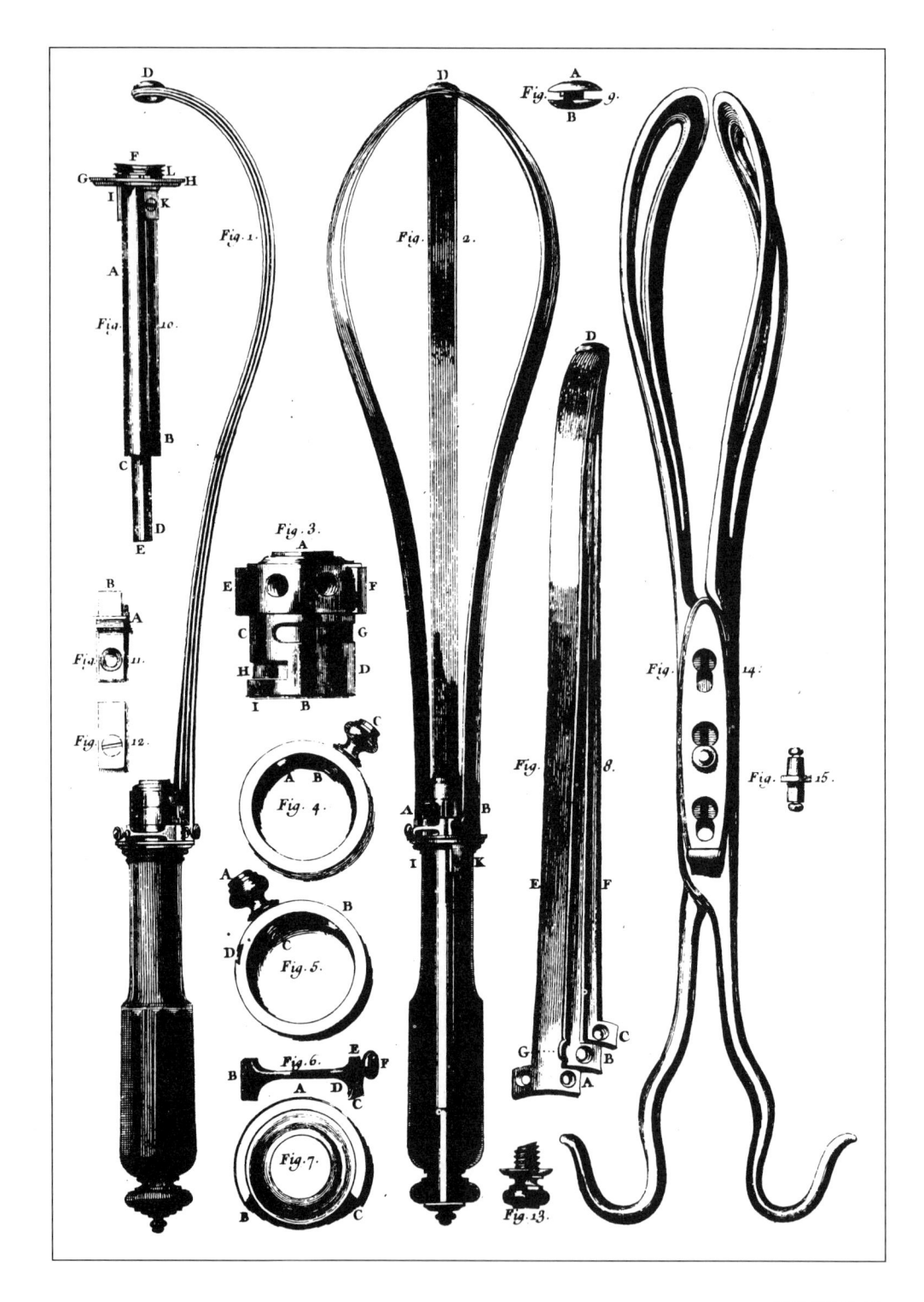

FIGURE 3.10.
Levret's *tire-tête* and Type I forceps. The *tire-tête* was used to extract the decapitated head. It was inserted with the blades folded (Figure 1) and the hinged blades were then opened out to encompass the head (Figure 2). The Type I forceps (Figure 14) were of heavy construction and had a triple articulation.

40 CHAPTER 3

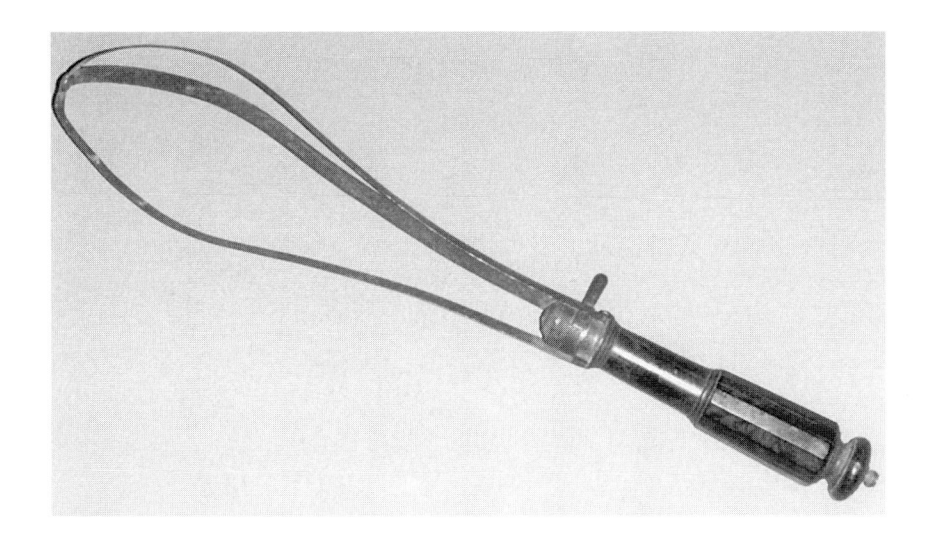

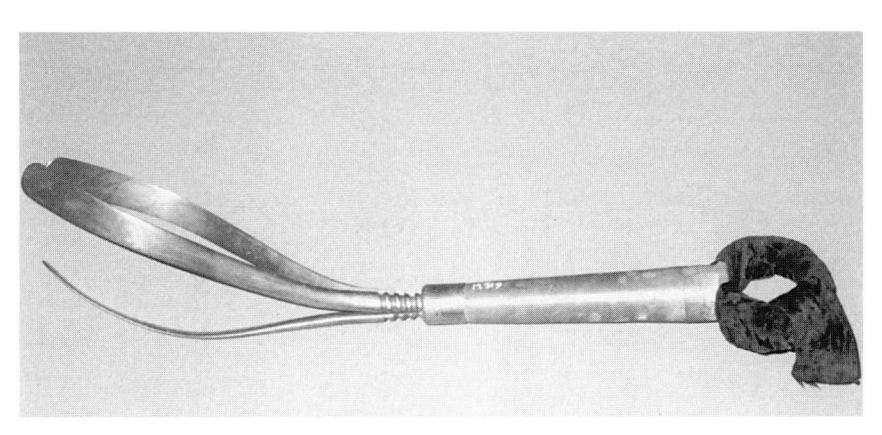

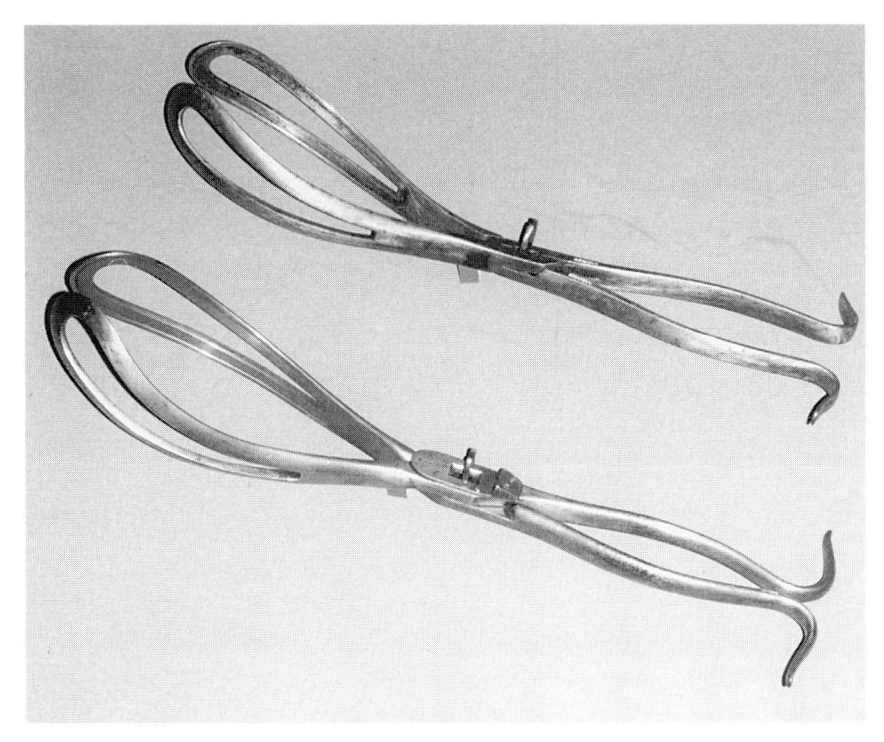

FIGURES 3.11, 3.12.
3.11: Levret's *tire-tête* from the Wellcome collection (Science Museum, London). 3.12: A simpler version in the RCOG collection.

FIGURE 3.13.
Levret's forceps, Types II and III. Note the progressive simplification of the articulation. (Science Museum, London)

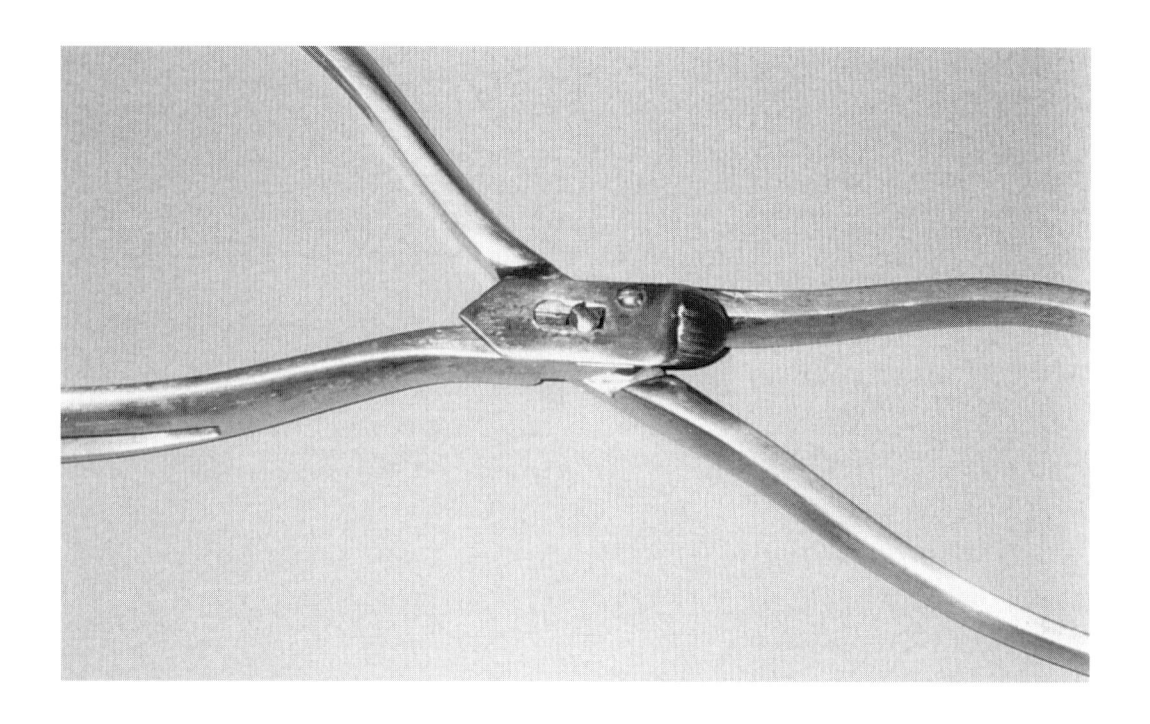

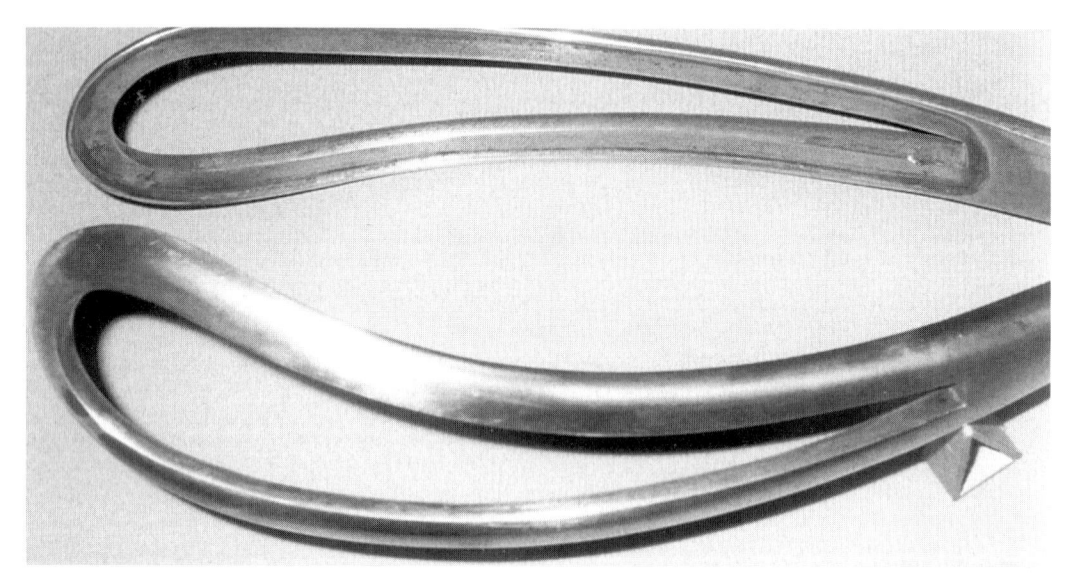

FIGURES 3.14, 3.15.
Levret's forceps. 3.14: Close-up of the simplified lock (RCOG). Figure 3.15: The hollowed out inner surface of the blades. (RCOG)

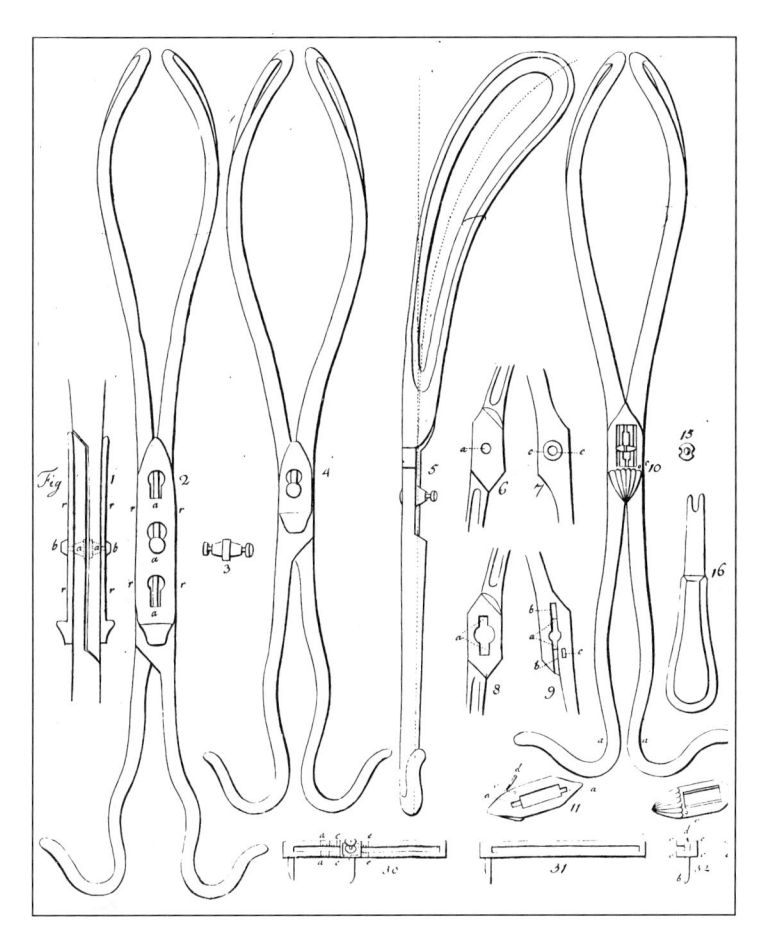

FIGURE 3.16.
Levret's forceps as illustrated by Mulder and Schlegel (1798). Left: Type I (1747) with three-position articulation and no pelvic curve. Center: Type II (1751) with simplified articulation and pelvic curve. Right: Type III (1760) with a new articulation requiring a key to lock it.

FIGURE 3.17 (BELOW).
Comparison of early British and Continental forceps. Left: Smellie. Right: Levret. (Hibbard, 1993)

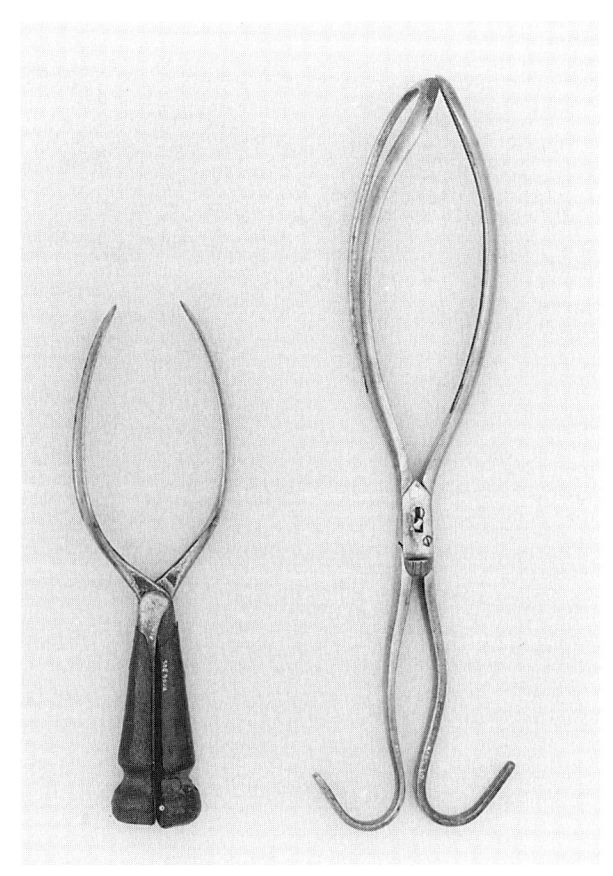

version also had a simpler keyhole-type lock and an additional refinement was a groove on the inside of the blades to obtain a firmer and better grip on the head. An illustration of his forceps incorporating these features did not appear until the third edition of his *Observations sur les causes et les accidens de plusieurs accouchemens laborieux* (1762). A later version (Mulder Type III), which was slightly shorter (418 millimeters [16.5 inches] compared with 483 millimeters [19 inches]) was described by Levret's pupil, Stein, and illustrated by Mulder and Schlegel (Figure 3.16, right).

The latter two models became the prototypes for subsequent Continental developments just as Smellie's forceps were the forerunners of later British forceps. They both used fenestrated blades and introduced a pelvic curve but differed significantly in their length, weight, and curvatures (Figure 3.17)

Levret was not reticent in extolling the virtues of his forceps. In the second edition of *L'Art des accouchemens* he claimed:

> The forceps made according to my last correction, is likewise useful in extracting in every case the head of the child, whether the face is turned toward the side of the pubis, whether it is facing the sacrum, whether

it is applied to one or the other of the ilia, whether it presents itself first in the birth canal, or whether it is the occipital region which was advanced first; for there is not a single one of these instances in which this instrument has not succeeded with me.... the head lends itself sufficiently to their passage without any necessity for using a force capable of harming either the mother or the child. (1761)

He also advised earlier intervention when the head was engaged so as to avoid the "pernicious effects" of delay in such cases as hemorrhage, convulsions, cessation of contractions, and maternal exhaustion—a common practice now but quite revolutionary in his time.

. . .

By the latter part of the eighteenth century men-midwives, or accoucheurs, were becoming firmly established, although fierce critics of them still abounded among midwives and the medical profession. Operative midwifery was beginning to be based on sounder foundations of objective anatomical studies, largely due to Smellie and William Hunter, and the role of forceps was being reappraised with some consideration for the life of the baby.

Although the thought processes underlying both British and Continental developments were similar, the solutions in terms of details of forceps design were different, as exemplified by the shorter, lighter forceps of Smellie and the heavier, longer forceps of Levret (Figure 3.17). It was from these beginnings in Britain and on the Continent that the divergent pattern of instruments and practice was established for the next hundred years.

BRITISH MAN-MIDWIVES AND THEIR CONSERVATISM: LATE EIGHTEENTH-CENTURY, EARLY NINETEENTH-CENTURY PRACTICE

In the latter part of the eighteenth century the public demand for better-trained midwives was increasing. However, the man-midwives were still meeting opposition from the midwives and were treated with some reservations by the public. The main concerns arose from female modesty and fears of the outcome of their interventions, for their services were still largely called upon only as a last resort. These views were encapsulated in a monograph by John Blunt (the pseudonym of S. W. Fores), *Man-Midwifery Dissected,* published in 1793. Blunt described himself as "A student under different teachers, but not a practitioner of the art." The subtitle of his book was *The Obstetric Family: Instructor for the Use of Married Couples and Single Adults of Both Sexes* and the contents on the title page were "A Display of Management of every Class of Labours by *Men* and *Boy*-mid*wives*; [*sic*] also of their cunning, indecent, and cruel Practices. Instructions to Husbands how to counteract them. A Plan for the complete Instruction of Women who possess promising Talents, in order to supersede Male-practice. Various Arguments and Quotations, proving that Man-midwifery is a personal, a domestic, and a National evil." The volume comprised a series of letters addressed to Alexander Hamilton (page 53), whom he saw as an active promoter of the use of the lever, and William Osborn (page 50), who was, in Blunt's eyes, an opponent. Blunt claimed that males were able to practice midwifery only in Christian communities and that this had started in Europe with the introduction of the lever, thereafter spreading to Britain. His criticisms were aimed initially at William Smellie, whom he accused of an indecent mode of teaching midwifery to young men and of advising the clandestine use of forceps. Smellie is probably the inspiration for the cartoon frontispiece of Blunt's monograph (Figure 4.1).

Blunt claimed that his principal aim was to stop the secret use of Lowder's lever (Chapter 16), thereby supporting Osborn, who was also against secrecy, but his underlying message was to promote modesty and the use of trained midwives, with a plea for "the proper education of sufficient number of decent women to supersede male practice in natural labours, and thus entirely prevent the needless use of destructive instruments and the practice of low, illiterate and half instructed females."

In illustration of attitudes and how at the time passions sometimes ran high on the use and abuse of forceps, A. R. Simpson quoted Dr. Joseph Clarke, Master of the Rotunda Hospital, Dublin, as saying that he would rather cut off his right hand than apply forceps in a primipara. When a Dr. Beatty quoted statistics in favor of forceps, Clarke challenged him to a duel. In spite of the widely differing opinions on operative midwifery spanning the turn of the century, better-qualified doctors were practicing midwifery and were giving careful consideration to some of the finer points of forceps design and improving upon the relationship between structure and function. In London and Edinburgh a number of developments occurred; changes were also beginning to appear in Dublin.

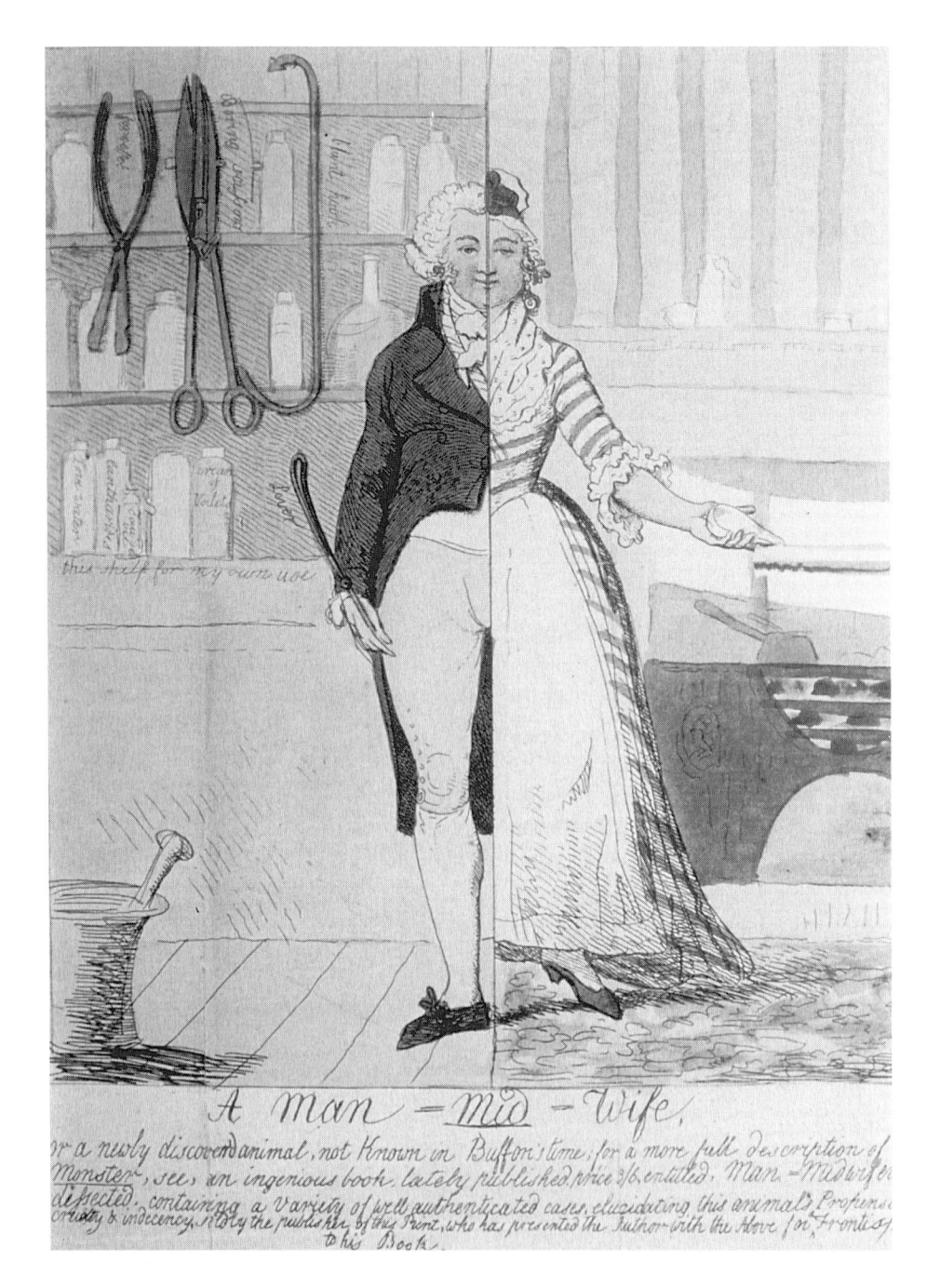

FIGURE 4.1.
A man-midwife from *Man-midwifery Dissected Addressed to Dr Alex Hamilton* by Thomas Blunt (1793). The legend reads: "A Man-<u>Mid</u>-Wife or a newly discovered animal, not known in Buffon's time; For a more full description of this <u>monster</u> see an ingenious book, lately published, price 3/6, entitled Man-Midwifery dissected, containing a variety of well authenticated cases, elucidating this animal's propensities to cruelty & indecency, sold by the publisher of this Print, who has presented the Author with the Above for a Frontispiece to his book."

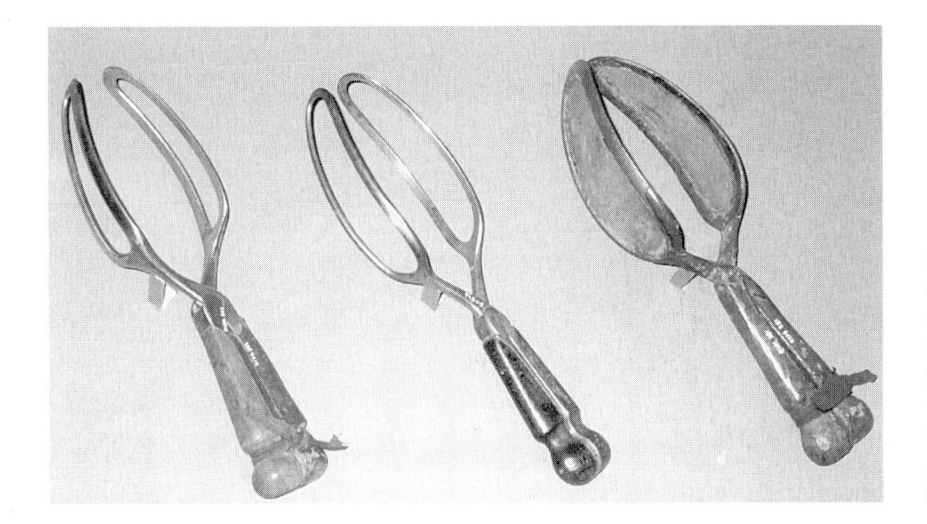

FIGURE 4.2.
Orme's, Lowder's, and Haighton's forceps. Orme's forceps (left: 256mm/10.25ins) were for use when the head was on the perineum. Lowder lengthened them (center: 287mm/11.25ins) for use when the head was higher. Haighton enlarged the fenestra to give a better grip and made them slightly longer (right: 292mm/11.5ins). (RCOG)

Late Eighteenth-Century London

Smellie retired to his native Lanark in 1759, by which time his former pupils, both medical practitioners and midwives, were practicing all over the country and abroad. Smellie was highly respected in Europe and his views continued to carry great weight away from London. Unfortunately his rational, conservative views left London with him, leaving the way open for a large number of undistinguished practitioners to shoot from the hip with their newfound weapons, often with disastrous results. So it was that a degree of polarization developed, with interventionists in the minority at one extreme and arch conservatives in the mold of William Hunter at the other, the most influential of the latter being Thomas Denman (below) and, later, James Blundell (page 49).

Straight Forceps

Orme, Lowder, and Haighton Because of lack of written contemporary records it is difficult to assign with certainty many of the refinements that occurred in the late eighteenth century. However, certain names do stand out. In the London scene the names of David Orme, William Lowder, and John Haighton are generally linked and it is difficult to distinguish among their forceps and the many look-alikes made by local cutlers and blacksmiths. The common feature was that they were all straight and short. They differed mainly in the shape of the blades, which were shorter, rounder, and wider than those of Smellie and the tips were farther apart

David Orme (1727–1812) moved to London after qualifying in Edinburgh, was appointed to the City of London Lying-In Hospital, and lectured at Guy's Hospital. Orme left no written description of his forceps (Figure 4.2, left). They were, however, described by Continental obstetricians and by Lowder. The former included J. Mulder, author of *Historia litteraria et critica forcipum et vectium obstetriciorium*, whom both Orme and Lowder taught when Mulder was in London. Lowder's descriptions gave lengths varying from between 254 and 267 millimeters (10 and 10.5 inches) long.

William Lowder (d. 1801), a graduate of Aberdeen, also lectured at Guy's and St. Thomas Hospitals, although he does not appear on the hospital staff lists. In his lecture notes he stated that he favored the Smellie type of straight forceps because they could be applied in any direction, whereas the French Levret type with the pelvic curve could only be applied in one direction, hence his preference for the forceps of his colleague Orme.

Orme used forceps only when the head was on the perineum but Lowder, who used them when the head was higher in the pelvis, found that the maternal tissues were liable to be caught in the articulation. He therefore lengthened the forceps by 25 millimeters (1 inch) and he also discarded the leather covering that was in general use at the time (Figure 4.2, center).

John Haighton (1755–1823) was the third member of the St. Thomas/Guy's group but also failed to leave any written description of his forceps, which were designed in about 1790. They were subsequently described by his nephew, James Blundell (page 49) in 1834. The main advance in his design was in the large size of the fenestra, which allowed the parietal eminences to project through them and afforded a better grip with less risk of undue compression and damage to the fetal head, compared with other forceps of the time, which had more slender blades (Figure 4.2, right).

Thomas Denman (1733–1815), was born in Bakewell in northern England. He trained in London and obtained his medical degree from the University of Aberdeen in 1764.

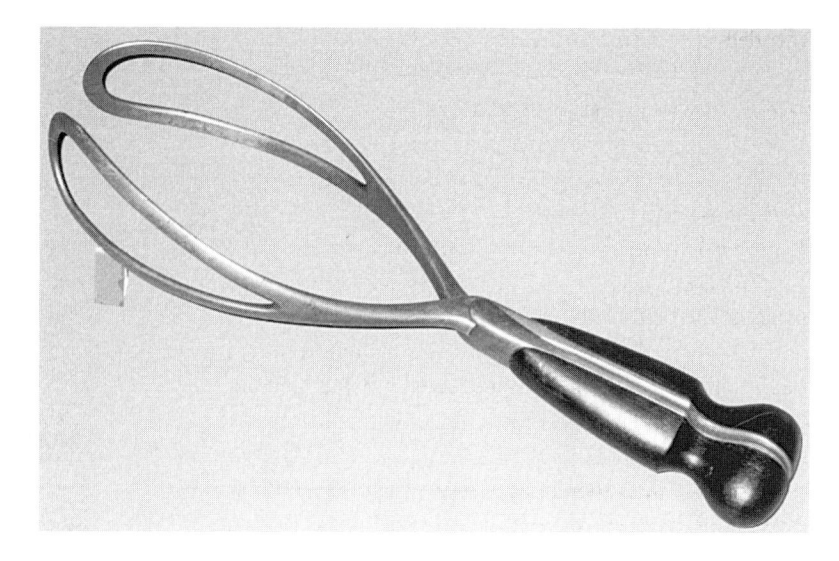

FIGURE 4.3.
Denman's forceps. These forceps (275mm/ 10.875ins), are of the Denman type, though he left no written description and there are many minor variants of the design. (RCOG)

Contrary to information often stated, Denman could not have studied under Smellie, who retired to Lanark in 1759, because Denman spent nine years as a ship's surgeon, mainly overseas, until 1763. Denman was eventually appointed *physician accoucheur* at the Middlesex Hospital in 1769. He established a large practice, which forced him to give up this post and his lecturing in 1783, about the time of the death of William Hunter, whom he succeeded as the leader in the field and took his place as Court Physician. He gradually handed over his practice to one of his sons-in-law, Richard Croft, and became mainly a consulting physician. His philosophy, as stated in his *Aphorisms* (1815), was that "The abuse of art produces more and greater evils than are occasioned by all the imperfections of nature."

Denman's treatise, *Introduction to the Practice of Midwifery*, was first published in 1788 and became a standard text that went into many editions. The fifth edition was published shortly before his death in 1815; two more editions were published posthumously, the last in 1832. His *Aphorisms on the Application of the Forceps and Vectis* ran to nine editions, the last being published in 1836, twenty-one years after his death. This pocket volume contains such admonitions as:

> It has long been established as a general rule, that instruments are never to be used in the practice of midwifery; the cases in which they are used are therefore to be considered merely as exceptions to this rule.
>
> [A]fter the cessation of the pains, the head of the child should have rested for six hours in such a situation as to allow the use of the forceps before they are used.

(Shades of William Hunter!)

As a means of avoiding operative delivery Denman introduced the concept of inducing labor prematurely so as to have a baby of smaller size who could negotiate a contracted pelvis (Chapter 17).

Denman favored the slender forceps of the Smellie pattern and although Das claimed that Denman designed his own forceps (Figure 4.3) there is no mention of this in his publications. He does mention the instrument designed by his colleague Osborn (see below), which at one time he appeared to favor, although later he was opposed to the pelvic curve. It is more likely that he merely had straight forceps for his own use made to the Smellie pattern, but with the tips more widely spaced, as in Orme's forceps. He remained a proponent of the lever, or vectis. In his *Practice* he expressed the belief "that the vectis, prudently used, is in every case an equally safe and efficacious instrument with the forceps, and a better adapted instrument in many cases which occur in practice." The fillet, he claimed, was now wholly neglected as having failed to meet its supposed particular advantage in assisting delivery when the head was too high to apply forceps or lever (Chapter 16). Denman taught that the forceps should be used only when there was "total want or deficiency of the natural pains of labour." In relation to the problem of concealed postpartum hemorrhage he said that he had "not even troubled [him]self with the state of the uterus. . . ." Both of these principles were destined to have dire consequences.

A. Milne's 1868 epitaph on Denman stated that he was "Simple minded, yet acute and experienced, and imbued in a peculiar way with everything obstetrical."

The conservatism of London obstetricians continued into the nineteenth century, mainly under the aegis of James

Blundell (1790–1878), a nephew of Haighton, who became Professor of Obstetric Medicine at Guy's Hospital. His *Lectures on Midwifery* (1832, 1839) and *Principles and Practice of Obstetricy* (1834) were written in an emotive and flowery style and, as well as being widely read in Britain and America, were translated into German and Italian. His *Principles and Practice of Obstetric Medicine* was subsequently revised and updated, most notably by A. L. Lee and N. Rogers in 1840, to make it "the best Work on Obstetric Medicine in the English language." Lee and Rogers added some four hundred pages derived from other major sources such as Denman, Osborn, David Davis (Chapter 6), F. C. Naegele (Chapter 8), and Hamilton.

Blundell, while cautioning against premature interference, especially if the cervix was insufficiently dilated, also warned of the dangers of undue delay. In reference to "turning" (internal podalic version) his advice was to

> [n]ever turn without need; never rashly have recourse to the operation, without considering whether it be, or be not safe; but if fully satisfied that turning will not be attended by more than ordinary danger, and if further satisfied that there is no reasonable hope of the child's coming away in any other manner, the sooner the operation is performed the better . . . Happy might it have been for women generally, and still happier for their offspring, if instruments had never been invented.

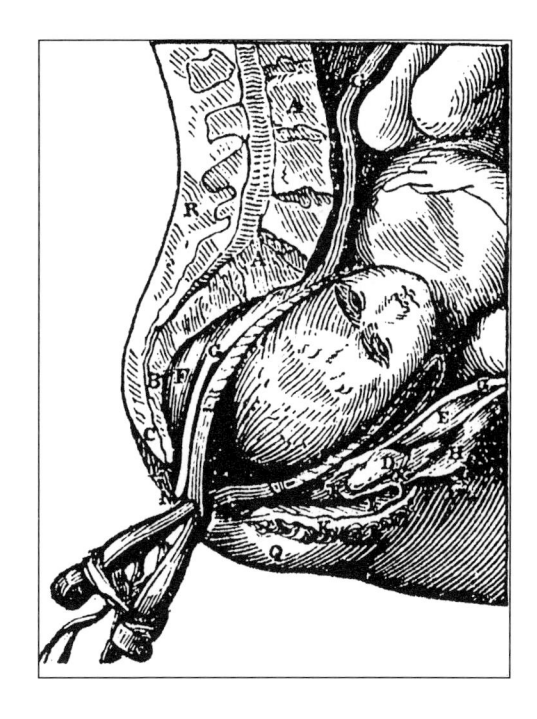

FIGURE 4.4.
An example of an illustration of forceps application from Blundell (1840). These were crude copies of Smellie's illustrations and do not fit the description in the text.

Blundell treated his obstetric instruments with respect and fear: "I do not like to see an elegant pair of forceps. Let the instrument look like what it is, a formidable weapon." He regarded obstetric instruments in general as "always a great obstetric evil, but not always to be avoided. Dreadful are the evils resulting from the employment of obstetric instruments! And dreadful, too, are those evils which result from neglecting their administration, when really required!"

If the head did not advance he was prepared to wait a few hours before attempting a further application of the forceps. Although he emphasized the need to cooperate with natural efforts he nevertheless used an oscillatory movement of the forceps to aid descent of the head when necessary. Once the head had descended to the outlet he generally preferred to remove "this dangerous instrument" and anticipate spontaneous delivery.

Thus Blundell continued to promote, with considerable influence, the English conservatism and undesirable practices of the preceding century which, with few exceptions, was typical of the London school of the time. This not only included his attitude to instruments but also to other archaic practices such as bloodletting, which he advocated before applying the long forceps, especially if the vagina or cervix was rigid, the soft parts were swollen, and/or the patient was overwrought.

Blundell claimed to have used both straight and curved forceps but favored the former because of their versatility in application to the head irrespective of its position, the usual application being over the forehead and occiput when the head was arrested at the brim. He believed that there was little place for short forceps on the grounds that if the head was low enough to apply them they were unnecessary and on rare occasions when assistance was required the lever was more appropriate. He was opposed to a pelvic curve and while he regarded the narrow blades of Orme as suitable he preferred the wider fenestra of Haighton, his mentor and uncle. He was against leather covering on hygienic grounds.

In none of his published works, including later editions with added material, did he describe forceps of his own design, although he enumerated the desirable features of long forceps: about 356 millimeters (14 inches) overall, without a pelvic curve; with a loose lock to give some tolerance; and

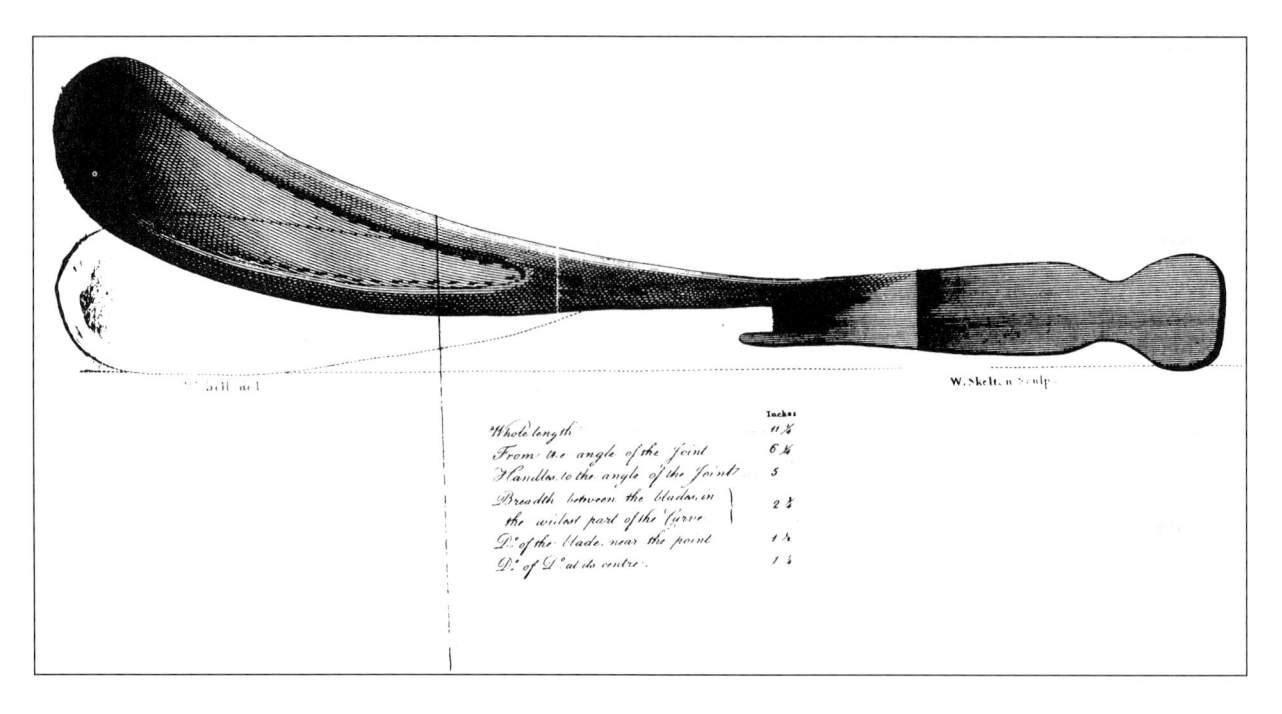

FIGURE 4.5.
Osborn's forceps. Design and measurements from his *Essays* (1792).

with a degree of elasticity to accommodate the shape of the fetal head. In spite of these recommendations the accompanying illustrations are crudely copied from Smellie and show leather-covered short forceps being used in cephalic application (Figure 4.4).

Whether or not Blundell had forceps specially designed to his specification is unclear. Doran (1921) described a long, straight forceps without finger rests ascribed to Blundell. Das (1929) quoted Doran but had an illustration of forceps with finger rests, and the main instrument makers' catalogues illustrate "Blundell's" forceps of both types. As late as 1911 the London instrument makers Montague still offered "Blundell's" forceps (without finger rests) in their catalogue.

Short Curved Forceps

William Osborn (1736–1808) trained with William Hunter in London and with Levret in Paris. He was a fellow lecturer with Denman, with whom he founded a school of midwifery in 1770. Denman gave up lecturing to pursue his large practice, as stated above, but he continued writing, expressing opinions at variance with those of Osborn, particularly in relation to the use of the vectis (Chapter 16). Osborn was incensed by this and stated in the Preface to his *Essays on the Practice of Midwifery* (1792) that he

was astonished, because the declaration was a direct dereliction of the opinions which he formerly held, of the doctrine which he always taught, and the practice which he had followed for thirty years. [Osborn was] mortified because of the considerable and extensive influence of Denman's authority which might provoke the general mischievous use of that instrument [the vectis].

Denman felt that he had been misrepresented and claimed that he was anxious to avoid abuse of instruments, which was largely true. However the important issue is that latterly he favored the vectis rather than forceps, when instrumental intervention was required, whereas Osborn became increasingly critical of the vectis, although he had himself designed one.

In his *Essays on the Practice of Midwifery* (1792) Osborn gave a good and balanced account of the pros and cons of the forceps and the vectis. Osborn claimed that the vectis was used excessively because it could be used secretly and therefore criteria for its use could be less stringent. He also claimed to have devised the "living lever," a vectis with a bending blade (see also Chapter 16, Aitken and Davis). Robert Bland's *Observations on Human and on Comparative Parturition* (1794) was a destructive dissection of Osborn's *Essays* and of his practices, particularly attacking Osborn's

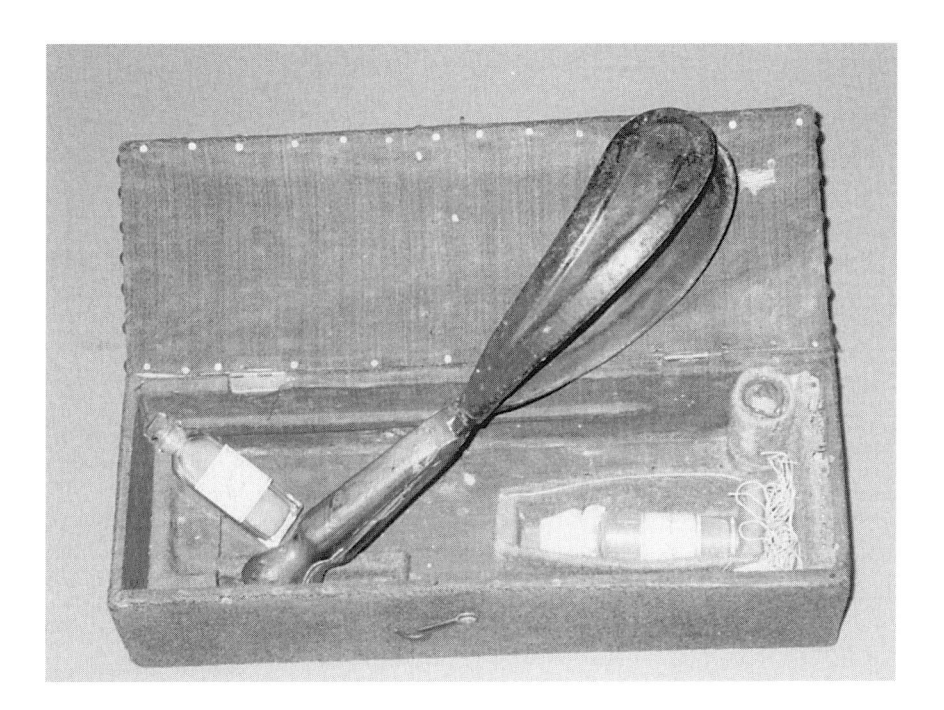

FIGURE 4.6.
Osborn's forceps (285mm/11.5ins). These forceps were found in a box of later date containing silk sutures and bottles of extract of ergot of rye and of chloroform, suggesting the use of these forceps after the advent of chloroform anesthesia. (RCOG)

support of forceps in preference to the vectis and supporting Denman and many other practitioners who, he claimed, had abandoned the forceps for the vectis. Bland estimated the need for use of the forceps or lever as no more than one in seven or eight hundred deliveries.

Osborn, like Denman, was strongly opposed to Caesarian section and to artificial means of stimulating uterine activity. "We possess no means of restoring the expulsive powers of the uterus . . . all medicines formerly recommended . . . are discarded in modern practice."

There is no written detail of his forceps design but he gave a clear diagram and basic measurements in his *Essays* (Figure 4.5). Denman had referred to them nine years previously but again without a written description. They were said to combine the principles of the Levret forceps with the lightness characteristic of English forceps of the time and were described by Denman as a miniature Levret, intended to combine the qualities of the long and the short forceps. They were similar to Smellie's curved forceps and were completely covered with leather, including the fenestra (Figure 4.6). He claimed they provided a good grip, with the blades resting on the mastoid processes so that they could not compress the parietal bones.

Osborn's prerequisites for forceps application were typical of the time: entire cessation of labor pains (although not specifying a six-hour delay as did Denman) and the head must be in the pelvic cavity, a useful criterion being the ability to feel an ear. He gave six clear rules for the actual delivery:

(1) The cervix must be fully dilated.
(2) The forceps must always be applied over the ears.
(3) During introduction the points of the blades must always be in contact with the head.
(4) Traction must be in the axis of the pelvis and the handles must not be tied together.
(5) Traction must be cautious and deliberate in manner, intermittent, and commensurate with the resistance.
(6) The left hand must be constantly applied to the perineum to minimize laceration.

Osborn was very conscious of minimizing trauma and in addition to his last rule he claimed that the pelvic curve on his forceps "reduced the pressure on the perineum by upwards of one inch."

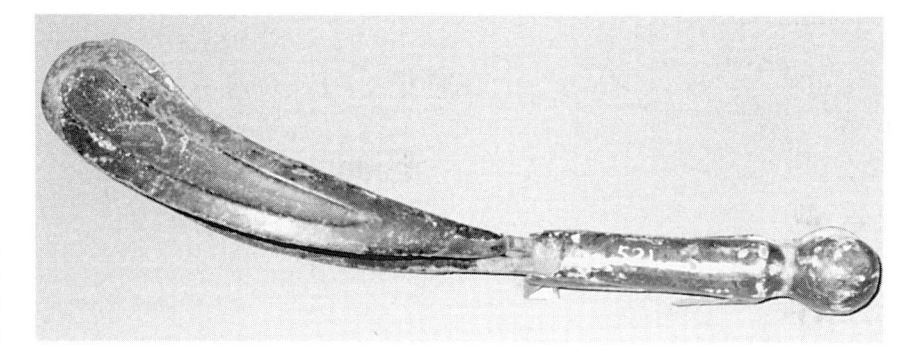

FIGURE 4.7.
Thynne's forceps (297mm/11.75ins). These forceps are similar to Osborn's but with longer blades. (RCOG)

There are many forceps bearing a close resemblance to Osborn's instrument, which is not surprising considering Osborn claimed that twelve hundred practitioners had attended his lectures. It is likely that many had their own versions made locally. One modified version that is reasonably well authenticated is that of Andrew Thynne (1749–1813), who was the first lecturer in midwifery at St. Bartholomew's Hospital. His forceps (Figure 4.7) closely resemble those of Osborn but the tips of the blades are wider apart and the blades are relatively longer.

The Edinburgh School

R. W. Johnson (1769) devised many novel instruments, including at least two designs of forceps, as well as a perforator, a director, and the embryulcus (or eductor, page 231), his principle aim being to stop the secret use of Lowder's lever. All his designs were the result of careful analysis of the problems related to delivery with forceps and he was the first person to describe oblique positions of the head in his 1769 work, *A New System of Midwifery*. He always showed marked concern for the relative comfort of the mother and addressed in particular the problem of perineal damage during forceps delivery. This discussion of perineal damage was to lead to the first significant deviation from the basic Smellie designs.

Johnson's first pair of forceps had a transverse slit in the root of one of the blades at the junction of the handle and blade and this blade was inserted first. The other blade was passed through the slit. Although he found these forceps satisfactory in a number of cases the failure rate was unacceptably high and he soon abandoned them. However, the same principle was revived later by John Beatty (circa 1829) of Dublin, and in the Scottish school by John Barclay of Aberdeen and by Alexander Ziegler of Edinburgh (Chapter 8).

In his generally known forceps (Figures 4.8, 4.9, left) Johnson reverted to the Smellie-type articulation but made the joint deeper. The blade had a pelvic curve but he added a terminal, turned-up tip to the blade, which he claimed facilitated insertion, gave a better hold on the head, and prevented slippage. This unique design became a characteristic feature of Scottish forceps in the second half of the eighteenth century. A further innovation was setting the long axis of the blades back with the addition of an inverted curve to minimize pressure on the perineum; this construction became known as the perineal curve. These and other carefully thought-out details and precise measurements were set out in the elaborate instructions for the instrument maker because Johnson was concerned that there were inferior inexact copies in use. The overall length was 280 millimeters (11 inches) and the maximum width between the blades a mere 64 millimeters (2.5 inches). As a covering material he insisted on morocco leather, because it was nonabsorbent, but was prepared to accept bare blades if they were well-finished and smooth. When a leather covering was used he insisted that it be changed after each use to avoid the problems of infection.

Johnson's prerequisites for forceps application were full dilatation of the cervix and the maximum diameter of the head through the pelvic brim. The blades were inserted in the hollow of the sacrum and then wandered laterally to achieve a bitemporal application. Although there is no record of how successful this design was presumably it satisfied the needs of the time, at least in Edinburgh, because Johnson's successors used similar instruments with only minor modifications.

Thomas Young (1726-1783) was Professor of Midwifery at the University of Edinburgh and is generally regarded as the founder of the obstetric school there. Although written notes of Young's lectures still exist in the Royal College of Obstetricians and Gynaecologists' library, there is no contemporary record of his forceps. However, both J. Mulder (1794)

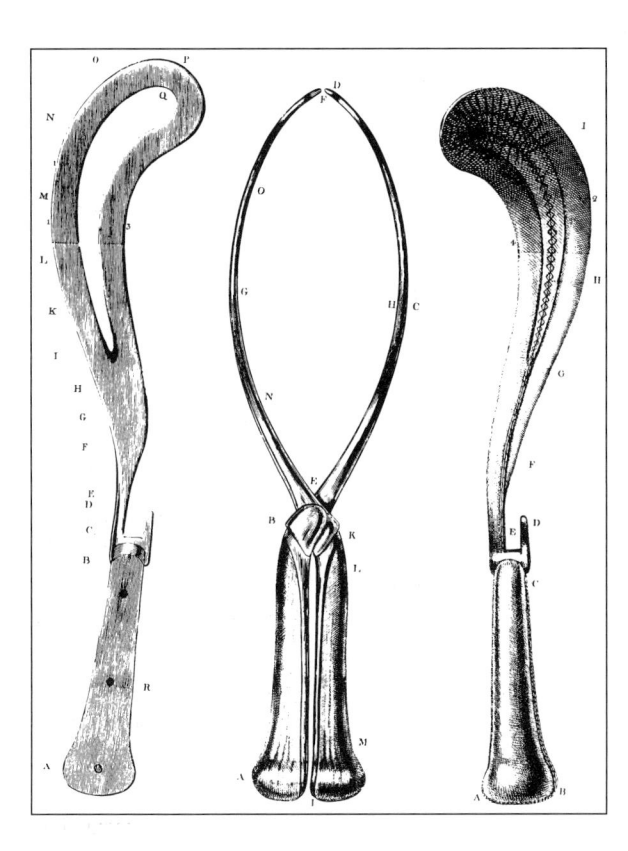

FIGURE 4.8.
Johnson's forceps. Plate VI from *A New System of Midwifery* (1769), showing the characteristic blade design and the perineal curve.

FIGURE 4.9.
Johnson's, Young's, Hamilton's forceps. Johnson's forceps (left) correspond with his own description. Young's forceps (center) are similar but slightly larger (302mm/11.75ins) and with more divergent blades. Hamilton's forceps are similar to Johnson's but with a hinged handle. (RCOG)

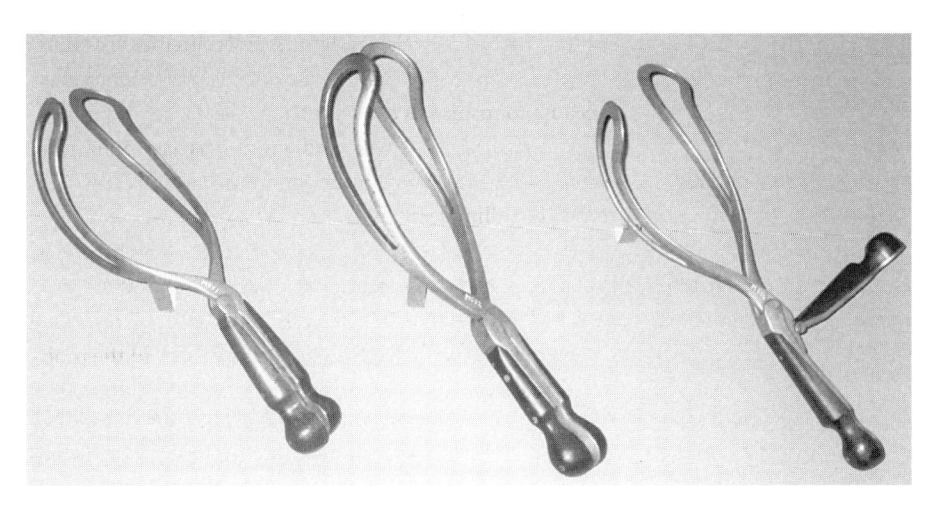

and H. F. Kilian give illustrations, showing them to be of the Edinburgh pattern of the time, with the turned-up tip to the blade (Figure 4.9, center). According to Das (1929) they were slightly bigger than Johnson's forceps and diverged at a wider angle.

Alexander Hamilton (1739–1802), who was appointed Joint Professor of Midwifery at Edinburgh in 1780, succeeded Young upon the latter's death in 1783. Hamilton was assisted by his son, James (d. 1839), who succeeded him in 1800 and probably contributed to the design of the forceps that bears their name by introducing a slightly elongated version. The forceps (Figure 4.9, right) were very similar to those of R. W. Johnson, with the blade shape typical of the time in Edinburgh. The original design (1794) was 292 millimeters (11.5 inches) long. The handle was 114 millimeters (4.5 inches) and the greatest width was 70 millimeters (2.75 inches). The right handle was hinged to facilitate introduction when the patient was lying on her left side (Chapter 8). The later version was 12.5 millimeters (.5 inches) longer.

Alexander Hamilton was always a protagonist of forceps, but for limited indications. In the second edition of his *Outlines on the Theory and Practice of Midwifery* (1787), he said

BRITISH MAN-MIDWIVES 53

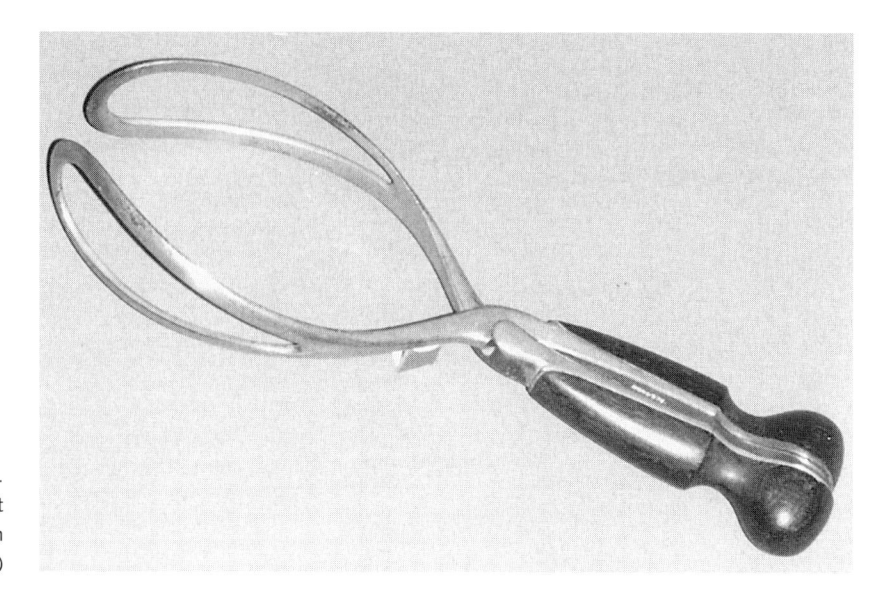

FIGURE 4.10.
Collins's forceps. One of the first short (254mm/10ins) straight forceps designs from Dublin. (Science Museum, London)

that the lever was "extremely limited in its means... and a dangerous expedient in the hands of a young practitioner," while the forceps in the hands of a prudent and cautious operator could "be employed without doing the least injury to mother or child." In the fifth edition of *Outlines* he advised that the forceps should only be used if the head was in the pelvis, while the lever was used when the head was less than half in the pelvis and in a "natural" (vertex) presentation and some contractions were present (1806). He also advocated the use of Leake's three-bladed forceps (Chapter 9) in cases of extreme difficulty.

James Hamilton broadly followed his father's teaching initially. In his publications of 1793 and 1794 he was clearly a protagonist of Lowder's lever (Chapter 16) where forceps were inappropriate, but by 1836 he was discounting the lever and strongly advocating forceps and their use earlier in the second stage of labor. He also taught that the forceps should always be applied in correct cephalic position and, if the head was not occipito-anterior, rotation should be performed with the forceps while traction was applied, except in the case of a full occipito-posterior position. For this, he advocated extraction without rotation.

Dublin

Conservatism was the general rule in Dublin through the first half of the nineteenth century, as is illustrated in the statistics discussed later in this chapter. No instruments of distinction emerged from Dublin until the middle of the century and these are discussed in later chapters, but it seems that prior to the mid 1800s both English short forceps and European long forceps were used. The first design to originate in Dublin was that of Robert Collins (Master of the Rotunda Hospital, 1826–1833). His short, light, straight forceps, developed about 1830, were 254 millimeters (10 inches) in length and had a larger-than-usual gap between the tips (38 millimeters [1.5 inches] instead of 25 millimeters [1 inch] or less) (Figure 4.10). But as Collins performed only twenty-four forceps deliveries during his seven-year mastership, and some of these before he invented his instrument, their flaws and virtues were probably never fully evaluated.

Other Developments

Two other notable advances in British forceps design came late in the eighteenth century. John Aitken of Edinburgh, in his *Principles of Midwifery, or Puerperal Medicine* (1784, 1786), introduced several novelties in his forceps designs, including parallel forceps (Chapter 10). He also incorporated a screw-regulating mechanism in the handle, which prevented the handles from coming together so that the compression force on the head could be controlled (Figure 4.11) (see also Chapter 5).

Also in 1784, Evans of Oswestry, Shropshire, added almost parallel shanks 25 millimeters (1 inch) in length and incorporated a screw in the handle that was remarkably similar to Aitken's. It is not clear whether these two practitioners had the same idea independently but Aitken, in the 1786 edition of his book, accused Evans of passing off the screw as his own invention. He did not comment on the similarity of the shanks.

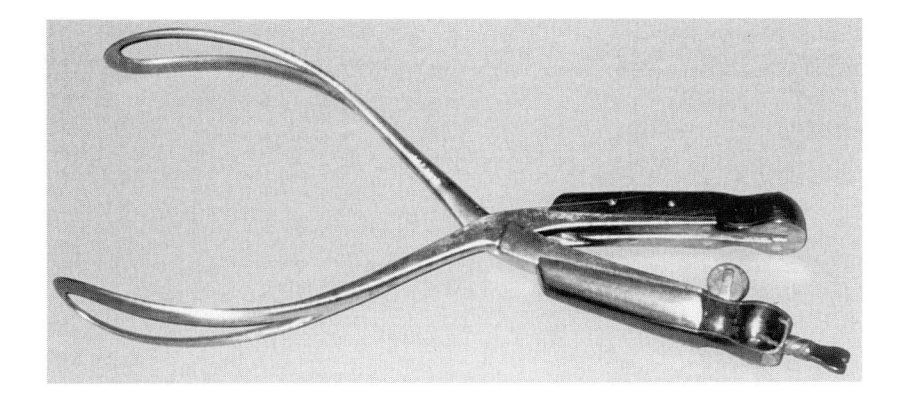

FIGURE 4.11.
John Aitken's forceps. Note the screw in the handle to regulate the compression force on the head, a feature that later became popular in Europe (*See* Chapter 6). (RCOG)

Attitudes to Operative Delivery in the Late Eighteenth and Nineteenth Centuries

The century of British conservatism, referred to previously, led James Hamilton to conclude, in a rather more conciliatory vein than some more outspoken writers, that "there is too much reason to believe that British practitioners, from their unwillingness to give pain or hurt the feelings of their patients, are apt to procrastinate and loose the favourable time for safe and effectual interference" (1836).

It is difficult to unravel and interpret such statistics for operative delivery that are available for the late eighteenth through early nineteenth century Britain because of differing populations studied, selection of cases, imprecise descriptions, ill-defined exclusions, and uncritical appraisal. Many authors, seeking to further their own causes, were selective in their sources and the conclusions they derived therefrom and gave data based on only those cases to which they had been called. Nevertheless an increasing number of practitioners were collecting statistical data, rather crudely by modern standards, but reasonably objectively, and these show the general trends in the management of dystocia even though the results, in terms of mortality and morbidity, may be dubious. The following information illustrates the pattern of operative intervention in Britain during this period, together with some European comparisons.

John Burns, who was Professor at the University of Glasgow, first published his *Principles of Midwifery* in 1809. This popular and enduring text ran to ten editions, the last being published in 1843. In early editions of his book he quoted such authorities as William Osborn, who said that the forceps were to be used only when "all the powers of life [were] exhausted," but over the years Burns's attitudes changed and his criticism of the prevailing conservatism increased. In the tenth edition Burns presented data collected from Dublin showing that maternal mortality increased with lengthening duration of labor (Table 4.1).

TABLE 4.1. Maternal Mortality Related to Duration of Labor (Burns, 1843)

Duration of labor	Maternal mortality
30–40h	1:34
40–50h	1:15
50–60h	1:9
60–70h	1:8

Burns also estimated that the incidence of forceps delivery had actually decreased since the time of Smellie (about 1 forceps delivery for every 125 births), who taught that interference was rarely indicated until at least twenty-four hours had elapsed, except in cases of fits or hemorrhage. In fact Smellie's forceps results were good and in the 1765 edition of his *Treatise* he described 52 forceps deliveries with only 2 maternal deaths, 8 dead babies, and 1 perineal laceration.

One of the first practitioners to collect statistics on an international basis was Fleetwood Churchill of Dublin, who published his results in 1841 in *Researches on Operative Midwifery*. A summary of his observations on practice at the end of the eighteenth and beginning of the nineteenth centuries is shown in Table 4.2. This table illustrates well the conservatism of the British as compared with the Continentals in the use of forceps, the rate in Britain being less than half that on the Continent. On the other hand perforation was used by the British nearly twice as often as forceps, although it was a very uncommon procedure in Europe. Data on maternal mortality were available in only a limited number of cases but for forceps delivery in Britain it was 4.8 percent (14 out of 294 deliveries) compared with 7.3 percent (35 out of 479 deliveries) in France and Germany. In Britain maternal mortality after perforation was 21 percent (52 deaths in 251 cases).

TABLE 4.2. Frequency of Forceps Use and Craniotomy in the Late Eighteenth–Early Nineteenth Centuries (Churchill, 1841)

Series	Deliveries	Operations (%)
Forceps		
British 1781–1840	42,196	120 (0.28)
French 1797–1831	44,736	277 (0.62)
German 1801–1837	261,224	1702 (0.65)
Perforator and crotchet		
British 1781–1819	41,434	181 (0.45)
French 1797–1811	36,169	30 (0.08)
German 1801–1837	256,655	132 (0.05)

T. More Madden, Assistant Physician at the Dublin Lying-in Hospital (the Rotunda), gave a comprehensive review of practice at the Rotunda Hospital in an address to the Dublin Obstetrical Society in 1875, based on two papers published previously (1874a,b). The data from seven masterships, spanning the years 1787 through 1874, are shown in Table 4.3 and illustrate the progression to interventionist attitudes after the middle of the century, from the conservatism of Collins (1826–1833), when forceps were applied in only 0.14 percent of cases, and then only if the cervix was fully dilated, the head was on the perineum, and an ear could be identified; to the interventionist approach of George T. Johnston (1868–1874). By then application of the forceps before full dilatation of the cervix was quite common, a widespread belief being that once the membranes had ruptured "inertia" (reduction or cessation of uterine activity) would ensue. For example, during Johnston's mastership in one year alone there were 35 forceps applications before full dilatation.

In More Madden's own series of 75 forceps deliveries seventeen (22.7 percent) were before full dilatation, of which only 6 were more than half dilated. His main indications were "rigidity" and "exhaustion" after labors lasting fifteen to eighty hours, with 6 women being in labor for over twenty-four hours.

TABLE 4.3. Operative Deliveries at the Dublin Lying-in Hospital under Various Masters: 1787–1874 (More Madden, 1875)

Mastership	Deliveries	Forceps (%)	Perforator (%)
Joseph Clarke 1787–1794	10,387	14 (0.13)	49 (0.47)
Samuel Labatt 1815–1822	21,867	0	0
Robert Collins 1826–1833	16,654	24 (0.14)	118 (0.71)
Charles Johnson 1842–1845	6,702	18 (0.27)	54 (0.80)
TOTALS	55,610	56 (0.10)	221 (0.40)
Robert Shekleton 1847–1854	13,748	220 (1.60)	54 (0.39)
A. H. McClintock 1854–61	3,700	76 (2.05)*	5 (0.14)
George T. Johnston 1868–1874	7027	639 (9.1)	29 (0.41)
TOTALS	24,475	935 (3.82)	88 (0.36)

*includes vectis

Although more active and liberal attitudes toward intervention, based on scientific observations, were becoming more common in the second quarter of the nineteenth century, the entrenched conservative practitioners continued to hold sway for a long time. As late as 1852 Edward Murphy, David Davis's (Chapter 6) successor at University College Hospital, London, recommended that, while temporizing and deciding on the method of delivery for feeble uterine action, treatment should be "free general depletion, followed by nauseating doses of tartar emetic, emollient enemata, and local fomentations and a moderate dose of liquor opii" in order to check the advance of inflammatory symptoms. After a period of rest ergot of rye could be given to stimulate uterine action, with due caution to avoid the death of the child. His recommendations were based on the experience of Dublin practitioners, where he had formerly practiced, and upon which his own practice was based. He also drew attention to the data of Hardy of Manchester, relating to forty-eight cases. Hardy was one of the first, if not the first, practitioners to observe "fetal distress" due to uterine hypertonus. He noted that in the majority of cases where ergot had been administered fetal bradycardia occurred fifteen to thirty minutes later, followed in many cases by cardiac irregularities. When there was a sustained bradycardia of less than 110 beats per minute the baby rarely survived. Only 14 babies were live born, of which 7 were delivered by forceps or vectis after receiving ergot. Of the 34 stillbirths, 19 required intervention with forceps, vectis, or crotchet—hardly a testimonial for the use of ergot!

Murphy also collected data from various other sources in Britain and on the Continent, more extensively covering the same period as Churchill and much of the data are derived from common sources. The findings are shown in Table 4.4. The trends are similar in both series but it is notable that the intervention rates for London practitioners quoted by Murphy are lower than those for Britain given by Churchill, and the forceps incidence in German practice is much higher in the Murphy series.

Even as late as 1878 Fordyce Barker (1819–1891) of Bellevue Hospital in New York also referred to the conservatism of British practitioners, especially the London school, until the change in teaching of Davis, Rigby, and Ramsbotham in England; Churchill in Ireland; and Dewees, Meigs, and Hodge in America. However, change was slow because even the progressives tempered their teaching with warnings of danger. Barker attributed the British horror of forceps to

(1) ignorance of the mechanism of labor, the practice and precepts of Smellie having been forgotten;

(2) exaggeration of the dangers of forceps delivery and failure to recognize the dangers of prolonged labor; and

(3) confounding the difficulties of (relatively rare) high forceps with low forceps application.

TABLE 4.4. The Frequency of Forceps Deliveries and Perforations (Murphy, 1852)

Date	Author	Cases n	Forceps n(%)	Deaths	Perforations n(%)	Deaths
London						
1781	R. Bland	1,897	4 (0.21)	-	8 (0.42)	-
	S. Merriman	2,947	21 (0.71)	-	9 (0.31)	-
1828–1843	F. Ramsbotham	35,745	49 (0.14)	3	38 (0.12)	6
TOTALS		40,589	74 (0.18)		55 (0.14)	
Dublin						
1787–1793	J. Clarke	10,387	14 (0.13)	2	49 (0.47)	16
1826–1833	R. Collins	16,414	24 (0.15)	4	79 (0.48)	15
1835–1837	J. Beatty	1,182	9 (0.76)	-	3 (0.25)	-
1835–1840	F. Churchill	1,640	3 (0.18)	-	12 (0.73)	-
1832–1835	E. Murphy	5,699	14 (0.26)	1	29 (0.51)	6
TOTALS		35,322	64 (0.18)		172 (0.49)	
France (Paris)						
1797–1811	Boivin	20,357	96 (0.47)	-	16 (0.08)	-
1812–1820	La Chapelle	22,243	77 (0.35)	-	12 (0.05)	-
TOTALS		42,600	173 (0.41)		28 (0.07)	
Germany						
1797–1827	Jansen	13,365	341 (2.5)	-	5 (0.04)	-
1801–1821	Boër	26,965	100 (0.37)	-	43 (0.16)	-
1811–1827	Moschner	12,329	120 (0.97)	-	4 (0.03)	1
1814–1827	Carus	2,549	184 (7.22)	-	9 (0.35)	-
1817–1828	Siebold	2,093	300 (14.3)	-	1 (0.05)	-
1821–1825	Riecke	221,923	2,740 (1.23)	127	98 (0.04)	35
1823–1827	Kluge	1,111	68 (6.1)	14	8 (0.72)	3
1825–1827	Kilian	9,392	120 (1.28)	-	4 (0.04)	-
?	Naegele	1,711	55 (3.21)	-	5 (0.29)	-
TOTALS		291,438	4,028 (1.38)		177 (0.06)	

Also in 1878 Arthur Edis, of the British Lying-In and Middlesex Hospitals, London, stated that many practitioners still urged giving a good dose of ergot, a practice that he regarded as both unscientific and unsafe. He quoted Robert Barnes (Chapter 6) as saying that "when you have given ergot you are likely to be in the position of Frankenstein, you have evoked a power which you cannot control." Edis emphasized the difference in British and Continental practice by quoting the incidence of forceps deliveries in Dublin given by Collins (1 in 600) with Stein of Marburg (1 in 5.5). His conclusions relating to good practice of the time, which seemed to be generally acceptable, were as follows:

A distinction had to be made between high and low applications.

Forceps could be employed safely for both mother and child in many cases where the cervix was not fully dilated but was not to be used simply to complete the first stage of labor.

When the first stage was very prolonged and the patient's powers were exhausted, forceps were to be applied without further delay, as an aid to parturition and not as a *dernier ressort.*

Forceps were preferred to ergot when the uterus had been allowed to pass into a state of inertia.

As a general rule forceps were to be employed to complete delivery, when there existed good grounds for believing the child to be dead, in those cases where the head was firmly impacted in the pelvis.

Statistics showed that resorting to the application of forceps, even as frequent as 1 time in 10, diminished the dangers of parturition to both mother and child. (1878)

A few years later, a scheme of dystocia management based on pelvic size that gave an indication of contemporary thought and teaching was set out by R. and F. Barnes (1885) (Table 4.5).
Even by the end of the nineteenth century W. M. Campbell, Consultant Surgeon at Liverpool Northern Hospital, showed in a comprehensive review of current practices that there were still widely divergent views on procrastination, the use of uterine stimulants, and the use of high forceps delivery before full dilatation. He gave data from sixteen practitioners scattered throughout the British Isles, covering 69,967 deliveries, and recorded forceps rates ranging from 0.52 percent to 30 percent (average 9.22 percent), although the higher incidences were probably based on only those cases to which the author had been called personally. Campbell also drew attention to the fact that toward the end of the century patients' attitudes were changing. They were more enlightened, less fearful of operative intervention, and, in some cases, even asked for instrumental delivery (1899).

In summary, although some data appear in more than one series, sometimes with discrepancies in the figures, a general picture of the frequency of operative deliveries can be obtained from the available data:

In the late eighteenth through early nineteenth centuries forceps were rarely used in British practice (about 1 in 400 deliveries), perforation being the preferred intervention.

There was a sudden rise in forceps delivery in Dublin from 1847 onward, which probably reflects a general trend in Britain.

The French applied forceps about twice as often as the British.

The Germans had the highest intervention rates, but with considerable variations between different centers.

In British practice most practitioners used the perforator more frequently than the forceps, whereas on the Continent the frequency of perforation was of the order of 1 in 2000 deliveries.

. . .

By the middle of the nineteenth century the conservative legacy of Hunter, Denman, and others was on the wane and more rational intervention policies were emerging, which will be discussed in Chapter 6.

TABLE 4.5. Plan for the Management of Dystocia (R. and F. Barnes, 1885)

Conjugate		Operations at term	Operations at 7 months
4.25–4 in.	May end in:	natural labor	
4–3.75 in.	"	forceps or turning	natural labor
3.75–3.50 in.	"	turning	forceps
3.50–2.25 in.	"	craniotomy	turning
2.25–1.75 in	"	craniotomy doubtful, Caesarean section	craniotomy, Caesarean section excluded

THE EVOLUTION OF EUROPEAN FORCEPS FROM THE LATE EIGHTEENTH TO THE MID NINETEENTH CENTURY

While conservatism remained the order of the day in England, on the Continent a more aggressive attitude persisted and the approach to difficult delivery was more intrepid and traumatic. The Continental approach to intervention was also reflected in the frequency of forceps delivery (Chapter 4), as shown in the collected data of Fleetwood Churchill (1841), with rates in the order of 6 forceps deliveries for every 1000, both on the Continent and in Edinburgh, which was two to four times the rate of England and Ireland. Straight forceps were rarely used in Continental practice, as a result of the tradition stemming from Levret's influence. The European forceps were generally longer and heavier with greater cephalic and pelvic curves and, in many cases, provided considerable compression and traction force. Heavier forceps were used particularly in Eastern European cities such as Prague, where instruments were notable for their heaviness rather than originality of design. The forceps used by the Prague School throughout the nineteenth century, as shown in Figures 5.1 and 5.2, are a good example of this heavy design. They were manufactured by a number of makers and are individually difficult to identify.

The Continentals possessed a remarkable ardor for inventing instruments that were, in the words of G.-J. Witkowski, "sometimes useless, often dangerous but always ingenious" (see Chapter 11). Many of the more novel designs and the emergence of axis traction are described in other parts of this book. This chapter discusses principally the mainstream developments, starting in the last quarter of the eighteenth century. This was a time of great inventive activity. There was a preoccupation with perfecting the articulation; with increasing traction force, particularly by the introduction of finger rests; and with means of controlling the compression force on the fetal head. By 1841 D. W. H. Busch, in his *Atlas*, was able to illustrate eighty-nine different forceps, mainly Continental; by 1887 Witkowski showed nearly two hundred different designs. The instruments described in this chapter are selected because they represent landmarks in design and/or were in widespread use. Many other less practical designs, minor variations of common instruments, or those of interest mainly from their curiosity are illustrated in the atlases of the time, such as Mulder (1794), Busch (1841), Kilian (1835, Figure 5.3), and Witkowski (1887).

French Developments from Levret's Designs

While in Europe there were many minor modifications in length and curvature of the Levret instruments, in the second half of the eighteenth century or more there seemed to be a preoccupation with the design of the articulation. In contrast, the English, or Smellie, articulation, with minor modifications, held sway in Britain. The Continental handles generally retained the earlier hooked design of the Levret type, permitting considerable traction force, especially if a cord or strap was looped on to them (Chapter 10). A few obstetricians adopted wooden handles, which tended to be long enough to grip with both hands.

Of the various locking devices, a button screw and pivot was the most favored but in the original Levret (Levret Type I) forceps the mortise was in the center of the female blade, which had to be raised to allow the pivot to pass through

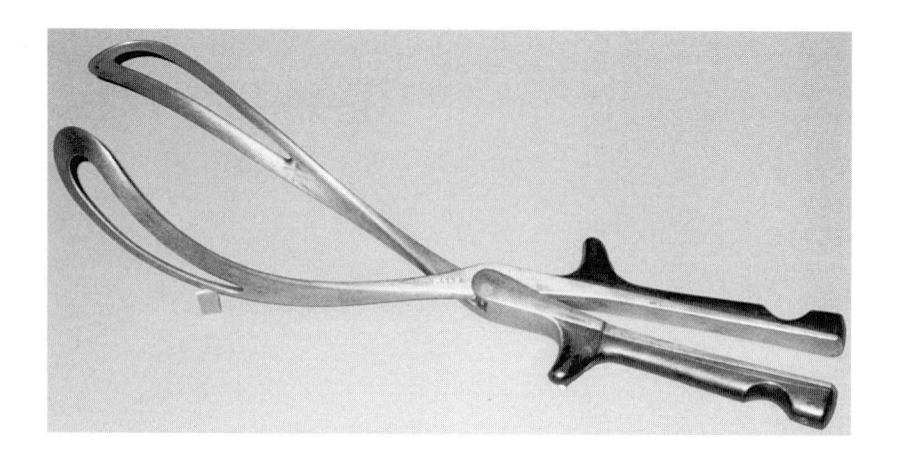

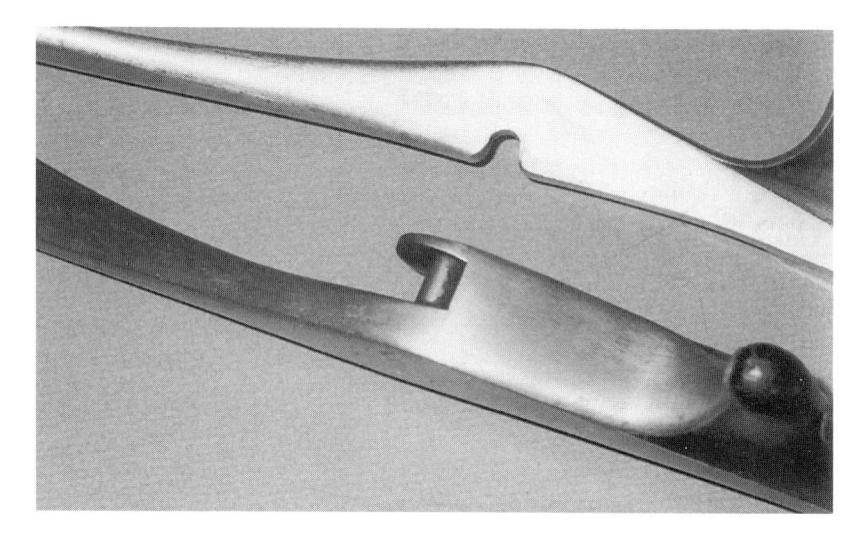

FIGURES 5.1, 5.2. Prague School. An example of late eighteenth-century forceps of the Prague school. Figure 5.2 shows an unusual articulation predating a similar improved design by Brunninghausen (see figures 5.11, 5.21). (RCOG)

the mortise. This type was eventually abandoned because it was too unstable to fit together, especially if the blades were not accurately apposed (as was common).

There were many other minor variations in the Levret patterns that were not significant contributions and were dependent on individual theorizing, preferences, and prejudices. Among others, M. Piet (d. 1807) altered the curvature of the blades (1767) and Péan elongated the blades (circa 1770).

P. V. Coutouly (1738–1814) devised several pairs of forceps of varying degrees of horror and complexity, some with screw devices joining the handles, which gave considerable mechanical advantage for crushing the head (Chapter 8). His first and more conventional design, dating from 1777, according to Das (Figure 5.4) was in the European style: long and heavy with marked curves, hooked handles, and the blade tips met when closed. In these features the Coutouly forceps were very similar to the Levret Type II (see Chapter 3, Figure 3.11), but lacked the inner groove on the blades. In addition, the lock was a simplification of and improvement upon the Levret lock. It comprised a pivot rising from the lower blade that passed through a hole in the upper blade. This was then secured by a sliding bolt.

The most detailed analysis of the use and design of forceps came from the influential Jean Louis Baudelocque (1746–1810). Baudelocque became Surgeon-in-Chief and accoucheur at the newly established Paris Maternité in 1798, as well as being accoucheur to Napoleon's wife. He described himself as perhaps the most ardent living proponent of the forceps yet said, "If it should be proved, and I am not very far from believing it, that the forceps have been more fatal than useful to society, that they have destroyed more than they have saved from inevitable death, I should nevertheless look upon them as the most important discovery that has ever been made in the art of midwifery" (1790).

Baudelocque gave equal credit to Smellie and Levret for the development of the forceps and especially for the introduction of the pelvic curve. A full description of his own

60 CHAPTER 5

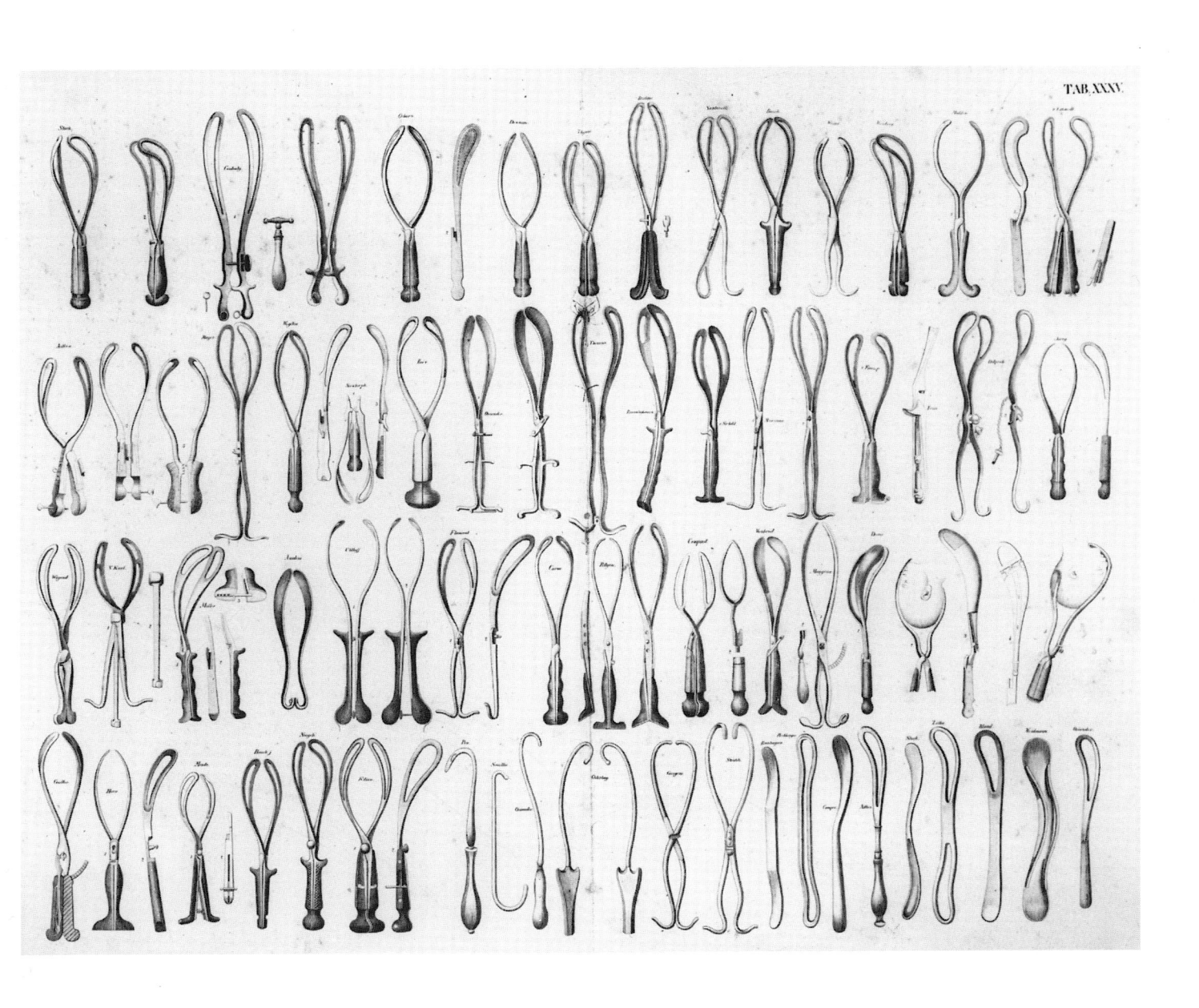

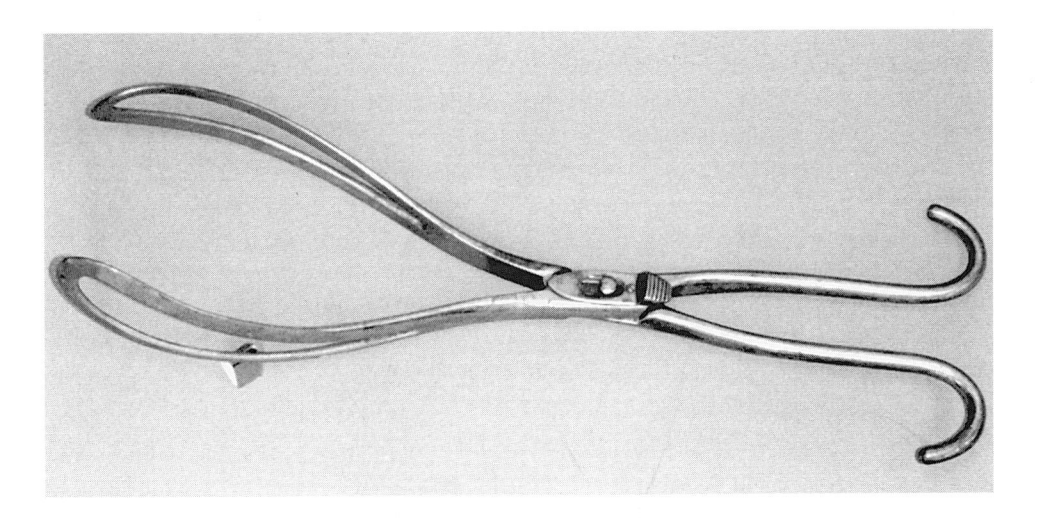

FIGURE 5.3.
Obstetrical instruments from Kilian's *Atlas* of 1835.

FIGURE 5.4.
Coutouly's original forceps. They are similar to those of Levret but have a simpler lock and are without the grooves in the blades. (University College Hospital, London)

EVOLUTION OF EUROPEAN FORCEPS 61

FIGURE 5.5.
J. L. Baudelocque's forceps. These forceps are of the basic Levret style without grooved blades but are heavier and 50 mm (2 ins) longer. (University College Hospital, London)

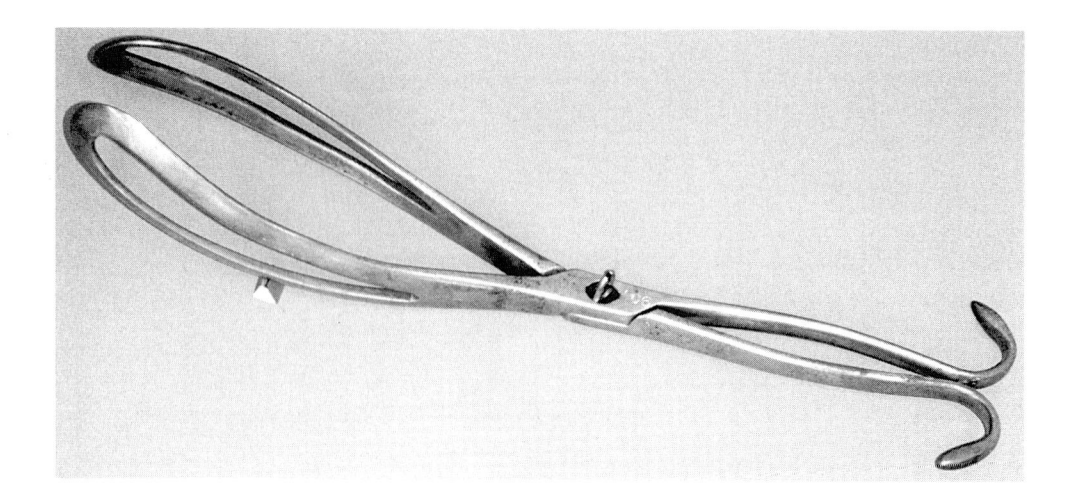

instrument is given in Heath's translation of his *L'Art des accouchemens* (*System of Midwifery*). Baudelocque favored, not surprisingly, the long forceps of the Levret type, since they were the standard instrument of the day in France. He increased the length of his own instrument (circa 1781) by 50 millimeters (2 inches) but omitted Levret's ridge on the inner surface of the blades (Figure 5.5). The additional length facilitated his practice, in common with many of his fellow countrymen (but, for some reason, not Levret), of applying the forceps when the head was still above the pelvic brim. This practice was rarely accepted in Britain although Smellie had acknowledged, if not advocated, it in his teaching when he used the longer, curved forceps of his own design. Baudelocque also advocated completing the delivery with the forceps after the head had been brought down into the pelvis rather than removing the blades and waiting for natural expulsion. Because of their heavy construction and shape the Baudelocque forceps were not well suited to delivery from the lower birth canal. Otherwise there was no obvious benefit from the delaying tactic and it may well have been detrimental, but at least the mother did give birth by her own efforts.

Baudelocque carried out a number of cadaver experiments to assess the degree of compression that could be achieved when the forceps were applied to different diameters of the head. He concluded that accoucheurs had exaggerated the degree of reduction that could be achieved safely and that this amounted to no more than 4 to 5 lines (1 line = 1/12 inch) when the blades were applied bitemporally and that there was minimal increase, if at all, in the diameter at right angles to that which was compressed. Although some accoucheurs believed that the forceps could be used safely to compress the head to the same degree achieved with natural molding, Baudelocque emphasized that with natural molding, the process occurred slowly and allowed time for the cranial contents to adapt to the space available, whereas with the forceps the process was sudden and allowed virtually no time for the head to adapt to the space.

Baudelocque's general rules for applying the forceps deviated from British practice and were very much in the Continental tradition, apart from always positioning the blades in correct cephalic orientation. He made a point of avoiding secrecy by showing and explaining the instruments to the mother, who would lie on her back with the buttocks over the end of the bed. He taught that the blades should, with very rare exceptions, be applied to the sides of the head, irrespective of its position. This was at variance with the more widely practiced method of inserting the blades and applying them to the head laterally, in correct pelvic orientation, irrespective of the position of the head. Levret had also advised a correct cephalic application but said that the blades should be introduced where there was the most room, usually the sides of the pelvis, and then "wandered" into position as necessary to achieve a correct cephalic application. When the head was in an oblique or transverse position in the pelvic cavity Baudelocque favored rotation with the for-

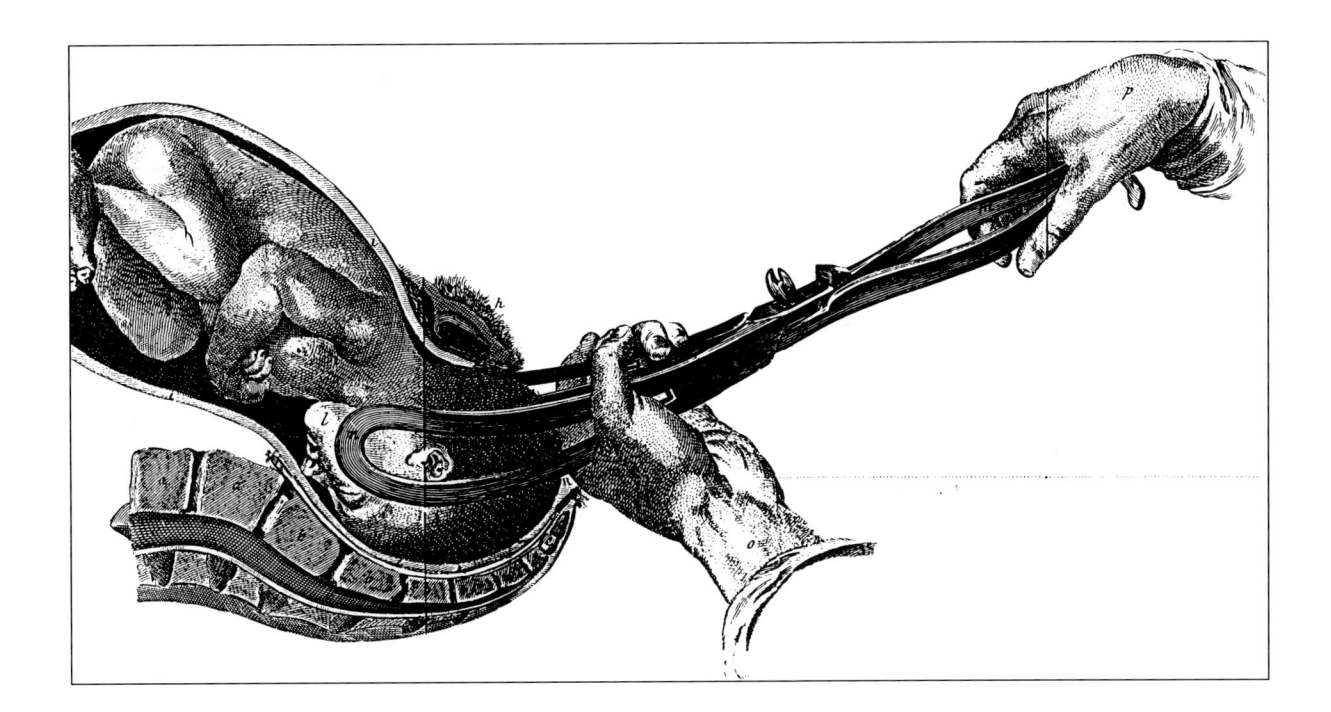

FIGURE 5.6.
J. L. Baudelocque's forceps showing the method of application and traction. (Baudelocque, 1789)

ceps, describing the maneuver of swinging the forceps handles around in an arc that was described again more than fifty years later by Friedrich Wilhelm Scanzoni (1821–1891) of the University of Würzburg in his *Lehrbuch der Geburtshilfe* (1853), and which thereafter bore Scanzoni's name.

Baudelocque's manner of holding the blades is shown in Plate VIII of his *L'Art des accouchemens* and it is notable that the left hand is used to grasp the base of the blades rather than being used on the handles (Figure 5.6). This allowed for application of great force.

Baudelocque's forceps also became popular in America and W. P. Dewees of Philadelphia had his own version made locally, from a Paris pattern, which did not differ greatly from the original (1811, 1825). Dewees's notes appended to his abridged version of Heath's translation of Baudelocque's *L'Art des accouchemens* (1811), included an advertisement for the American instrument maker Eberle, who had worked in Paris under the direction of Baudelocque (see also Chapter 7).

J. L. Baudelocque's less illustrious nephew, A.-C. Baudelocque, who worked in the Faculty of Medicine at the University of Paris, made some minor modifications to his uncle's design in about 1833. These were described in 1853 by J. P. Bethell in his article entitled "Description of a New Obstetric Forceps." He concluded that the nephew's version was totally unsuited to the purposes for which it was intended, mainly because the widest distance between the blades was close to the distal ends, and as a consequence when the forceps were applied the tips were separated by a distance of about 75 millimeters (3 inches).

Antoine Dubois (1756–1837), Senior Surgeon and Professor at the Maternité in Paris, delivered the Empress Marie-Louise using forceps for an occipito-posterior position and succeeded in resuscitating an apparently dead baby, for which he was immediately rewarded with a barony by Napoleon. A. Dubois's forceps, invented in 1791, were illustrated by both Mulder (1798, Table VII) and Kilian (1856, Table XX). They were of the Levret pattern with a slot-and-screw lock (Figure 5.7, bottom). The tip of one handle had a screw cap that concealed a sharp hook to be used for the extraction of a dead child. In the original model, as illustrated by Kilian, this handle, and sometimes both handles, were covered by removable wooden sheaths that facilitated the grip (Figure 5.8, bottom). Later models were more refined. It is said that Charles Pajot, also a professor in Paris (Chapters 12, 13), taught his pupils that the hook was placed there as a reminder that it should never be employed.

Paul Dubois (1795–1871) was Antoine's son and succeeded him as Senior Surgeon and Professor at the Maternité. Paul Dubois made various modifications to the basic Levret pattern, including a lateral mortise joint (circa 1850) (Figure

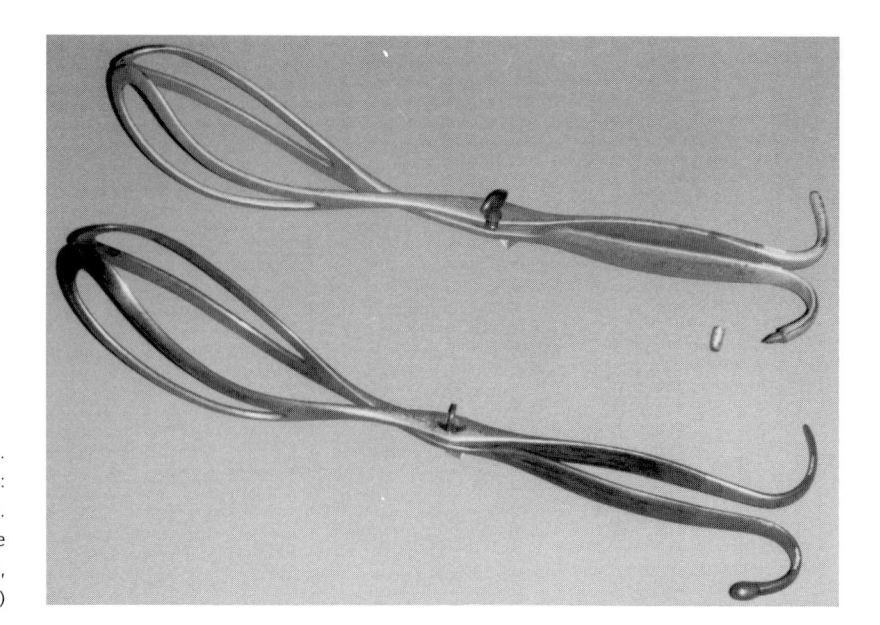

FIGURE 5.7.
Antoine and Paul Dubois's forceps. Bottom: A. Dubois's forceps. Top: P. Dubois's forceps. Note the sharp point at the end of one handle covered by a screw cap. (Science Museum, London)

FIGURE 5.8.
Antoine and Paul Dubois's forceps. These versions have detachable wooden handles, as illustrated by Kilian (1856). (Science Museum, London)

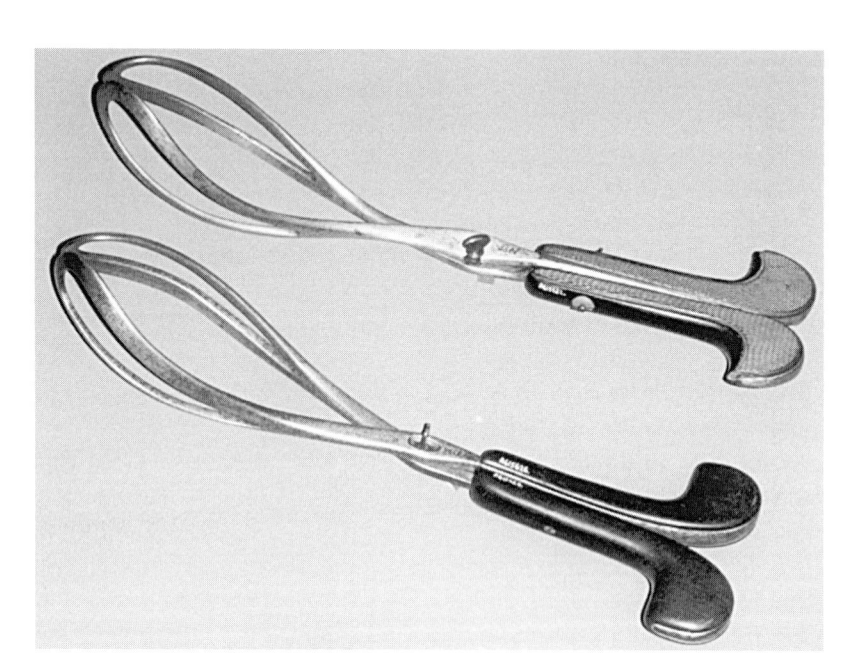

5.7, top). One version of his forceps, with no wood on the handle, was illustrated by Kilian (1856, Table XXXII). Although wooden handles were uncommon on European forceps of the time, some examples of P. Dubois's forceps did have ebony handles and he incorporated the protected spike in the handle, as his father had done (Figure 5.8, top). In another version, made by the instrument maker Charrière, a toothed ratchet was incorporated in the handles to lock the blades together. P. Dubois also had a version with a jointed handle.

Parisian obstetricians continued to modify the Levret-type forceps. Péan described an elongated version (see Baudelocque, 1790; Moreau, 1837) and F. J. Moreau, a professor in the Faculty of Medicine, made further modifications to the Péan instrument, which he described in his *Traité pratique des accouchemens* (1837). This instrument is described in detail in the English translation of Moreau's work (Betton, 1844). It was 419 millimeters (16.5 inches) long and the blades were closer together near the pivot to reduce the risk of perineal laceration (Figure 5.9). The crotchet-shaped

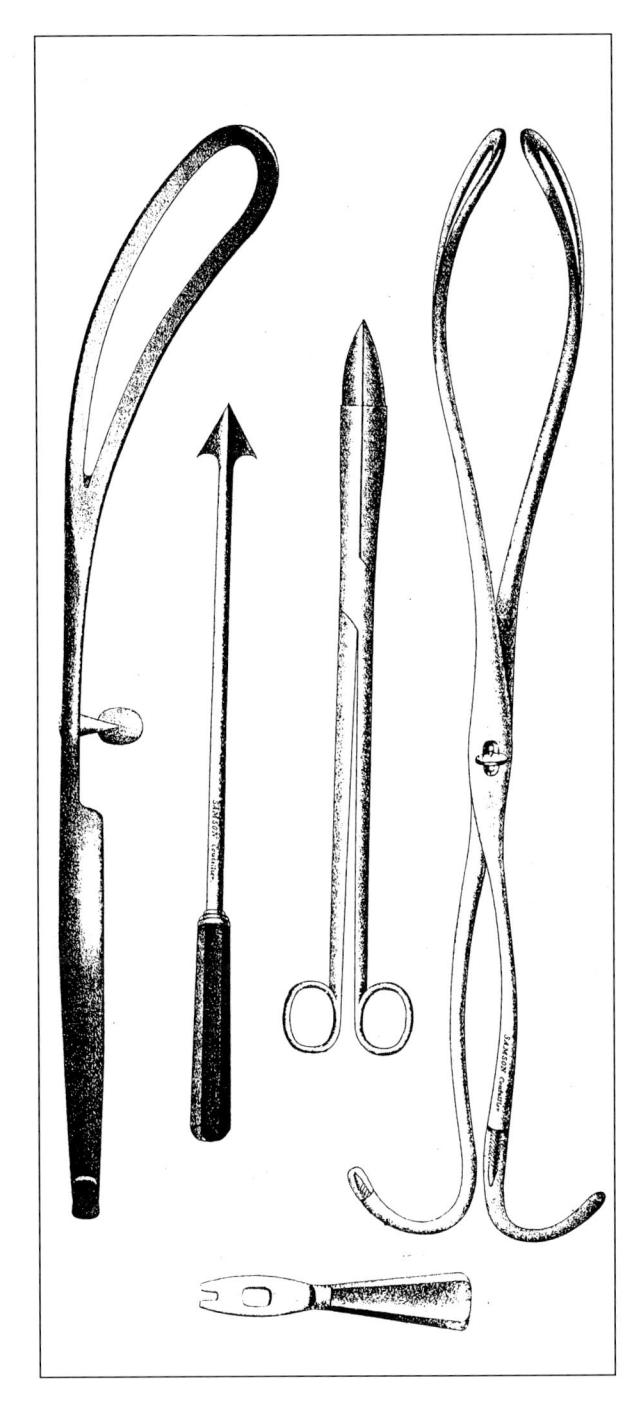

FIGURE 5.9.
Moreau's forceps. Another elongated modification of Levret's forceps. The screw caps on the handles conceal a sharp hook and a perforator. A separate key is used to tighten the screw joint and to remove the ends of the handles. (Moreau, 1837)

FIGURE 5.10.
Cazeaux's forceps. The forceps have detachable wooden handles, similar to those of Dubois. A key to tighten the joint is provided. (Cazeaux, 1850)

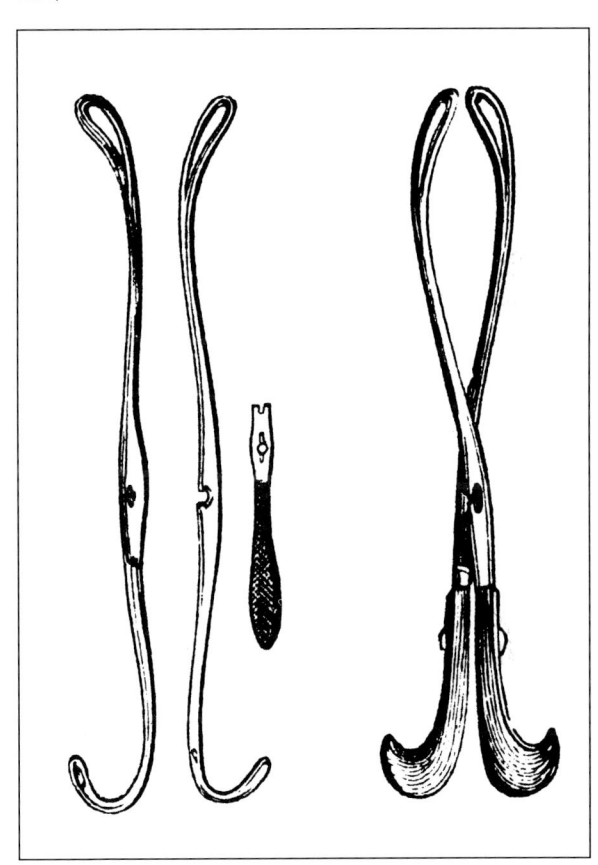

handles had screw-capped ends, one of which concealed a sharp hook and the other a perforator. In addition a key was provided to tighten the screw joint and to unscrew the ends of the handles.

P. Cazeaux is known particularly for his *Traité théorique et pratique de l'art des accouchments*, first published in 1840, later editions of which were revised by E. S. Tarnier. It was also translated into English by W. R. Bullock of Philadelphia (1868). Cazeaux's forceps (circa 1835) were very similar to the Levret instruments but in one illustration they are shown with wooden handles (Figure 5.10). Cazeaux also provided a key for tightening the screw lock, which was a common feature in French design.

R. P. Flamant (d.1833) was Professor at the Faculty of Medicine in Strasbourg. He described his forceps in 1816 in his *Mémoire pratique sur les forceps* but gave no measurements or illustrations. However, they are shown in Kilian's *Armamentarium* (Table XXVI). They were of the Levret style but the articulation was a pin-and-socket type with a sliding lock on the female blade to hold the pin in place.

EVOLUTION OF EUROPEAN FORCEPS 65

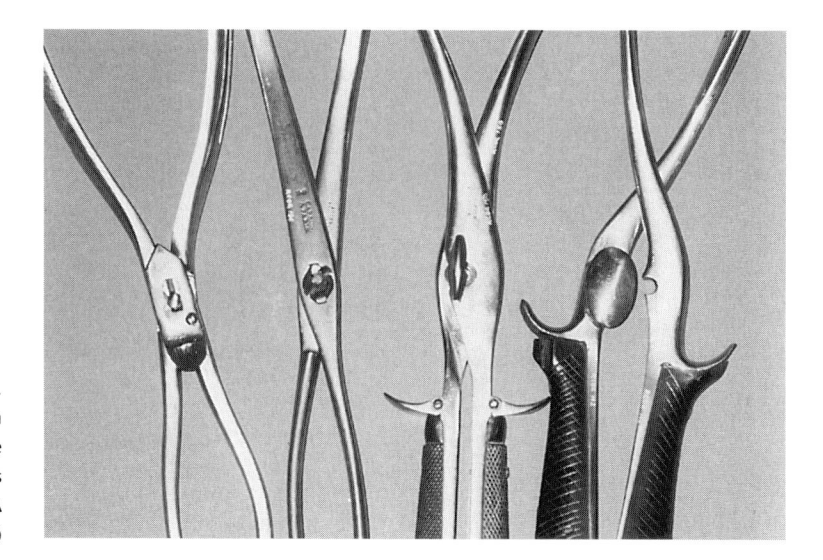

FIGURE 5.11.
Comparison of European locks. European accoucheurs were more inventive than the British in their design of joints. Examples illustrated are from left to right: Coutouly, A Dubois, Stolz, Brunninghausen. (RCOG)

FIGURE 5.12.
Tarsitani's forceps. The joint is made with a pivot on both aspects of the male blade so that either blade can be introduced first. (Science Museum, London)

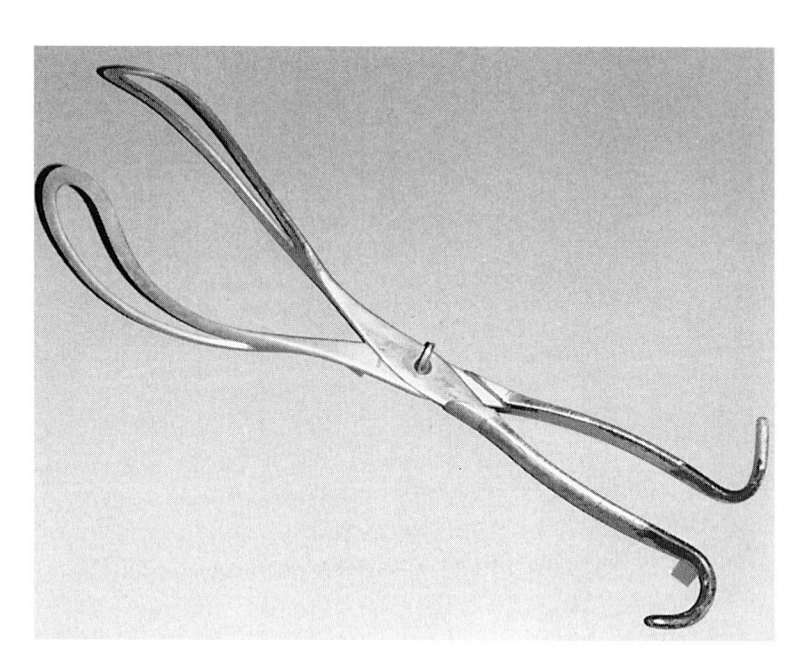

The variations on the Levret theme over this period were generally not significant but they were indicative of unease about the designs, particularly about the articulations, and this continued far into the nineteenth century, with trials of various other locking mechanisms, including the reversible lock, the block lock, and the lateral mortise and, occasionally, the English lock.

Other Modifications to Articulations

The Reversible Lock
A problem common to most Continental crossover articulations (Figure 5.11), the necessity of positioning the male blade below the female to allow the pivot to enter the mortise, was addressed by D. Tarsitani of Naples. He presented the simple solution of putting a pivot on both the upper and lower surfaces of the male blade so that locking could be achieved without further manipulation even if the female blade was applied first (Figure 5.12). Although he made further modifications it seems that these did not meet his needs for he later devised parallel forceps (Chapter 11.) His original instrument was exhibited at the Academy of Medicine in Paris in 1843 by the makers Tureau and Davan (Capuron, 1842–1843) and was discussed further by Capuron at a later meeting of the Academy (1843–1844).

The same problem was tackled in a different way by the Lyons School. Jean-Simon Thenance introduced a parallel forceps in 1781. The main feature of Thenance's forceps was that the blades did not cross and the articulation was at the

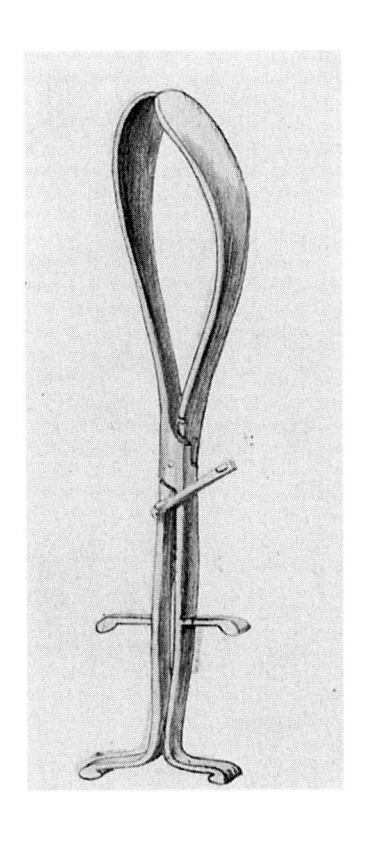

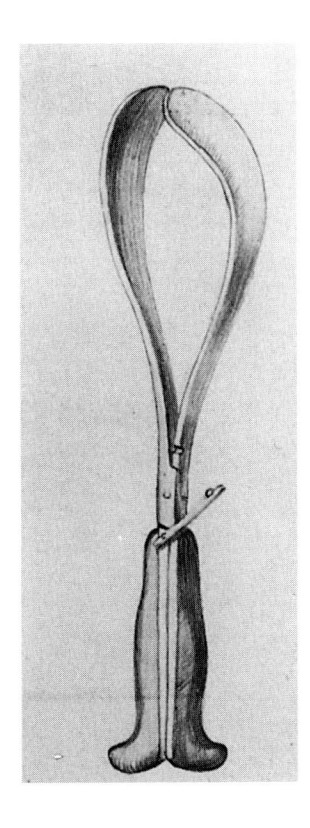

FIGURE 5.13.
F. B. Osiander's forceps, second pattern. This shows the block-lock and groove in the left blade. (Doran, 1913c)

FIGURE 5.14.
Weissbrod's forceps. The lock is similar to that of Osiander. (Doran, 1913c)

ends of the handles. This type of forceps came to be known as the *forceps Lyonnais* and is discussed in detail in Chapter 11. In Germany there was more novelty in design rather than minor variations on old themes, particularly in relation to the articulation and in attempts to combine ease of use with stability.

The "Block-Lock"

The "block-lock," a term coined by A. Doran, was devised by F. B. Osiander (1759–1822) a controversial figure who became a distinguished professor at the University of Göttingen. His professional career is well documented by Doran (1913c). Osiander was a vociferous advocate for the free use of the forceps. By 1792 he had used them 39 times in 168 deliveries; the forceps incidence at Göttingen during his reign was 40 percent. He carried out one perforation, which was his first and last. He preferred to perform Caesarian section if forceps delivery was not possible, a very avant-garde practice in his day. Although it was generally taught that 40 pulls on the forceps was the limit before abandoning the procedure, Osiander claimed that he had pulled as many as 175 times, in some cases with no harm to the mother or baby! There was a literary war between Osiander and his most open opponent, L. J. Boër of Vienna (see below), who was very critical of Osiander's high rate of operative intervention. J. F. Osiander, F. B.'s son and a pupil of Boër, continued the war after his father's death. However, it seems that father and son both became more moderate in their views in later life.

F. B. Osiander invented a number of obstetric instruments but none, including his forceps, found wide favor and soon fell into disuse because they were too heavy and unwieldy. His forceps were devised between 1798 and 1803. Some were coated with India rubber to prevent corrosion. They were of considerable stature, bigger than many cephalotribes (Figure 5.13). The blades were solid and each handle had two finger rests. An early model had a ratchet and lock at the free end. The other notable feature was the articulation. A pin in one blade fit into a hole in the right blade and was secured by a block-lock. This system was only known to be used by two other obstetricians, J. B. Weissbrod and C. L. Mursinna.

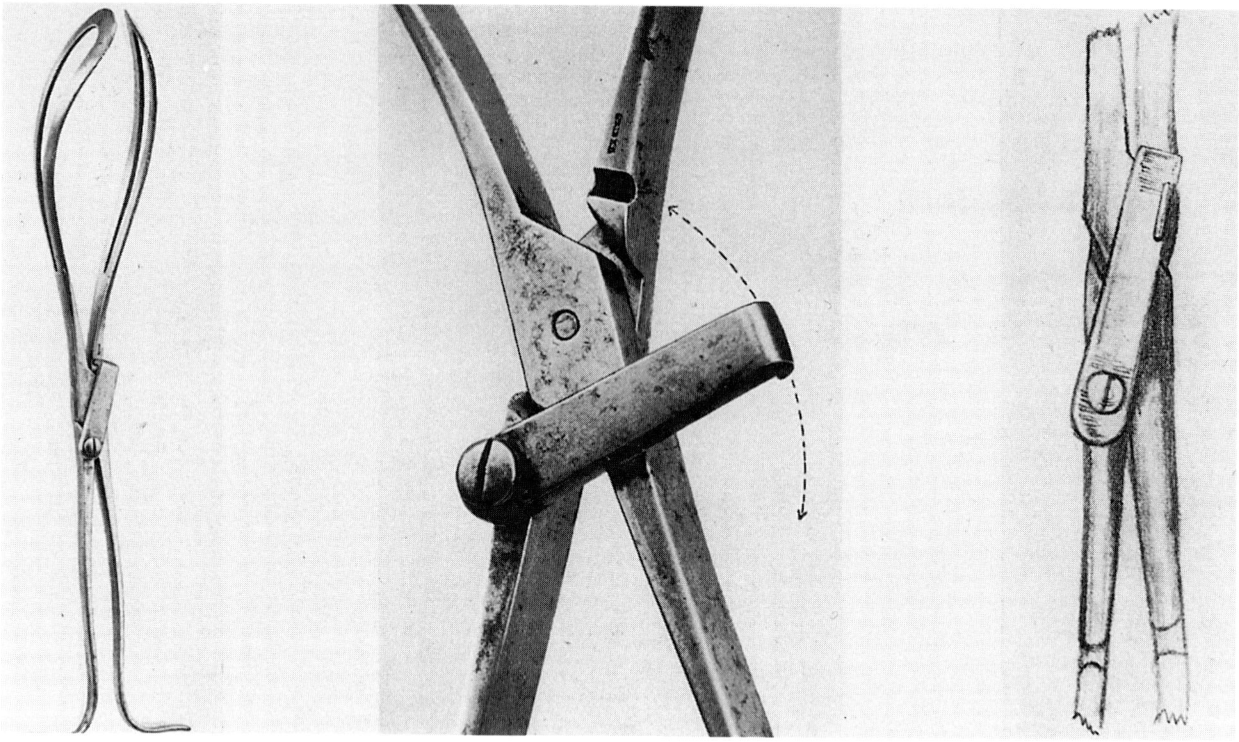

FIGURE 5.15.
Mursinna's forceps. Close-up views showing the locking mechanism. In the right illustration a small thumb piece has been added. (Doran, 1913c)

J. B. Weissbrod was Director of the Munich Lying-in Hospital. His forceps (circa 1825, Figure 5.14) were described by Doran (1913c) and differed from Osiander's only in the handles, which were made of wood and terminated in a knob, a compromise between the English smooth, wooden, rounded end to the handle, or palm rest, and the Continental traction hooks.

C. L. Mursinna (1734–1823) had a fascinating life story, which is detailed by Doran (1913c). He began life as a barber-surgeon in his native Pomerania. He had a varied career, much of it spent intermittently as an army surgeon, although he eventually held a chair in surgery at the University of Berlin. His forceps, which were a modification of Levret's, were first described in 1803, and the details of their construction were given in detail by Doran (1913c). Unlike Osiander he was relatively conservative in their use (5 applications in 260 labors) and said that he only used them when the patient's condition was so grave that no other measure would ensure speedy delivery. Different examples of his forceps show minor variations. Essentially they were modeled on the Levret pattern but were 50 millimeters (2 inches) longer, with the extra length mainly in the handles to facilitate a good grip (Figure 5.15). The articulation had a block-lock and was adapted from Osiander. However, unlike Osiander, Mursinna retained the fenestra in the blades.

The English Lock in Europe

Outside France the English lock appears to have been quite well known and was adopted by some German obstetricians over a long period. It may be that this concept led to the development of lateral mortises in that country. One of the first Germans of note to adopt the English lock was J. D. Busch in 1796 (see "Finger Rests" below). A. F. Hohl (b. 1794) was a professor in Halle. He described his own forceps design in his *Lehrbuch der Geburtshülfe* (1855) (Figure 5.16). The interesting features were: the lock, of the English type, which he acknowledged as a modification from Smellie; long handles with terminal finger rests, in the style of Adam Elias von Siebold (page 71); and solid blades, which were hollowed out in the normal site for the fenestra. Hohl also illustrated the application of the forceps obliquely on the head and used Pajot's method of holding the blades and applying traction (Figures 5.17, 5.18).

Eduard Martin (1809–1875), a pupil of F. C. Naegele, was Busch's successor in Berlin, where he became the leading obstetric authority and was accoucheur to the Crown Prin-

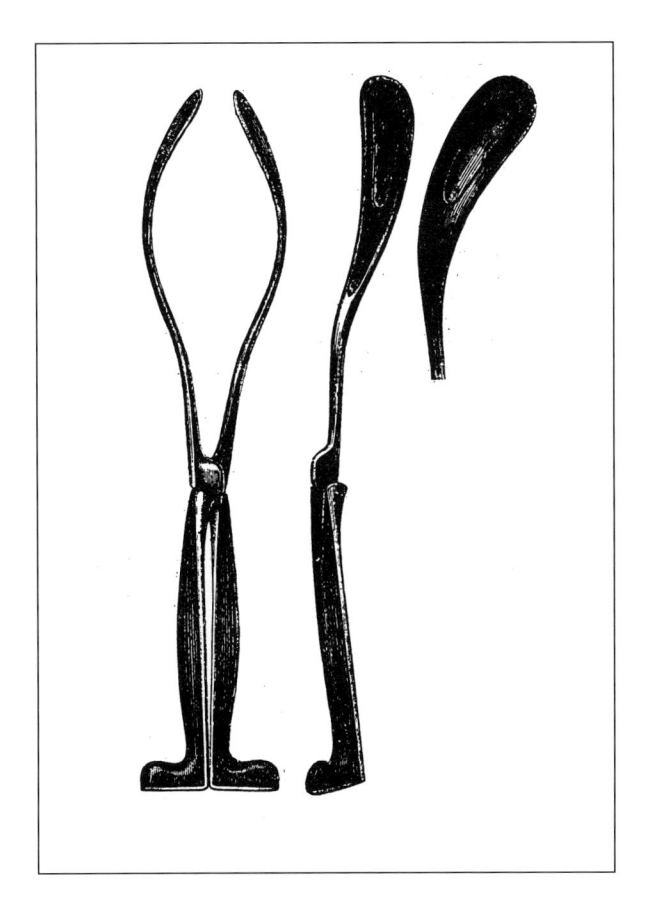

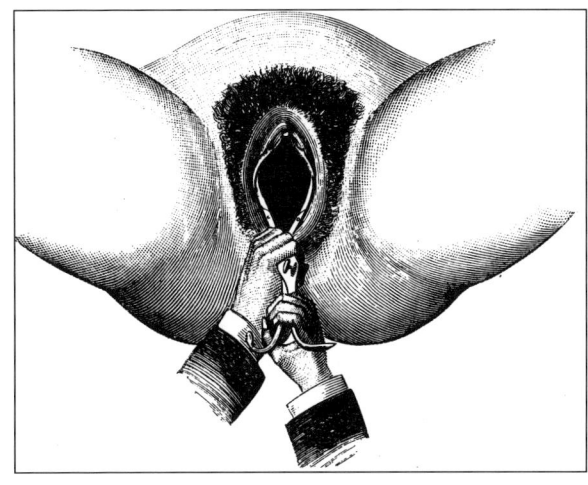

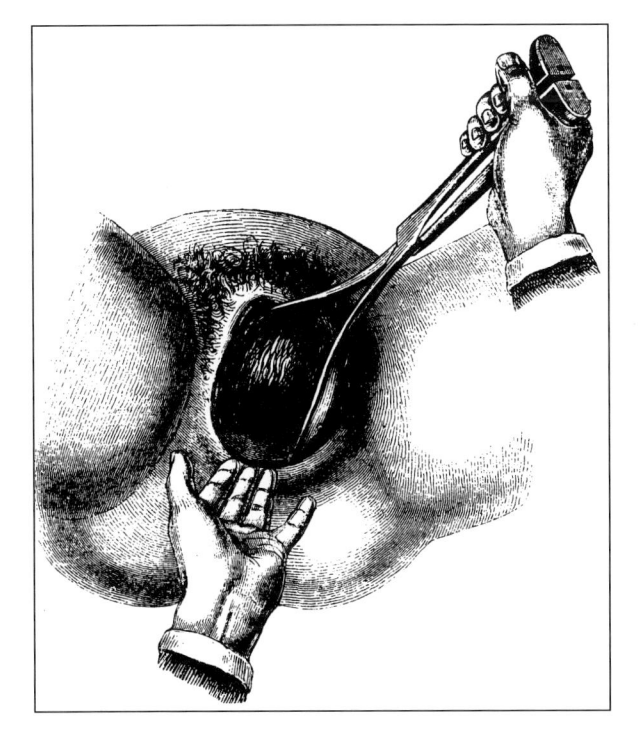

FIGURES 5.16–5.18.
Hohl's forceps. 5.16 (above left): Note the English lock, the terminal finger rests, and the hollowed out solid blades. 5.17 (below left): Oblique application of the forceps. 5.18 (above): Pajot's maneuver. (Hohl, 1855)

EVOLUTION OF EUROPEAN FORCEPS 69

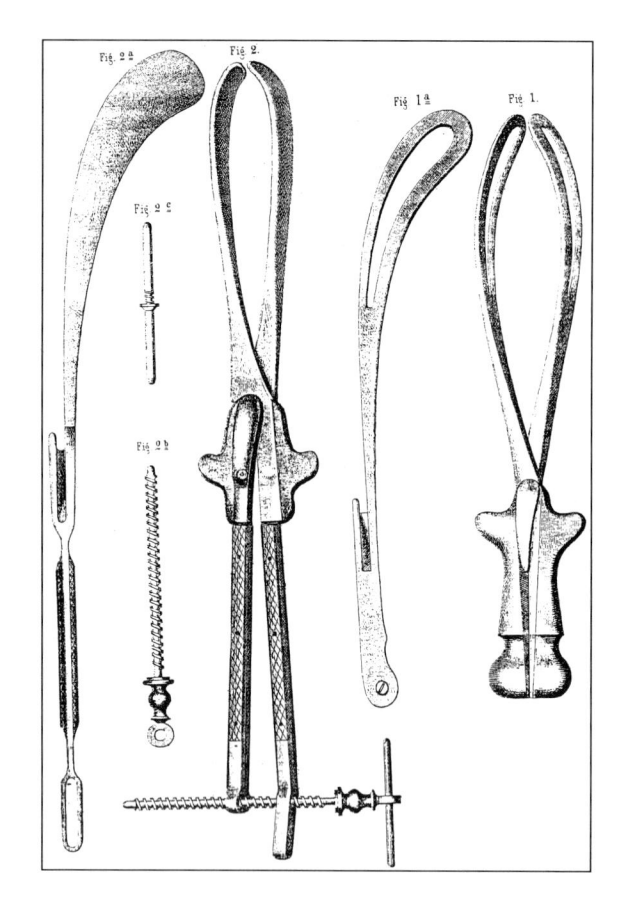

FIGURE 5.19.
Martin's forceps and kephalotryptor. The forceps (right) are of the heavy Continental type and have a marked pelvic curve, they have English features in the relative shortness, the lock, and the finger rests. The kephalotryptor is shown on the left. (Martin, 1862)

FIGURE 5.20.
E. von Siebold's forceps. Note the recessed notch to accept the pivot, thereby adding to the stability. The terminal finger hooks facilitate an increased leverage force. (E. von Siebold, 1802)

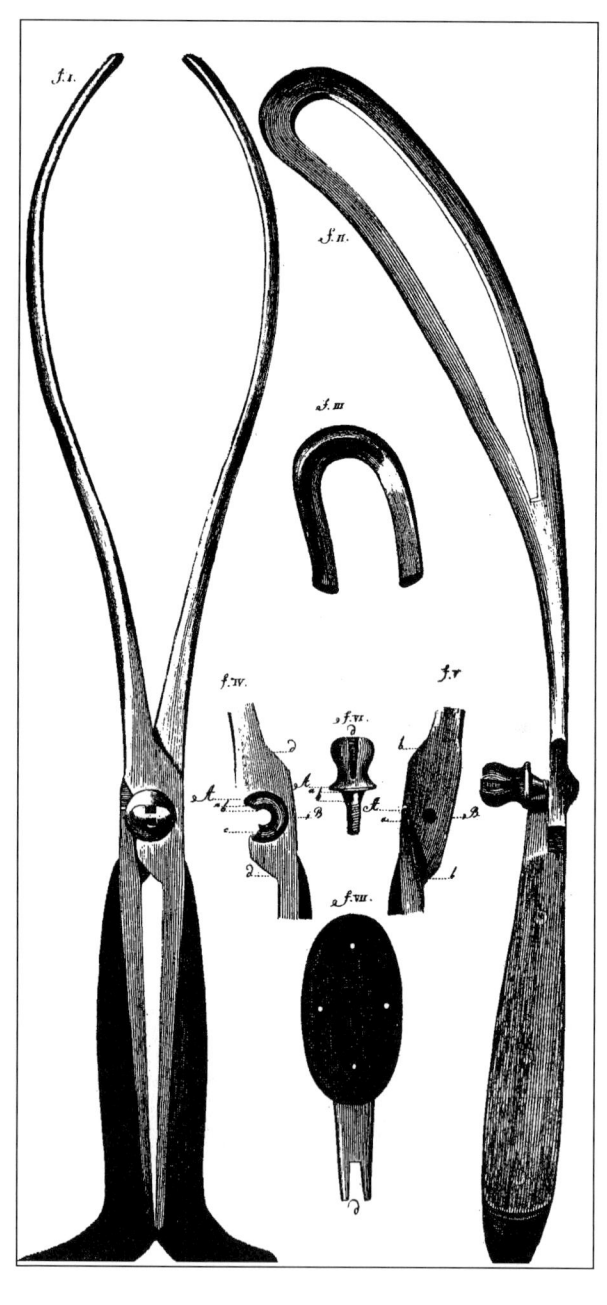

cess of Prussia (Princess Irene of England). He introduced his forceps in 1839 and they, together with his other instruments, are illustrated in his *Atlas* of 1862 (Figure 5.19). They were shorter (355 millimeters/14 inches) than most Continental instruments of the time and showed considerable British influence, with an English lock and palm rests, but also had finger rests. However, they had the Continental heaviness and marked pelvic curve.

The Lateral Mortise

A major improvement to the articulation was made by Elias von Siebold, from Würzburg, and was described in the journal *Lucina* in 1802 and by Eduard C. J. von Siebold in his textbook, *Lehrbuch der Geburtshülfe* (1854). Elias von Siebold made the mortise with a notch in the side of the blade so that the pivot could be slid directly into position; this construction was widely adopted in Europe. The pivot was

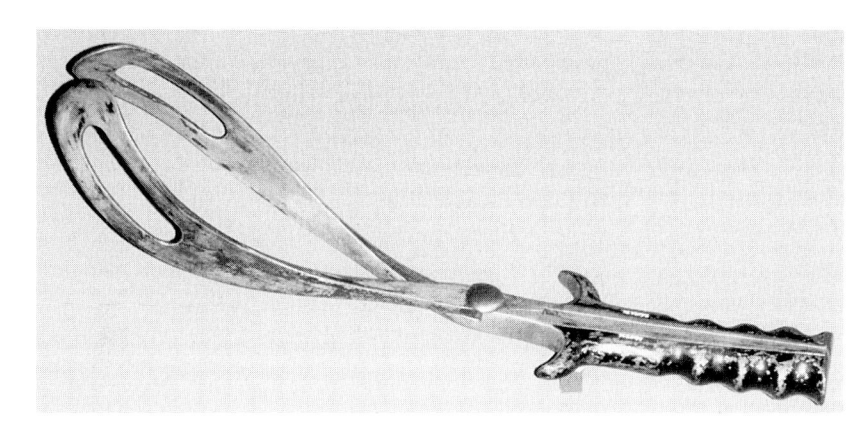

FIGURE 5.21.
Brunninghausen's forceps. The articulation is a compromise between French and English patterns, combining stability with ease of use. For detail see figure 5.11. (Science Museum, London)

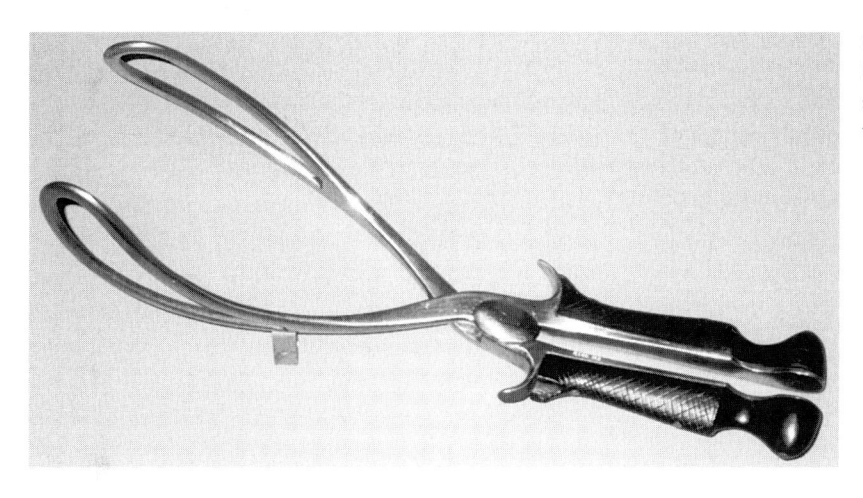

FIGURE 5.22.
Naegele's forceps. Modifications from various sources were incorporated but the important feature was the Brunninghausen lock. (RCOG)

screwed down with a key (Figure 5.20). The design of the pivot was similar to that of Cazeaux (Figure 5.10).

Adam Elias von Siebold regarded the main function of the forceps as a compressor rather than a tractor and therefore a firm and stable articulation was required (1810–1812). This was achieved by having a screw pivot sliding into a notch, as referred to above. The notch was recessed so that when the pivot was screwed down it fit into the recess, thus making a stable closure. In addition, and also as an aid to more effective compression force, he moved the finger rests, which had been introduced by Busch (page 72), from the proximal to the distal end of the handle, thereby increasing the leverage. A. E. von Siebold's forceps were also known in America and Dewees illustrated a pair shown to him by the instrument maker Eberle (page 63) in relation to Baudelocque's forceps. However they differed from the instrument illustrated by Siebold, having hooked, metal handles like Baudelocque's rather than the wooden handles shown in the original Siebold instrument. The important point was that the lock was that of Siebold and it found favor with the influential Dewees.

Another major improvement in the overall design of the forceps that became very popular and had a long and widespread effect outside France came from Hermann Joseph Brunninghausen (1761–1834), Professor of Surgery, University of Würzburg. His forceps (1802) were heavy, with long blades and small fenestra. The long handles were of wood applied to metal and had finger rests. The most notable feature, and a major advance, was in the construction of the articulation, which was quite elegant because of its simple design and construction and also quite stable. His design comprised a simple fixed pin pivot surmounted by a large mushroom-shaped head on the left blade that fit firmly into a notch on the right blade. (Figure 5.21). This compromise between the stable but difficult–to-handle French locks and the less stable but easily closed English lock turned out to be highly successful and was widely adopted.

Franz Carl Naegele (1778–1851) was Chief Obstetrician for the Neckar, Main, and Tauber regions. His forceps (circa 1830) (Figure 5.22) incorporated modifications that he had picked up from various sources, the greatest influence being that of Brunninghausen. Indeed, W. Kuhn and U. Tröhler

(1987) were reluctant to credit Naegele with a design of his own, the only significant difference from Brunninghausen's forceps being an additional knob at the end of the handle. A detailed description, including minor variations, was given by Adolphe Pinard (1844–1934) in his *Dictionnaire encyclopaedique* (1879). The weight was 652 grams (23 ounces), the overall length 379 millimeters (15 inches) and the maximum distance between the blades 67 millimeters (2.6 inches). The handles were of wood with a terminal notch, mounted on metal, with strong metal finger rests backed by lateral extensions of the wooden handles. The articulation was copied from Brunninghausen and was also elegantly designed to facilitate locking.

Although the credit for the concept of the lateral-mortise articulation must go to Brunninghausen there is no doubt that Naegele's achievement was to popularize the design throughout Europe. By the second half of the nineteenth century Naegele's forceps were in general use in Germany. In Britain the Naegele pattern influenced J. Y. Simpson in the design of his long forceps and Edward Rigby the Younger (1804–1861), lecturer at St. Thomas's and St. Bartholomew's Hospitals, London, introduced an Anglicized version, lighter in construction without finger rests, in which he was faithful to the Brunninghausen lock, which he described as "the most perfect lock" (1841)

Forceps of the Brunninghausen-Naegele type continued to be used for at least a century, often with other names attached. For example, K. Schroeder (d. 1887), a professor at the university in Erlanger, in his textbook of 1870 favored the Brunninghausen-Naegele design. Though he made no original contribution and gave no description of a personal design in his book, his name has been ascribed to forceps that appear in most instrument catalogues of the time.

Thus it was that, after decades of experimenting with articulations of varying complexity and practical limitations, the simple and efficient Brunninghausen-type lock began to dominate European practice.

Finger Rests

Europe was divided over the relative roles of the forceps for compression and traction. It is clear from the heaviness and the proximity of the blades that compression was a major consideration with many obstetricians. However an increasing number were searching for improved traction efficiency. One way of accomplishing this was to add finger rests rather than relying on the attachment of tapes or hooks, especially when using forceps with hooked handles, as had been the practice. Elias von Siebold added finger rests at the ends of the handles but this was not mechanically very efficient and forceps began to appear with finger rests at the proximal end of the handles. Although J. Aitken had described rudimentary finger rests in 1786 (see Figure 10.23), their primary purpose was to facilitate placement of the fingers to protect the lower birth canal from injury rather than to provide traction.

Johan David Busch (1755–1833) is usually given credit as the first to introduce the finger rests, or flanges, at the proximal end of the handles to facilitate oscillating traction, a feature subsequently taken up by many European and British obstetricians who designed instruments, notably J. Y. Simpson. Busch was a professor at the University of Marburg and had used both Levret's and Smellie's forceps but found neither entirely satisfactory. He, unlike many of his contemporaries, rejected forceps as an instrument for skull compression and used them solely for traction. He introduced his own forceps with finger rests (Figure 5.23) and they featured in Stark's *Archiv für die Geburtshülfe* (1794). The example of Busch's forceps described by Doran (1914) was heavy (567 grams/20 ounces) and 350 millimeters (13.75 inches) in length, with a marked pelvic curve. The handles were long enough for a two-handed grip and the fenestra had slots to permit the use of traction tapes if necessary. Busch's forceps had a protective coating of rubber, a feature probably introduced by Osiander (see above) toward the end of the eighteenth century that continued intermittently until the use of hardened steels, nickel, and chromium plating became widespread toward the end of the nineteenth century. Another notable feature for a German instrument was the use of the English lock, a novelty for European designers.

D. W. H. Busch (1788–1858), at the University of Marburg, Johan David's son, became better known than his father and popularized his father's forceps, to which he made a few minor modifications, including lengthening the handle. Doran (1914) gave a translation of the description of the forceps from D. W. H.'s *Atlas*. The forceps were 400 millimeters (15.75 inches) long, of typical heavy German construction, which was in general heavier than the French, and with a marked pelvic curve.

Joseph Alexis Stolz (1803–1896) was a successor to Flamant as a professor at the University of Strasbourg in the Faculty of Medicine, which was transferred to Nancy following the Franco-Prussian war in 1870. Stolz achieved recognition for his discourse entitled *Induction of Premature Labour* (1835), a procedure that was at the time opposed in France but as the result of his paper gradually found favor.

Stolz's forceps (circa 1839) (Figure 5.24), although based on the Levret pattern, embraced several innovative features and were a turning point in Continental design. 420 millimeters (16.5 inches) in length, they were intermediate between the longer forceps in use in Paris and the shorter German instruments. The blades were large and wide and the

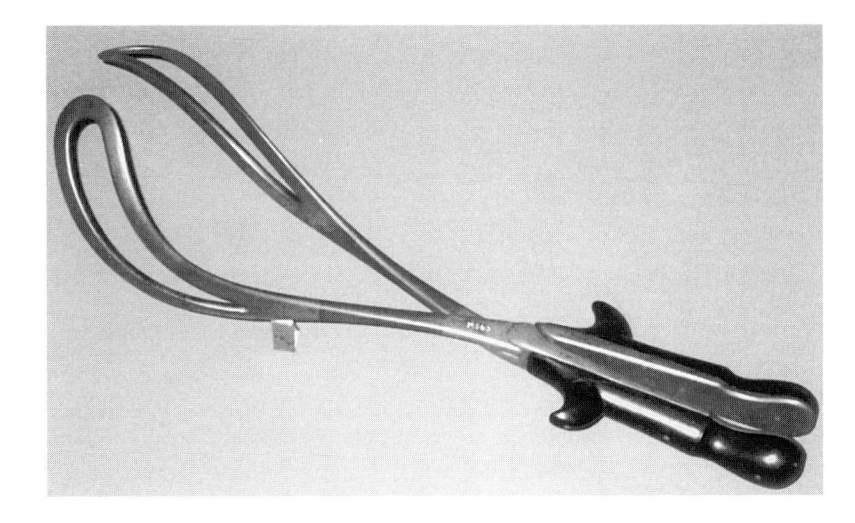

FIGURE 5.23.
J. D. Busch's forceps. The finger rests were introduced to facilitate oscillating traction. (RCOG)

FIGURE 5.24.
Stolz's forceps. The lock is similar to that of E. von Siebold. Note the folding finger rests. (RCOG)

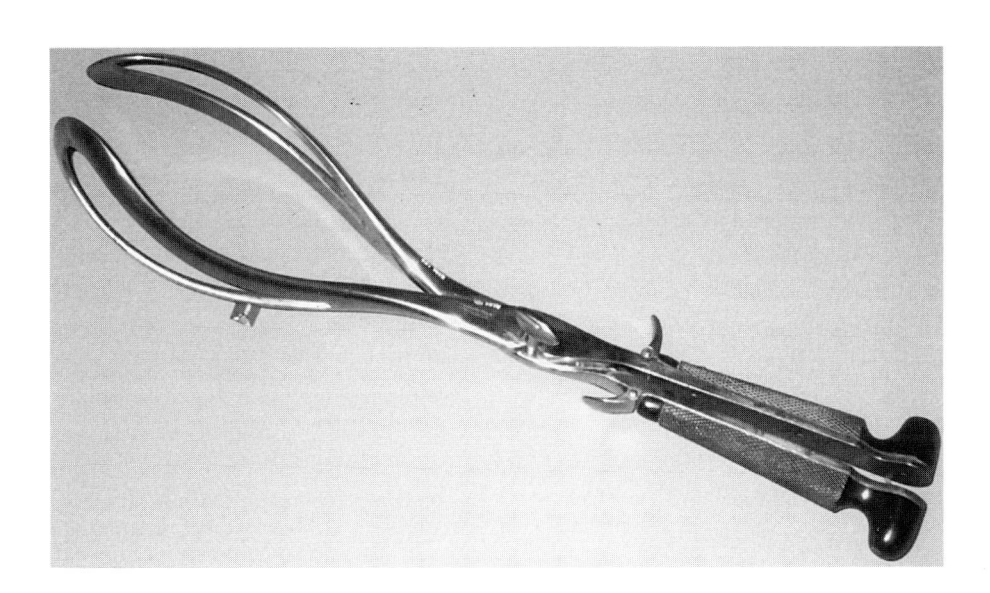

distance between them was greater than in many previous designs, resulting in less compression of the head. The joint comprised a notch and screw pivot that enabled the blades to be firmly fixed together. The handles were of ebony, with palm rests in the English style but larger, and with hinged finger rests, which, Stolz claimed, provided greater traction force without fatiguing the fingers. In addition the proximal siting of the finger rests gave a better direction of traction The finger rests were hinged because Stolz claimed that fixed rests, as in the Busch instrument (page 72) made insertion of the blades more difficult and spoiled the instrument's elegance.

Stolz, in the introduction to the tenth edition of H. F. J. Naegele and W. L. Grenser's *Traité pratique*, which he edited, extolled the virtues of his instrument and praised the well-known maker, Charrière, for

perfectly meeting the intention of the inventor. Two ears or mobile hooks were joined to the upper parts of the handles by solid hinges in such a way that when folded the hooks formed a continuation of the handle; lowered they presented two large slightly concave projections, with very rounded edges, on which could rest the fingers of one hand, and exert not only a great traction force but also transmit it easily in a suitable direction for the instrument and the head, without fatigue to the [operator's] hand.

Otto von Spiegelberg (1830–1881) was a peripatetic professor from Breslau who traveled widely in Europe and the United Kingdom while occupying four chairs at different institutions in Germany in the space of five years (1860–1865). His highly popular *Lehrbuch der Geburtshülfe* did not ap-

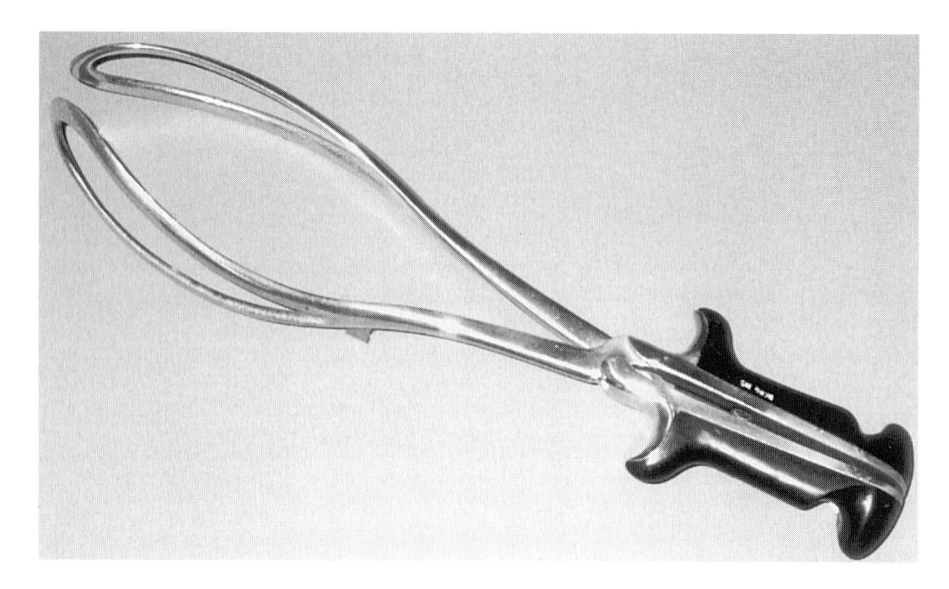

FIGURE 5.25.
Forceps ascribed to Spiegelberg. They were probably originally designed by Trefurt in 1844. (RCOG)

pear until 1878 (English translation, 1887), late in his career, and in this work he gave a detailed critique of the desirable qualities of forceps. He was one of the few Continental obstetricians who accepted a place for short straight forceps for outlet deliveries. He decried high forceps application (with the head above the brim) and therefore length in the forceps was not a desirable feature (he set the upper limit at 400 millimeters [15.75 inches]). He was also critical of long handles because they were capable of producing undue compressive force. In a somewhat arrogant and nationalistic style he declared, "The instrument and the operation have reached their highest development in Germany... The German forceps combine the best points in the French and English, and have now been brought to a degree of perfection that leaves nothing to be desired."

In relation to the forceps bearing his name, Spiegelberg claimed no originality. He said that he used the modification made by Trefurt (1844), which was in principle a combination of the instruments of Busch, F. C. Naegele, and Joseph Servazius d'Outrepent (1775–1845) of Würzburg. But because Spiegelberg set out in such detail how forceps should be made it seems that the Trefurt pattern subsequently came to bear Spiegelberg's name. The forceps illustrated (Figure 5.25), from the collection of the Royal College of Obstetricians and Gynaecologists, were made in Dublin in 1860 following a visit Spiegelberg had made there.

Based on his extensive travel on the Continent and in London, Edinburgh, and Dublin, Lucas Johann Boër (1751–1835), Professor and Director of Midwifery at the Vienna Lying-In Hospital, devised his own forceps (described by C. G. Carus [1828]), which differed from contemporary German instruments in being in the style of Smellie and relatively short (305 millimeters/12 inches). The blades had a slight pelvic curve and the joint was a modification of Smellie's in that only one blade had a mortise that received the shank of the other blade, rather than mirror-image interlocking mortises on the two blades.

It is evident that in Europe during this period instruments were being designed with compression force in mind and these designs often differed only in detail. At the same time the recognition of the potentially harmful effects of compressing the baby's skull led to consideration of how to regulate the compression force.

Pressure-regulating Devices and Labimeters

The considerable potential compressive force inherent in the design of most Continental forceps was further compounded by the lack of flexibility in the steel from which they were made. Although the forceps were regarded mainly as a compressive instrument, some practitioners recognized that there was a limit to the degree to which the head could be compressed without killing the baby, as was evidenced by the aforementioned experiments by J. L. Baudelocque on the skulls of dead babies. From these observations arose a desire to control or limit the amount of compression; this was achieved in various ways. One was the widening of the distance between the blades. However, the most common method was to limit the closure of the handles, either by merely inserting a cloth or wooden wedge between them or

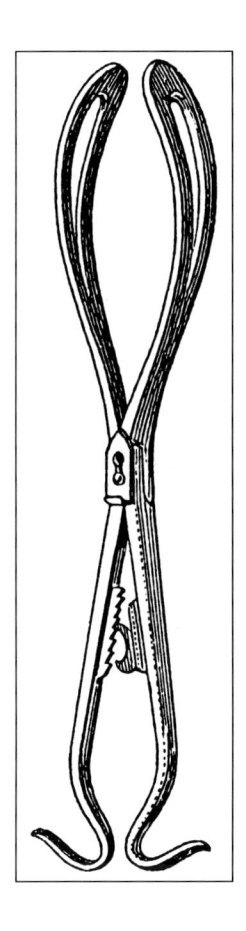

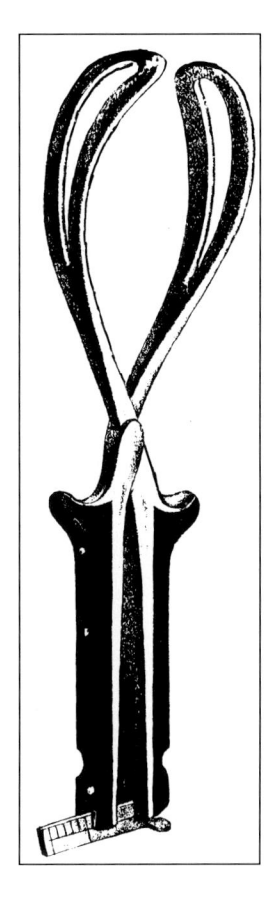

FIGURE 5.26.
Petit's forceps. This was probably the first design to incorporate a pressure-regulating device in the form of a ratchet-and-tooth mechanism. (Tarnier and Budin, 1901)

FIGURE 5.27.
J. D. Busch's labimeter. This was an addition to his earlier forceps. (D. W. H. Busch, 1841)

by more sophisticated devices incorporated in the design. Many of the attachments had a measuring scale so that the bitemporal diameter (assuming correct cephalic application of the forceps) and the degree of compression achieved could be measured. The earlier devices appeared in the 1770s but by the early nineteenth century interest waned as the philosophy of the forceps being primarily a traction rather than a compression instrument took hold. In the early nineteenth century there was renewed interest in and further development of parallel forceps (that is, forceps without crossover articulations), particularly those that had a terminal articulation (Assalini) that also limited compression force, and these are discussed in Chapter 10. Labimeters were rarely described after about 1820, although they continued to be illustrated in textbooks until the middle of the century.

In Britain, J. Aitken (1784) and Evans (1784) both incorporated pressure-regulating devices in the handles of their forceps (Chapter 4) but the concept never found wide favor in the British Isles, probably because the lighter British forceps with shorter handles permitted less compression force than Continental instruments.

Jean Louis Petit (1774) was probably the first to incorporate a regulator in the forceps. The instrument that he described was essentially the same as one of the many versions of Grégoire's forceps with the addition of a ratchet-and-tooth mechanism inside the handles. This mechanism prevented the approximation of the handles and hence the blades (Figure 5.26), thus limiting the compression of the head.

J. D. Busch (1801–1802) added a labimeter to his earlier forceps, described previously (page 72) and this pair was illustrated, together with nine other forceps (by other inventors) incorporating labimeters, in his son's *Atlas* (D. W. H. Busch, 1841) (Figure 5.27).

G. W. Stein (d. 1803) at the University of Marburg was, according to Doran (1913c), a staunch supporter of Levret's forceps, rejecting all modifications as *missgestaltete Bastarde*—"deformed bastards"—referring to many variations conceived during his lifetime, a notable one being the forceps of his pupil Osiander. His belief, as stated in his *Practische Anleitung zur Geburtshülfe* (1793), was that compression should be the chief action of the forceps. He invented a simple labimeter device that was placed between the forceps handles and could be used with any forceps without any modification to the instrument (Figure 5.28) (1728). His son and successor in the chair, G. G. Stein, also gave a description of his father's labimeter (1804).

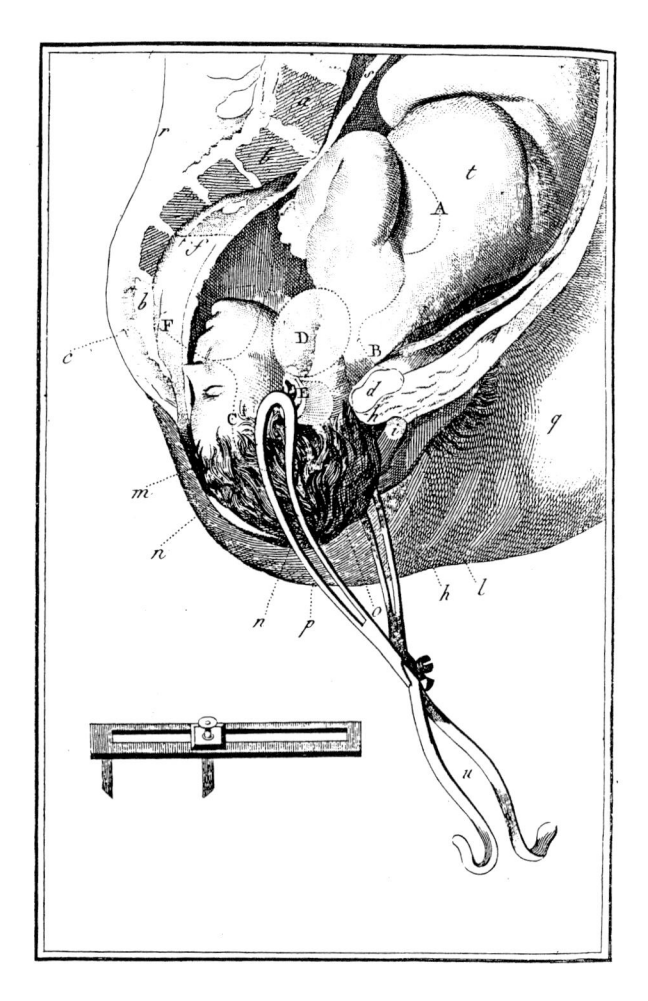

FIGURE 5.28.
G. W. Stein's labimeter. A simple device that could be used with any forceps. (G. G. Stein, 1804)

FIGURE 5.29 (BELOW).
Mende's forceps. The wedge slides in a groove in one handle. The inner surface of the other handle has a graduated scale from which the cephalic diameter can be read. (Kuhn and Tröhler, 1987)

FIGURE 5.30 (OPPOSITE TOP).
Von Froriep's forceps. The sliding metal bar in the handle prevents approximation of the handles. (Von Froriep, 1804)

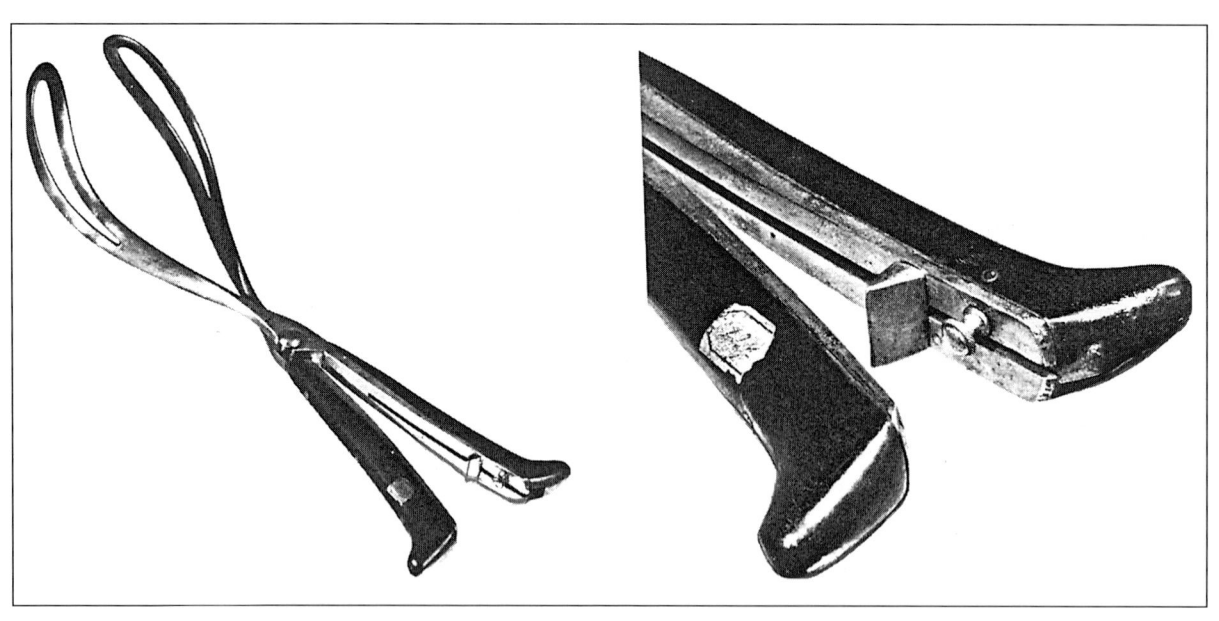

76 CHAPTER 5

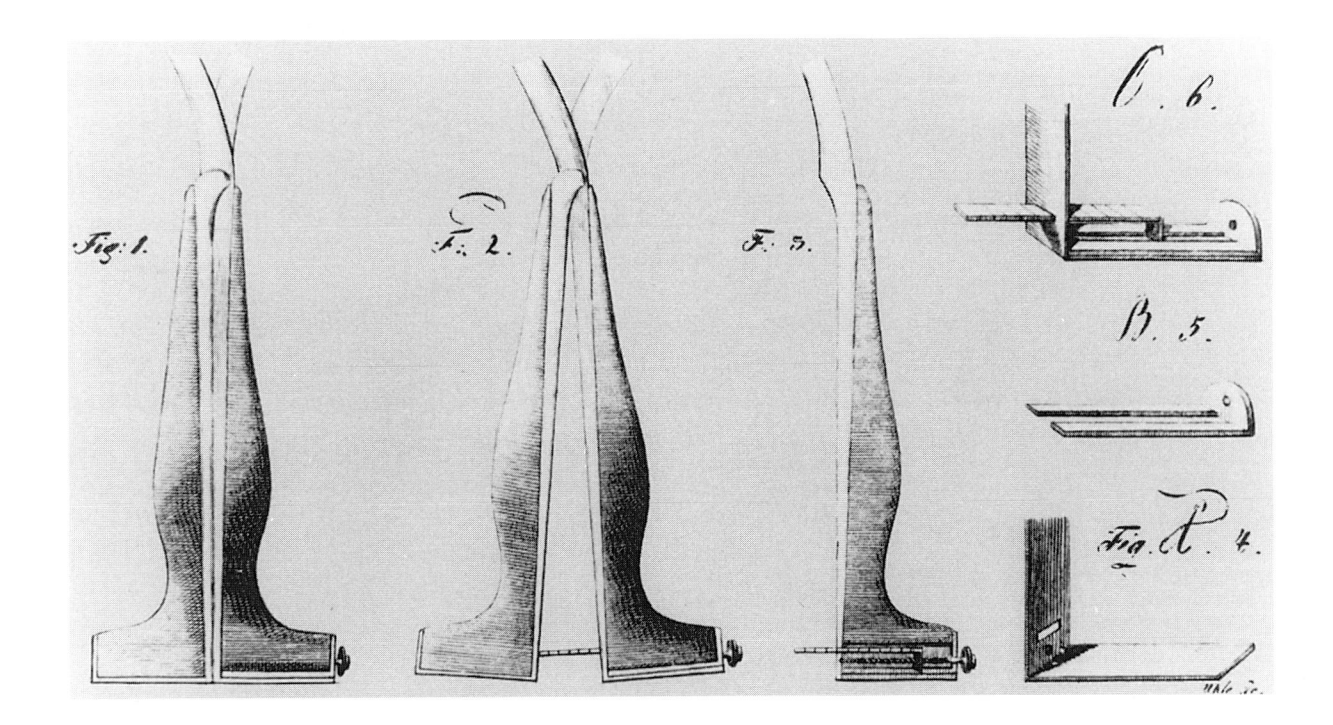

L. J. K. Mende (b. 1779) a professor at the University of Göttingen, invented separate forceps for high and low operations. Both had Siebold-type handles with finger rests and the Brunninghausen lock, but those used for high operations were longer and had a more marked pelvic curve. However, his more notable contribution (circa 1828) was the addition of a labimeter, which comprised a movable wedge on the inner surface of one handle that controlled the space between the blades (Figure 5.29). On the inner surface of the other handle was a groove with a graduated scale for measuring the head.

Ludwig Friedrich von Froriep (1779–1847), who was a professor of obstetrics in Jena, Halle, Tübingen, and Weimar, invented forceps in 1804 that incorporated a screw in the distal end of the handle (1804, 1832). This screw controlled the projection of a metal bar from the inner surface, limiting the approximation of the other handle (Figure 5.30). This was a simple and effective mechanical design that deserved attention and was illustrated in many of the texts of the time.

A more sophisticated design was that of Fries, a professor in Münster, which incorporated a screw mechanism in one handle from which projected a peg (Figure 5.31), the degree of closure being adjusted by screwing the peg up or down (1806).

FIGURE 5.31.
Fries's forceps. The peg projecting from the inner surface of one handle is moved up or down by a screw mechanism. (D. W. H. Busch, 1841)

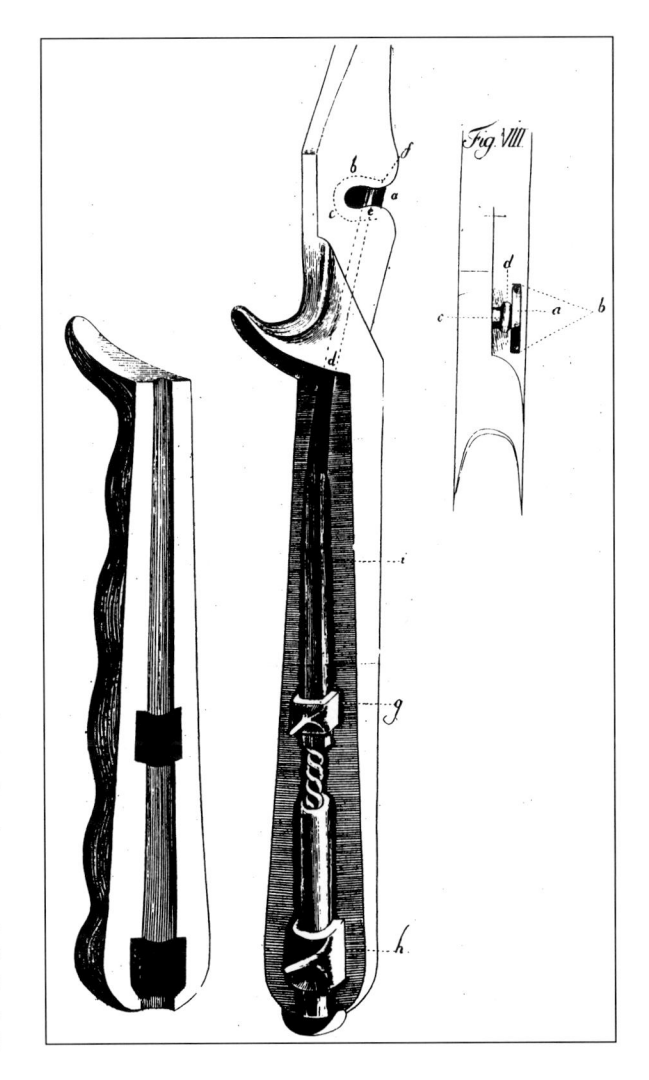

EVOLUTION OF EUROPEAN FORCEPS 77

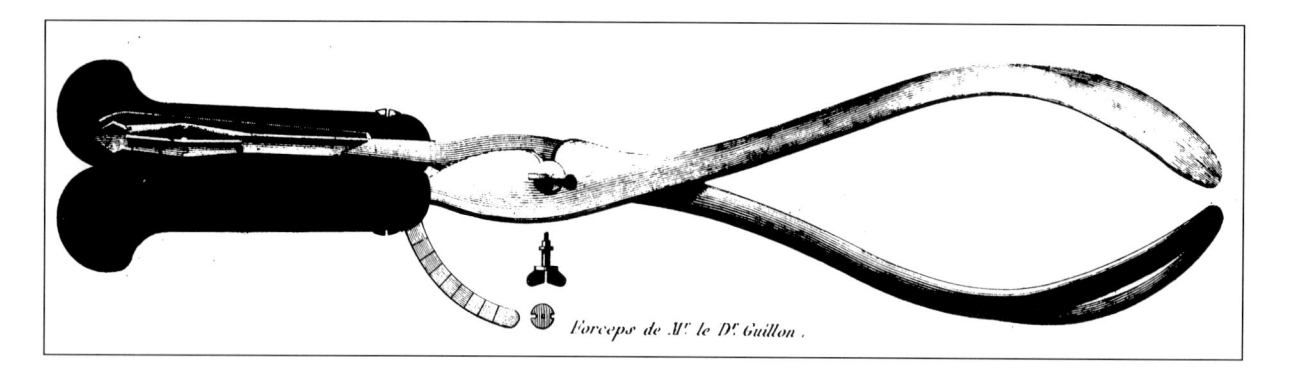

FIGURE 5.32.
Guillon's forceps. A graduated quadrant on one handle slides through a slot in the other handle. (Maygrier, 1822)

Two very similar simple devices originated in Paris. J. B. Guillon of the Hôtel Dieu in Paris invented forceps (circa 1820) that were long and heavy with a slot and screw lock and wooden handles. The labimeter was a graduated quadrant that hinged on the proximal end of one handle and slid through a slot in the other handle (Figure 5.32). Soon after this, in 1822, Jacques Pierre Maygrier of Paris (1771–1834) used the same principle for the labimeter but added it to forceps with hooked metal handles (1822, 1833). These designs had no particular merit other than simplicity but seemed to meet the personal preferences of their originators. Although they gave a certain scientific gloss to the art of operative delivery they probably had little practical value and interest in them waned by the second quarter of the nineteenth century.

. . .

Although effective compression had been a dominant factor in European forceps design, increasing thought was being given to forceps as traction instruments, hence changes in the design of handles and the introduction of finger grips or lugs. Other aids to traction are discussed in Chapter 11.

There was throughout this period a preoccupation with finding an ideal articulation, with varying degrees of success, while meanwhile the British had generally settled for the simple and effective lock based on the Smellie design. The Continental difficulties arose mainly because of unnecessary complexity of design, until the turning point was reached with the introduction of the Brunninghausen lock.

THE BRITISH RENAISSANCE OF THE NINETEENTH CENTURY

The Princess Charlotte Tragedy

The culmination of British conservatism was epitomized in the obstetric management of Charlotte Augusta, daughter of George, Prince of Wales (later George IV) and Princess Caroline, during her pregnancy in 1817, which was expected to produce an heir to the throne. The events have been well described by J. Dewhurst (1980) and detailed and scholarly analyses of the relevant papers and letters have been made by Eardley Holland (1951) and F. Crainz (1977).

The backgrounds of Charlotte's three medical attendants, Sir Richard Croft, Mathew Baillie, and John Sims are both interesting and relevant. The first two were married to the twin daughters of Thomas Denman. Croft, whom Holland described as diffident and lacking in self-confidence, by all accounts adhered slavishly to his father-in-law's conservative teaching. He had a large and fashionable practice that he had inherited from his father-in-law. Baillie was also from Lanarkshire and a son of the manse and was initially a morbid anatomist. He was a nephew of William and John Hunter and thus had an entrée into Court circles. Sims's involvement was minimal, but none the less relevant, since his advanced age and lack of expertise enhanced the influence of Croft and Baillie. Although he was a Court physician he was sixty-eight at the time in question and his expertise was in botany.

Charlotte's antenatal course was relatively uneventful but Dewhurst suggests that she was probably anemic, evidenced by repeated bloodlettings for headaches and a diet poor in iron content. Labor commenced at 7:00 P.M. on Monday, November 3, 1817. Progress in the first stage was slow, lasting twenty-six hours, but she reached the second stage at 9:00 P.M. on Tuesday, November 4. After twenty-four hours in the second stage of labor, she delivered a large stillborn boy at 9:00 P.M. on Wednesday, November 5. There was difficulty with the placenta, which had to be removed by exploring the uterus. Binders, probably made of linen, were applied, as was the custom of the day. At 11:45 P.M. she became unwell, deteriorated steadily, and died at 2:30 A.M. Death was apparently due to concealed hemorrhage, probably aggravated by preexisting anemia, prolonged labor, and exhaustion. Earlier intervention and forceps delivery would have reduced the risks of the complications that followed and more detailed observation after the delivery, including expressing the blood clots from the uterus, might have saved her life. The whole episode proved too much of a strain for Sir Richard Croft and three months later he shot himself with pistols to each temple while in attendance at another confinement.

Thus, at the end of the second decade of the nineteenth century the shadow of the Princess Charlotte tragedy persisted, and was likely to do so until the royal succession was safe, for George IV's twelve living children had shown themselves to be particularly incompetent at producing legitimate offspring.

At last in 1819 the Duchess of Kent became pregnant and David Davis (see below) was appointed by the Duke of Kent as royal accoucheur. In the event his intervention was not required, and the normal delivery was conducted by Madame Siebold (no relation to the Von Siebold discussed in Chapter 5), the doctor-midwife whom the Duchess had brought to England with her. Davis's appointment helped to enhance his career and he brought a fresh approach to obstetric problems. Had he been royal accoucheur two years earlier the British royal succession might have been very different.

So it was that, following the Charlotte tragedy, the Hunterian legacy of conservatism was about to be challenged. In Britain, the desire to improve the prospects of live birth, particularly when the head was arrested at the pelvic brim, led to more radical rethinking of standard practice and instrument construction in the first half of the nineteenth century, including forceps design. Thus long forceps gained increasing popularity in the British Isles by the mid-nineteenth century as an alternative to craniotomy or version when the head was arrested at the pelvic brim, although the use of the long forceps was largely confined to cases where the baby was still believed to be alive. Their adoption was facilitated by the advent of anesthesia and they were frequently employed before full dilatation of the cervix if the membranes had ruptured.

David Davis and His Influence

David Daniel Davis (1777–1841), a largely unsung hero of British obstetrics, was born in West Wales, the son of a farmer. He started to train for the nonconformist ministry but turned to medicine because of his deep concern for the social problems of the day. He graduated from the University of Glasgow in 1801 and practiced as a physician in Sheffield for ten years. Why he turned to midwifery is not certain but he was probably influenced by the brain damage that his first son suffered as the result of a traumatic instrumental delivery. With the help of Thomas Denman, he settled in London in 1813, where he was appointed to Queen Charlotte's Hospital as physician accoucheur and to the Royal Maternity Charity in 1816 on the testimony, *inter alia*, of Croft and Sims. In 1827 he became the first Professor in Midwifery at the University of London at University College. However, fortune was not on his side. From 1831 he suffered recurrent ill health and eventually this forced his retirement from the chair in 1841. He died just four weeks later. As an epitaph it would be difficult to better the words of Glynne Jones: "A man of sound judgment and wide clinical experience, he combined clarity and precision as a teacher with dexterity and caution as an operator. Although he lived before the advent of anaesthesia, asepsis and modern surgery, nevertheless he was able by his teaching and example to revolutionise the practice of midwifery in this country" (1972).

Davis's magnum opus was *Elements of Operative Midwifery*, first published in 1825. His writings show clearly how different he was from those who had started him on his career. He pleaded for better training, better design of instruments, and more ready recourse to intervention in the interests of both mother and baby, claiming that "the entire subject of Operative Midwifery has been in a state of the most abject neglect for the last fifty years."

Davis designed numerous pairs of forceps for use in various circumstances and was particularly concerned with minimizing injury to the baby. His forceps were destined to be used throughout Britain and in America, as well as in several European centers. His destructive instruments were constructed to reduce the risk of maternal trauma. "The changes of forms, or additional parts are . . . intended to add to the security and facility of the operations to be performed with them. . . .   . . .it is of great importance to act rather in aid of nature than in opposition to her efforts. . . ."

With the publication of *Elements of Operative Midwifery*, a new era had begun, one with a return to balanced management and selective instrumental delivery, which would have gladdened the heart of William Smellie and would at least have been acceptable to William Hunter.

The collection of the Royal College of Obstetricians and Gynaecologists includes all the obstetric forceps and destructive instruments illustrated in Davis's *Elements of Operative Midwifery*. They were all made by Joseph Botschan of Finsbury and the forceps (Figure 6.1) are stamped DR. DAVIS'S FORCEPS. In addition a number of previously undescribed instruments, including two pairs of forceps, have recently come to light at University College Hospital and appear to be experimental designs.

The Common Forceps (Davis I)

Davis's "Common Forceps," as he called them (Figures 6.1 ["common"]–6.3), were designed to occupy the least possible space in the pelvis and to "compress the head more equably, and therefore in a manner less calculated to do it injury." Davis's common forceps had broad blades that were lightly constructed of steel with large fenestra and hollowed interiorly in order "to lie in close contact to every part of the child's head to which they are applied, and to admit of the reception, and firm purchase, of extensive portions of its lateral parietes." The cephalic curve was reduced, because the wide fenestra facilitated contact with all parts of the head. The shanks were parallel and longer than most contemporary forceps. The right blade was hinged to facilitate introduction with the patient lying on her left side (*pruderie britannique*).

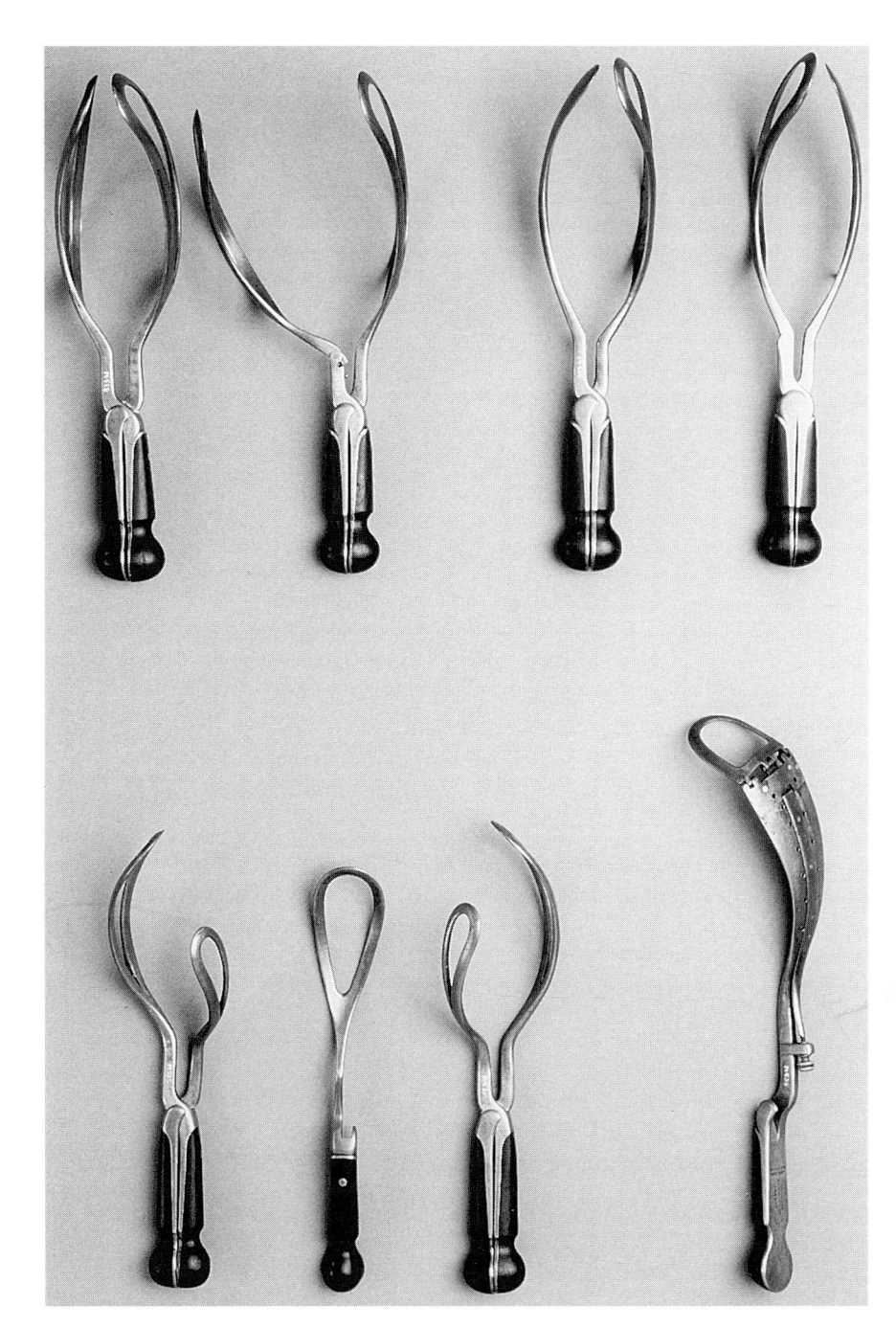

FIGURE 6.1.
David Davis's forceps set. A complete set of the forceps illustrated by Davis. Top row, left to right: The first two are examples of "common" forceps, with unhinged and hinged handles, respectively. The last two are Davis II, unequal breadth, two versions. Bottom row, left to right: The first three are examples of Davis III and IV, unequal length; the last is Davis V, jointed blade. All of the blades were made to be interchangeable so that different combinations could be used. (RCOG)

FIGURES 6.2, 6.3.
Davis's "common" hinged forceps. 6.2: The main features are the broad, light blades with large fenestra hollowed interiorly to fit the contour of the head. 6.3: The hinged right blade is to facilitate application with the patient in the left lateral position. (Plates II and III, Davis, 1825)

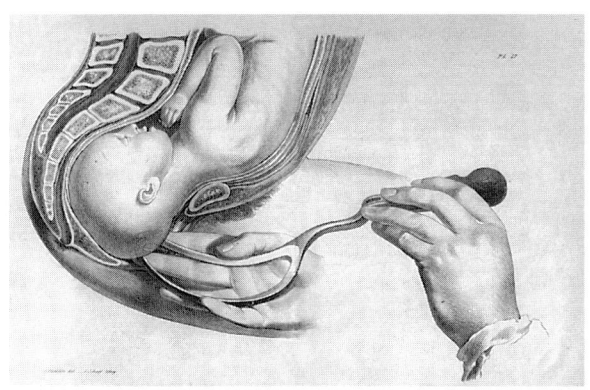

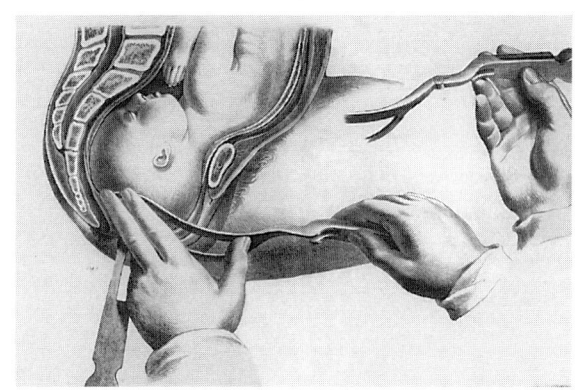

BRITISH RENAISSANCE: 19TH CENTURY

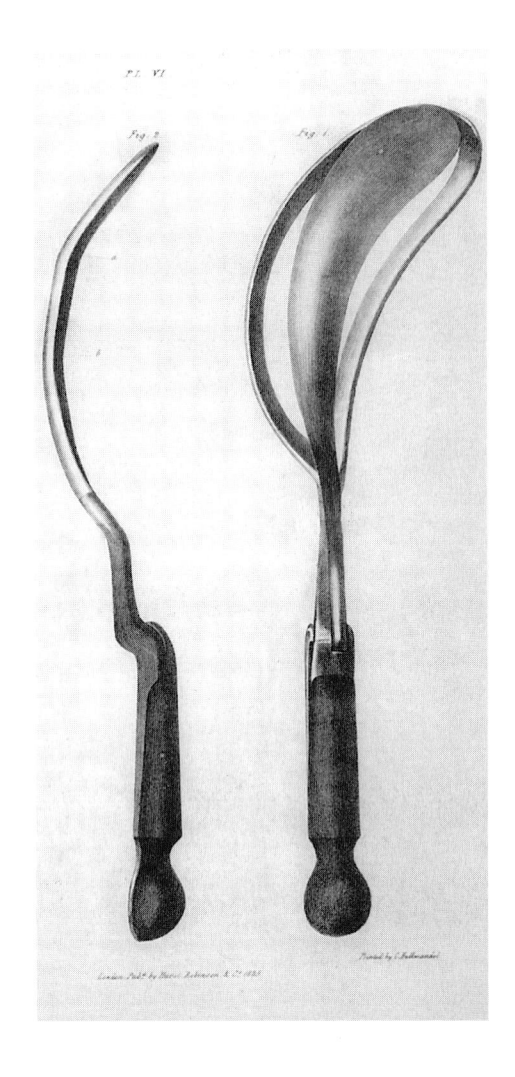

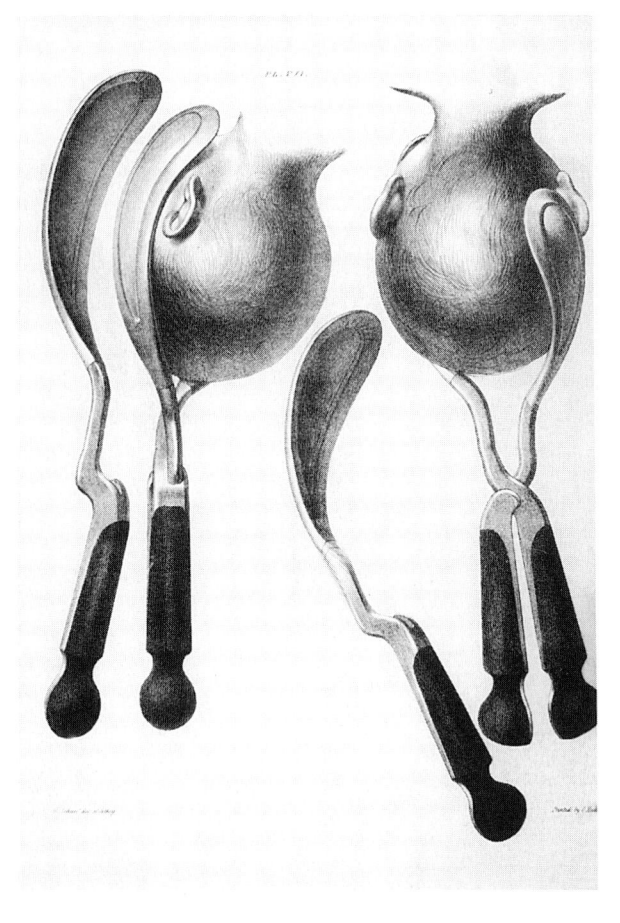

FIGURE 6.4 (LEFT).
Davis's unequal breadth forceps (Davis II) and jointed blade (Davis V). The right forceps shows the narrow blade for use when space was too limited to allow introduction of the normal blade. The left forceps shows a blade with two hinges that allowed limited flexibility when introduction of the blade was difficult (See also Figure 6.9). (Plate VI, Davis, 1825)

FIGURES 6.5, 6.6 (RIGHT).
Davis's unequal length forceps (Davis III and IV). 6.5: These forceps have a pelvic curve and were intended to be applied obliquely to the head. They could be used for rotation. 6.6: The straight blade was intended for use when the head was low in the birth canal and could be applied conventionally or antero-posteriorly. (Plates VII and IX, Davis, 1825)

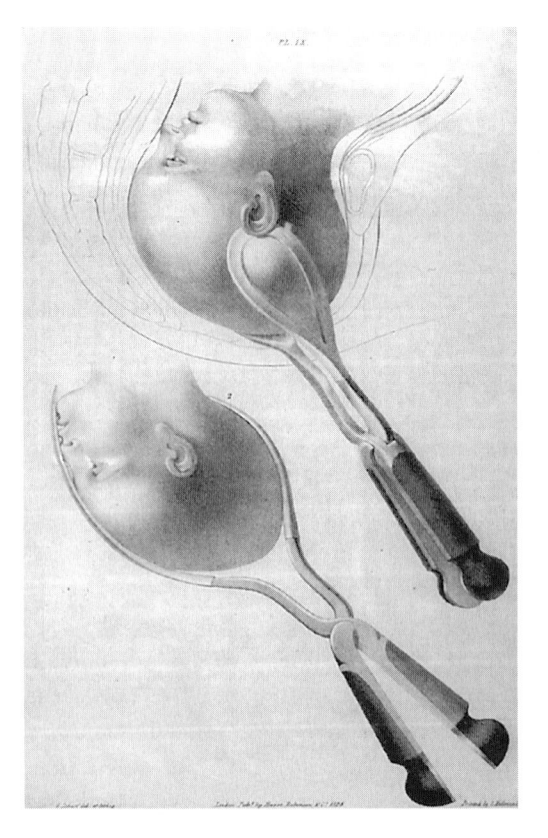

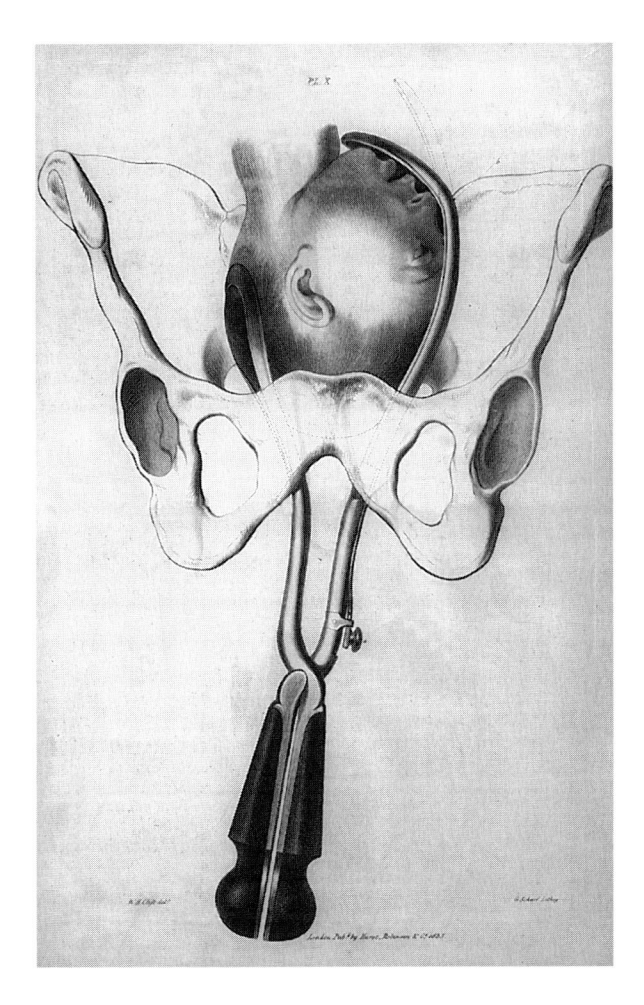

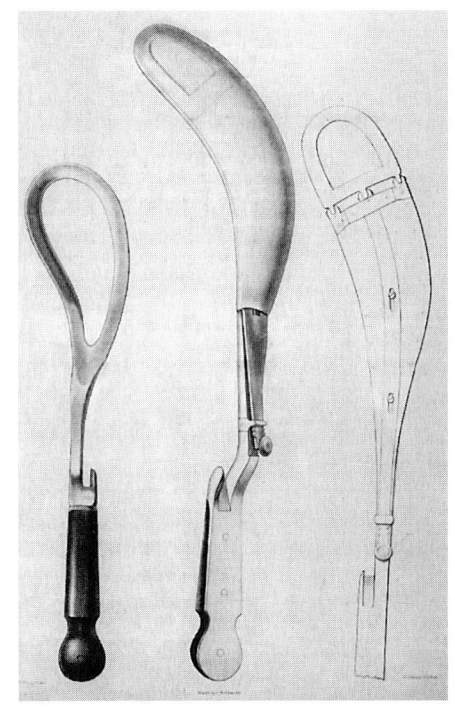

FIGURES 6.7, 6.8.
Davis's flexible jointed blade (Davis V). 6.7: The jointed blade was intended as a substitute for long forceps when delivering a high head. The angle can be adjusted by either a screw mechanism or, as in this illustration, a ratchet. 6.8: This illustration shows the construction of the blade and the leather covering, together with the short blade with which it would be used. (Plates X and XI, Davis, 1825)

Blades of Unequal Breadth (Davis II)

These narrower blades (Figures 6.1 "Davis II," 6.4) were designed for "certain inconvenient positions," that is, when the head was lying abnormally in the pelvis. Each of the blades (right and left) was also intended to be used with the opposite blade of the common forceps. Indeed Davis emphasized that all forceps should be made to match so that blades could be interchangeable: "In giving an order for the construction of a set of forceps, it should always form part of the instructions that all the several counterparts should be made to act together in pairs."

Blades of Unequal Length (Davis III and IV)

These forceps were intended for use in the third and fourth positions (left occipito-lateral and right occipito-lateral). The longer blade was applied to the latero-frontal parts of the head and face, in the anterior oblique pelvic diameter (Figures 6.1 "Davis III and IV," 6.5, 6.6). The shorter blade was applied occipito-laterally (behind the ear) in the posterior oblique pelvic diameter. The short blade could be straight or have a pelvic curve. The latter is believed to be the first forceps specifically designed for instrumental rotation of the fetal head: "[A] gentle rotary movement of the head is then to be effected from left to right, i.e. in the same direction with the sun's course . . . so as to bring the occipito vertical part of the head into the arch of the pubes. . ." (1825).

The straight blade (Davis IV) was intended for use with the Davis III set.

The Jointed Blade (Davis V)

Davis was not an enthusiastic supporter of the British long forceps for arrest at the pelvic brim, especially when the head was in the transverse position. His jointed blade was intended to replace the conventional British long forceps in such cases (Figures 6.1 "Davis V," 6.7, 6.8). The blade, covered with soft

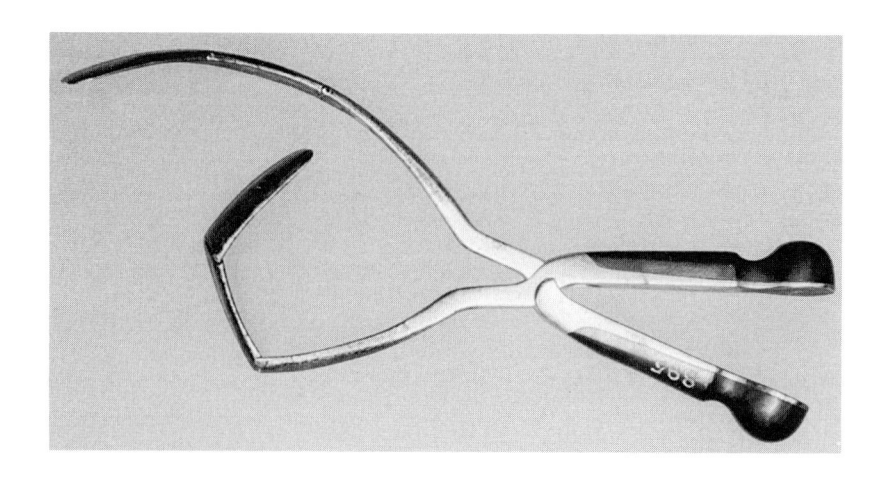

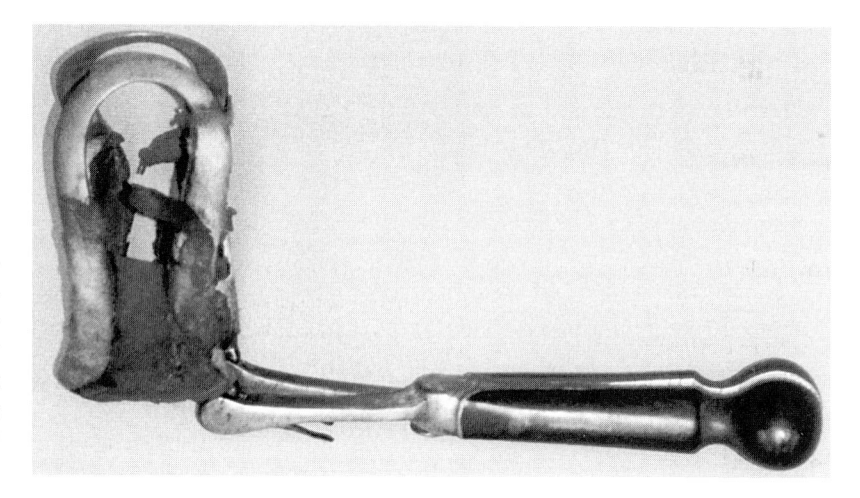

FIGURES 6.9, 6.10. Undescribed forceps found at University College Hospital, London. 6.9: This pair of forceps has one hinged blade similar to that shown in Figure 6.4 (left) but the degree of flexibility is greater than that suggested by the text. 6.10: Short vertically hinged blades with a ratchet mechanism. Their use is unclear. (University College Hospital, London)

flannel and leather to minimize trauma, was applied over the face. By use of a ratchet or a screw, the distal part of the blade was flexed to give better purchase. It was normally paired with a short blade and was intended for occipito-facial application. The jointed blade was applied over the face and, when in correct position, the terminal part was flexed to give a firm application over the face and chin. When combined with the small blade over the occiput there was only partial counter-pressure so that it worked partly as a forceps and partly as a lever.

An interesting further development was the recent discovery in the University College Hospital obstetric department of two pairs of forceps (Figures 6.9, 6.10) clearly made for Davis and stamped but not previously identified in his publications. They are both unusual and were probably experimental. The pair illustrated in Figure 6.9, labeled "Cat No. 895," had narrow blades without fenestra, each of which had two transverse hinges enabling the blades to fold inward. This is probably a prototype for the flexible blade illustrated in Davis's book. "Cat No. 879," (Figure 6.10), had short hinged blades with a ratchet mechanism that allowed the blades to rotate vertically through a right angle. The blades were fenestrated and covered with flannelette and leather. Davis was one of the last obstetricians to use coverings, a practice that he subsequently abandoned. It is likely that this was a pair of forceps he referred to in his book that were specifically intended for delivery of face presentation but never used: "[A] peculiar modification of a pair of forceps. But not having had the opportunity of trying it on a living subject. . . . I do not feel myself at liberty, at present, to give any account of its mechanism."

David Davis was thus in the vanguard of a new era of obstetric practice with his thoughtful and careful construction of instruments, which facilitated their use and helped to minimize trauma to both mother and baby. The simplicity and functional efficiency of his "Common Forceps" ensured that they achieved world-wide acclaim and, in particular, the blade design was incorporated in many other forceps,

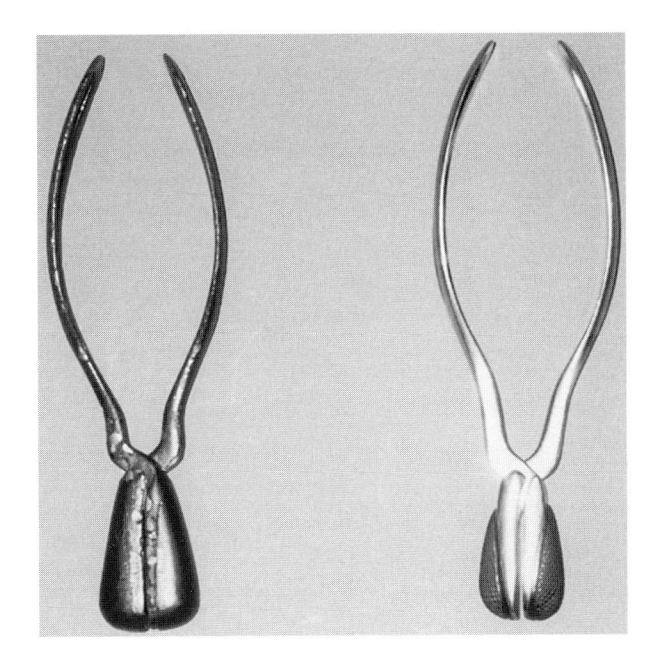

FIGURE 6.11.
J. Y. Simpson's short forceps. Note the short handle and separated short parallel shank. One pair has a protective covering of gutta percha. (RCOG)

especially in America (Chapter 7). However, his other designs, innovative as they were, did not achieve the same degree of popularity.

Short and Intermediate Forceps in the Mid-Nineteenth Century

Although longer forceps were becoming more popular in Britain by the mid-nineteenth century, thought was also being given to improving the design of short forceps. Most practitioners had at least one short and one long pair. However, elongated short forceps, intended to be multipurpose, also became common and other refinements appeared. Many of these, which were shown at the *Conversazione* of the Obstetrical Society of London in 1866 and were detailed in their *Catalogue and Report* (Meadows, 1867), were sufficiently popular to be made by a number of instrument makers and therefore many minor variations in design were encountered. Some of the more important examples are discussed here but an almost infinite number of variations are to be seen in the instrument catalogues of the latter part of the century, for example, in London: John Weiss and Son London (1863), S. Maw and Son (1866), Arnold and Sons (1873), and Down Brothers (1889); and in America, George Tiemann of New York (1889). Forceps with special features (such as hinged and detachable handles and blades and asymmetric forceps) are described in other chapters.

The epitome of small, light forceps for outlet deliveries was the design of James Young Simpson (1811–1870), a man of great ability with a dominant personality whose many achievements have been documented in his *Collected Works* (1871). Simpson was the youngest of seven sons of a Bathgate baker. Having completed his medical courses in Edinburgh in 1829 at the age of eighteen he had to wait two years before he could obtain his license to practice. He spent much of the intervening time studying obstetrics and visiting clinics in England and France. By the age of twenty-eight he had become a professor at the University of Edinburgh. Although he is best known for his long forceps (see below), he also designed a short straight forceps and the first functional vacuum extractor (Chapter 15).

The outstanding feature of his short forceps (Figure 6.11) was the very short handle, as in the modern Wrigley's forceps, and some versions had a protective coat of gutta percha (Figure 6.11, left). They were only 241 millimeters (9.5 inches) long and the handles were only 63.5 millimeters (2.5 inches) long. Although there was no finger ring as seen in several other forceps, such as those of Greenhalgh and Hopkins (below), with short handles, the short shanks were separated to allow placement of a finger between them for traction. The greatest distance between the blades was 60 millimeters (2.375 inches) and the tips almost touched when the blades were closed.

John Clark (1761–1815), who was a lecturer with Denman and Osborn, used a short, curved forceps, typical of the early nineteenth-century British instruments, the distinguishing feature being a stout blunt pin in one palm rest that fit into a socket in the opposite handle (Figure 6.12).

J. Hopkins, Surgeon to the Duke of Kent, invented forceps that were 362 millimeters (14.25 inches) long and incorpo-

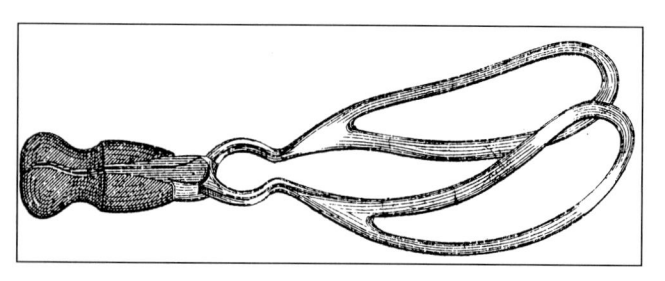

FIGURE 6.12 (LEFT).
Clark's forceps. There is a pin-and-socket arrangement in the palm rests. (Science Museum, London)

FIGURE 6.13 (RIGHT).
Hopkins's forceps. These are the earliest forceps to have a finger ring in the shank, later popularized by Barnes. (Weiss, 1889)

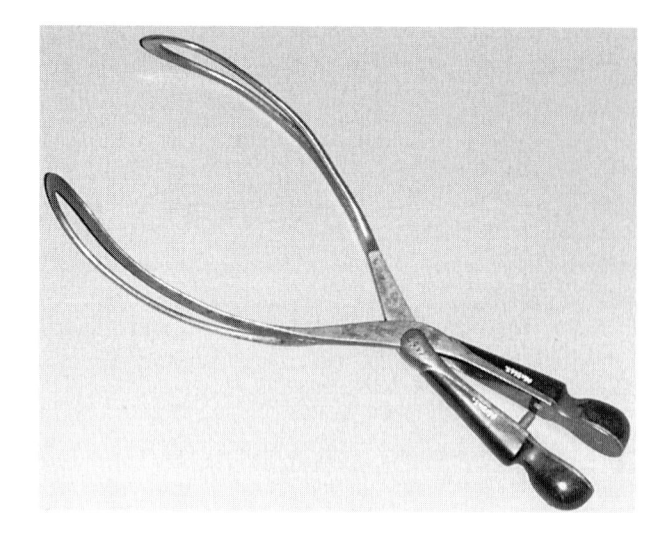

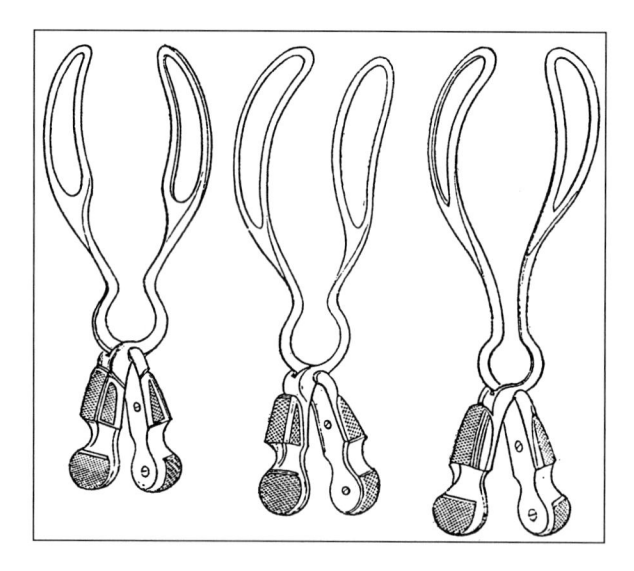

FIGURE 6.14.
Greenhalgh's forceps. The three pairs, short straight, short curved, and long curved, were shown at the 1866 *Conversazione*. They all incorporated a finger ring. (Meadows, 1867)

rated a finger ring in a rudimentary shank, effectively lengthening the handle (1826) (Figure 6.13), a feature novel at the time but later popularized by Robert Barnes (page 94) in his long forceps. The blades were better designed to fit the head, with an elongated oval, wide fenestra and a slight pelvic curve. The forceps were exhibited at the 1866 *Conversazione*.

Robert Greenhalgh (d. 1887), Lecturer and Physician Accoucheur at St. Bartholomew's Hospital, also favored the finger ring, which he incorporated into three designs that were all shown at the *Conversazione* (Figures 6.14, 6.15) The first two pairs (Figure 6.14), created in 1839, were short forceps, one with straight blades (280 millimeters/11 inches) and the other with a pelvic curve (292 millimeters/11.5 inches). In 1852 he introduced a shank, increasing the overall length to 330 millimeters (13 inches). He described the forceps as "strong, light and wieldly and suited to any and all cases requiring the use of the forceps" (Meadows, 1867). The blades were similar to those of Davis but those in the short forceps were narrower at their extremities and were rounded out internally. The short handles limited the grip and traction force but this was compensated for by the finger ring, through which, if desired, a traction tape could be passed.

The usual practice of the time was to hold the blades together by a ligature or tape that bound the handles and thus caused sustained pressure to the head. William Gayton of the North Western Hospital in London believed this to be undesirable and his forceps (Figure 6.16) incorporated a spring rack and lock so that the pressure could quickly be released between contractions (1863). He later (1866) added

86 CHAPTER 6

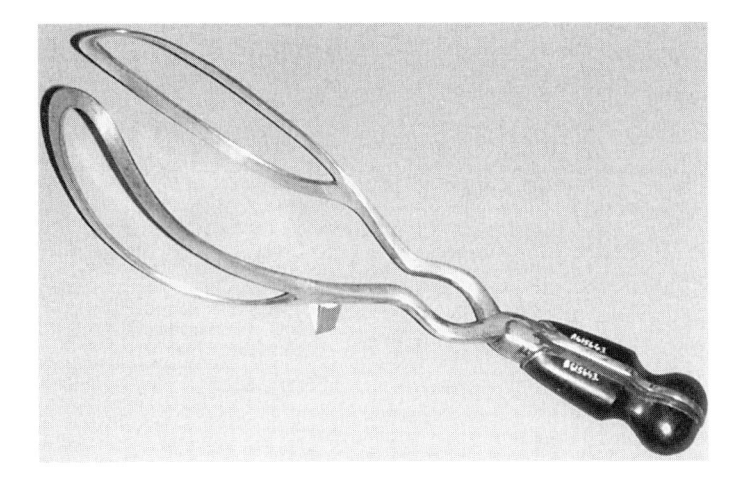

FIGURE 6.15.
Greenhalgh's short curved forceps. The forceps are light but strong. The blades are similar to Davis's, with a convex inner contour. (Science Museum, London)

finger rests to the handles. Later designers took this lead and added various securing devices, usually hinged screws and wing nuts, either to the tip of the handle or close to the articulation. These are seen particularly in association with axis-traction forceps (Chapter 14).

Diverging Shanks

Although by the middle of the eighteenth century the generally favored method of elongation was the parallel shank, before this lengthened divergent shanks were often used, as originally seen in Smellie's long forceps. Tapered blades with a long, thin section between the lock and the fenestra was characteristic of Dublin instruments in the early part of the nineteenth century. However, the elongation was modest compared with European instruments and later British forceps with parallel shanks. The overall lengths of the Irish instruments in the Royal College of Obstetricians and Gynaecologists' collection range from 305 millimeters (12 inches) (T. E. Beatty) to 348 millimeters (13.75 inches) (Churchill).

Fleetwood Churchill (1808–1878) was described by Dr. Charles West, President of the Obstetrical Society of London, in his Annual Address to the Society in 1879 as "an Englishman by birth, an Irishman by adoption, cosmopolite by his erudition"(West, 1880). His forceps, first described in 1840, underwent minor modifications over the next twenty years. They were about 305 millimeters (12 inches) long, without a pelvic curve (Figure 6.17, left). The blades were long (203 millimeters/8 inches) and slender, parting at the lock

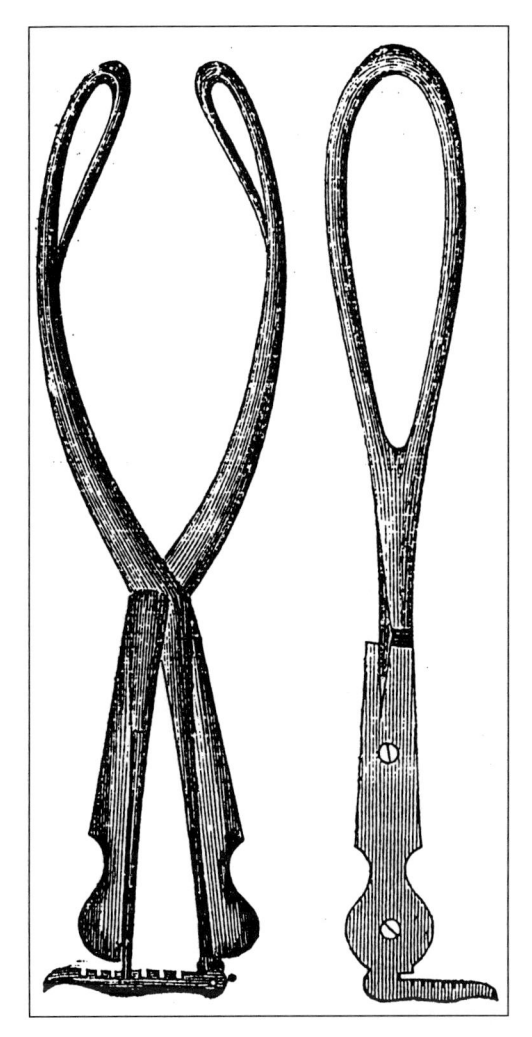

FIGURE 6.16.
Gayton's forceps. Gayton was the first to incorporate a spring rack and lock in his design to hold the blades in apposition. (Gayton, 1863)

BRITISH RENAISSANCE: 19TH CENTURY   87

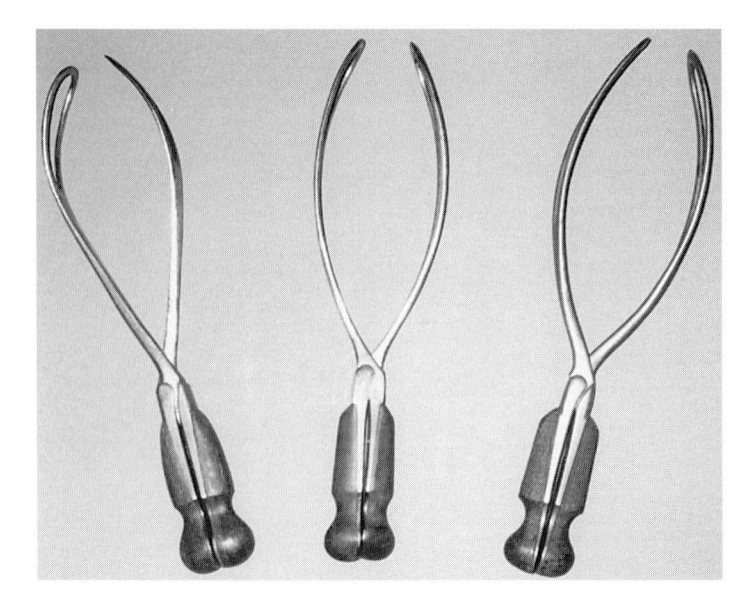

FIGURE 6.17.
Forceps with diverging shanks. Left: Churchill. Center: T. E. Beatty. Right: Hewitt. The Churchill/Beatty type of forceps was popular in Ireland but Hewitt introduced his version to the London scene. (RCOG)

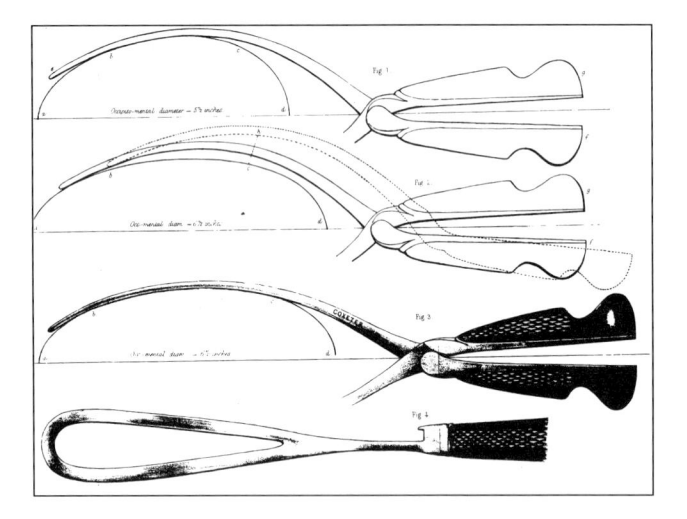

FIGURE 6.18.
Hewitt's forceps. Details of the design. These forceps were longer and narrow, specifically for application to elongated, molded heads. (Hewitt, 1861)

without any definite shank and with the cephalic curve increasing toward the point. The fenestra were small and the blades strong to prevent springing. The cephalic curve was increased toward the tip and did not start until about 90 millimeters (3.5 inches) from the joint.

Thomas E. Beatty (1800–1872), a close friend of Oscar Wilde and Professor of Obstetrics and President of the Royal College of Surgeons of Ireland, produced his forceps in about 1842, with the typical elongated blade of the Dublin school. (Figure 6.17, center); these came into widespread use. Doran (1921) referred to them as "medium forceps" and described them as being like Denman's forceps with long, slender blades and no pelvic curve. They were regarded as remarkable for their lightness (weight 313 grams [11 ounces]), slenderness, and strength (Meadows, 1867).

Graily Hewitt (1828–1893) was Physician to the Samaritan and British Lying-In Hospitals and was a lecturer and an assistant physician at St. Mary's Hospital, London. His forceps (1861) (Figures 6.17, right; 6.18) were specifically designed for cases in which the head was unduly elongated and conventional blades did not easily fit. The overall length was 313 millimeters (12.25 inches) and the blades were long (203 millimeters/8 inches) and narrow, with no true shank but an unusually wide cephalic curve (diameter 366 millimeters/14 inches).

Thomas More Madden (1838–1902), who held appointments at the Rotunda, the National Lying-In, and the Misericordae Hospitals in Dublin, went to extremes in his forceps designs and described a very light, short pair in the Simpson style, 254 millimeters (10 inches) in length and with short handles (1874a). In a later description (1875) he mentioned the addition of a finger ring. The greatest distance

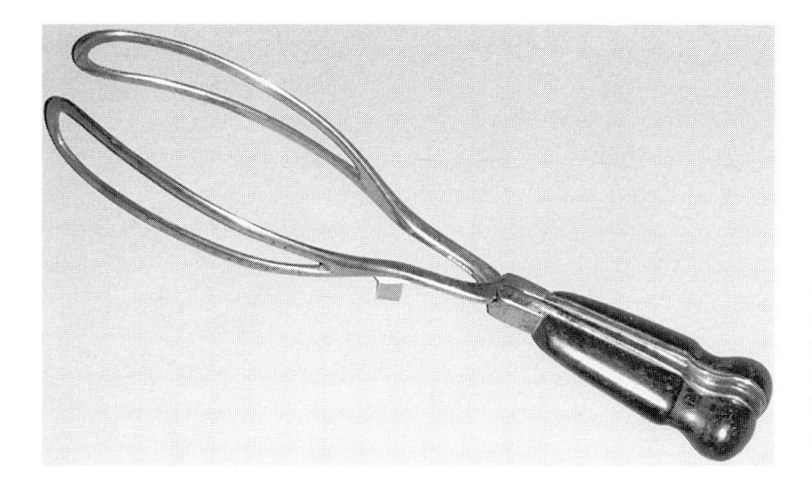

FIGURE 6.19.
Murphy's forceps. His blades were a compromise between the narrow and broad blades then in use and were a modification of T. E. Beatty's forceps, showing the influence of Murphy's Dublin background. (Science Museum, London)

between the blades was 73 millimeters (2.875 inches) and between the tips 32 millimeters (1.25 inches). His claim that it was a most efficient tractor suitable for nine out of ten cases in which instrumental assistance was required seems extravagant in the context of the time and the usual indications for forceps delivery, unless he was performing a large proportion of very easy deliveries. His long forceps, which he himself described as "somewhat formidable looking, but of great power" are discussed in Chapter 9.

Short Straight Shanks

Edward Murphy (1802–1877), who had been Assistant Physician at the Dublin Lying-in Hospital, succeeded David Davis as Professor of Midwifery at University College Hospital. He was generally more conservative than his predecessor, who he regarded as being much bolder in advocating application of the forceps.

Murphy emphasized that forceps were for compression as well as extraction and that for the former procedure their power was very limited. He cited the experiments of Baudelocque (1789) on stillborn babies using Levret's forceps, where he applied increasing degrees of compression force until the forceps bent (Chapter 5). Even so the degree of compression achieved was small, of the order of 2 lines (12 lines = 1 inch) or, where the head was particularly soft, of up to 4 lines. Because of his belief that the forceps could have little compressive force Murphy was skeptical about their value in overcoming obstruction, and if the fetus was dead he preferred extraction with the crotchet as a safer alternative.

In his *Lectures on the Principles and Practice of Midwifery* (1862) Murphy illustrated all the forceps in common use at the time. For low forceps deliveries he favored the blade shape of Collins and of Aitken, with the distance between the blades of about 76 millimeters (3 inches) and between the tips of about 38 millimeters (1.5 inches), rather than those of Denman, in which he regarded the blades as being too close together and the handles too short; or those of Conquest (Chapter 8), with their wide fenestra. He helped to popularize the Dublin pattern, using a modification of T. E. Beatty's design and advocated their use for "intermediate" operations, later modifying them by making a short parallel shank (Figure 6.19).

Murphy also described his criteria for application of the forceps. When the head was arrested in the pelvic cavity, careful assessment of the degree of impaction was essential. As a general rule it should be possible to feel an ear but other criteria included the ability to pass the fingers between the head and the pelvic wall, to press the head back easily, to pass a catheter easily, and for there to be no gross swelling of the vagina. With regard to timing, Murphy considered that four hours without progress was quite long enough but this could be reduced if adverse factors such as "pain, swelling or heat in the passages" was observed. Unlike many of his contemporaries, such as F. H. Ramsbotham, he did not consider reduced or absent uterine activity as a criterion and would apply the forceps even in the presence of good uterine action if the indications as specified above were there. Murphy also advocated the asymmetric forceps of Radford or the more refined interchangeable blades of Davis as giving a better fit over the face and occiput.

James Braithwaite (d. 1919), the first obstetric physician of the Leeds General Infirmary, in 1869 described a short, straight forceps with short parallel shanks made so that the convexity of one blade accurately fit inside the concavity of the other blade, with the idea of introducing both blades simultaneously, one blade sitting inside the other (Figure 6.20) The handles were held together by a metal sheath, most

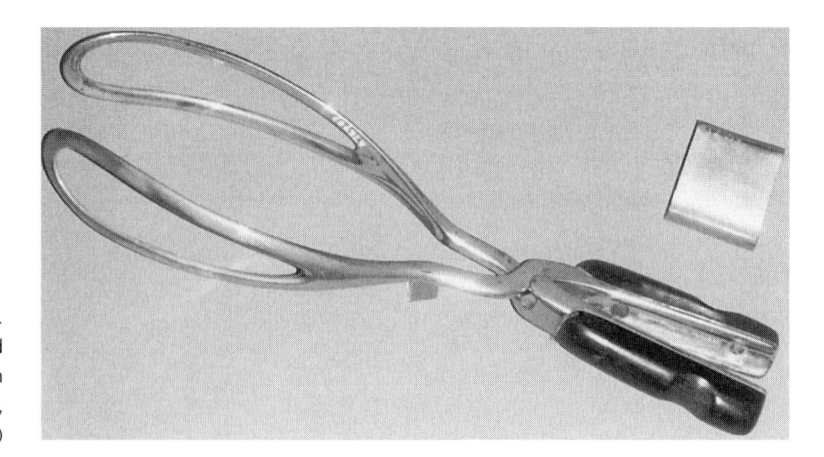

FIGURE 6.20.
Braithwaite's forceps. The forceps were inserted with one blade inside the other and then "wandered" into position. (Science Museum, London)

likely a unique feature. The blades were inserted together into the hollow of the sacrum and then "wandered" into position. Braithwaite claimed the major advantages to be: rapid and painless application; safer for the child than ergot; and light, portable, and able to be "carried in the breast-pocket where it is invisible and where it cannot be lost in travelling."

Long Forceps in Nineteenth-Century British Practice

Many of the British instruments described thus far have been called "long" forceps, a term that originated at the time of Smellie. These instruments were still short by Continental standards. As a generalization "short" forceps were rarely over 300 millimeters (11.75 inches) long, while "long" instruments were up to about 340 millimeters (13.5 inches) in length.

There were sporadic references to the use of long forceps in the late eighteenth and early nineteenth centuries. Although James Hamilton of Edinburgh reported the successful use of long forceps in the case of Sally Gray in 1795, he did not give details of the instrument he used (see Radford, 1839). John Haighton (1755–1823) of Guy's Hospital, according to Radford (1839), who attended his lectures, advocated double-curved, long forceps. Unfortunately Haighton left no written description of them but Radford gave their overall length as 343 millimeters (13.5 inches), which is longer than forceps ascribed to Haighton in museum collections. For example, the four pairs in the collection of the Royal College of Obstetricians and Gynaecologists range from 280 to 314 millimeters (11 to 12.5 inches) in length. Conquest (1820a) also advocated long forceps, his original description giving the length as 355 millimeters (14 inches).

By the middle of the nineteenth century attitudes were changing and high forceps applications were becoming more common. This was facilitated by the advent of anesthesia. In consequence longer forceps became more desirable and the new designs were at least 345 millimeters (13.5 inches) and even up to 380 millimeters (15 inches). These could truly be designated as long forceps. To avoid confusion later writers sometimes referred to the earlier generations of "long" forceps as "medium" or "intermediate."

Long Straight Forceps

Credit is usually given to James Blundell for introducing forceps with parallel shanks to the London scene (Chapter 4). Charles Waller (1802–1862) of St. Thomas's Hospital made at least two modifications of Blundell's long forceps in about 1831 but did not describe them in the second edition (1831) of his textbook *Elements of Practical Midwifery; or, Companion to the Lying-in Room*. They were illustrated in Witkowski's *Armamentarium* and Doran's *Descriptive Catalogue*. Waller's instrument differed from Blundell's instrument in that the handles were more slender, the parallel shanks were closer together, and the blades were wider with smaller fenestra (Figure 6.21).

Straight, long forceps were a misadventure. The were intended for high forceps deliveries but without a pelvic curve it must have been almost impossible to apply them accurately, if at all, to a high head.

Long Curved Forceps

Thomas Radford (1793–1881) of the Manchester Lying-In Hospital was an outstanding leader in obstetric innovation and teaching in the middle of the nineteenth century. He was one of the new wave of obstetricians advocating earlier intervention and the more liberal use of Caesarian section, although even at the end of his career the mortality rate from

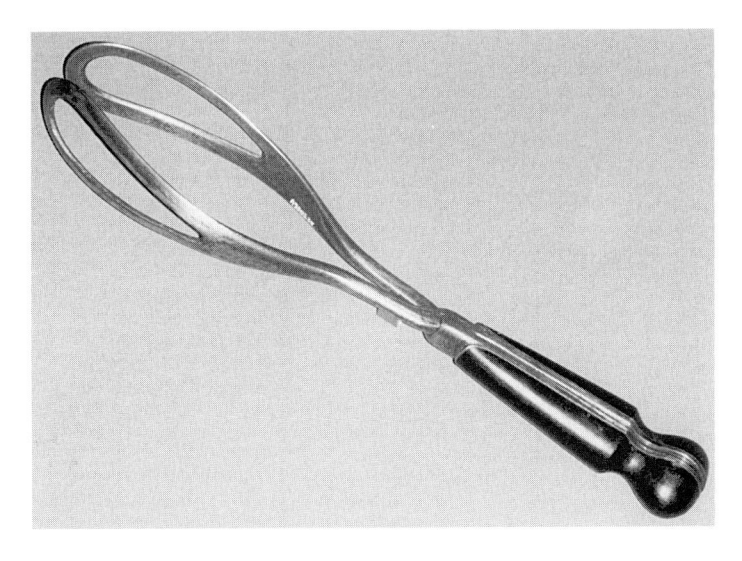

FIGURE 6.21.
Waller's forceps. A development of Blundell's long forceps. (Science Museum, London)

FIGURE 6.22.
Radford's curved forceps. This is one of the earliest British true long forceps, breaking from traditional conservatism. (RCOG)

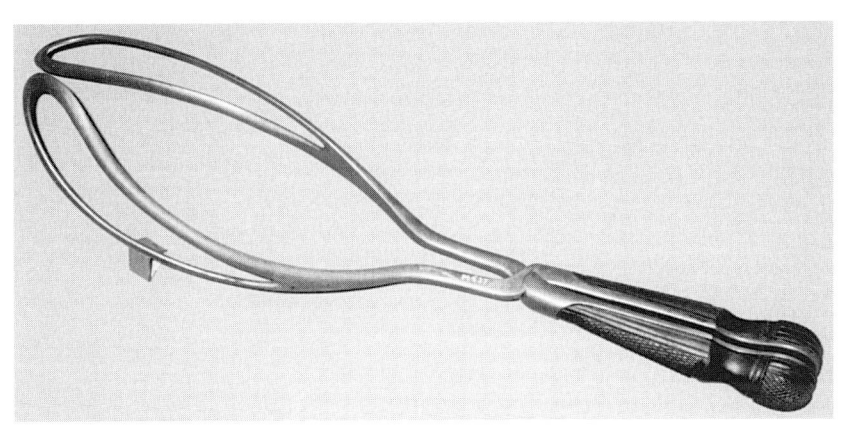

this operation was close to 80 percent. Thus, with David Davis and others, he helped to break the conservative traditions of the previous century. He published widely and in his *Essays on Various Subjects Connected with Midwifery* (1839), he critically appraised the forceps of his predecessors and contemporaries. This led to his own designs for long forceps (356 millimeters/14 inches), starting with his long curved forceps (Figure 6.22). However, it had been his experience that the high head was most commonly in an oblique position and the straight forceps produced "disagreeable effects" because they could not be applied in correct cephalic orientation (biparietally) and therefore increased the risk of damage to the baby. To counteract this problem he developed his asymmetric forceps (Chapter 9).

J. Ramsbotham (1767–1847), a lecture in midwifery at the London Hospital (1832), and John Burns of Glasgow (1843), in company with other British authorities of the time, recommended correct pelvic application of the forceps, irrespective of the orientation of the head. It was generally agreed that the guidelines were different from those for the use of the short forceps, for with the latter the blades should be applied over the transverse diameter of the head. However, for the long forceps the pelvic orientation ruled their application. A dissenter from this view was David Davis (page 80), who claimed that the long forceps in common use at the time were not suitable for all positions of the head at the brim, and that they could only be applied with safety to the sides of the head. It was for this reason that Davis introduced his asymmetric and jointed forceps, referred to above, which could be effectively and safely applied to the oblique or transverse head in correct pelvic application (Chapter 9).

F. H. Ramsbotham (1801–1868) an obstetric physician and lecturer at the London Hospital, described the long forceps as one of the most valuable instruments employed in midwifery "if formed according to the size and dimensions which I shall presently demonstrate, and used in the cases to which it is particularly appropriate" (1841). His instrument (Figure 6.23) was 324 millimeters (12.75 inches long) and was based on Osborn's forceps (Chapter 4) but heavier, with a

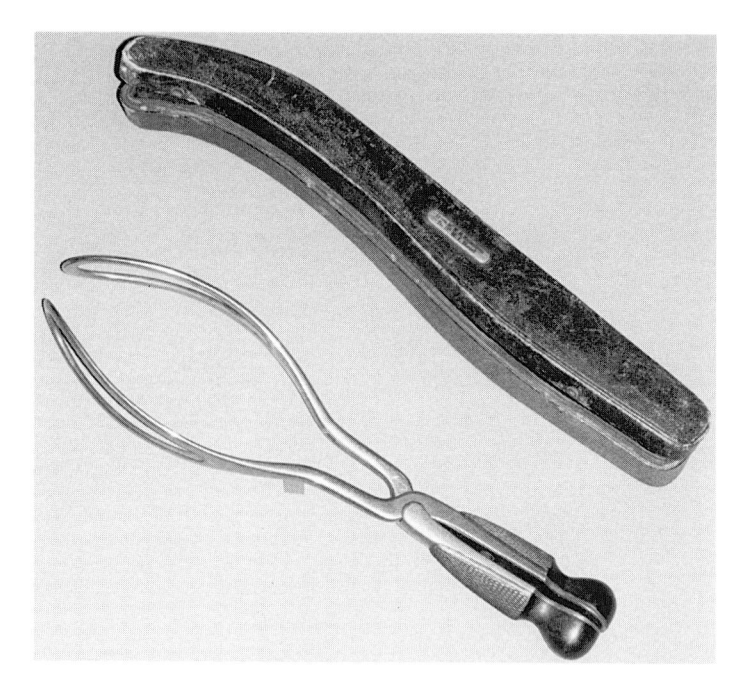

FIGURE 6.23.
F. H. Ramsbotham's forceps with case. They were intended for use when the head was just engaged and turning was not feasible. (Science Museum, London)

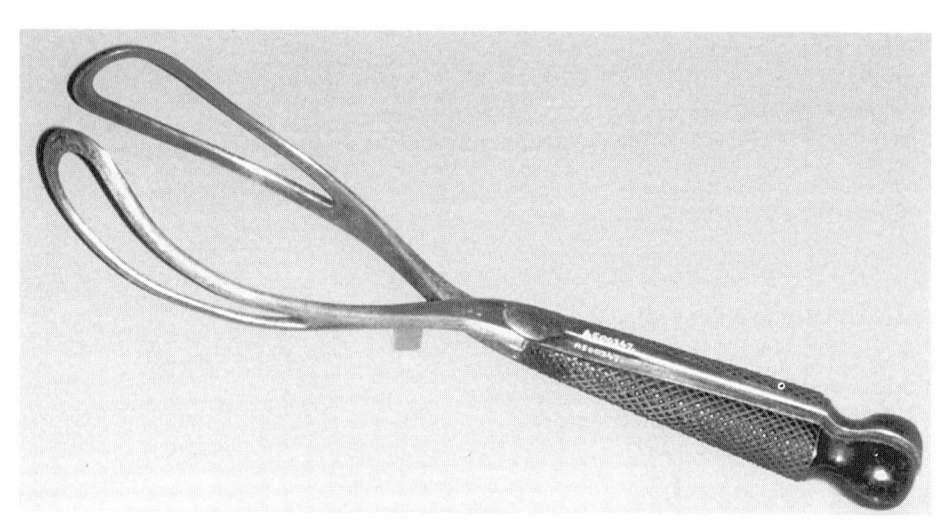

FIGURES 6.24, 6.25.
Edward Rigby the Younger's forceps. A lighter modification of Naegele's forceps, with a Brunninghausen lock. (Science Museum, London)

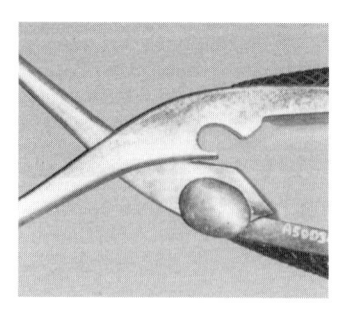

reduced pelvic curve and the addition of parallel straight shanks of 38 millimeters (1.5 inches), as in Radford's instrument. He stressed the value of the long straight shanks in avoiding perineal laceration and also emphasized that the internal surfaces of the blades should be slightly convex and the joint loose to allow for some lateral play.

Ramsbotham described the instrument as particularly serviceable when the head was partly engaged in the pelvic brim, too low for the practitioner to turn the head but not low enough to feel an ear. The application of the blades should be in a correct pelvic relationship irrespective of the orientation of the head. He gave the credit for this concept to a Frenchman, de Leurie, who published a paper in 1779 and to whom Ramsbotham refers to as "a French Physician of some eminence" (1834). De Leurie's concept was in contradiction to the preference of Smellie and his successors, who maintained that the blades should be applied in correct cephalic relationship, as with the low forceps, so that the blades would commonly lie in the hollow of the sacrum and behind the pubes. However, it was generally accepted that there were occasions when, because of pelvic contracture, an oblique application might be required.

Edward Rigby the Younger (Chapter 5) was an activist and original thinker of the time. He was for many years Lecturer in Midwifery at both St. Bartholomew's and St. Thomas's Hospitals and was the first president of the Obstetrical Society of London. He was a strong advocate of the forceps: "The forceps is by far the simplest and safest means of artificial delivery, and is therefore an operation which should always be had recourse to in preference to any of the others wherever it is possible" (1841). In 1829 Rigby translated into English Naegele's *Essay on the Mechanism of Parturition*. He favored Naegele's forceps with the Brunninghausen lock, which he introduced into Britain and described as "the most perfect lock," being easier to articulate and disarticulate than the English lock while maintaining the firmness of a pivot joint. His forceps were a lighter modification of Naegele's instrument and did not have finger rests (Figures 6.24, 6.25)

Rigby's general rules for forceps design were that the distance between the blades should never be less than 51 millimeters (2 inches); the tips should be at least 13 millimeters (.5 inches) apart (In Britain they tended to be wider and on the Continent narrower than this.); the fenestra should be wide and ample, as in the forceps of Hopkins and Davis; the fenestra should be oval in shape, unlike the Orme/Lowder types where the greatest breadth was near the lock. The blades nearest to these criteria were those of Hopkins (page 85). Rigby also differed from many of his contemporaries in advocating tying the handles of the forceps together and gradually tightening them in order to compress the head.

James Young Simpson's Long Forceps and Their Modifications

The deficiencies of existing long, double-curved forceps as tractors became more apparent after the advent of anesthesia, which gave obstetricians much greater scope in the use of instruments. The greater the pelvic curve, the greater the degree of inefficiency and this was particularly evident in European forceps of the Levret type. The inappropriate direction of traction was partly overcome by the introduction of the perineal curve. Many obstetricians took to using tapes, or *lacs*, passed through the fenestra, or tried to compensate by use of what came to be known as Pajot's maneuver (Chapters 12, 13).

Although J. Y. Simpson's short forceps were, and have remained, the model for simplicity and safety, his long curved forceps of 1848 were of far greater importance in British practice and, like his short forceps, became the prototype for many subsequent designs. It may be more than coincidence that led him to describe the forceps to the Edinburgh Obstetrical Society the year after he first used ether in obstetrics, for anesthesia made difficult forceps operations, including high forceps, more feasible.

Simpson's long forceps (Figure 6.26, right) were heavier than those previously used in Britain and owed something to the Continental designs of the period. Simpson used

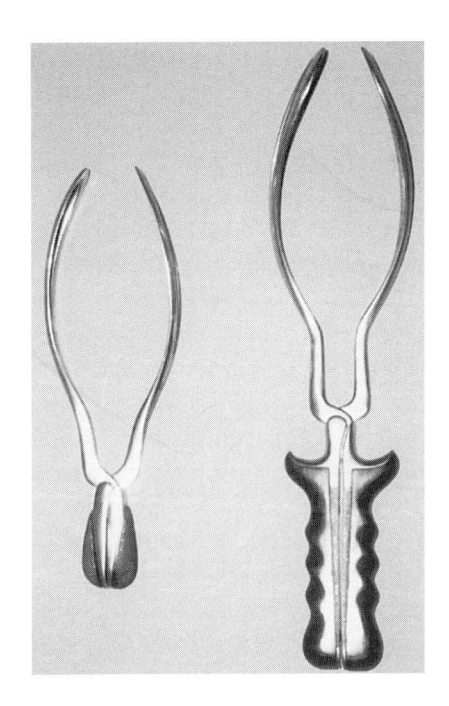

FIGURE 6.26.
J. Y. Simpson's short and long forceps. The long forceps are 350mm (14.75ins) long, 115mm (4.5ins) longer than his short forceps. (RCOG)

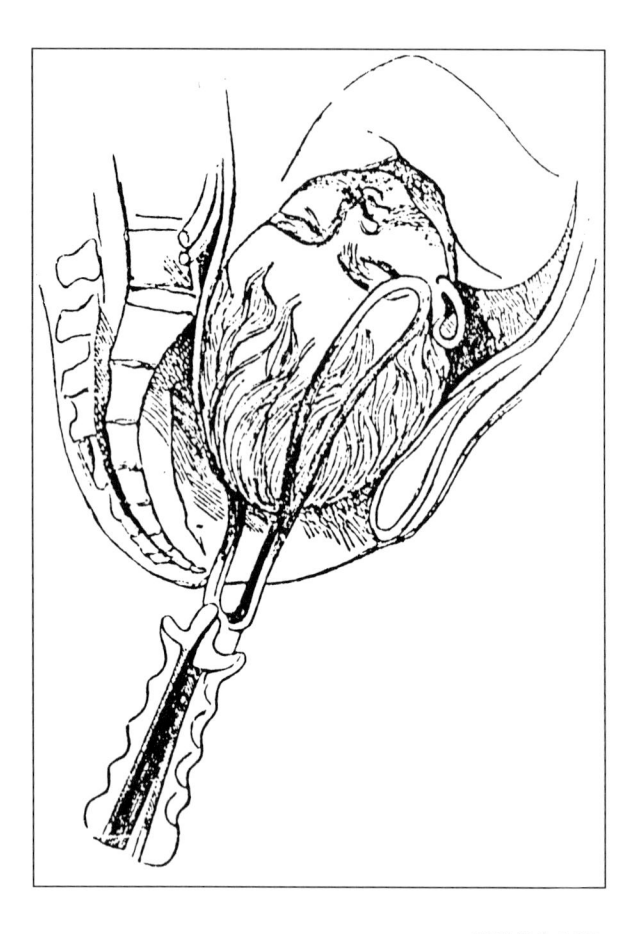

FIGURE 6.27.
J. Y. Simpson's long forceps. He favored an oblique application. (From *Selected Works*, ed. Black, 1871)

Ramsbotham's forceps as the basis for his design and incorporated many of the ideas he had picked up on his European travels. Their overall length was 350 millimeters (13.75 inches) and the blades were long and large (160 millimeters/ 6.25 inches). The articulation was of the English type, but larger than was common at the time, in order to prevent the blades readily unlocking between contractions, thus giving the advantages of the Continental locks without their complexity. The joints were loose to allow more lateral motion, thus facilitating their application. The handle, which had a roughened upper surface to indicate the direction of the pelvic curve, was similar to those seen in many Continental patterns, and with the addition of transverse finger rests after the style of J. D. Busch (page 72) to facilitate oscillating traction; and deep finger rests along the handle, first seen in Brunninghausen's forceps (page 71). The parallel shanks were described by Simpson as indispensable in the prevention of injury to the outlet.

Although Simpson advocated forceps delivery for many purposes, as did his contemporaries, he regarded the most common indication as disproportion due to a contracted pelvic brim, with a reduced antero-posterior diameter. He advised something nearer a correct pelvic rather than cephalic application, so that one blade of the forceps was over the side of the fetal occiput and the other obliquely over the brow (Figure 6.27). He considered that the oblique position in relation to the pelvis was desirable as providing the most room and reducing risk of injury to the urethra.

There were many minor variants of Simpson's long forceps over the years. J. Mathews Duncan (1826–1890), who had been a private assistant to J. Y. Simpson and was the first person to inhale chloroform in Simpson's experiments, was passed over as Simpson's successor by the Edinburgh Town Council, in favor of J. Y. Simpson's nephew, A. R. Simpson. As a result Duncan moved to St. Bartholomew's Hospital. Duncan's forceps (circa 1860) were a modification of Simpson's, but with shorter handles and no finger rests. (Figure 6.28). It is probable that he shortened the handles because his method of forceps use was different from that of Simpson, for he was strongly opposed to the oscillatory, or pendulum, method of traction then in general use in Britain and on the Continent and advocated by Simpson (Duncan, 1876).

H. Oldham (1815–1902), an obstetric physician and lecturer at Guy's Hospital, London, also modified the handle, making it smooth and straight (circa 1850) (Figure 6.29). Neither these nor similar variants can be regarded as major contributions to the obstetric armamentarium and were usually inferior to Simpson's carefully and thoughtfully designed instrument. The most important and enduring of the variations of Simpson's forceps were those designed by Robert Barnes (1817–1907), probably the most influential of the London obstetricians in the second half of the nineteenth century, with appointments successively at the London, St. Thomas's and St. George's Hospitals, as well as being on the staff of the Royal Maternity Charity. He was a founder of the Obstetrical Society of London and, subsequently, of the British Gynaecological Society. His *Lectures on Obstetric Operations* (1870) was translated into several languages and won him an international reputation. Barnes gave much consideration to the design of forceps and devised his modification of J. Y. Simpson's forceps in about 1862, exhibiting them in 1866 at the Obstetrical Society of London *Conversazione* (Meadows, 1867) (Figure 6.30). He described what he considered to be the essential features in *A System of Obstetric Medicine and Surgery* (1885), emphasizing that the lock and handles should be clearly outside the vulva even when the blades were applied to the head at the pelvic brim. His forceps had the parallel shanks of the Simpson forceps but with a ring at the handle end of the shank, thereby ef-

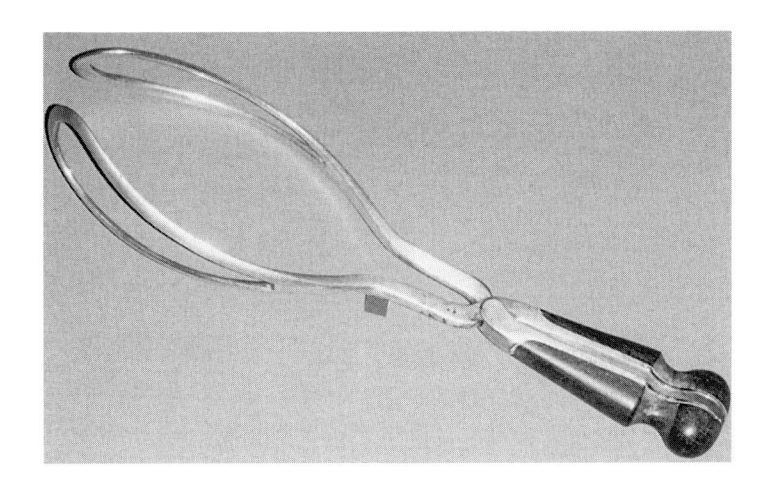

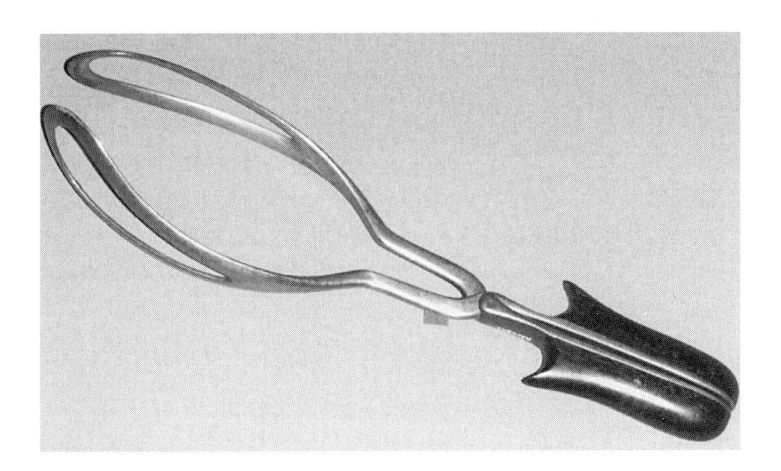

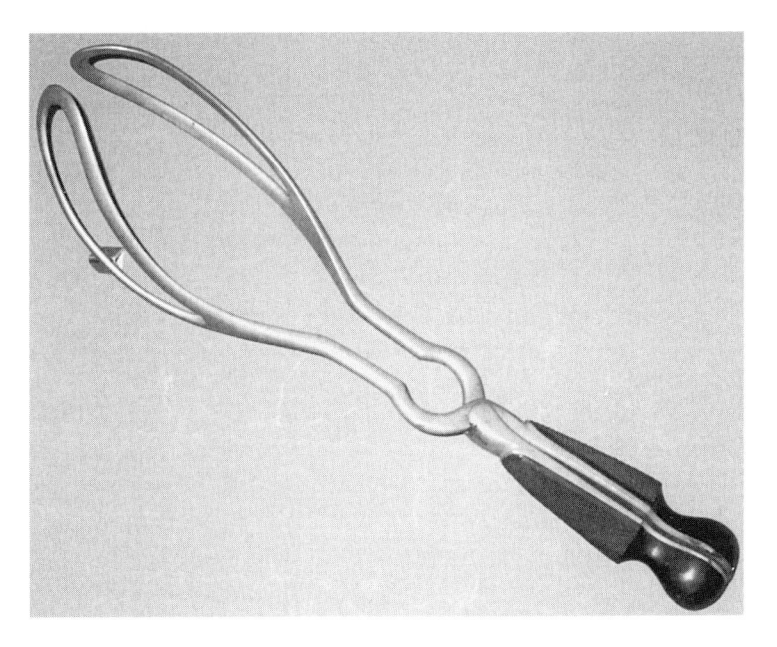

FIGURE 6.28.
Mathews Duncan's forceps. The blades are similar to Simpson's but the handles are shorter and without finger rests, reflecting his method of use. (Science Museum, London)

FIGURE 6.29.
Oldham's forceps. These are another variant of Simpson's forceps, differing only in the handle. (Science Museum, London)

FIGURE 6.30.
Barnes's forceps. Note the finger ring. The forceps are slightly longer than those of Simpson. (RCOG)

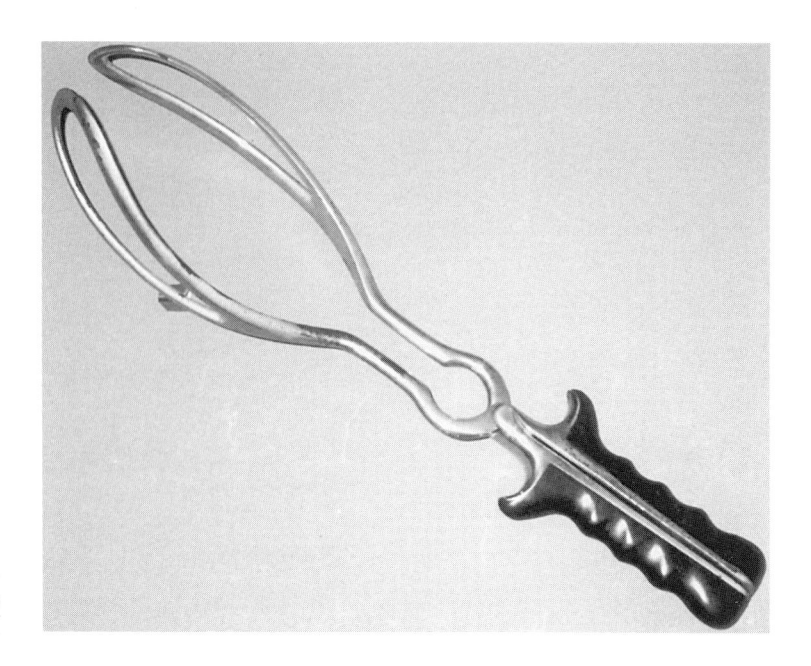

FIGURE 6.31.
Anderson's forceps. He combined the features of Simpson and Barnes in the handle design.

fectively lengthening the handle as well as facilitating finger traction. He also discarded the transverse finger rests and had smooth handles. He pointed out that British forceps had some "spring" in the blades while European designs were more rigid and therefore had greater compressive power. In the use of the forceps he favored an oscillatory action, described by Simpson, but one performed gently and imperceptibly, which he claimed mimicked nature. This technique was widely used for the next hundred years. Robert Barnes later designed an axis-traction forceps based on Tarnier's instrument but it was Neville's modification of the original Barnes forceps that achieved enduring popularity (Chapter 14).

C. L. Anderson (1843–1900), Honorary Assistant Surgeon at the Liverpool Ladies Charity and Lying-In Hospital, endeavored to combine the merits of Simpson's and Barnes's forceps (1879). He used Simpson's handle, omitting the roughened upper surfaces and included Barnes's long shank with the finger ring (Figure 6.31). The cephalic curve was less than that in the Simpson and Barnes designs and the distance between the tips was less. George H. Kidd (1878) considered this to be a disadvantage that would increase the danger to the child. Anderson's forceps are often erroneously referred to as Barnes's forceps, even in instrument makers' catalogues.

A remarkable but not very praiseworthy fact is that the Simpson/Barnes/Anderson designs, with modifications such as the addition of compression screws to the handle and axis-traction devices such as that of Neville, have continued to be used more or less uncritically for over a century. The long relatively flat curve of the blades and the limited maximum distance (75 millimeters/3 inches) between the blades were intended to fit the greatly molded head that might occur after several days in labor. Thus in modern practice these forceps would be expected to have a reduced area of contact and the localization of the traction force would predispose the child to unnecessary intracranial stresses. There was also the possibility of blade slippage and thus abrasive trauma. Under ordinary circumstances in modern practice the handles, because of the closeness of the blades, would not approximate, thus creating a temptation to apply excessive compression force, which was one of the objectives and desirable features of the forceps when they were conceived. Furthermore, in current practice there are wide variations in the measurements of instruments of the same type, even from the same manufacturer. These problems have been addressed by Forster (1971) and by Hibbard and McKenna (1990) (Figures 6.32–6.34).

. . .

Although the changes in British practice in the nineteenth century were slow to evolve they were inevitable and long lasting. They resulted from the inspiration of a number of obstetricians, often with considerable influence, applying an intellectual approach to the problems of the day. Notable among these were David Davis, F. H. Ramsbotham, J. Y. Simpson, and Robert Barnes, whose influence became world-wide, as is seen, for example, in their effect on subsequent American designs.

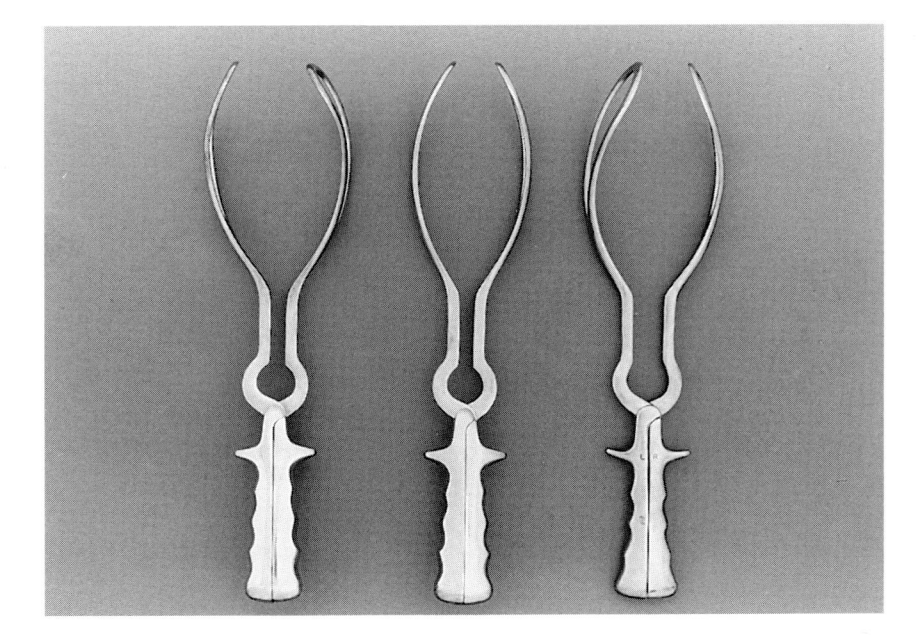

FIGURE 6.32.
Anderson's forceps. Variations in the shape of the blades in use in one delivery unit. (Hibbard and McKenna, 1990) (RCOG)

FIGURES 6.33, 6.34.
6.33 Anderson's and 6.34 Wrigley's forceps, showing the fit to the fetal head. (Hibbard and McKenna, 1990) (RCOG)

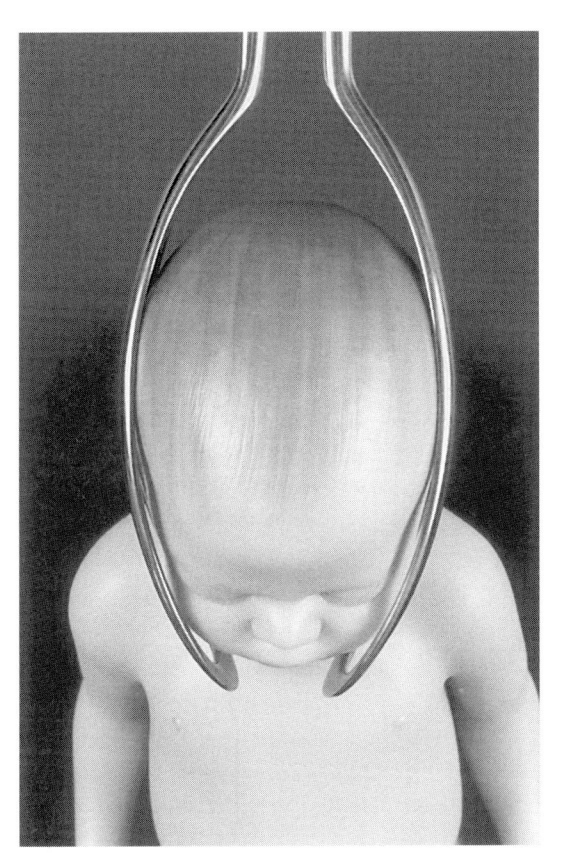

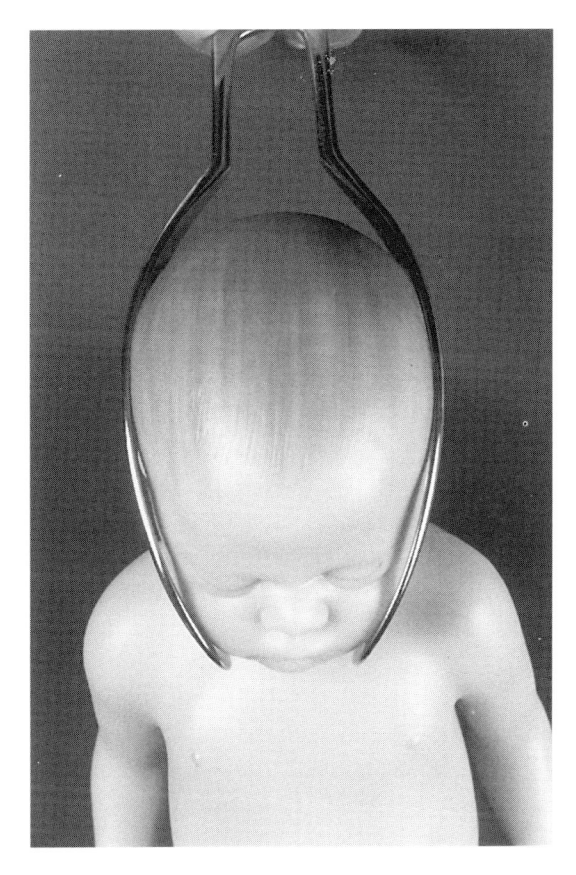

Early development of long forceps was tentative; merely lengthening the forceps while not adopting a pelvic curve was impractical. Soon Continental influence became evident but British forceps remained lighter in construction and more refined in design, appropriate to their use more as tractors than compressors. By the middle of the nineteenth century operative procedures and manipulations were being facilitated by the advent of anesthesia. Axis traction and other mechanical additions were yet to come but the general configuration of the forceps in Britain endured for at least another 150 years.

BRITISH RENAISSANCE: 19TH CENTURY **97**

AMERICAN FORCEPS OF THE NINETEENTH CENTURY

7

Medical involvement in midwifery, which was slow to develop in the New World, has been well described by H. Thoms (1933). The first medical practitioner, Deacon Samuel Fuller, a serge maker by trade, arrived aboard the Mayflower in 1620. His third wife, Bridget Lee Fuller, was held in great esteem as a midwife and was probably involved in the three births that occurred during the Mayflower's voyage. Thereafter traditional midwives were in general use and were usually immigrants, although there is an early record of at least one man-midwife, John Dupuy (1717–1745).

In the late eighteenth century courses for man-midwives were being conducted in Philadelphia by William Shippen, Jr. (1736–1808). The son of the founder of the University of Pennsylvania, he had studied in Europe under Smellie and Hunter. Shippen, Jr., gave his first course of lectures on medicine, surgery, and midwifery from his father's house in 1762 and started a more advanced course in 1765. In New York, J. V. B. Tennent was the first Professor of Midwifery in America at King's College, which later became Columbia University. However the first American textbook, *A Compendium of the Theory and Practice of Midwifery, for Midwives, Students and Young Practitioners*, was not published until 1808 in New York. It was written by Samuel Bard (1742–1821), who had trained in Edinburgh and taught in the British tradition. In the second edition, published in 1817, it is recorded that he was solicited to include a chapter on the use of instruments but decided against it.

The attitude to instrumental delivery was traditionally conservative and at that time stimulation of labor to assist delivery was being championed in New York by John Stearns (1770–1848). Stearns was a physician from Saratoga County who later moved to New York City. After using ergot, which he called *pulvis parturiens*, for several years he claimed that he "seldom found a case that detained me more than three hours." His letter detailing his observations was published in the *New York Medical Repository* in 1808 and this led to widespread use of the substance but, unfortunately, without observance of the obvious precautions. By 1822 Stearns was still advocating the use of ergot, but only when used with extreme caution. He also recommended it for abortion, retained placenta, and postpartum hemorrhage. However, the fatalities associated with its use in labor were such that prescription was restricted to use for abortion and after delivery only.

The nature and development of obstetric practice and the tools of the trade were mainly dependent on the origins of the colonists and subsequent immigrants, with some areas of predominantly British practice and some predominantly Continental. The first forceps in America had been brought from England and France and this custom of importing instruments from these countries predominated for many decades although, as instruments started to be made in America, many modifications crept in. Indeed, later in the century so called "Simpson's long forceps" were very popular but many of local manufacture bore little resemblance to the original instrument (Chapter 6) and some were of crude construction. R. P. Harris (1872a) related the story of a practitioner using a crude and inaccurate copy of Davis's forceps who caused such lacerations with them that the mother died. In a subsequent malpractice suit brought by the husband five thousand dollars in damages were awarded—one of the earliest examples of obstetric litigation in America.

In this chapter only mainstream developments of conventional American forceps will be considered. Special features will be discussed in the appropriate chapters that follow.

Early Nineteenth Century

In early years British forceps, especially Haighton's (Chapter 4), were very popular and were also manufactured in Philadelphia (Harris, 1872b). Later David Davis's forceps were popularized by Charles D. Meigs (1792–1869), a professor of midwifery at Jefferson Medical College in Philadelphia, through his book, *Obstetrics—The Science and the Art* (1849) and Davis blades were featured in many subsequent American designs, followed by Simpson's long forceps. Meigs's philosophy was that the forceps was the child's instrument, to be used as a tractor, not a compressor, and that the shape of the Davis blades in relation to the shape of the head was such that "I think it is almost out of the bounds of possibility to injure the foetus with it." He condemned, although not completely, the Baudelocque forceps then in common use: "This powerful instrument, in skilful hands, may be made use of to overcome very great obstacles: but, in careless or unskilful application, may be the cause of great mischief." Meigs was strongly, and often erroneously, opinionated and though his book was popular and influential for a brief time, it was eventually overshadowed by Dewees's text (see below). However he did acknowledge a place for the (Elias von) Siebold type of forceps and in particular the lighter version designed by Robert M. Huston (1795–1864) (Figure 7.1) of Jefferson Medical College. Huston had illustrated his forceps in his edition of Fleetwood Churchill's *On the Theory and Practice of Midwifery*. Meigs described them as a modification of Siebold's forceps, weighing only 588 grams (21 ounces), compared with 756 grams (27 ounces) for a pair of Siebold's forceps made in Berlin.

Later, Continental influences resulted in the introduction of heavy, long curved forceps of the Levret/Baudelocque pattern, followed by other popular European designs such as those of Elias von Siebold (Chapter 5) and, subsequently, Tarnier's axis-traction forceps (Chapter 13). However, innovative American designs were slow to appear and many of these were minor variations of traditional instruments.

Thomas C. James (1798–1861), who studied in London under Osborn and Clark, was reputedly, with John Church of Philadelphia, the first to regularly teach obstetrics. He became the first Professor of Obstetrics at the University of Pennsylvania and was instrumental in getting the subject recognized as a compulsory part of undergraduate education. Soon after graduating at the age of twenty in 1812, he designed his own forceps. The following story is related by Harris (1872a) and by Thoms (1961): In Chester County there were two elderly practitioners who had never used forceps, their instruments for obstructed labor being limited to the crotchet and embryotomy scissors. The young James was called to a case in which a destructive operation was pro-

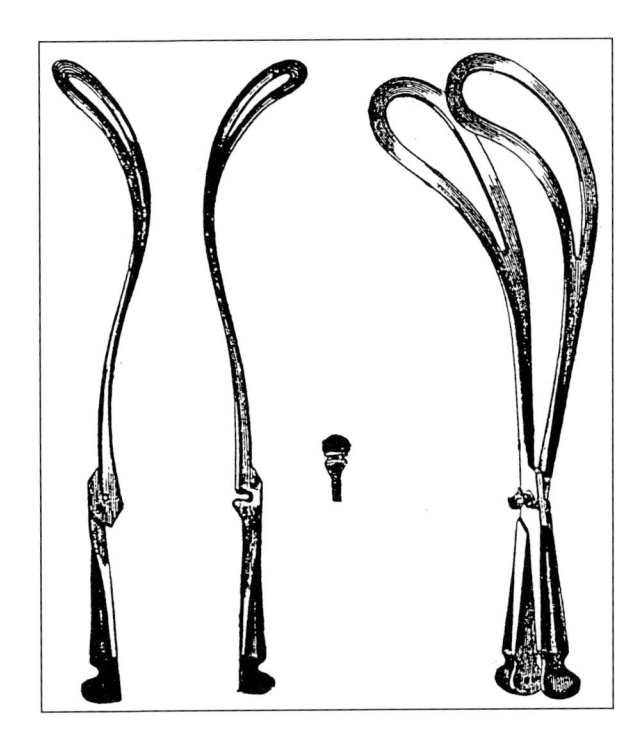

FIGURE 7.1.
Huston's forceps. A lighter version of Siebold's forceps with a screw lock. (Meigs, 1849)

posed and successfully delivered the baby with his forceps, thereby beginning a successful career for himself.

James's curved forceps were in the London style of the time (Figure 7.2), with narrow blades, short wooden handles, and a maximum distance between the blades of 69 millimeters (2.75 inches). However, the blades were of crude construction and the narrow fenestra were sharp-edged, with the potential for lacerating the fetal head.

By the 1820s there was an outstanding practitioner in Philadelphia: William Potts Dewees (b. 1768), who was of Swedish descent and promoted the principles of Baudelocque. Thoms claimed that he exerted a greater influence on American obstetrics than anyone before him. His *Compendious System of Midwifery*, first published in Philadelphia in 1824 and then in London in 1825, ran to twelve editions. Dewees advocated much practice on the manikin, or "obstetric machine," and the use of the lithotomy position for assisted delivery. He, in the European tradition, was more of an interventionist than his British contemporaries and declared that "[a]pplication of instruments should not be too long delayed from an imaginary fear that the woman might suffer from their use or from an ill-grounded hope that the woman might deliver herself."

Dewees recorded in his book that he used short forceps for many years but abandoned them because of their limitations. He combined this with severe criticisms of Denman

FIGURE 7.2.
James's forceps. The blades were sharp-edged and the widest distance between them was only 64 mm (2.5ins). (Harris, 1872a)

FIGURE 7.3.
Dewees's forceps. This is the later pattern, after Siebold. (Dewees, 1824)

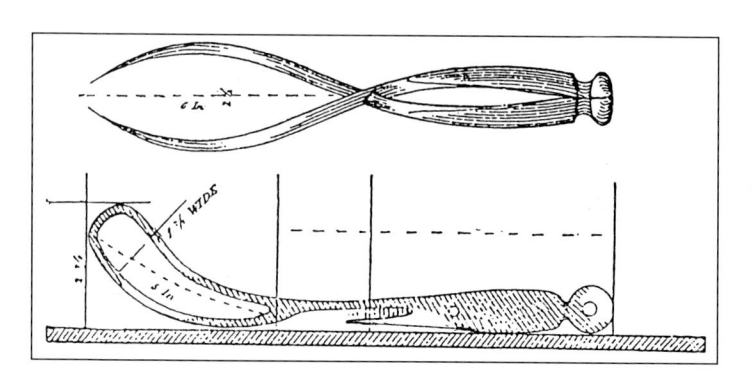

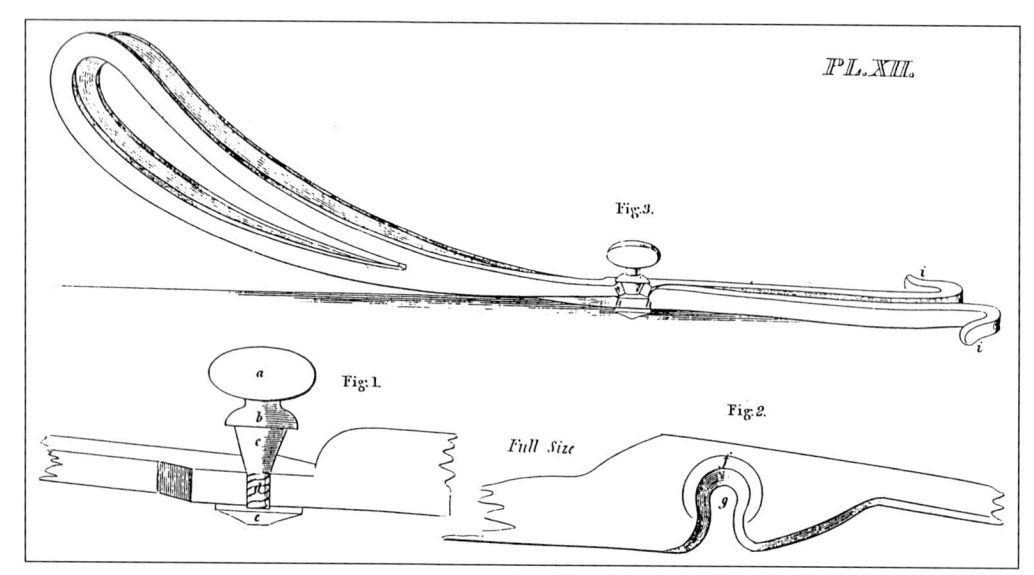

and his *Aphorisms*, and of Osborn. Of Denman he said that "[he], more perhaps than any other man, is chargeable with perpetuating errors in the use of forceps, because, he is considered the highest British authority upon the subject. In his attempt at precision he has created confusion; and, in his desire to generalise, he has so many exceptions, that his Aphorisms are no longer rules."

He accused Osborn of furthering Denman's reluctance to use forceps. Dewees subsequently had two types of forceps made by local instrument makers. The first, made from a Paris pattern, was of the Baudelocque type; the second was in the style of Siebold from a pair that Mr. Eberle (Chapter 5) had shown to Dewees (Figure 7.3).

Hugh L. Hodge (1796–1873), a professor of obstetrics at the University of Pennsylvania, was a major influence on American obstetrics, largely stemming from his classic work *The Principles and Practice of Obstetrics*, first published in 1864. In this he gave a detailed critique of forceps design and use, favoring the long forceps as "being adapted to every emergency, equally applicable, whether the head be at the inferior or the superior strait, or in the cavity of the pelvis. Hence there is no necessity for the practitioner to accustom himself to different instruments." He also supported the European practice of attempting correct cephalic application rather than pelvic orientation, which was common in Britain.

He described his forceps, invented around 1833, as "eclectic," as indeed they were, showing in their design the mixed European influences. He took as his basic model Baudelocque's forceps and over the years, with the assistance of his instrument maker John Rorer, modified them to reach his final design (Figures 7.4, 7.5). The blades were similar to

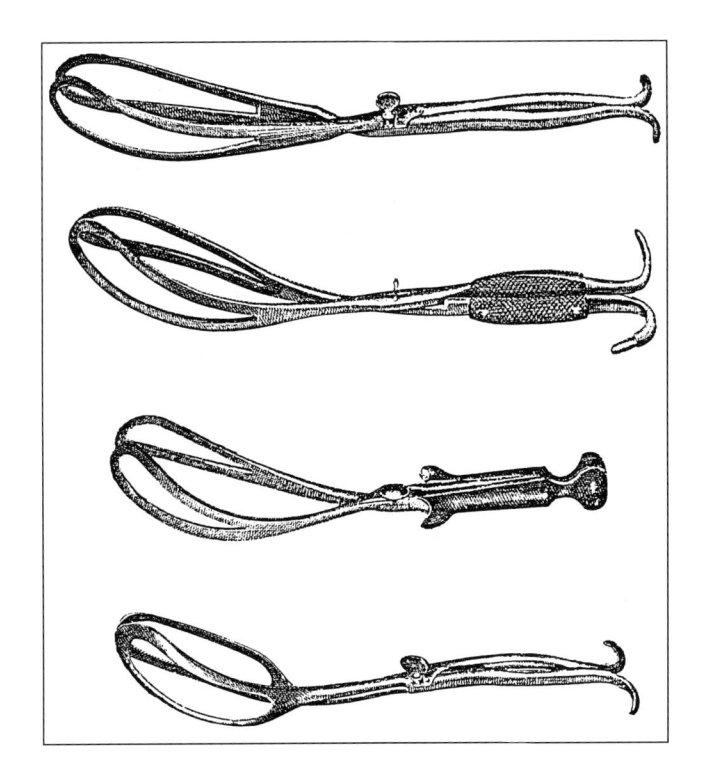

FIGURE 7.4.
Evolution of Hodge's forceps. Top to bottom: Baudelocque, Dubois, German, Hodge. (Hodge, 1864)

FIGURE 7.5.
Hodge's forceps. (University of Liverpool)

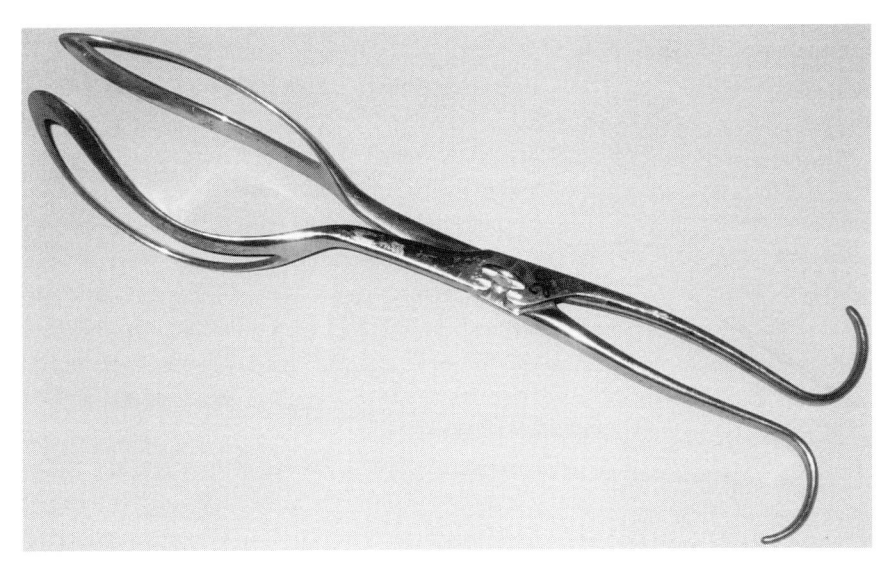

those of David Davis, the handles were hooked in the French style, and the pivot and screw lock was similar to that of Siebold.

Hodge's criticisms of Baudelocque's instrument were

(1) it was unnecessarily heavy;

(2) the pelvic curve was inadequate;

(3) the blades diverged from the joint, resulting in unnecessary risk of perineal laceration;

(4) the fenestra were too small, resulting in a poor cephalic grip;

(5) the cephalic surface of the blades was too flat so that they occupied too much space and thus there was an increased risk of scalp damage; and

(6) the lock was inferior to the English and German types.

AMERICAN FORCEPS: 19TH CENTURY **101**

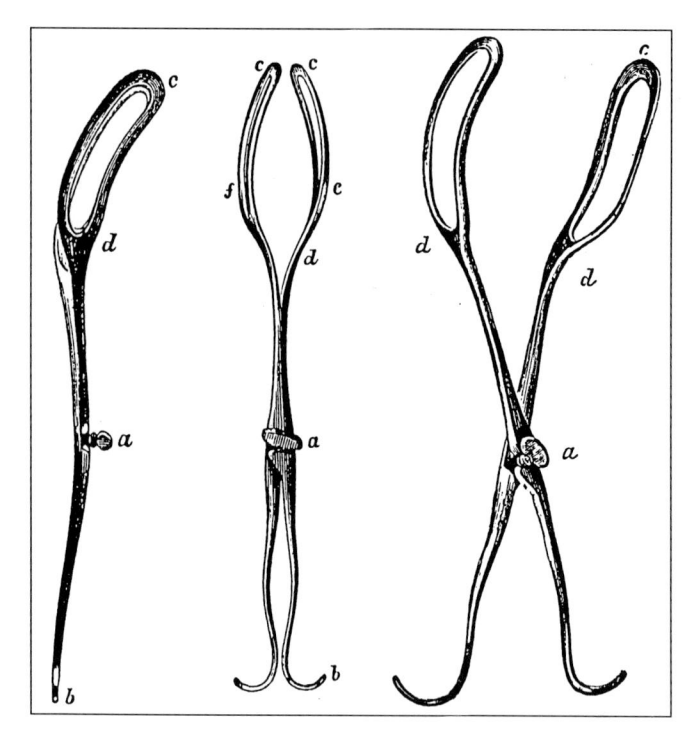

FIGURE 7.6.
Measurements of Hodge's forceps:
Overall b-c: 406mm (16ins); Handle a-b: 173mm (6.8ins); Shank a-d: 89mm (3.5ins); Blade d-c: 91mm (3.6ins); Between tips c-c: 13mm (0.5ins); Max between blades e-f: 63mm (2.5ins). (Hodge 1833)

This would seem to leave little left of Baudelocque's design but Hodge did in fact retain the overall concept. The essential features of his modifications were

(1) the weight was reduced from Baudelocque's 735 grams (26 ounces) to 485 grams (17 ounces), the strength being conserved by using steel of a better temper;

(2) the pelvic curve was slightly increased but to preserve the traction line and compensate for any loss of power the handles were slightly curved in the opposite direction;

(3) the shanks were nearly parallel;

(4) the fenestra were larger and the cephalic surfaces of the blades had a double concavity better to fit the fetal head; and

(5) the lock was of the conical screw-pivot type described by Siebold.

The measurements are shown in Figure 7.6.

Mid and Late Nineteenth Century

By 1889 George Tiemann, the major instrument maker in New York, listed and illustrated sixty-three different patterns of forceps, the majority being of American design. Many of these achieved little more than local popularity, having been presented at local society meetings, with written descriptions in the transactions of those bodies. The influence of David Davis was evident in many of the designs, especially in the shape of the blades (see Bethell, Wallace, and Sawyer below).

J. P. Bethell, Physician to the City Hospital, Philadelphia, as evidenced by his 1853 article, endeavored to design forceps "on philosophical principles," which gave an optimal fit in relation to both the maternal pelvis and the fetal head. The blades resembled those of David Davis but the shank was elongated to facilitate high application. The lock was similar to Siebold's and the blades were set back on the shanks to improve the mechanics of traction from high in the pelvis (Figure 7.7).

William Wallace (1835–1896) was an English medical educator who moved to Brooklyn in 1864. Although at the time short, light forceps were not popular, Wallace introduced a forceps (1865) of light construction with broader Davis-type blades and Hodge-type hooked metal handles (Figure 7.8). They were used extensively in America and particularly by graduates of Jefferson Medical College.

In 1876 Edward Warren Sawyer (b. 1848) of Rush Medical College in Chicago introduced a pair of slightly curved forceps for outlet extractions that were less than 250 millimeters (10 inches) in length and weighed only 150 grams (5 ounces). He combined Davis's blades, Hodge's shanks, and the English lock. The handles had hard rubber plates (Figure 7.9). The intended uses were to save the perineum when rupture was imminent and to rotate the fetus from the occipito-posterior position (Sawyer, 1876, 1885; see also Dorland, 1896).

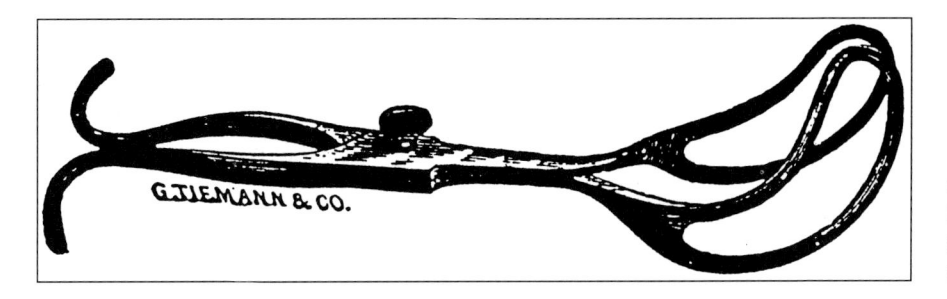

FIGURE 7.7.
Bethell's forceps. A synthesis of Davis's and Siebold's forceps, with the blades set back. (Tiemann, 1889)

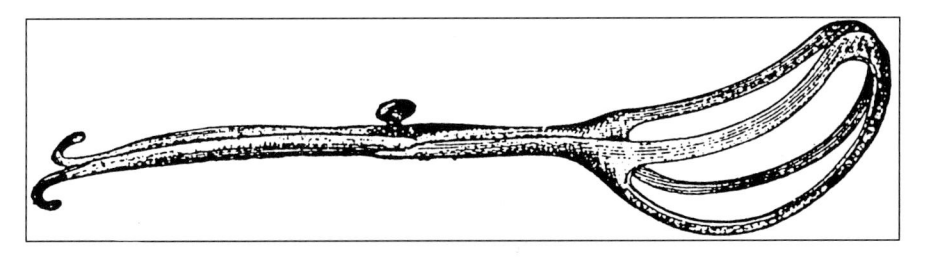

FIGURE 7.8.
Wallace's forceps. A combination of Davis-type blades and Hodge-type handles. (Mann and Hirst, 1889)

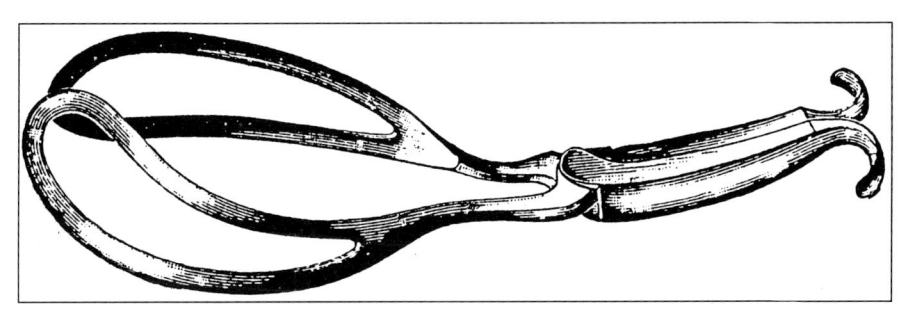

FIGURE 7.9.
Sawyer's forceps. A light forceps, slightly curved, for outlet delivery, again adopting Davis's blades. (Dorland, 1896)

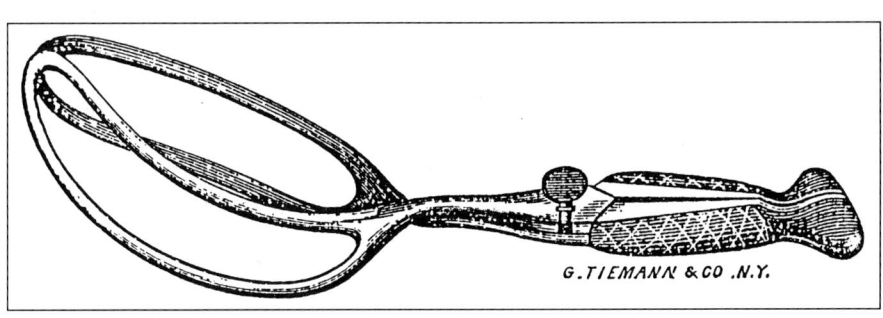

FIGURE 7.10.
Robertson's forceps. A modification of Hodge's forceps with shorter handles. (Robertson, 1872)

Francis Marion Robertson (1807–1892), Professor of Gynaecology and Clinical Obstetrics at the Medical College of South Carolina in Charleston, had experience of all the forceps commonly in use at the time and preferred Hodge's, with some reservations, although he had earlier used Davis's on the recommendation of Meigs. Robertson adopted the Hodge blades but replaced the handles with shorter, wooden handles of the Davis design, thus making the instrument 343 millimeters (13.5 inches) long, 63 millimeters (2.5 inches) shorter than Hodge's forceps (Figure 7.10). Because of the Civil War he was not able to have his forceps made until 1868 and did not describe them until 1872 in his article in the *American Journal of Obstetrics*.

The primary consideration of William David Schuyler (1834–1887) of New York (1884) was to reduce outlet trauma by optimizing the traction line. He endeavored to achieve this by increasing the pelvic curve, bringing the shanks together at the root of the blades, adding an upward curve to the handle and, of greatest importance, introducing a perineal curve, or "step" (Figure 7.11).

Gunning S. Bedford (1806–1870), having previously worked in South Carolina, was a major influence in the foundation of the Medical College at the University of New York, where he became the Foundation Professor of Obstetrics and was a well-known teacher. In his *Principles and Practice of Obstetrics* (1861) he illustrated his obstetric case, comprised of forceps, vectis, perforator, and guarded crotchet.

He claimed that the forceps, shown in Figure 7.12, embodied some important improvements, particularly in regard to the lightness and thinness of the blades. He adopted

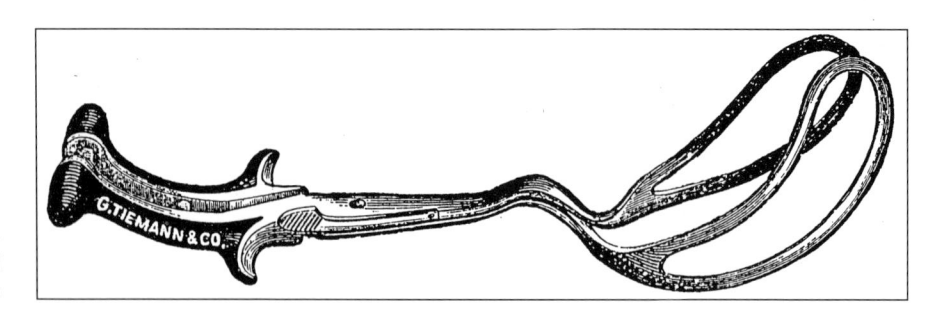

FIGURE 7.11.
Schuyler's forceps. Note particularly the perineal step. (Schuyler, 1884)

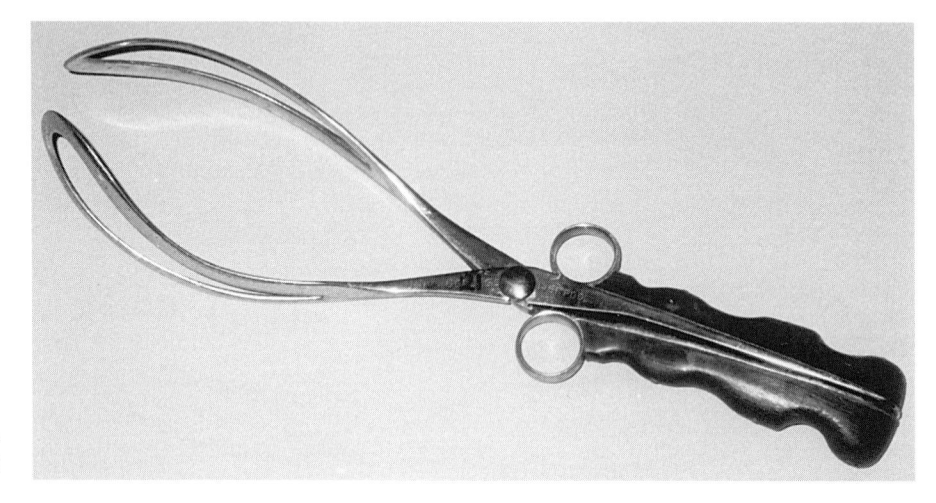

FIGURE 7.12.
Bedford's forceps. (University of Liverpool)

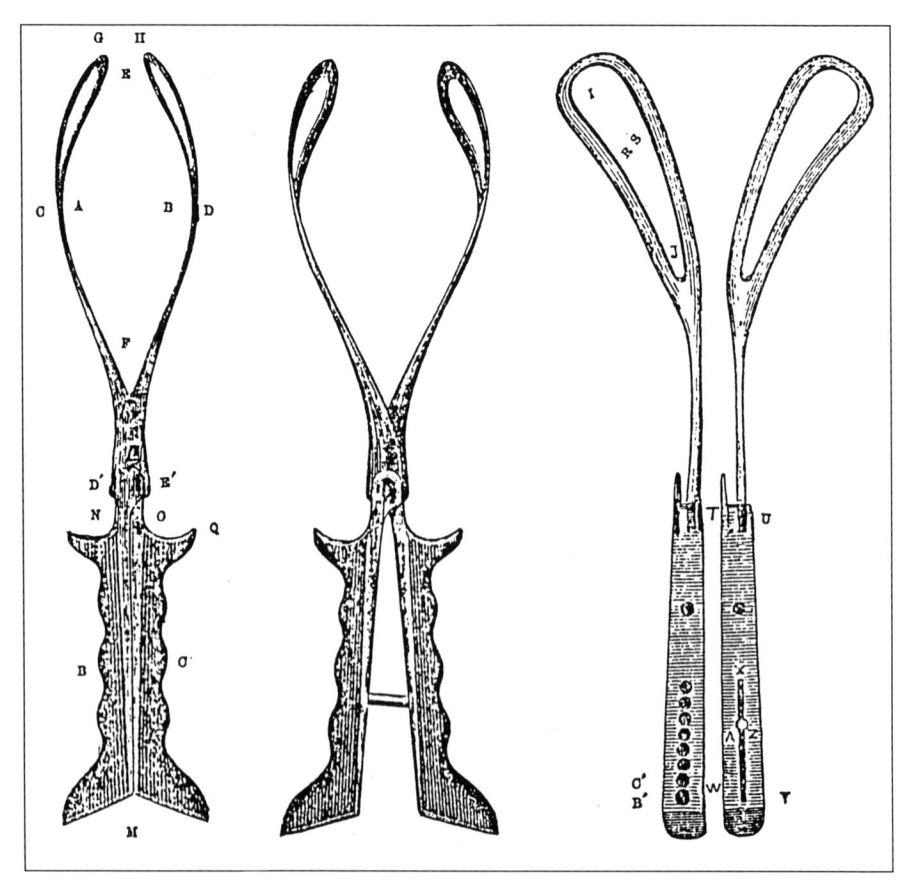

FIGURE 7.13.
Elliot's forceps. His design was based on J. Y. Simpson's long forceps but with modified handles incorporating a pressure-regulating device. (Elliot, 1858)

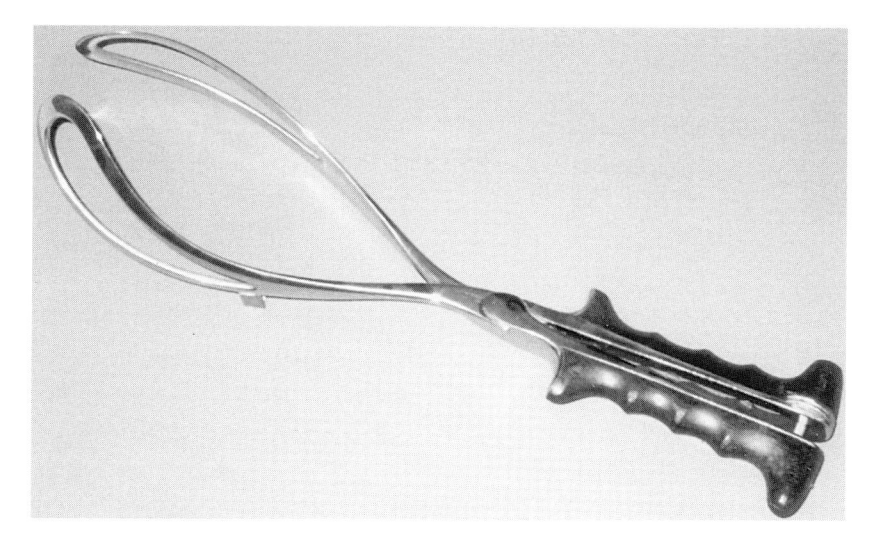

FIGURES 7.14, 7.15.
Elliot's forceps. Figure 7.15 shows the detail of the later pressure-regulating mechanism. (RCOG)

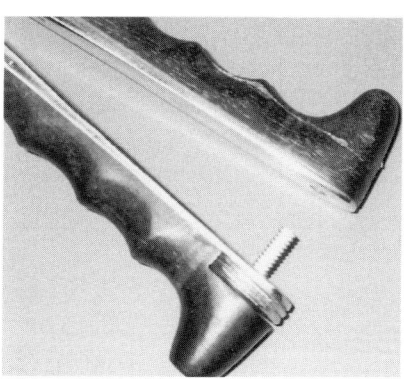

the Brunninghausen lock with a pin and pivot articulation, which had been popularized by F. C. Naegele (Chapter 5), and the handles had a terminal curve and proximal finger rings to give better direction and more traction power. He certainly did not lack confidence in the value or popularity of his instrument and claimed that the principal instrument makers informed him that they received more orders for his forceps than for any other. Later, in 1874, E. O. F. Roler, a founder of the Chicago Gynecological Society, designed a similar but heavier forceps with finger rings; this instrument was illustrated by Tiemann.

Parallel Shanks

Parallel shanks of the Simpson type were relatively uncommon in American designs, most examples originating from New York practitioners. William Alexander Norman Dorland (1864–1956) of Philadelphia, Assistant Demonstrator of Obstetrics at the University of Pennsylvania, claimed in his 1896 textbook that while the instruments of Hodge and Wallace were long and slender, and therefore had more compressing power, in Philadelphia, where the European tradition of practice dominated, Simpson's forceps were steadily gaining favor in spite of their shorter length. Although Tarnier's forceps were most often used for axis traction Dorland took the view that one could just as well use tapes on Simpson's or any other long forceps.

G. T. Elliot (1827–1871), a physician at Bellevue Hospital in New York, had started his training in Dublin in 1849 and was well experienced in practical obstetrics. He recorded that he had owned ten different forceps and used others loaned by friends, as well as Simpson's Air-Tractor (Chapter 15) on two occasions. He expressed a preference for Simpson's long forceps but in 1858 he gave a lecture on the desirable features of forceps and a Mr. Ford offered to make a model for him, which turned out to be useful and eventually came into common use in New York.

The instrument was 385 millimeters (15.25 inches) long and was based on Simpson's long forceps but was of lighter construction and had wooden handles, with both proximal and distal finger grips that were large enough to be grasped by both hands (Figure 7.13). The most innovative feature, as far as American design was concerned, was the sliding pivot

AMERICAN FORCEPS: 19TH CENTURY **105**

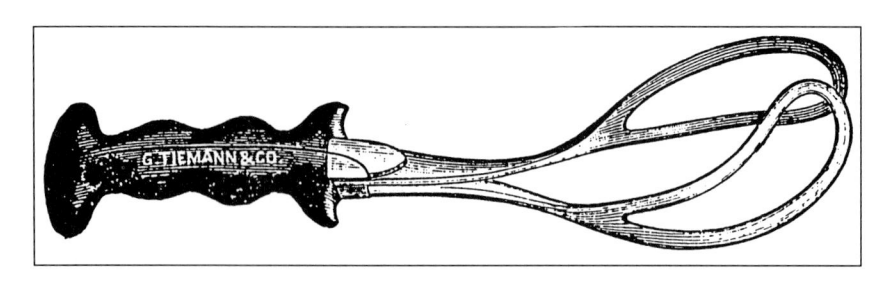

FIGURE 7.16.
Jewett's forceps. An updated version of Elliot's forceps without the pressure-regulating device. The handles are sheathed with vulcanized rubber. (Jewett, 1885)

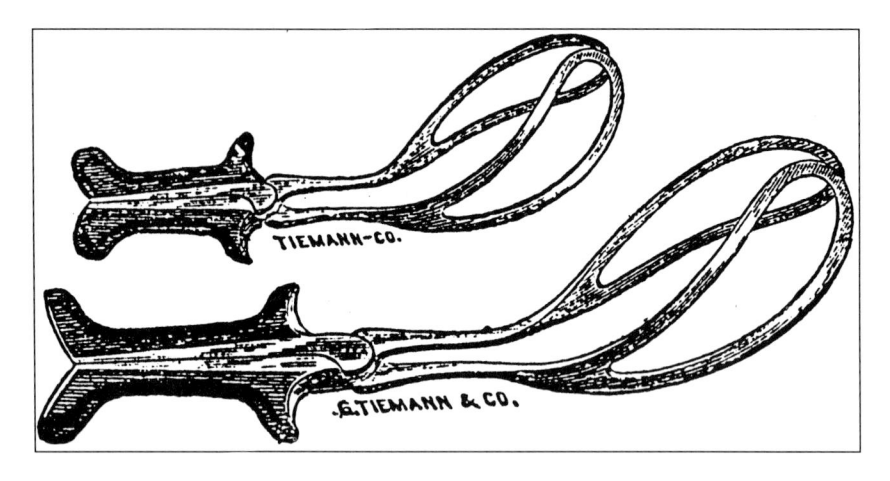

FIGURE 7.17.
Jenks's short and long forceps. The long forceps had exceptionally long blades. The handles are also of hard rubber. (Jenks, 1879)

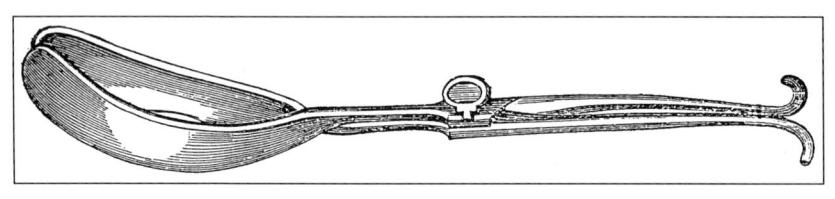

FIGURE 7.18.
Knight's forceps. The main features are the slender nonfenestrated blades with a reduced pelvic curve (1860).

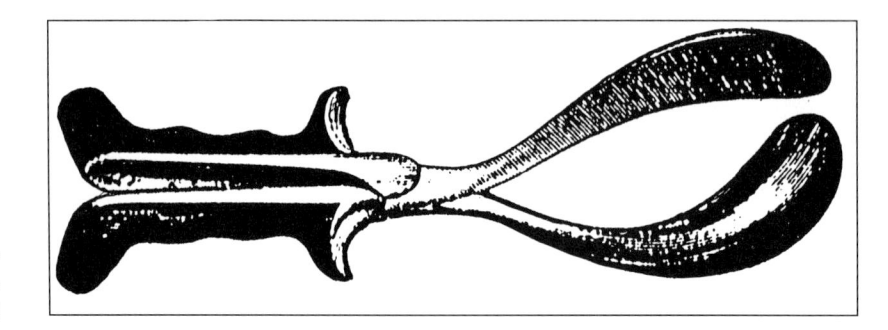

FIGURE 7.19.
McLane's forceps (original design). (Tiemann, 1889)

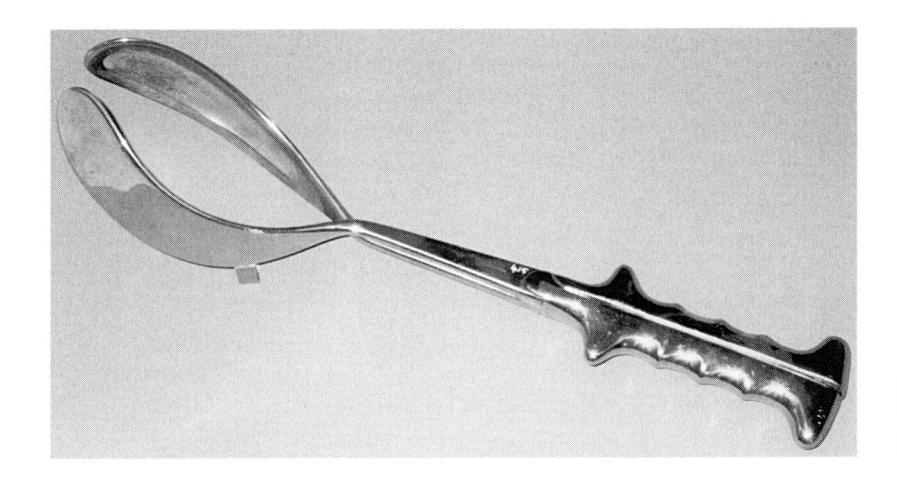

FIGURE 7.20.
Tucker-McLane forceps. Note the elongation of the shank. (RCOG)

that could be moved along a groove in the handle to fit into sockets in the other handle, thus limiting the approximation of the blades and the pressure exerted on the fetal head, even when a two-handed grip was used. A later model had an extending screw that fit into a socket in the other handle (Figures 7.14–7.15). This model was similar to the labimeters of Aitken and von Froriep that had been popular in Europe but by this time had largely been abandoned (Chapter 5). However, Elliot did not give any acknowledgment to these predecessors.

Charles Jewett (1839–1910), a professor of obstetrics and diseases of children at Long Island College Hospital, New York, updated Elliot's forceps in 1885 to meet modern sanitary needs by enveloping the handles with a sheath of vulcanized rubber (Figure 7.16). He also did away with the pressure-regulating pivot. Jewett subsequently designed his own axis-traction forceps (Chapter 13).

William Lusk (1838–1897) of Bellevue Hospital Medical College, New York, used a modified Simpson's long forceps, made for him in New York, that were based on a pair he brought with him from Edinburgh in 1865. His comment in his textbook of 1882 was that "A good pair of long forceps renders the possession of short forceps a superfluous luxury." He also noted that the forceps of Hodge, Wallace, and White were extensively used in America. He later improved and modified Tarnier's axis-traction forceps (Chapter 13).

Edward W. Jenks (1833–1903), also from New York, who was, among other things, the founder and first president of the Detroit College of Medicine, constructed both long and short forceps with parallel shanks (1879) (Figure 7.17). The long forceps (406 millimeters/16 inches) had exceptionally long blades and had finger rests at both ends of the handles.

Solid Blades
Samuel Thomas Knight (1817–1881) of Baltimore claimed in his 1860 article that the forceps in general use at that time were deficient for several reasons:

(1) the pelvic curve was excessive;

(2) the fenestra created a need for too much metal at the point of curvature, increasing the risk of perineal trauma;

(3) the large size of the fenestra allowed too free a protrusion of the parietal eminences through them (contrary to current perceived wisdom in relation to Davis's blades as related by Meigs); and

(4) the fenestra unnecessarily increased the width of the blades.

He also noted that the only forceps kept in stock by the instrument makers at that time were Davis's and Hodge's, a definite indication of their popularity.

Knight therefore designed his forceps with long, slender, nonfenestrated blades, with an increased convexity but a reduced pelvic curve, and a gradual taper from the handles to the blades (Figure 7.18).

James W. McLane (1839–1912), who was instrumental in getting the Sloane Maternity Hospital built in New York, favored long forceps with solid blades. His first design appeared in 1868 but he never published a description and an illustration did not appear in Tiemann's catalogue until 1880 (Figure 7.19). In the 1891 *Report of the Sloane Hospital* McLane's forceps had been used in 81 of the 83 forceps cases, including the first one ever performed at Sloane (Speert, 1963). Their subsequent popularity was enhanced when a resident physician at Sloane, Ervin A. Tucker (1862–1902), increased the length of the shank. In the twentieth century Ralph Herbert Luikart of Nebraska (b. 1889) made further modifications (Figure 7.20).

. . .

At the beginning of the nineteenth century obstetricians in America had been mainly dependent on instruments imported from Europe, the types of instruments used being influenced by their own origins and those of their forebears. The designs soon came to be copied locally, with modifications introduced by the obstetricians or instrument makers so that instruments often showed both British and Continental influences. Original designs that had the most influence on subsequent developments were, in the early years, Haighton's, followed by that of David Davis from Britain; and those of Baudelocque and Siebold from Continental Europe.

Later in the century, a number of European innovations, such as hinged and detachable handles, asymmetric forceps, and parallel forceps had their influence on American design and these are discussed in the appropriate chapters that follow. The most important advance was the development of axis traction. American obstetricians initially took up the designs from Europe but subsequently made their own modifications, which will be discussed in Chapters 13 and 14.

HINGED AND DETACHABLE HANDLES AND BLADES AND OTHER ARTICULATIONS

Modifications intended to make forceps more convenient and easier to use, in the context of contemporary practice but incorporating existing well-tried features of blade design, appeared sporadically from the late eighteenth century onward. To achieve these objectives, most of the changes involved making blades or handles demountable or hinged.

The first mention of a forceps with a jointed blade is in William Giffard's *Cases in Midwifery* (1734), where he illustrated a hinged forceps ascribed to John Freke (or Freake) (1688–1756). of St. Bartholomew's Hospital but there is no mention of the purpose or function of the hinge (Chapter 2, Figures 2.7, 2.8).

In Britain toward the end of the eighteenth century the problems encountered with inserting the right blade of the forceps with the patient in the left lateral position prompted the introduction of handles that were hinged or jointed at the shank. In Europe jointed blades were adopted to provide versatility in combinations of blades and handles of different length. In other cases the articulation was primarily to provide convenience and portability. Later, handles were jointed in the vertical plane to provide a perineal curve and/or to improve axis traction. The latter are described in the chapter on the development of axis traction (Chapter 12).

Hinged and Detachable Handles

Primarily for Transport and Storage

In about 1791 Mathias Saxtorph (1740–1800), a professor of obstetrics in Copenhagen, introduced a long forceps that combined Levret's blades with Smellie's handles, but in addition the handles were hinged and folded on to the blades specifically to facilitate transport (Figure 8.1). They were described in his works, which were edited by his son, Johan Sylvester, in 1804. The Saxtorph type of forceps continued to be used by Danish obstetricians during the early nineteenth century and a number of instrument makers took up the idea.

C. E. M. Levy succeeded the younger Saxtorph in Copenhagen in 1840 and modified the original design, combining Saxtorph's handle with Naegele's blades and added folding finger rests (Figure 8.2). Levy's forceps came to be widely used in Denmark for many years and were exhibited at the Obstetrical Society *Conversazione* in London in 1866 (Chapter 6). Doran (1921) gives a detailed description of this large instrument, which was 420 millimeters (16.5 inches) long and weighed 666 grams (1 pound, 8 ounces).

In Britain folding forceps primarily for the sake of facilitating portability only began to appear with the commoner use of long forceps in the second half of the nineteenth century; many of these were modified Simpson's or Barnes's forceps, without identification of the modifiers (Chapter 6). The hinges in the shanks were sometimes oriented to fold horizontally (Figures 8.3, 8.4) and sometimes vertically, as in Pearse's (1887) forceps (Figure 8.5).

John Noble Bredin of Kent also inserted hinges in the shanks to allow the blades to be folded back on the handles for ease of transport (Figure 8.6). In addition he added a winged screw nut on the end of the handle to avoid the need for a bandage or tape to keep the blades in apposition. He also concealed in one handle a stylet for rupturing the membranes. He claimed that such an instrument "must certainly prove a boon, at least to the country practitioner who has

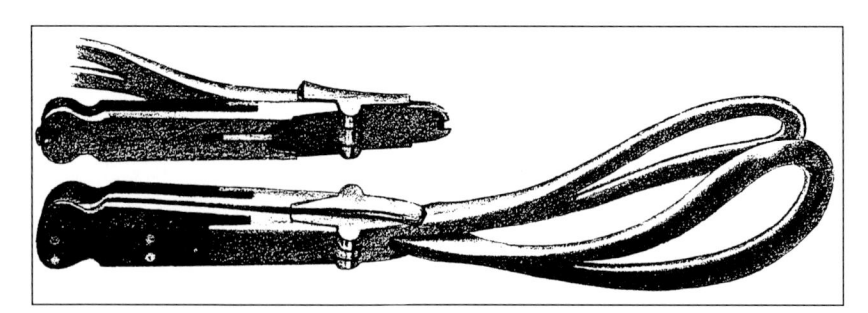

FIGURE 8.1.
Saxtorph's forceps. An early example of European forceps, hinged to facilitate transport. (D. W. H. Busch, 1841)

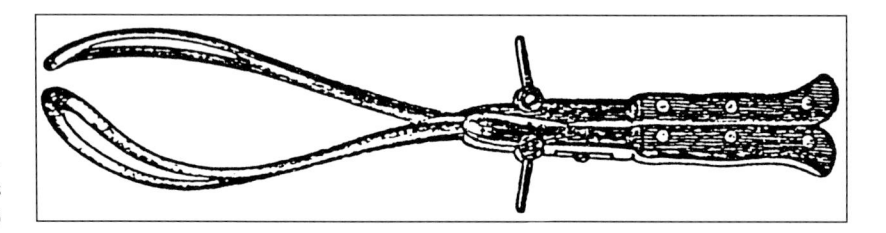

FIGURE 8.2.
Levy's forceps. A combination of Saxtorph's handles and Naegele's blades. (Meadows, 1867)

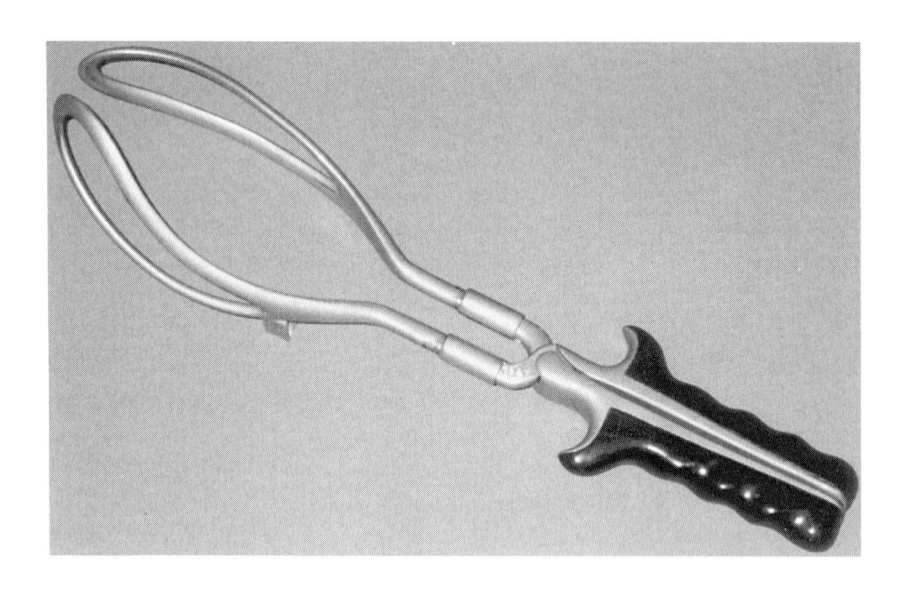

FIGURES 8.3, 8.4.
Hinged modification of Simpson's forceps (origin unidentified). Sliding collars conceal the hinges and serve as locks to give rigidity to the shanks. (RCOG)

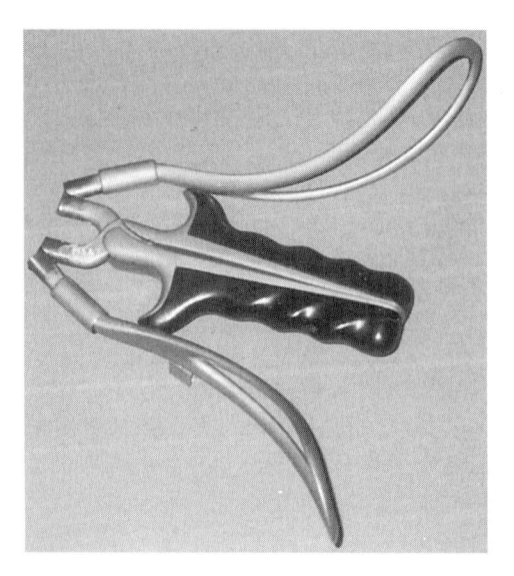

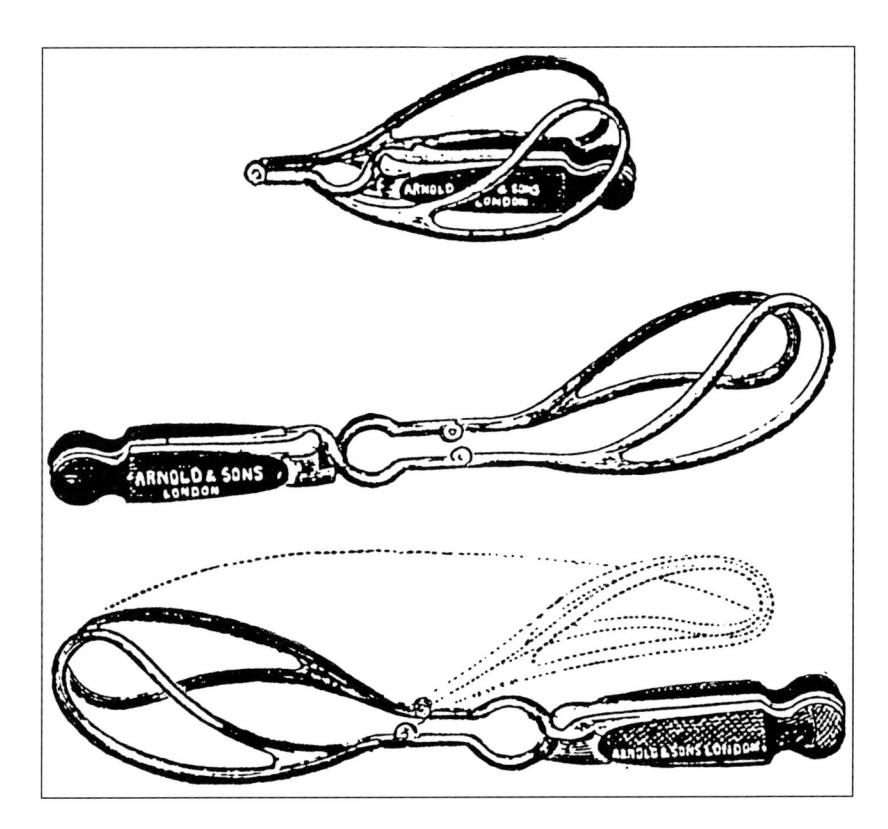

FIGURE 8.5.
Pearse's forceps. A vertically hinged modification of Barnes's forceps to facilitate transport. (Arnold and Sons, 1885)

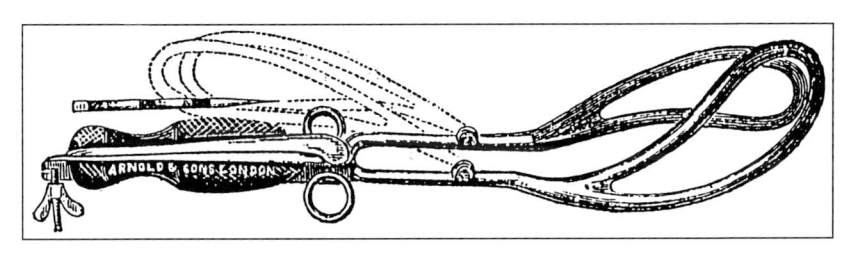

FIGURE 8.6.
Bredin's forceps. A similar hinge to that of Pearse, but with finger rings and a winged screw to keep the blades in apposition. Note the stylet for rupturing membranes, lodged in the handle. (Bredin, 1889)

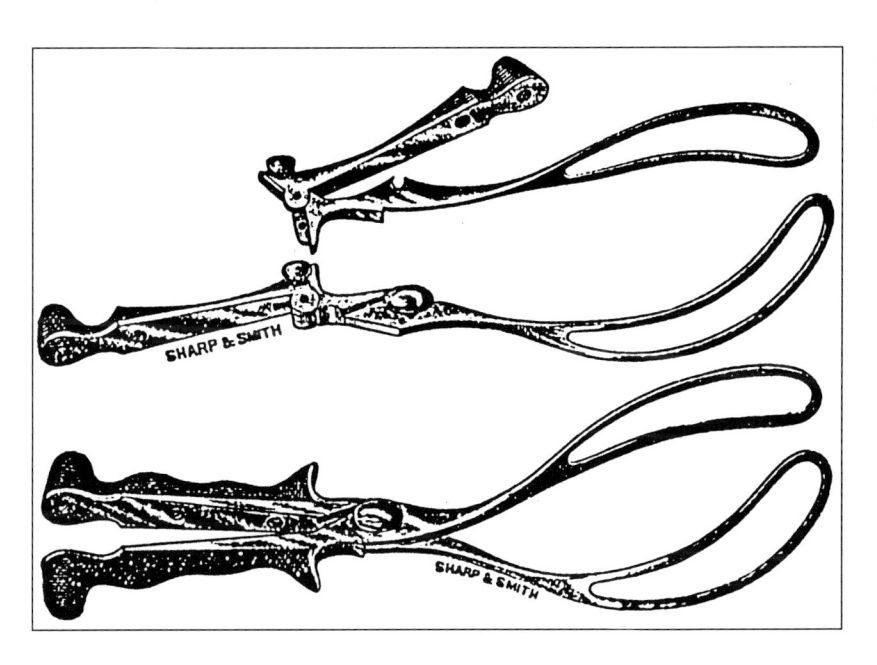

FIGURE 8.7.
Miller's jointed forceps. Laterally folding handles, also designed for portability. (Parvin, 1890)

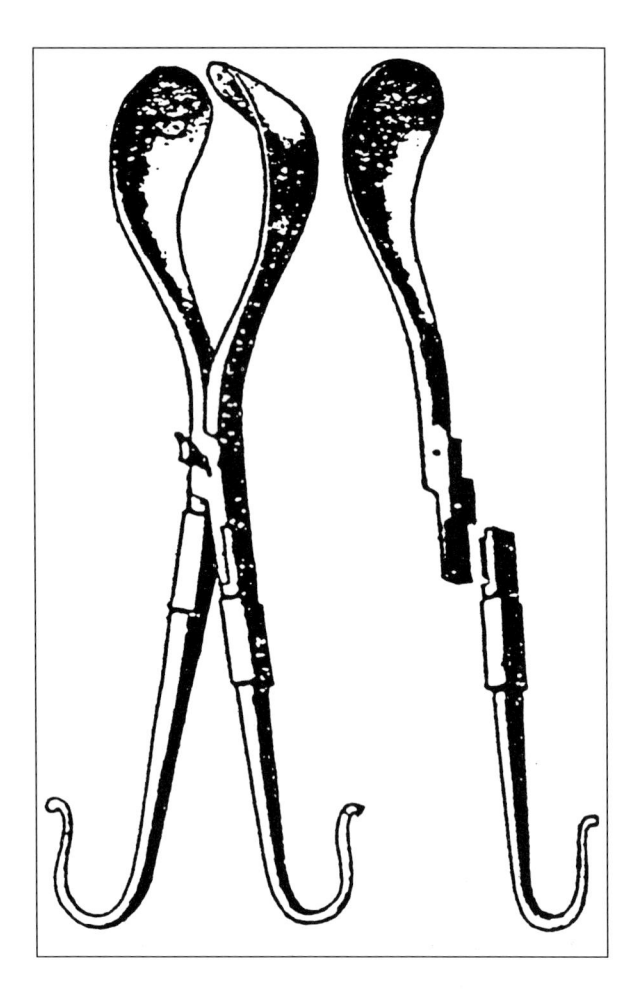

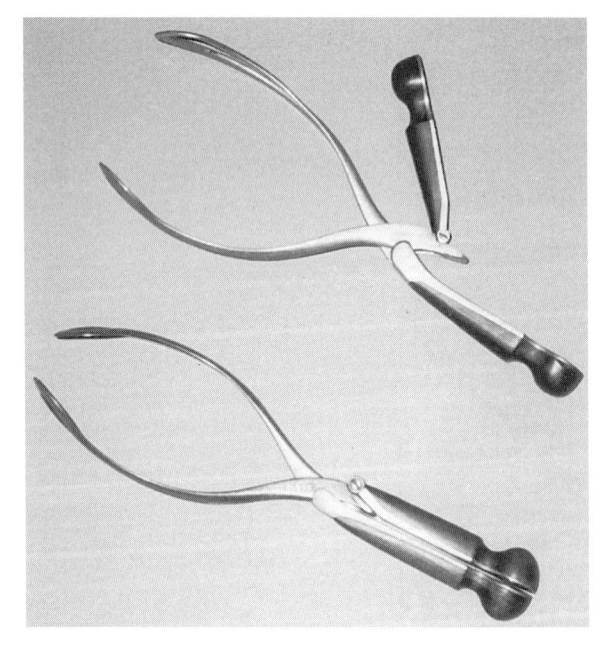

no doubt like myself, found himself seated perhaps on a restive horse with a long forceps dangling against its sides, on a dark night and on a dangerous road." (1889)

In America De Laskie Miller (1880; see Parvin, 1890) of Rush Medical College in Chicago designed a folding long forceps with a Brunninghausen-type articulation and folding handles. The finger lugs were split and hinged so that the handles folded inward for portability (Figure 8.7).

The virtues of detachable handles for portability were extolled by James Cappie (see below), although his forceps were designed primarily to facilitate insertion. Valette of Lyons also had detachable handles for his parallel forceps, which are described in Chapter 10.

Joints to Facilitate Insertion of the Forceps

Probably the earliest forceps made with separate blades and handles to facilitate insertion of the blades were designed by Jens Bing and were described by his pupil, Johan Gottfried Janck (1724–1763) in 1750 (Figure 8.8). The very long handles were attached after insertion of the nonfenestrated blades, which were similar in design to Palfyn's *mains de fer* and included a screw articulation. Janck said that Bing's objective was not so much ease of application as the sparing of the feelings of the patient since unnecessary exposure was avoided. Doran (1913d) reviewed the literature and concluded that the instrument was unfavorably received and never used outside Bing's own clinic. Levret, in particular, gave a long and unfavorable critique, denying the advantages that had been claimed by Janck (1751).

Alexander and James Hamilton introduced forceps with a hinged handle, based on the well-established Edinburgh design of R. W. Johnson (Chapter 4). There were numerous modifications of Hamilton's forceps and these have been described by Doran (1913d). The common feature was a hinged joint on one handle, close to the lock, with a pin or screw mechanism for fixing the handle in position. In some examples the hinge was in the left blade and in others the right. Most commonly, and probably Hamilton's original design and intention, the right blade was hinged outward to facilitate its insertion with the patient on her left side (Figures 8.9; 8.11, right). But the purpose of some of the other variations that originated from various makers, such as a hinged left blade or one blade hinged inward, are not easy to explain. Hinges on both blades may have been used to aid portability (see under "Primarily for Transport and Storage" above).

Although handles that were hinged or detachable for ease of insertion were in vogue for a relatively short time they continued to be used in Britain into the first half of the nineteenth century. David Davis (1825) added a hinge with a spring catch to the shank of the right blade of his common forceps (Figures 8.10; 8.11, left; see also Chapter 5). However, his successor at University College, Edward Murphy, claimed in 1862 that "it was quite unsuited for practitioners and obstetricians unless of long experience," an attitude difficult to understand in relation to a modification that clearly facilitated its insertion.

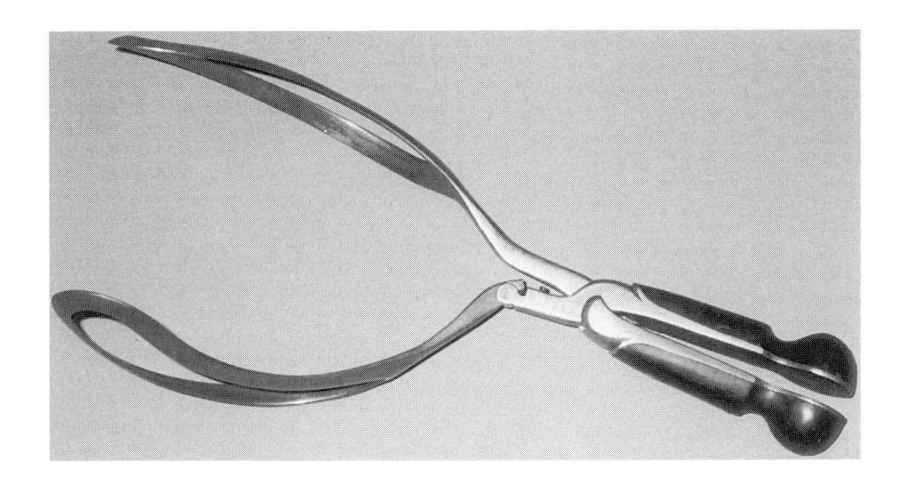

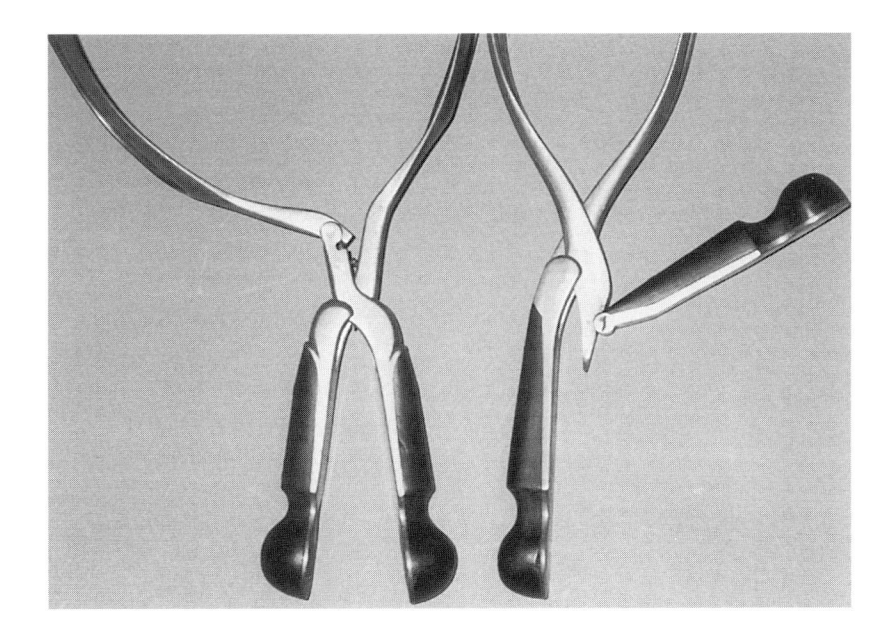

J. T. Conquest (1789–1866), who was Obstetric Physician to the City of London Lying-in Hospital and a lecturer at St. Bartholomew's Hospital, redesigned the short forceps, based on Haighton's forceps with wide fenestra and a perineal curve (1820) (Figure 8.12). His notable innovation was a screw joint on the handle of the blade that was applied uppermost. "One will at once acknowledge that extreme difficulty often presents itself to the introduction of the upper blade, in conse-

FIGURE 8.8 (OPPOSITE TOP).
Bing's forceps. The long detachable handles were to facilitate insertion and "to spare the patient's feelings." (Kilian, 1835)

FIGURE 8.9 (OPPOSITE).
Hamilton's forceps. In this version the right blade is hinged outward. (RCOG)

FIGURE 8.10 (TOP).
Davis's hinged forceps. The hinge is in the shank. There is a sliding pin locking mechanism. (RCOG)

FIGURE 8.11 (ABOVE).
Davis's and Hamilton's forceps. Detail of the joints. Left: Davis. Right: Hamilton. (RCOG)

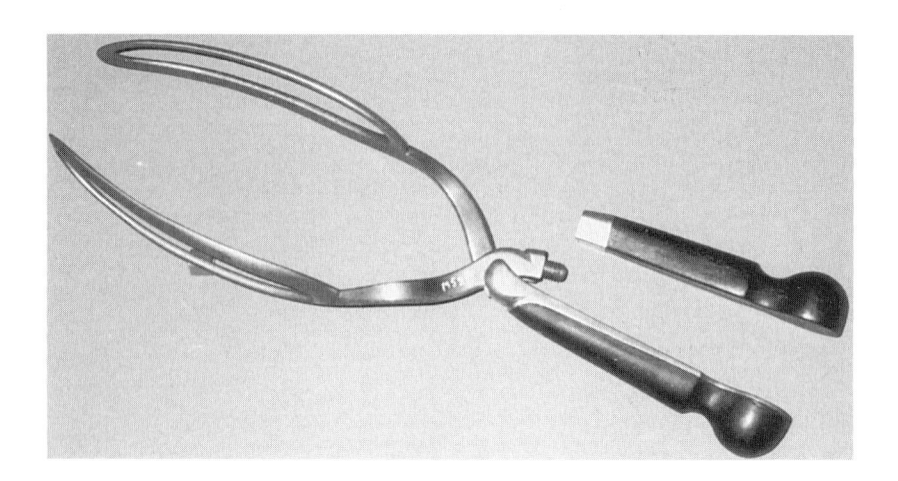

FIGURE 8.12.
Conquest's forceps. These forceps are based on Haighton's but have a detachable handle with a screw joint on the blade to be applied uppermost. (RCOG)

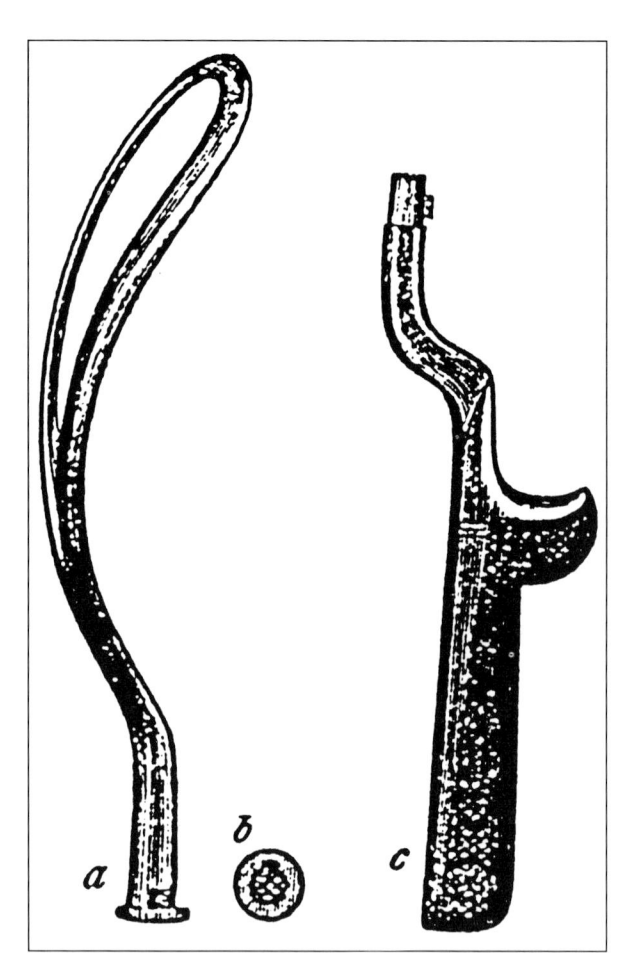

FIGURE 8.13.
Cappie's forceps. A Simpson-type forceps with a bayonet joint in the shank. It was intended to facilitate insertion and to improve portability. (Cappie, 1872)

114   CHAPTER 8

quence of the bed and mattress below preventing that depression of the handle which is essential to the elevation of the point of the blade, to carry it over the vertex." He considered that the alternatives, either to insert the blade in the hollow of the sacrum and "wander" it or to reposition the woman on her back, were unacceptable. The latter he described as "a disgusting and inelegant position, because the woman must stare her accoucheur in the face." His solution, the idea for which he acknowledged came from levers designed with movable handles, was "a moveable handle, by means of a screw . . . with the handle detached, there can be no difficulty in introducing the upper blade of the short forceps, directly over the side of the head, without changing the position of the patient. After the blade is fixed, of course the handle is to be screwed on, and the instrument used as any other."

James Cappie (d. 1889) of Edinburgh described a modification of Simpson's long forceps in which the handles and shanks were detachable from the roots of the blades (1863, 1872). In his later version the shanks had a bayonet joint with a nipple that fit into a socket at the root of the blade and was locked in position by a spring-loaded collar that fit into a lip on the nipple (Figure 8.13). While the instrument was designed to facilitate insertion, the virtue of its portability, as compared with other long forceps, was also emphasized, "the blades to be conveniently carried in one coat pocket, and the handles in the other" (1863). In the following discussion Cappie pointed out that Hamilton's forceps had soon fallen into disuse, while Alexander Keiller feared that the blades might "roll about in the vagina" or even pass right up into the uterine cavity and in both circumstances it would be difficult to attach the handles. A. R. Simpson disliked instruments that were vulnerable to damage, especially at the joints, and could get out of repair more easily than others. He favored inserting the right blade into the hollow of the sacrum and wandering it into position, or even putting the patient on her back! In spite of this cool reception Cappie was still promoting his forceps with a simplified bayonet joint in a paper in 1872, with much the same response in the discussion among the members of the Edinburgh Obstetric Society that followed the presentation of the original paper. In the same year David Gordon (1816–1886) also promoted a short forceps with detachable handles at a meeting of the Edinburgh Obstetrical Society, but they likewise received a cool reception and do not seem to have been used by anyone else.

A European multipurpose variant was designed by J. Carof of Brest (1869). The blades and handles were separate, as were the articulations, so that different combinations were possible (Figure 8.14). Thus they could be used as either a

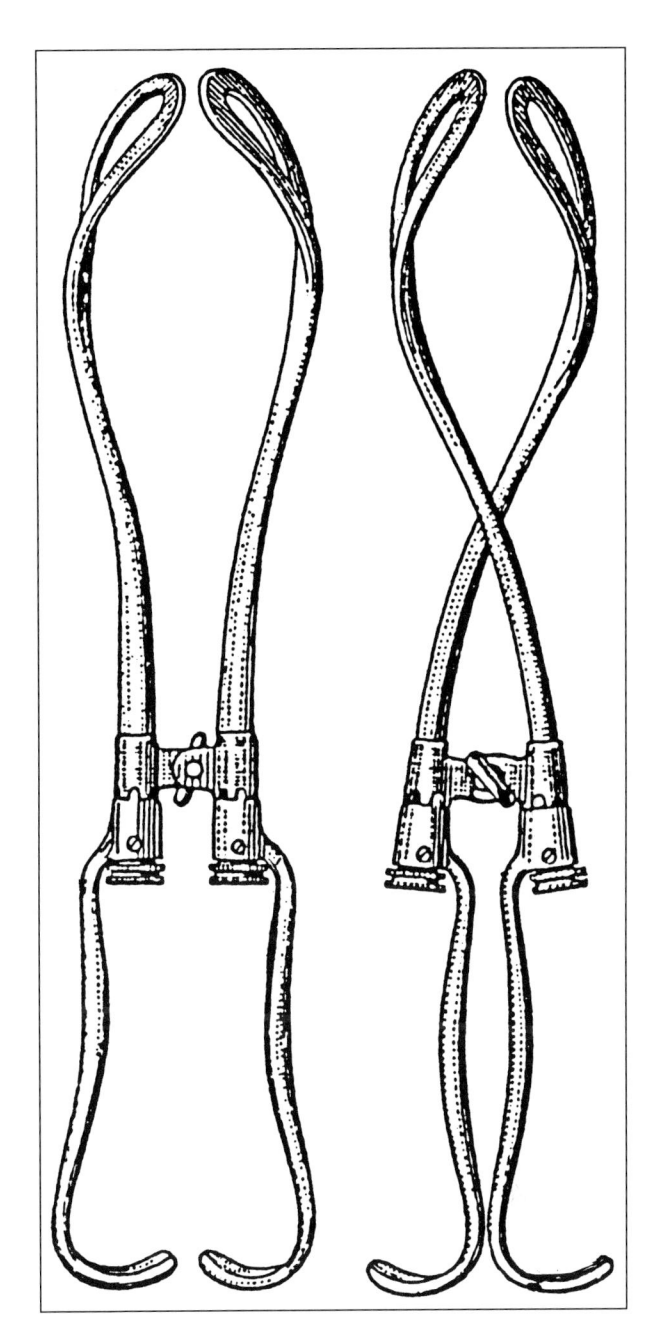

FIGURE 8.14.
Carof's forceps. This complex and impractical design was intended to be used in a variety of modes. (Tarnier and Budin, 1901)

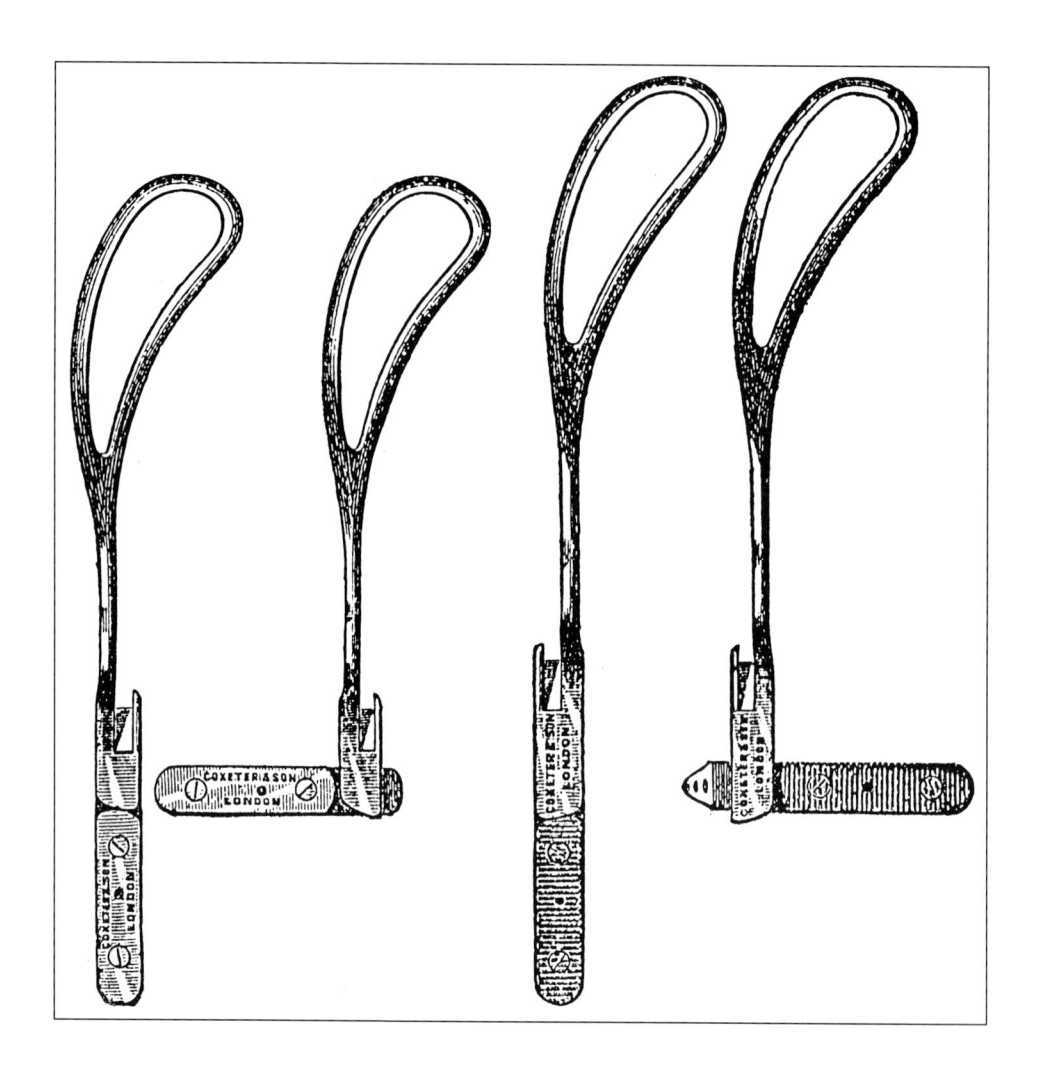

FIGURE 8.15.
Haslam's and Blenkarne's forceps. Left: Haslam. The lock is reversed and the handle of the right blade hinges backward. Right: Blenkarne. A similar design but longer and with the handle hinged forward. (Blenkarne, 1889)

crossed or parallel forceps or the blades could be introduced together. However, they met with much criticism and little favor. Das quotes from a paper by Wasseige in which the latter states that they were too complicated, too difficult to clean, and too expensive, and that the multifunctional uses were rarely required.

In 1887 W. D. Haslam of University College Hospital, London, also attempted to facilitate the introduction of the upper blade by reversing the crossover lock and inserting a hinge at the root of the handle on the right, or upper, blade, which enabled it to be turned backward to an angle of 90 degrees (Figure 8.15, left). The original model was a shortened version of Simpson's forceps but later (1889) Aveling-type handles were attached, which reputedly improved their function (Chapter 12).

W. L'Heureux Blenkarne of Birmingham was critical of the Haslam type of forceps when used by practitioners who preferred the application of the lower blade first and claimed that as the handle hinged toward the perineum it was obstructive (1889). His minor contribution was to lengthen the

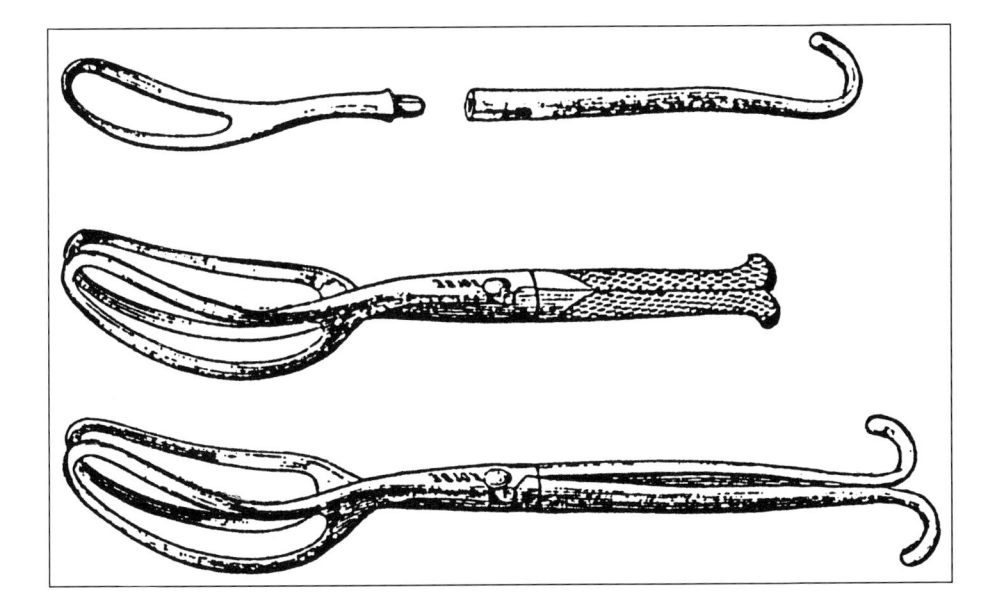

FIGURE 8.16.
Smith's forceps with interchangeable long and short handles. The joint is a pivot and ratchet. (Mann and Hirst, 1889)

FIGURE 8.17.
Stuart's forceps. The basic design is a pair of short forceps with Simpson blades and a ratchet closure. The long handles have a groove *D* with a pin *B*, which fit over the short handles. They are held in place by a thumb screw. (Stuart, 1877)

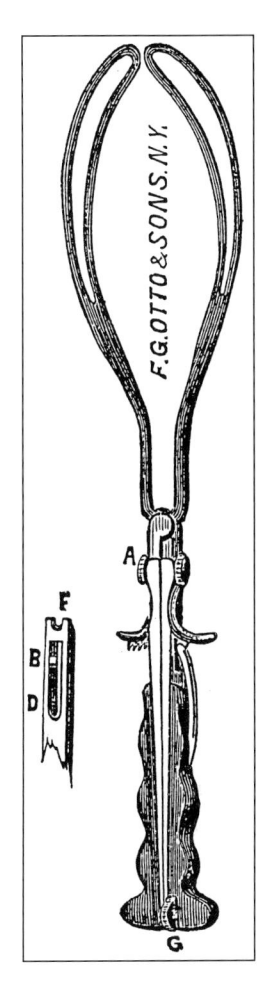

forceps and alter the hinge to allow the handle to be turned forward toward the pubes rather than backward (Figure 8.15, right). He maintained that this was nonobstructive and gave a good grasp for the hand when adjusting the position of the blade.

Forceps with Short and Long Handles
Albert Holmes Smith (1835–1885) of Philadelphia, better known for his modification of the Hodge pessary, constructed a forceps with two sets of handles (1879). They were also described by M. D. Mann and B. C. Hirst (1889) (Figure 8.16) and were based on Davis's blades. The handles were attached to the blades by a pivot and ratchet. The main purpose of the long handles was to increase the compression power.

Another American instrument with interchangeable handles was devised by Francis H. Stuart of Brooklyn, who described a pair of multipurpose forceps in 1877 (Figure 8.17). They were based on Simpson's long blades but had an Elliott-type lock and short handles, the overall length being 305 millimeters (12 inches). When long forceps were required longer handles could be fit over the short handles, increasing the overall length to 420 millimeters (16.5 inches). The extension handle was attached by means of a pin that fit into a slot on the short handle and was secured by a countersunk end fitting under a thumbscrew. Additional features were a ratchet catch on the handle and a terminal compression screw.

Interchangeable Blades
The idea of having detachable blades so that different blades could be used on the same handles originated with the French and descriptions of these *forceps brisés* are given in the textbooks of Charpentier (1883) and Tarnier and Budin (1901) and by Doran (1921).

The first dismountable handles were described by P. V. Coutouly (1738–1814) in 1777. He was a prolific designer and refiner of his own instruments and he published an account of his jointed *forceps brisé* in 1808. These are illustrated in Figure 8.18. They were of heavy construction and carefully

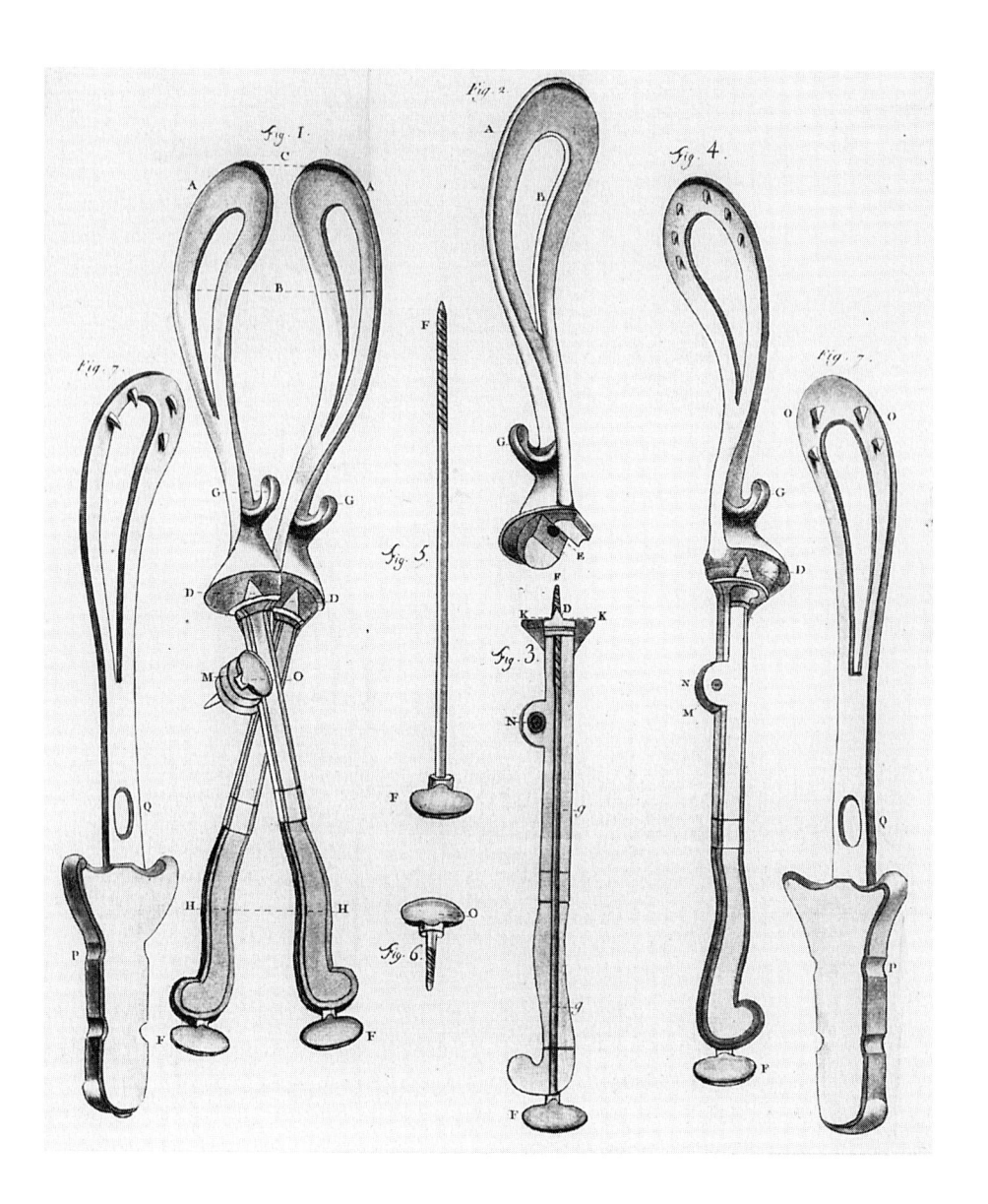

FIGURE 8.18.
Coutouly's *forceps brisé* and *crochets à dents*. Figures 1–6 show the forceps with alternative blades. Figure 7 shows the toothed crotchets. (Coutouly, 1808)

engineered (Figures 1–4), with the handles attached to the blades by a slotted and grooved joint, fixed by a long screw passing the length of the handle (Figure 5). The hinge is also of unusual heavy construction, with a wing nut (Figure 6). As well as the hooks at the ends of the handles, two heavy hooks were incorporated in the bases of the blades. Clearly they were intended for considerable tractive force and the reason for the detachable handles appears to be to enable the use of alternative blades that had internal teeth (Figure 4) and would be used for extracting the dead fetus. Also shown are his *crochets à dents* (Figure 7).

In 1817 Brulatour, Professor of Medicine at the University of Bordeaux, introduced a forceps based on the Levret design, with long heavy blades and a marked pelvic curve. They had three sets of interchangeable blades in which the roots

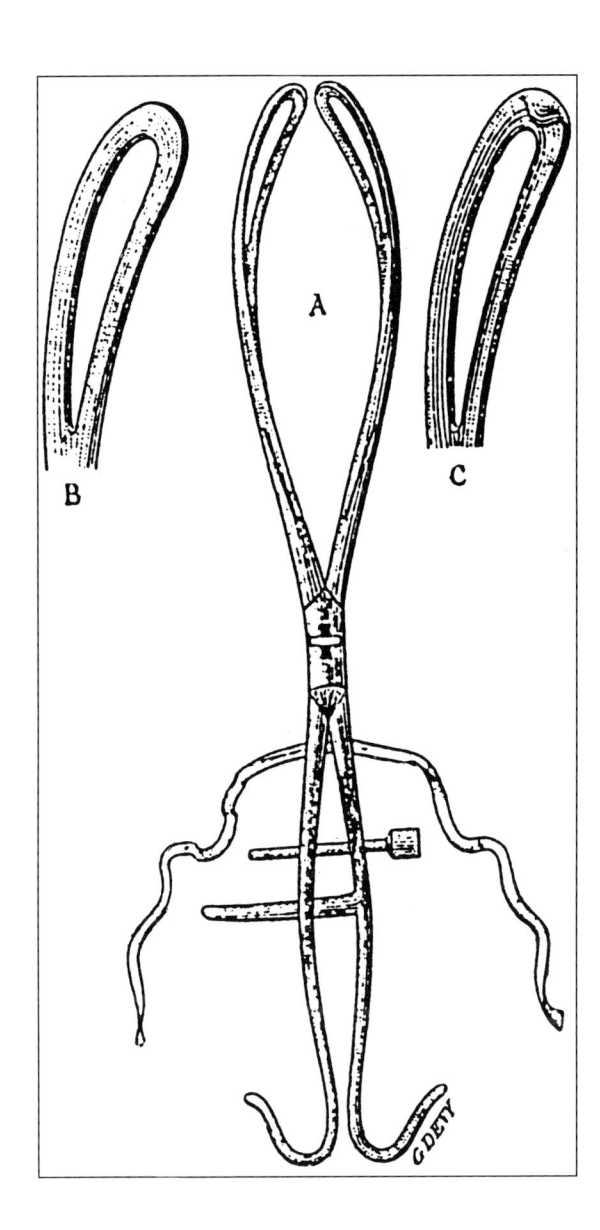

FIGURE 8.19.
Brulatour's forceps with interchangeable blades. Basically a Levret-type forceps with three different interchangeable blades. Note the pressure-regulating device (see also Chapter 6). (Tarnier and Budin, 1901)

FIGURE 8.20.
Pajot's *forceps brisés*. The blades were intended to be interchangeable but because of their great length (420mm/16ins) the joint was also a benefit to portability. Note also the protected point of the crotchet at the end of one handle. (Science Museum, London)

of the blades dovetailed into the shanks (Figure 8.19). Additional features were a tape passing through openings in the handles, a pressure-regulating screw, and a scale to show the degree of separation of the blades.

Charles Pajot (1816–1896), a professor at the University of Paris, invented *forceps à branches désarticulées (forceps brisé)* that were described by Charpentier and appeared in several catalogues of the day (Figure 8.20). They achieved great popularity, largely because of the simple articulation known as "Péan's aseptic joint" (Figure 8.21), which subsequently came to be used on forceps of many different patterns, such as the *forceps brisé à quatre cuillières modèle de la Charité de Lyon,* manufactured by Maison Mathieu of Paris and Lyons. Although these forceps were designed with interchangeable blades, most commentaries on them extol the virtue of portability, an important consideration with an instrument that was 420 millimeters (16.5 inches) long.

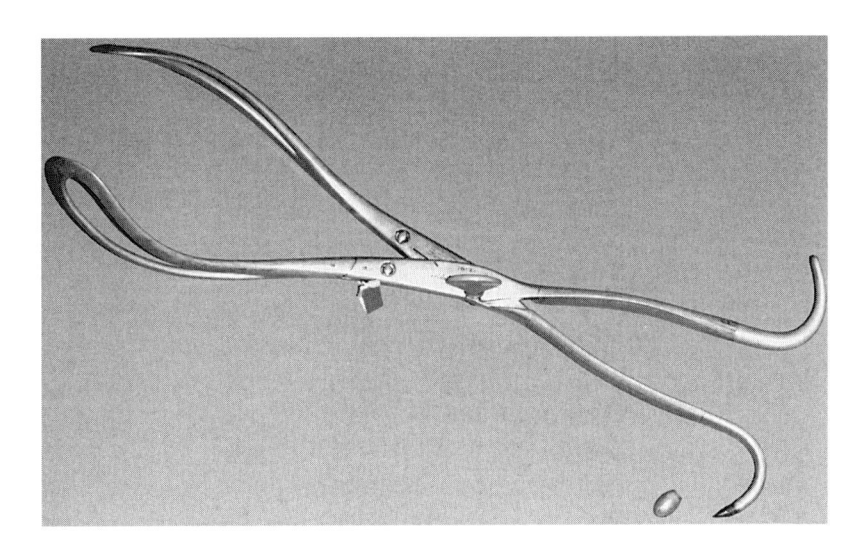

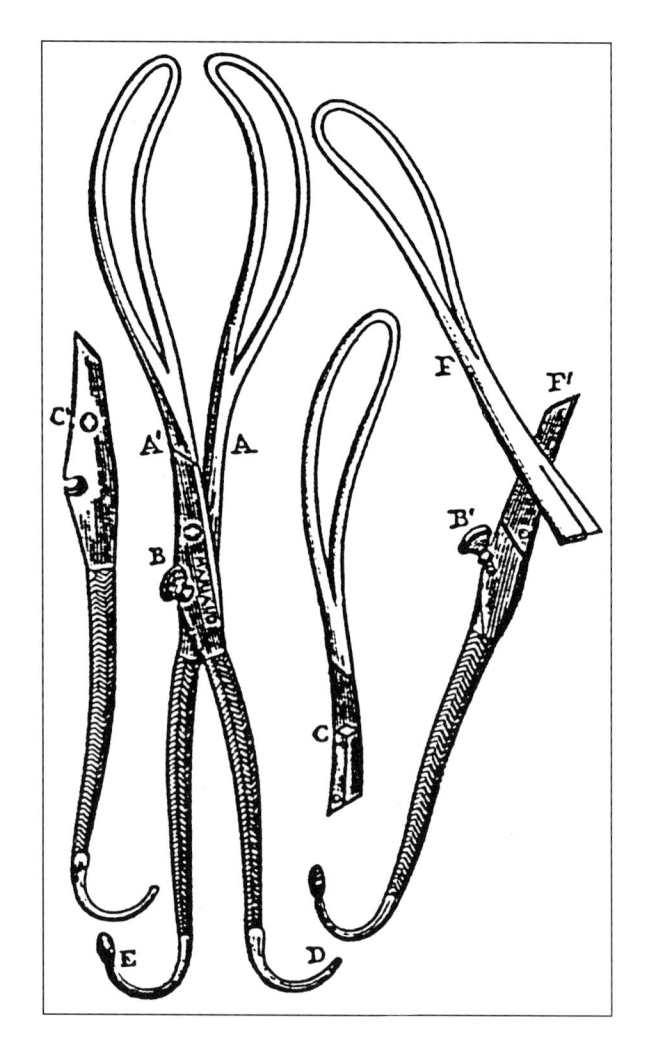

FIGURE 8.21.
Pajot's *forceps brisés*. The aseptic joint and alternative blades are shown. (Mariaud, circa 1875)

FIGURE 8.22.
Burge's forceps. The blades are interchangeable and the knurled wheel controls the distance between them. (Tiemann, 1889)

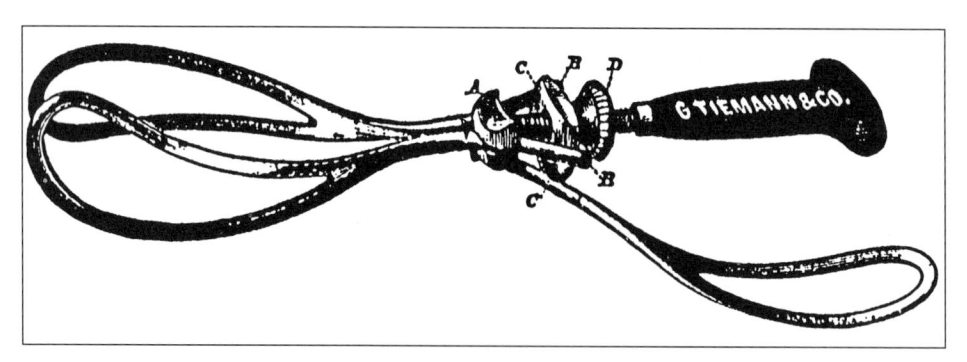

In 1880 in America, John Henry Hobart Burge (b. 1823) of Brooklyn described his "new obstetric forceps, multiple, adjustable and readjustable" (1880–1881) (Figure 8.22). A variety of blades could be attached to a single handle by an ingeniously designed lock that allowed the distance between the blades to be adjusted by rotation of a knurled nut, thus regulating the degree of compression on the head. These forceps are sometimes referred to as axis-traction instruments but this was not their primary purpose.

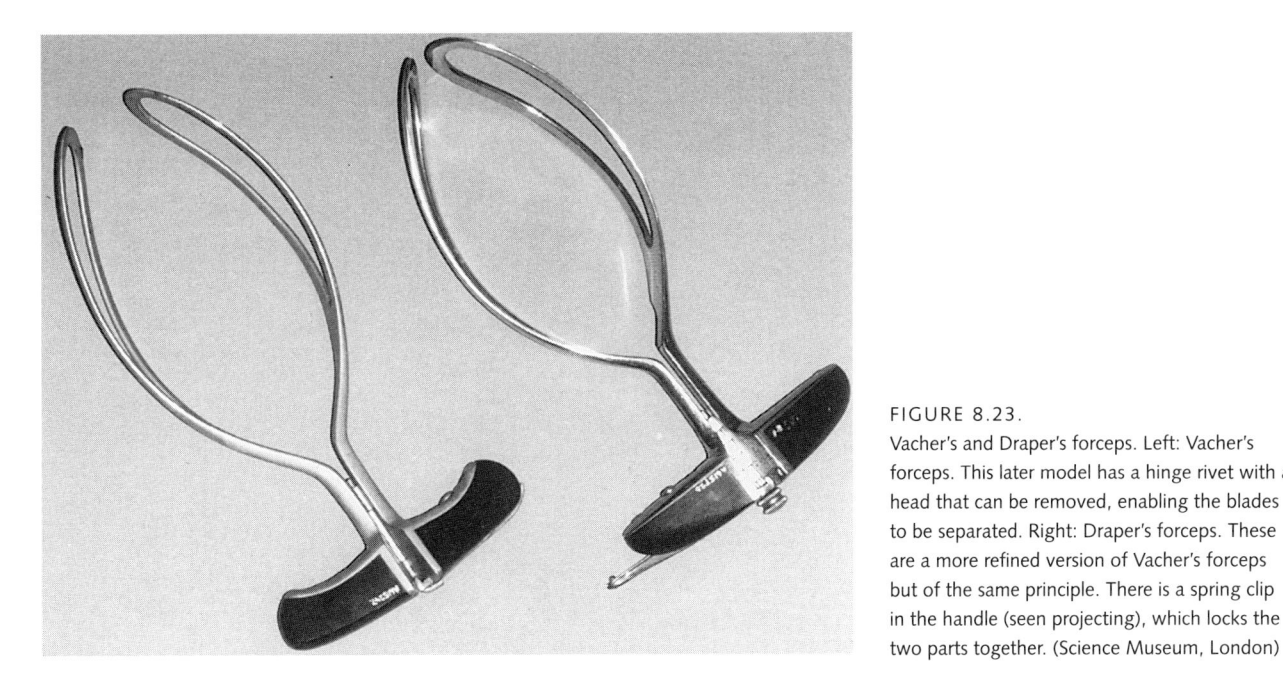

FIGURE 8.23.
Vacher's and Draper's forceps. Left: Vacher's forceps. This later model has a hinge rivet with a head that can be removed, enabling the blades to be separated. Right: Draper's forceps. These are a more refined version of Vacher's forceps but of the same principle. There is a spring clip in the handle (seen projecting), which locks the two parts together. (Science Museum, London)

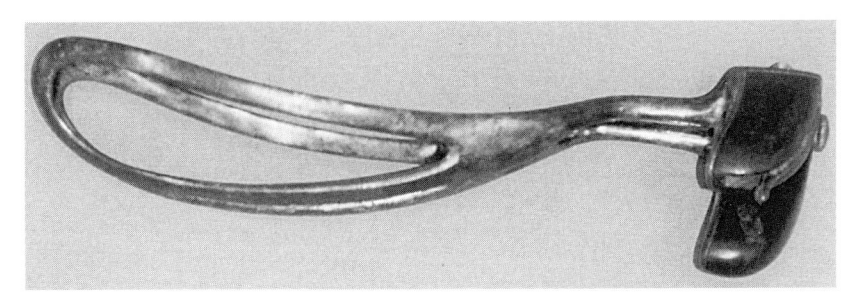

FIGURE 8.24.
Draper's forceps. They are shown here folded for introduction, or for use as a vectis. The blades, hinged longitudinally, were introduced with one inside the other and then opened out to "wander" to a correct cephalic application. (University College Hospital, London)

Folding and Rotating Blades

The idea of introducing both blades simultaneously, with one blade sitting inside the other, appears to have been introduced by James Braithwaite of Leeds in 1869 and he designed a forceps for this purpose (Chapter 6). Using the same principle for application, in 1873 Francis Vacher of Birkenhead designed a forceps in which the handles were connected by a longitudinal hinge so that after insertion the blades could be opened out to embrace the head (Figure 8.23, left). Vacher's forceps were light (255 grams/9 ounces) and had a small, spindle-shaped handle and a lever and catch to lock the handles when they were open. Vacher also advocated the use of the instrument as a vectis, with the blades closed.

W. Draper of York was attracted by the principle of Vacher's instrument but was critical of the design detail. He made a more refined version, described in his article in the *Obstetrical Journal of Great Britain and Ireland* (1875–1876), with a better handle shape and concealed catches (Figures 8.23, right; 8.24). These forceps were even lighter (235 grams/8 ounces) than the Vacher instrument and were intended for cases requiring "slight assistance." Other advantages claimed by Draper were that the instrument was small and portable and could be carried in the breast pocket. It could also be used under the bedclothes, without the patient's or attendants' knowledge. In fact neither Vacher's nor Draper's instrument was satisfactory in practice because the handles were too close to the perineum and when the blades were opened they caused trauma to the birth canal and the baby.

H. Löwenthal of New York concerned himself with improving the facility of locking the blades and produced a novel solution that he claimed to be superior to all others because it functioned as a tractor, compressor, and lever!

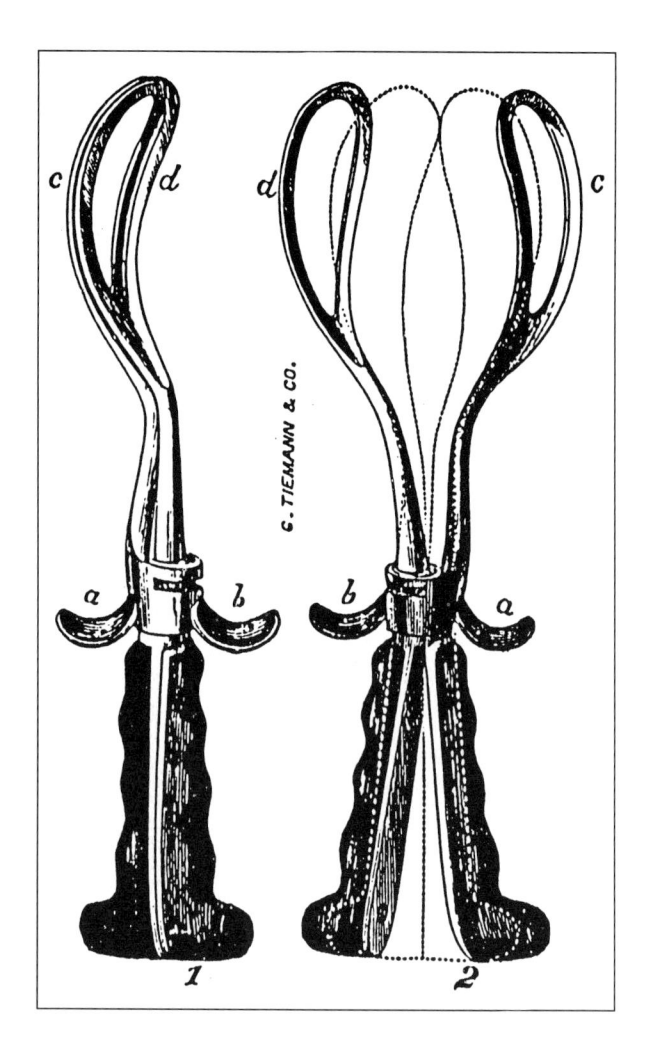

FIGURE 8.25.
Löwenthal's forceps. The articulation is a fixed longitudinally rotating lock. (Tiemann, 1889)

(Figure 8.25) (1873). The novelty was in the articulation, which was in the form of a fixed rotating lock. For insertion the blades (which had no pelvic curve) were rotated one inside the other (Figure 1) and after insertion were opened out (Figure 2). With this arrangement he claimed that as the blades were rotated they produced a higher degree of compression than with other instruments. However, he covered himself by saying that compression could not be excessive because with a large head the blades could not be made to rotate. Not surprisingly, there is no evidence of them achieving great popularity and they are not mentioned in the standard texts of the time.

Jointed Blades

The inventive David Davis devised forceps for almost every contingency (Chapter 6) and the blades of different pairs were interchangeable. Perhaps the most ingenious pattern was a blade that was transversely hinged 44.5 millimeters (1.75 inches) from the tip. The terminal part of the blade could be set at an angle by rotating a screw on the handle or, in some later models, by a sliding lever. It has been described in more detail in Chapter 6. The blade and mechanism were covered with layers of flannel and leather. It is also of some interest that a lever with a jointed blade and a forceps blade of similar construction was illustrated by the instrument maker John Weiss in 1831 in his first catalogue. It was labeled "Weiss's improved forceps and lever." There was no reference to Davis and it is not clear who was the originator of the idea, but Weiss certainly showed great ingenuity and novelty in the design of instruments generally and it is possible that Davis's instrument maker, Botschan, had copied the design if it had been available at an earlier date, that is, before the 1831 Weiss catalogue was published.

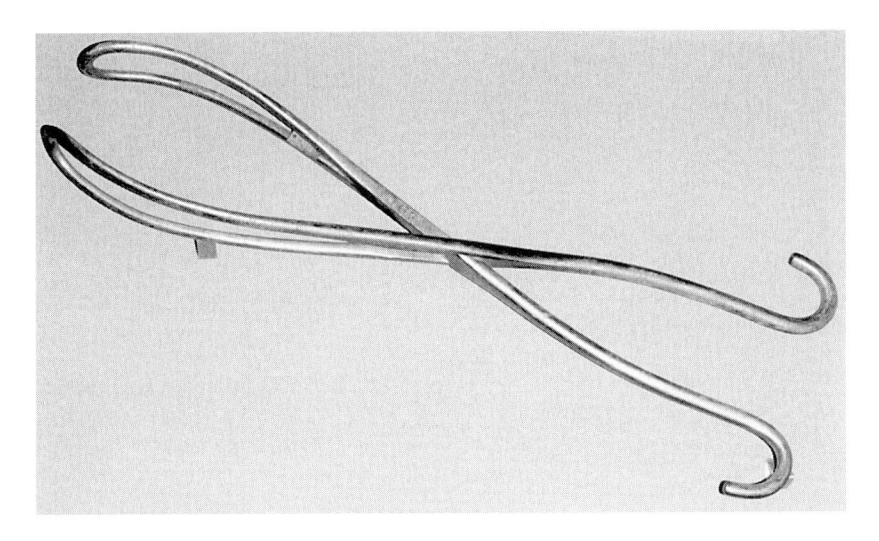

FIGURE 8.26.
Early unidentified interlocking forceps. University College Hospital, London. (University College Hospital, London)

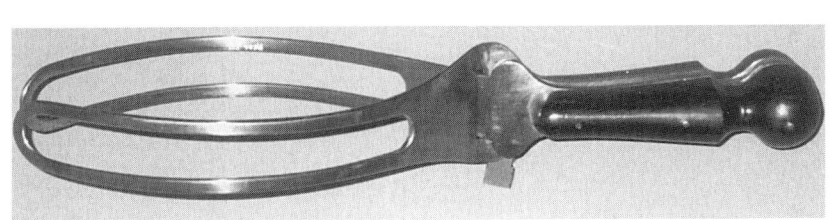

FIGURE 8.27.
J. Beatty's forceps. The female blade has only a slit to accept the male blade. (RCOG)

Interlocking Male and Female Blades

These forceps are all characterized by having one blade with a double shank through which the blade and shank of the other blade passed. An early unidentified pair are in the collection of University College Hospital, London (Figure 8.26).

John Beatty of Dublin (d. 1831) was a strong advocate of forceps in a city where their use was almost unknown at the end of the eighteenth century as a result of the conservatism of the master of the Dublin Lying-in Hospital, Joseph Clarke, under whom Beatty had worked. Beatty briefly described his forceps and their use in a paper to the Association of the College of Physicians (Dublin) in 1829 (see Beatty, T. E., 1866, for a reprint of the address). The unique feature of these straight forceps was the articulation, in which a transverse slit in the root of the female blade was wide enough to accept the narrower male blade (Figures 8.27, 8.29, right). He described the application as follows:

> I proceed by introducing the female blade of the forceps, slowly and carefully, over the upper side of the head of the child [the patient would be in the left lateral position], until it reaches beyond the ear; this being accomplished, the chief difficulty is overcome, for the male blade being passed through the slit in the female blade, readily applies itself in the proper position, by gently urging it forward under the inferior side of the head.

Alexander Ziegler (d. 1863), Consultant Surgeon of the Edinburgh Maternity Hospital and General Lying-in Hospital, designed at least three pairs of forceps (circa 1850) with a distinctive lock (Figures 8.28, 8.29, left): straight, curved, and one pair with a laterally directed pelvic curve (asymmetric) to facilitate correct cephalic application to the head lying transversely (see also Chapter 9). It is not clear whether he was aware of Beatty's earlier design but his version allowed more room for maneuvering when applying the blades. Apart from the articulation the other features are in common with those of Denman's forceps with slender blades and short handles, a popular instrument of the time. Although the application of the blades must have been quite difficult many instrument makers listed Ziegler's forceps and other obstetricians devised their own modifications.

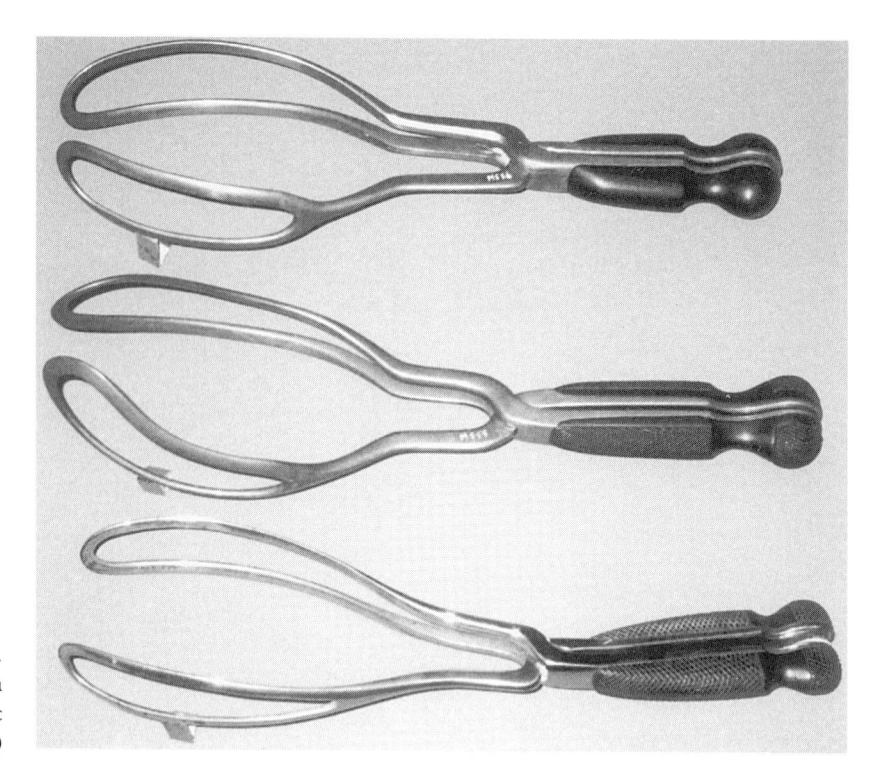

FIGURE 8.28.
Ziegler's forceps. Top to bottom: Straight; with a conventional pelvic curve; with a lateral pelvic curve (asymmetric). (RCOG)

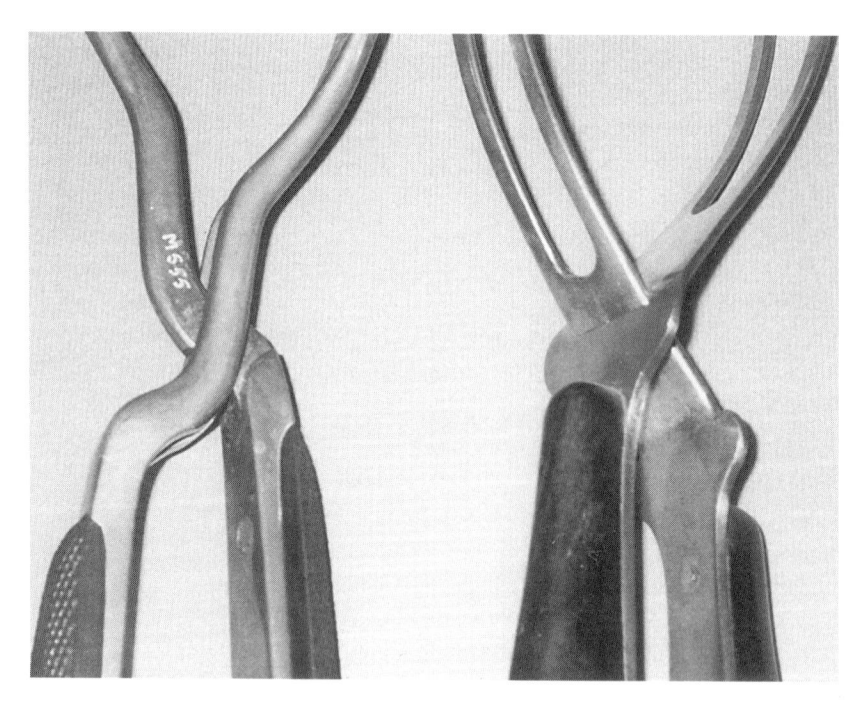

FIGURE 8.29.
J. Beatty's and Ziegler's forceps. Detail of the articulations. Left: Ziegler. Right: Beatty. (RCOG)

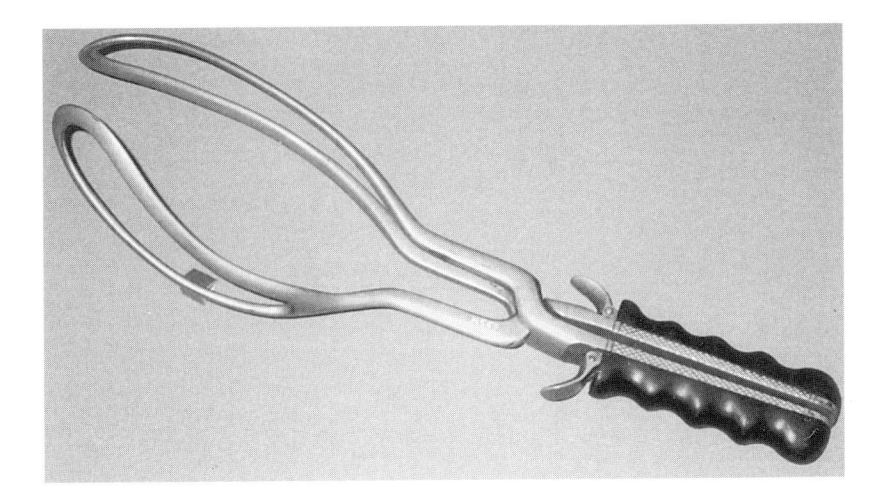

FIGURE 8.30.
Barclay's forceps. They are similar to Ziegler's but have Simpson's blades and hinged finger lugs. (RCOG)

Phillip H. Harper, Assistant Surgeon at the Surgical Home for Diseases of Women and a founding member of the Obstetrical Society of London, was highly regarded as a proponent for more frequent use of forceps (Harper, 1859). His novel forceps (1859) were long (355 millimeters/14 inches), with a pelvic curve and parallel shanks and the Ziegler-type articulation.

John Barclay, an assistant professor at the University of Aberdeen, combined the principle of Ziegler's articulation with the strength of Simpson's long forceps as well as adding hinged finger lugs (Figure 8.30) (1872). The method of application was to introduce the male blade first; the fenestra of the female blade was then slipped over the handle of the male blade and inserted along the curve of the sacrum. Following Barclay's publication in the *Lancet* Mark Long, a surgeon at the Poplar Hospital in London, announced in 1872 that he had used an essentially similar instrument for the past four years and that he had obtained the design from a Mr. Garman of Devonshire. The only differences were that Long's handle was 25 millimeters (1 inch) longer and the finger rests were fixed rather than hinged.

· · ·

Hinges and joints were adopted for a variety of reasons, including portability, facility of introduction, and to improve traction. However, the perceived needs for these devices diminished with changes in practice. Even detachable and hinged handles, which had practical benefits in portability and facilitating application of the blades when the patient was in the common English left lateral position, became less necessary as the lithotomy position for operative delivery came into more common use. So it was that the instruments described in this chapter had a limited vogue and were used less and less toward the end of the nineteenth century, gradually disappearing from instrument-makers' catalogues.

ANTERO-POSTERIOR AND ASYMMETRIC FORCEPS

9 The concept of using forceps with asymmetric blades in special situations developed in the early nineteenth century. However, it did not receive widespread attention until the second half of the century and even then was only in fashion for a brief time. According to Ignace Rist (1818), G. A. Fried of Strasbourg was probably the first person to promote the concept of asymmetric forceps around 1770, with an instrument in which the handle could be rotated on its long axis.

The first person to address seriously the problem of forceps for use on the high, transversely positioned head was J. Leake (1729–1792), who founded the Westminster Lying-In Hospital. He was a strong advocate of high forceps application at a time when this was unfashionable, especially in London. At the same time he was well aware of the difficulties that could accompany such a procedure, especially when the pelvis was flat, the head was lying transversely, and the occiput was lodged above the pubis, since the forceps tended to slip downward over the face; he accepted that occipitofrontal application would be necessary in such cases. He considered the lever to be a useful but dangerous instrument to assist the descent of the head past the pelvic brim. However, when it was introduced anteriorly, pressure damage to the urinary tract was a major hazard. Leake therefore tried to obtain the benefit of the lever without its dangers by combining the principle of its construction with that of the forceps in the form of a third blade. This third blade was attached to conventional forceps and functioned partly as a lever, the fulcrum for the additional blade then being the joint of the forceps rather than the maternal tissues (Figures 9.1, 9.2). With this combination it was possible to ease the head down anteriorly with the third blade and thereby prevent the main blades from slipping off (1773, 1787).

The concept of a pair of forceps curved on the flat, with long posterior and short anterior blades, is believed to have originated with André Uytterhoven (1799–1866), Chief Surgeon at St. John's Hospital, Brussels, around 1805 (see Poullet, 1883; Fry, 1889b). The purpose of this construction was to achieve a correct biparietal application when the head was lying transversely in the superior strait. A similar, if not identical, instrument was described, or as J. Poullet claimed, was reinvented, by M. R. Baumers of Lyons (1849). He took the basic design of the large, heavy Levret blades but put the pelvic curve on the flat, with the posterior blade following the sacral curve (Figure 9.3). Of the latter, Poullet is quoted as saying "no one claims to have ever succeeded in applying them to the living child; the instrument is therefore purely a theoretical one" (1883). Although Cazeaux claimed to have used them successfully, they did not meet with general approval.

In Britain David Davis was the pioneer, at the beginning of the nineteenth century, of designing forceps with unequal blades for special purposes, including blades of unequal length for application in the oblique pelvic diameter; unequal breadth for difficult malpresentations; and a jointed blade to use in place of high forceps, the blade being applied over the face. These are illustrated and discussed in detail in Chapter 6.

In the middle of the nineteenth century there was considerable diversity of opinion on the correct position in which to apply forceps to the high head lying in a transverse or oblique position. Henry D. Fry (1853–1919), a professor of obstetrics at Georgetown University, Washington, DC, concluded that the "the lack of uniformity [of opinion] proves the non-existence of a scientific basis" (1889a). In France one of the best known and enduring textbooks of the nineteenth

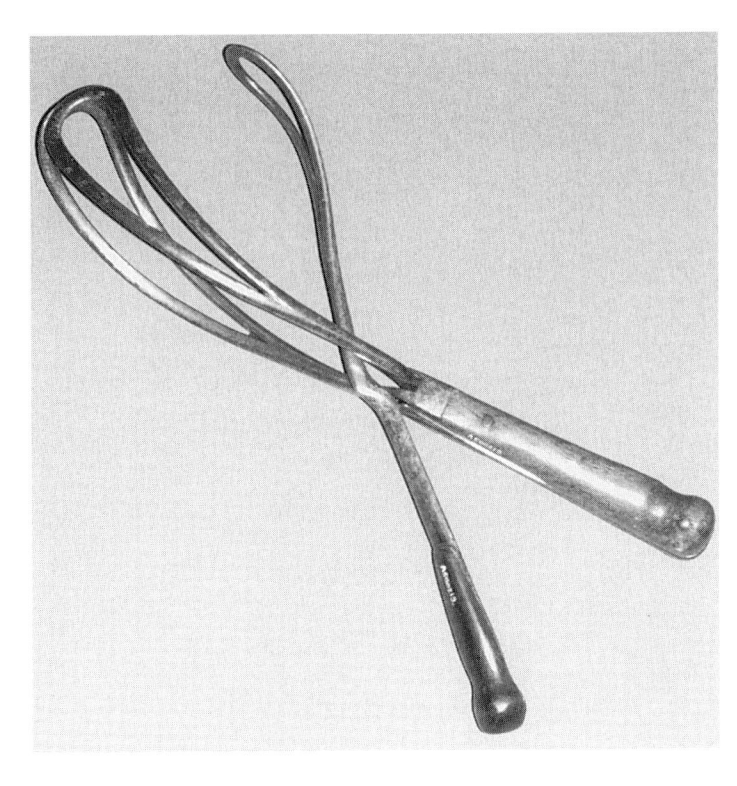

FIGURE 9.1.
Leake's three-bladed forceps. A conventional pair of curved forceps with an additional blade to be inserted anteriorly and used as a lever. (Science Museum, London)

FIGURE 9.2.
Leake's forceps. His original description and method of use. (Leake, 1773)

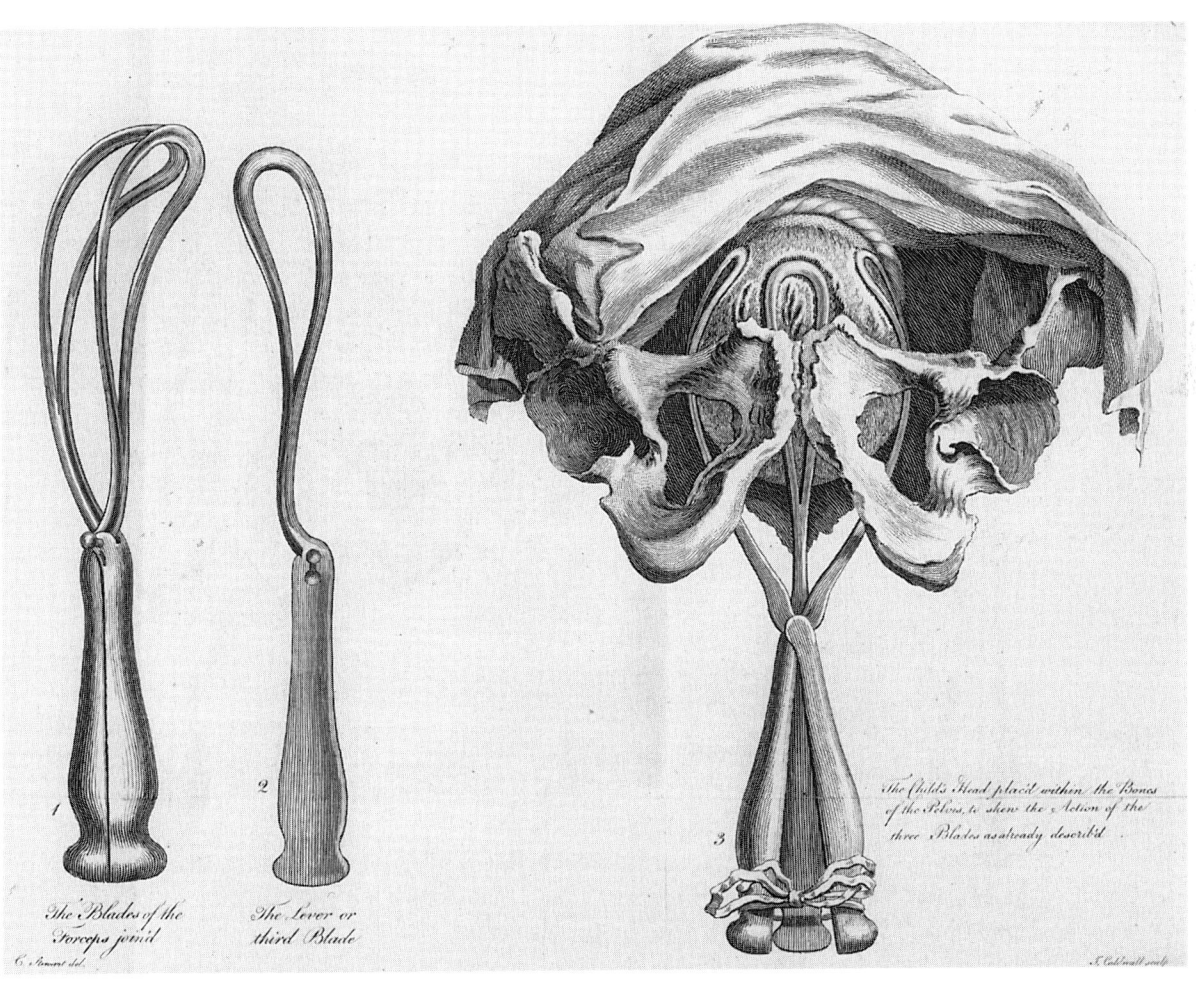

ANTERO-POSTERIOR AND ASYMMETRIC FORCEPS 127

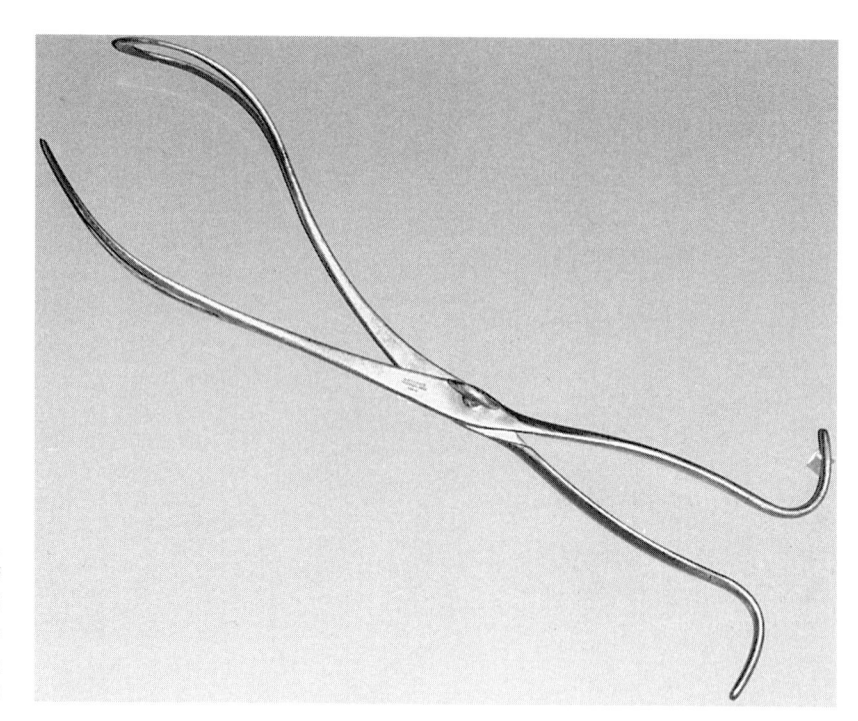

FIGURE 9.3.
Uytterhoven/Baumers forceps. This pair of forceps has a lesser lateral pelvic curve and thinner handles than the pair illustrated by Poullet. They may be the original Uytterhoven design. (Science Museum, London)

century was *Traité théorique et pratique de l'art des accouchements* by Cazeaux, first published in 1840 but continued, latterly under the pen of E. S. Tarnier, for a span of forty-five years. Cazeaux and Tarnier consistently recommended correct cephalic application, although this was not universal practice in France. However, in England, Germany, and Austria, correct application in relation to the pelvis was generally preferred. This discordance was also evident in American practice, which led Fry to carry out a survey among eighty-two American practitioners with the following results:

TABLE 9.1.   Cephalic or Pelvic Application? Nineteenth-Century American Practice

Application to sides of head whenever possible	42 (51%)
Application in relation to pelvis	31 (38%)
No rule—used both methods	9 (11%)

The main objection to the biparietal application was the difficulty in achieving it when the head was lying transversely (a situation that he and many of his respondents believed to be rare!). Fry believed that this difficulty arose from the lack of a suitable instrument since "forceps with the usual pelvic curve placed on edge [were] valueless." He was also critical of the significant number of obstetricians who generated an "an evil influence" by advocating that one pair of forceps should answer for all types of work. In another survey of eighty-three obstetricians he found that thirty (36 percent) used only one type of forceps; of those who used more than one type, thirty used axis traction for high operations. As a result of this survey Fry designed a forceps with the pelvic curve on the flat that he claimed enabled biparietal application whether the head was high or low, lying obliquely or transversely. The instrument was 407 millimeters (16 inches) long and also had a compression screw and the option of a traction rod that could be hooked into the fenestra of the anterior blade (Figure 9.4) (see also Chapter 14).

Fry presented his paper to the American Medical Association in 1889 and in the ensuing discussion criticism was unanimous. It was generally agreed that, whatever else, his forceps did not fulfill the functions of an axis-traction forceps. Theophilus Parvin (1820–1898) of Jefferson Medical College described its action as "being like drawing a wagon by one shaft."

In Britain most of the interest in antero-posterior forceps came from Glasgow, possibly because of a high incidence of rachitic flat pelves. William Reid (1878), in a lengthy dissertation on the use of long forceps when the head was at the brim, analyzed the parallelograms of forces involved with different degrees of pelvic curvature of the blades and how this angle influenced the force expended against the pubis. In Britain the angle of the blades of the curved forceps was commonly 30 degrees (Barnes's) whereas in Europe 40 degrees was more common; in America one widely used forceps (Meigs's) was 50 degrees. Using a traction force of 50 pounds Reid estimated that the force "doing mischief to the soft parts of the pubis" would be 11.4 kilograms (25 pounds) in the case of Barnes's forceps and 17.4 kilograms (38.3 pounds) with Meigs's forceps. Also, the greater the angle of the blades, the more difficult was the rotation of the head from a posterior position. However, when an increased angle was used there was less risk of perineal trauma.

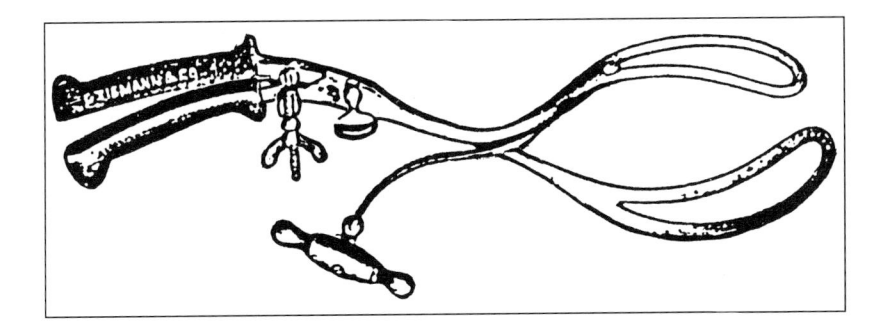

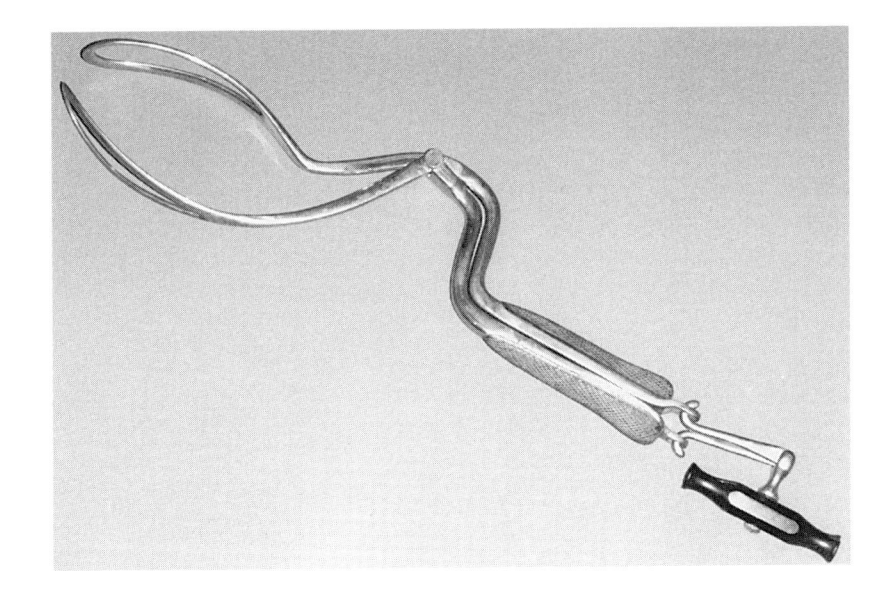

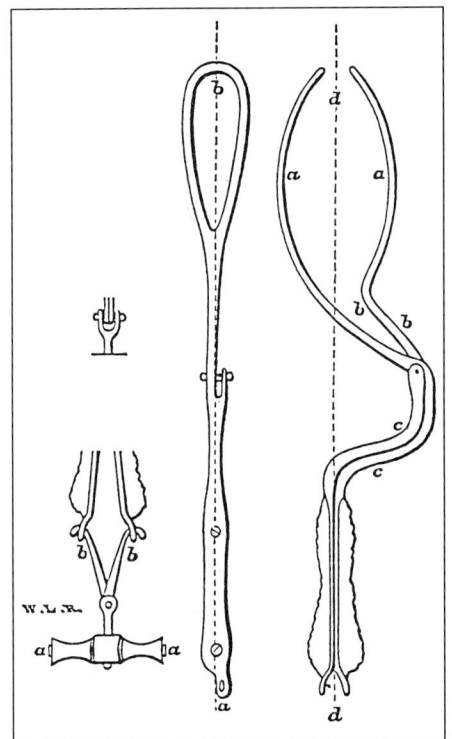

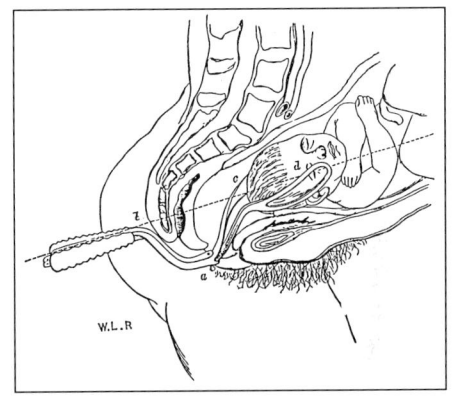

After a number of experiments Reid ended up with a pair of antero-posterior forceps (Figures 9.5–9.7) with a perineal step in the same manner as A. L. Galabin (see Chapters 12 and 13), although Reid said that he was unaware of Galabin's forceps at the time. Thus the handles were in the same long axis as the blades and effectively acted as straight forceps

FIGURE 9.4 (TOP LEFT).
Fry's forceps. He claimed an improvement on Baumer's design and added a compression screw and an optional single traction rod. (Fry, 1889b)

FIGURE 9.5 (ABOVE LEFT).
Reid's forceps. Note the perineal step. The traction handle facilitated autorotation of the head as it descended. (Science Museum, London)

FIGURES 9.6 (TOP RIGHT), 9.7 (ABOVE RIGHT).
Reid's forceps. Figure 9.6 shows Reid's original design details. Figure 9.7 shows the method of use. (Reid, 1878)

FIGURE 9.8 (RIGHT).
Dick's forceps. This appears to be the maker's (Dick) interpretation of Reid's forceps, with a greater perineal step and no traction handle. (Science Museum, London)

FIGURE 9.9 (BELOW LEFT).
Sloan's forceps. The blades are set at an angle of 30°. Note the closeness of the blades, with a maximum space of only 38mm (1.5ins). (Sloan, 1889)

FIGURE 9.10 (BELOW RIGHT).
Sloan's forceps. Application of forceps to a high transverse head in a flat pelvis. Left: Simpson. Right: Sloan.

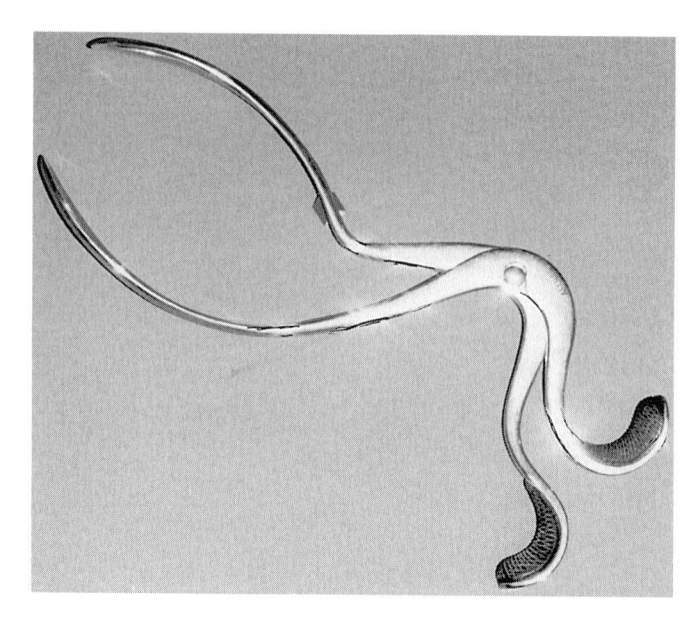

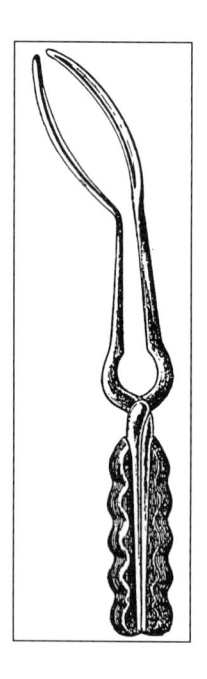

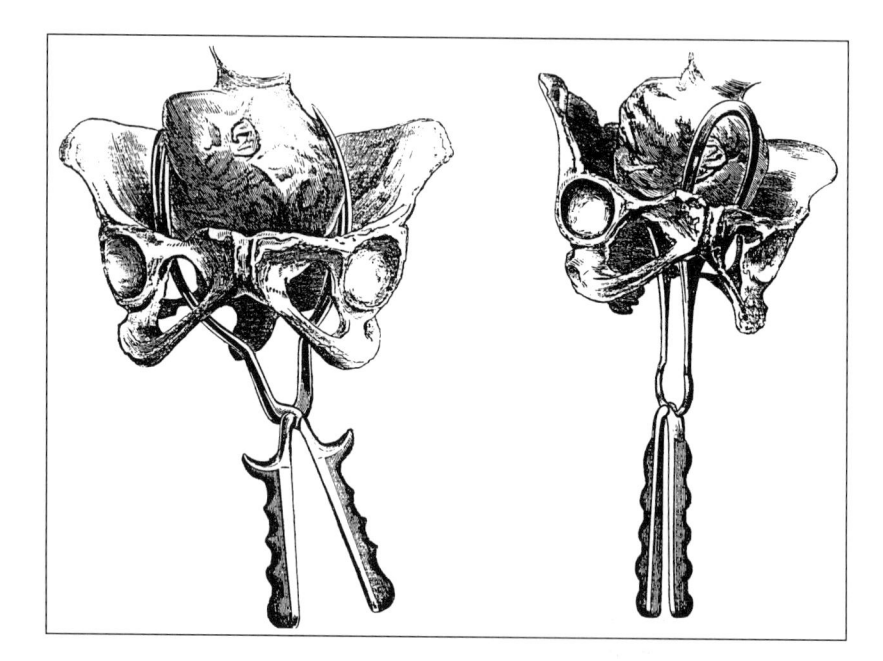

without the risk of perineal damage. The extremities of the handles were perforated to accommodate hooks attached to a transverse traction handle so that the head was free to rotate while traction was being applied. A forceps of similar design, manufactured by Dick of Glasgow, is in the Wellcome collection (Figure 9.8).

The antero-posterior compression forceps of Samuel Sloan (1842–1920), Obstetric Physician at Glasgow Maternity Hospital, were intended for use in cases of obstruction at the pelvic brim with the head transversely placed (1889) (Figure 9.9). Sloan conducted numerous cadaver experiments using pelves with a true conjugate of only 64 millimeters (2.5 inches). With the hope of a live birth, use of antero-posterior compression forceps was an alternative to craniotomy when attempted delivery with other forceps had failed. The overall length was 380 millimeters (15 inches). The blades were short but had wide fenestra; when closed the maximum distance between the blades was only 38 millimeters

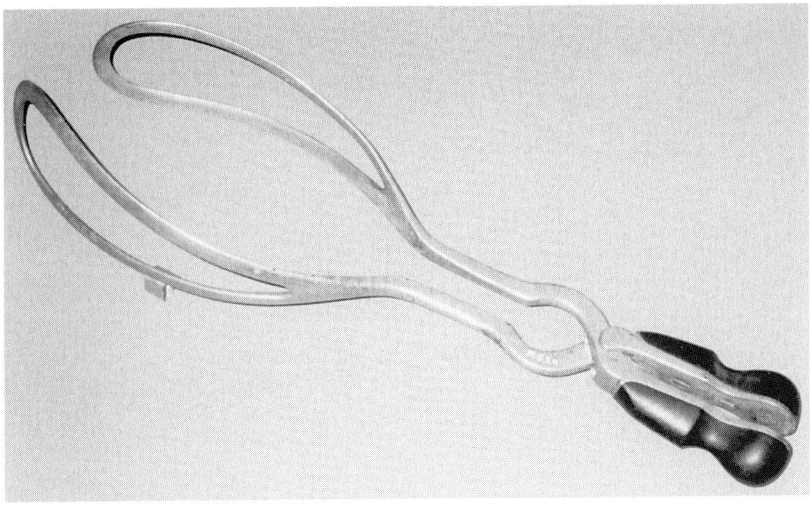

FIGURE 9.11.
Radford's straight asymmetric forceps. The short handles were intended to reduce potential compressive and leverage forces. (RCOG)

(1.5 inches). The long shanks terminated in a finger ring of the Barnes type. The lock was loose-fitting to allow for some tolerance in handle alignment. The favorable fit of the forceps in Sloan's experiments on flat pelves, compared with Simpson's forceps, is shown in Figure 9.10.

In the discussion that followed Sloan's presentation of his paper to the Obstetric Medicine Section at the Annual Meeting of the British Medical Association in 1888, most concern related to the use of forceps for compression, while Reid was still advocating his forceps that had not been well received after his original description of them in 1878.

Thomas Radford of Manchester described, *inter alia*, a long straight forceps with blades of unequal length. Although they were invented at an earlier date a detailed description of their use and benefits was given by him at the Obstetric Society *Conversazione* in 1866 (see Chapter 6; Meadows, 1867). In Radford's view the high head most commonly was in an oblique position and in his experience Haighton's forceps, with their large fenestra, which were in common use at the time, were ill-adapted for such situations for several reasons:

(1) one blade would overlie the orbit, with consequent risk of injury;
(2) the handles were too long, allowing undue leverage force;
(3) the blades would not close completely; and
(4) the lower birth canal was unduly stretched and contused.

He also had great difficulties in his attempts to use Davis's Type V forceps with a jointed blade. This led to the design of his asymmetric forceps (Figure 9.11), described in 1839 in his *Essays on Various Subjects Connected with Midwifery*. In these forceps the longer blade measured 349 millimeters (13.75 inches) overall and were reputedly a better fit and safer in use on the obliquely positioned head.

Radford continued the current practice of aiming for insertion of the blades at the sides of the pelvis. To facilitate this he adopted a reverse lock, which was a mirror image of the English lock, so that the right blade could be inserted first. He condemned the use of undue compressive force and in particular binding the handles together with a tight ligature. Evidently he found the instrument highly satisfactory, as he continued to promote its virtues enthusiastically over the next forty years (1865, 1878). In the latter paper he took issue with Galabin, whose view was that "[i]t has not been shown that the majority, or any considerable proportion, of the stillbirths which now occur in Britain would be preventable by a more timely resort to forceps" (1877a). J. G. Swayne (1819–1903), Physician Accoucheur to Bristol General Hospital, supported Galabin's contention, quoting from his own experience (1878). However, Radford pointed out that in several of Swayne's cases ergot had been administered to stimulate uterine activity, which in itself might have been detrimental.

Radford's forceps were unlike most asymmetric forceps in that the long blade was intended to be applied over the face and the short blade over the occiput. The short handles were to avoid undue compression of the head and traction was applied by using a silk handkerchief passed through the shanks by which "the practitioner can exercise as much tractile force as his powers will allow, and certainly to a greater extent than is compatible with the safety of the maternal structures" (1839).

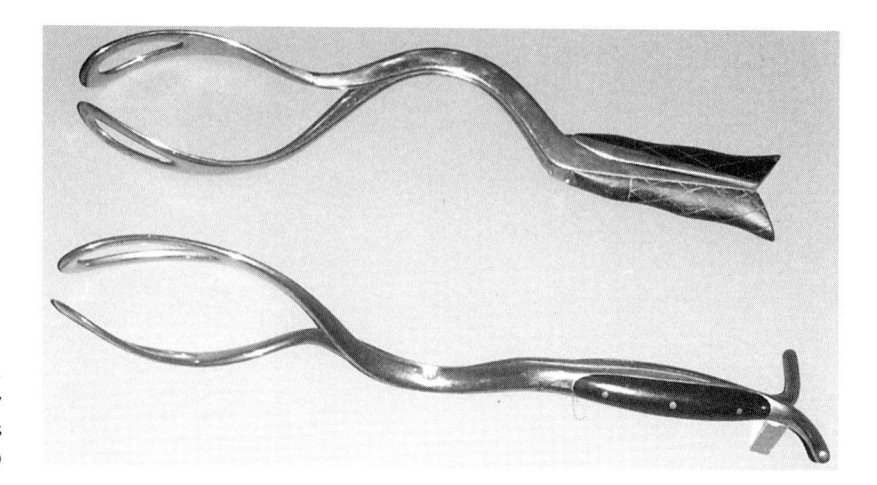

FIGURES 9.12, 9.13.
Asymmetric and oblique forceps made by Sandborg and Vedler. No further information is available. (Science Museum, London)

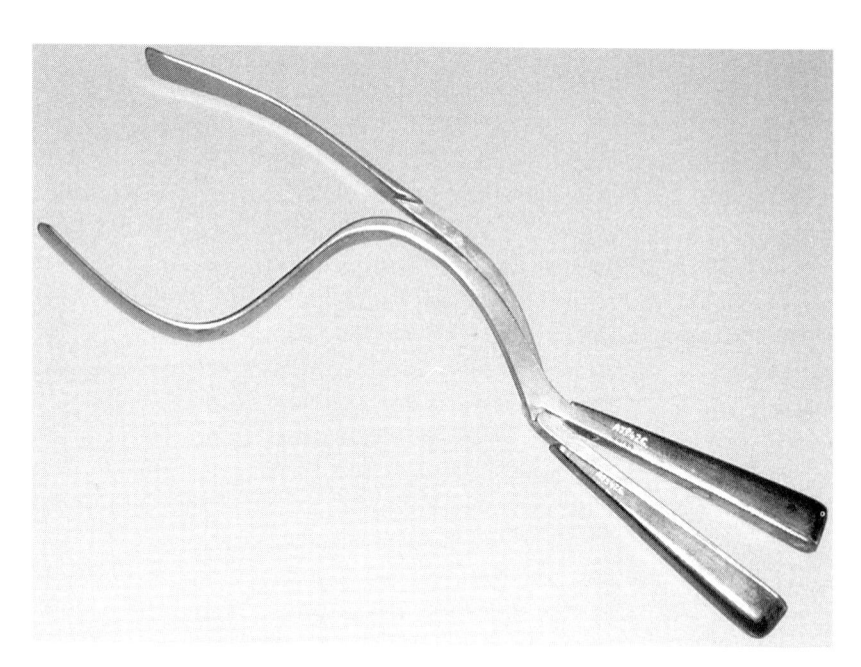

As well as the types of forceps described above, the Wellcome collection in the Science Museum contains a number of antero-posterior and oblique forceps by Sandborg and Vedler of Norway, some of which are shown in Figures 9.12 and 9.13; no further information about them is available.

Adjustable Joints to Produce Asymmetric Blades

One of Levret's early forceps had a lock with three alternative positions that was believed to allow for variation in the ratio of the length of the blade to the handle while preserving symmetry. It is possible that Levret had a place for an asymmetric forceps in mind but he never specifically referred to this option.

A multiposition joint was proposed by F. F. Ritgen (1787–1867), Professor of Midwifery at the University of Giefsen, in 1829, and his instrument was illustrated by Busch in his *Atlas* (1841), who designated it as "Ritgen II" (Figure 9.14). The long, flat shanks were superimposed with a simple pin-and-socket articulation. The single pin on one shank could be engaged in one of three sockets on the other shank, thus allowing either blade to be relatively shorter. A very similar idea was proposed over half a century later by Isaac E. Taylor (1812–1889) of Bellevue Hospital in New York, although he gave no recognition to Ritgen. Taylor's narrow-bladed forceps were intended specifically for use before full dilata-

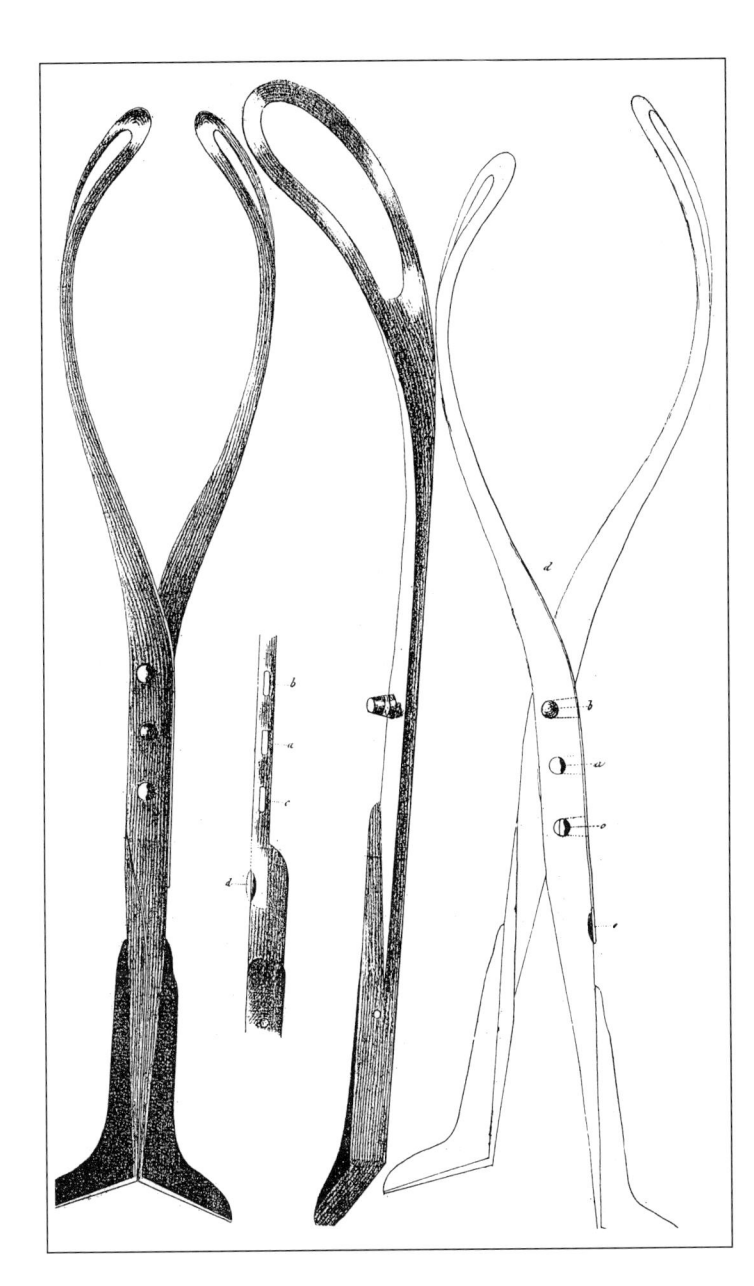

FIGURE 9.14.
Ritgen's forceps. This instrument with a multiposition joint was described by D. W. H. Busch as "Ritgen II." (D. W. H. Busch, 1841)

FIGURE 9.15.
Taylor's forceps. The narrow blades could be inserted before full dilatation of the cervix. As the head descended the blades could be adjusted to become symmetrical without having to remove them. (Tiemann, 1889)

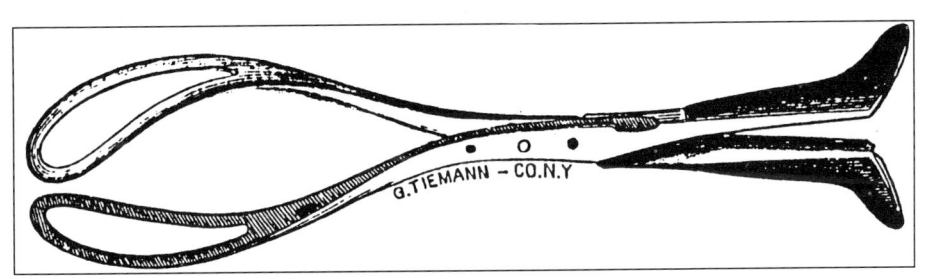

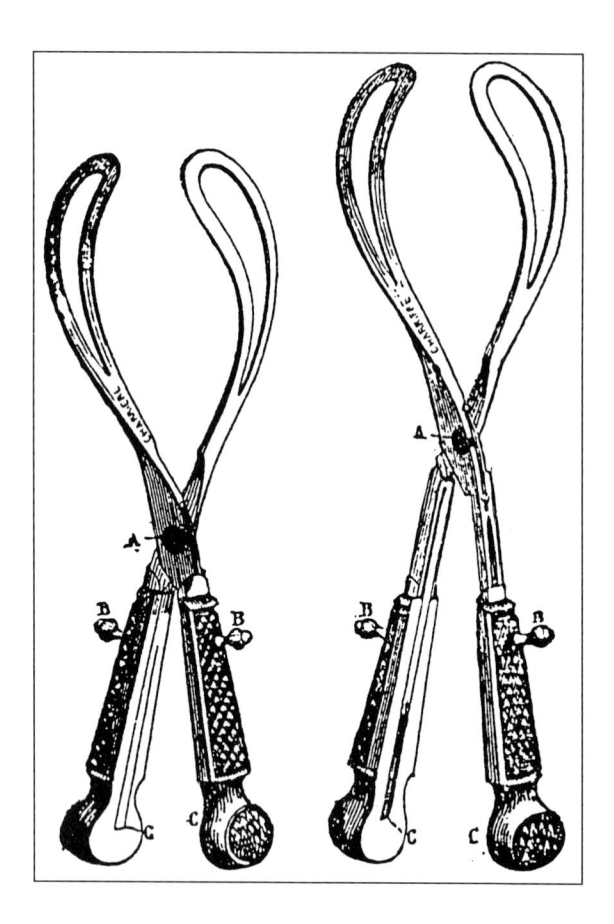

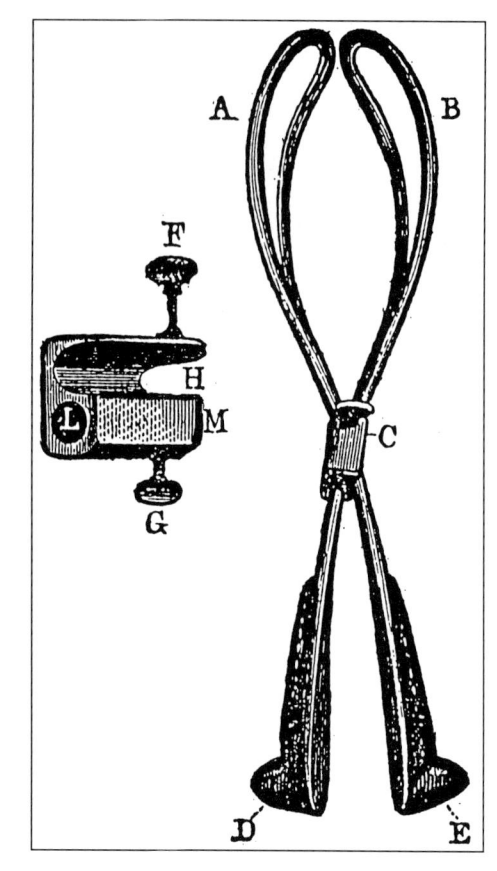

tion of the cervix and with the head high and oblique (Figure 9.15). The pivot on the male blade could be engaged temporarily in one of a series of three holes in the female blade. When the cervix was sufficiently dilated and the head had been brought down into the pelvis, the blades were readjusted symmetrically (1876).

Another instrument adjustable for asymmetry was described by C. J. Campbell (1820–1879), an Englishman who spent his whole professional life in Paris, was *chef de clinique* at the Maternité, and was one of the first obstetricians in France to use anesthesia. His novel instrument, dating from 1855 (Figure 9.16), had sliding extendable handles, with a range of 70 millimeters (2.75 inches), and could thus be used as long, short, or asymmetric forceps. The screws by which the handles were fixed were intended to serve as finger rests.

A unique joint to achieve asymmetry was described in 1855 by A. Mattei (Figure 9.17) (1855, 1856). The two branches of the forceps were symmetrical but the crossover articulation was achieved with a separate sliding block ensheathing one shank and a groove in the block to receive the shank of the other blade. The shanks were held in position with thumb screws.

In 1883 the innovative J. Poullet (1870–1915), who was head of the obstetrical clinic at the Faculté de Médecine in Lyons, described his *forceps général*, intended for application to the head in any position but especially, like the forceps of Uytterhoven, for antero-posterior pelvic application (Figure 9.18). The sliding articulation allowed for adjustment and asymmetric application of the blades. In his publication Poullet admitted that he had never actually used the instrument and he soon moved on to other concepts. As with many of the ingenious mechanical innovations of the time it seems to have had a brief life, if any life at all, and does not even receive a mention in the popular contemporary textbooks of Charpentier (1883) and Tarnier and Budin (1901).

. . .

Asymmetric forceps were an ingenious attempt to overcome a serious problem: the application of forceps when the head was at or above the brim of the pelvis in an occipito-lateral position. Previously in such cases "turning" (internal podalic version) might have been used, or long forceps applied with the blades over the face and occiput. There was a growing awareness of the potential danger to the baby of such an application, but a correct cephalic application would have been impossible using conventional long, curved forceps.

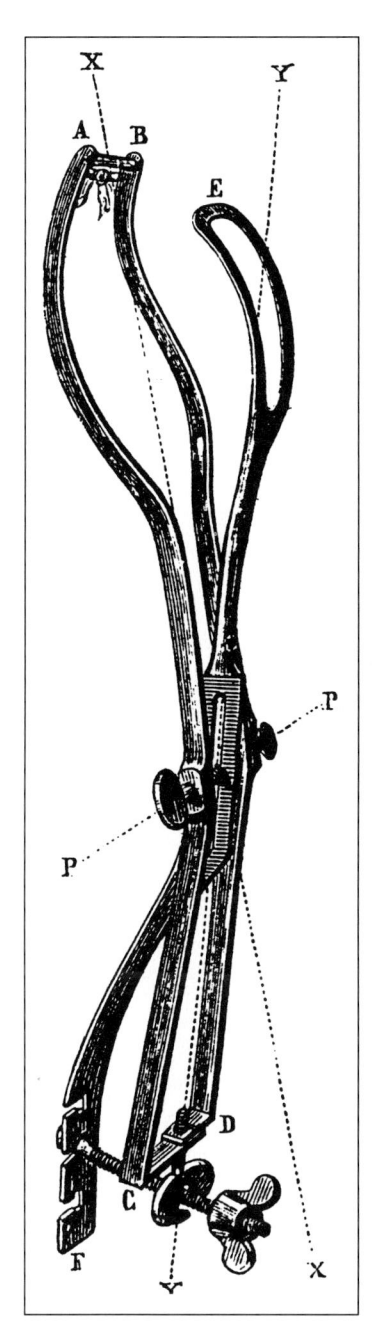

FIGURE 9.16 (OPPOSITE LEFT).
C. J. Campbell's forceps. The handles are extendable. The fixing screws act as finger lugs. (Poullet, 1883)

FIGURE 9.17 (OPPOSITE RIGHT).
Mattei's forceps. The novel joint comprises a drilled and grooved block in which the round shanks can slide, being fixed with thumb screws. (Mattei, 1856)

FIGURE 9.18.
Poullet's *forceps général*. They were intended for application to the head in any position and have a sliding articulation. (Poullet, 1883)

Although it is not clear how effective these instruments were in practice it is notable that many of them were designed by some of the most experienced and respected obstetricians of the day who had clearly identified the problem and logically approached a possible solution. There were many other variations of asymmetric forceps but some, such as the instruments of McLaurin and Murdoch Cameron, as well as those of Fry referred to above, were designed specifically for axis traction and will be described in Chapter 14.

NONCROSSED, OR PARALLEL, FORCEPS

10

Although crossover articulations have dominated the design of forceps throughout their history, "parallel," or noncrossing, blades have had steady minority support for over two hundred years. Apart from Palfyn's *mains de fer*, or spoons, tied together with a napkin, and the crude instruments of Schlichting (1747), Rathlauw (1747), and de Wind (1751) (Chapter 1), in the early eighteenth century, the first definite records of parallel forceps are those described by John Aitken of Edinburgh (1786) (see below) and Jean-Simon Thenance of Lyons (1802). For the next hundred years Lyons obstetricians continued the endeavor to improve upon parallel forceps designs. In fact Jacques Mesnard (1685–1746), an accoucheur at Rouen, published descriptions of several instruments (Figure 10.1) in his *Guide des accoucheurs* (1753). These included *une tenette en cuiller* (first described in 1741), which he described as an anticrotchet, comprised of a parallel forceps with the blades held together by a screw and wing nut and a pin and socket (Figure 10.2).

The Lyons Noncrossed Forceps

In Thenance's forceps the parallel branches were articulated by a hinge with a loose pin (Figures 10.3, 10.4). In addition, perforations in the shank were intended to accommodate a napkin that was wrapped round the handles to fix the blades together. The description of the forceps, which was reproduced by M. Rolland (1905), was remarkable for the attention to detail and very precise measurements. Although the design was based on Levret's forceps the blades were longer and wider, the overall length being 457 millimeters (18 inches). Thenance's objective was to overcome the difficulty in locking the branches in difficult cases. However, they did not seem to be very satisfactory, judging by the comment of Poullet, also from Lyons, who said that "[Thenance's] instrument, with its colossal dimensions is just an instrument of curiosity in the show cases of museums" (1883).

Valette (1857) revived the Lyons forceps of Thenance but made them smaller and of lighter steel (406 millimeters/16 inches) (Figures 10.5, 10.6). The blades were detachable and were attached to the handles by bayonet locks. A hinge joint united the ends of the handles and a sliding ring was added to accommodate the napkin.

Another Lyons accoucheur and a prolific designer of forceps, M. Chassagny (1813–1890), returned to the Thenance principle in the late nineteenth century. Over a period of thirty years or more he carried out numerous experiments on models, using pressure gauges and dynamometers, each experiment leading to further design modifications. His earlier long forceps were made of flexible steel and were truly parallel, with slight incurving of the terminal parts of the blades. One branch terminated in a rounded hook that had a sharp point at the tip, covered by an olive-shaped screw cap. The branches were joined near the end of the handle by a detachable crossbar and screw that kept them 60 millimeters (2.375 inches) apart. In addition the blades were drawn together near their root either by an adjustable leather strap (Figure 10.7) or by an adjustable metal clip. Various other articulations, such as ratchet crossbars, were also described. In addition lacs, or traction tapes, were attached in various ways in different versions. These versions included features such as holes in the fenestra, notches on the bottom edge of the blades, or a notched bar across the fenestra, and these features were also used on his later designs (1885, 1891).

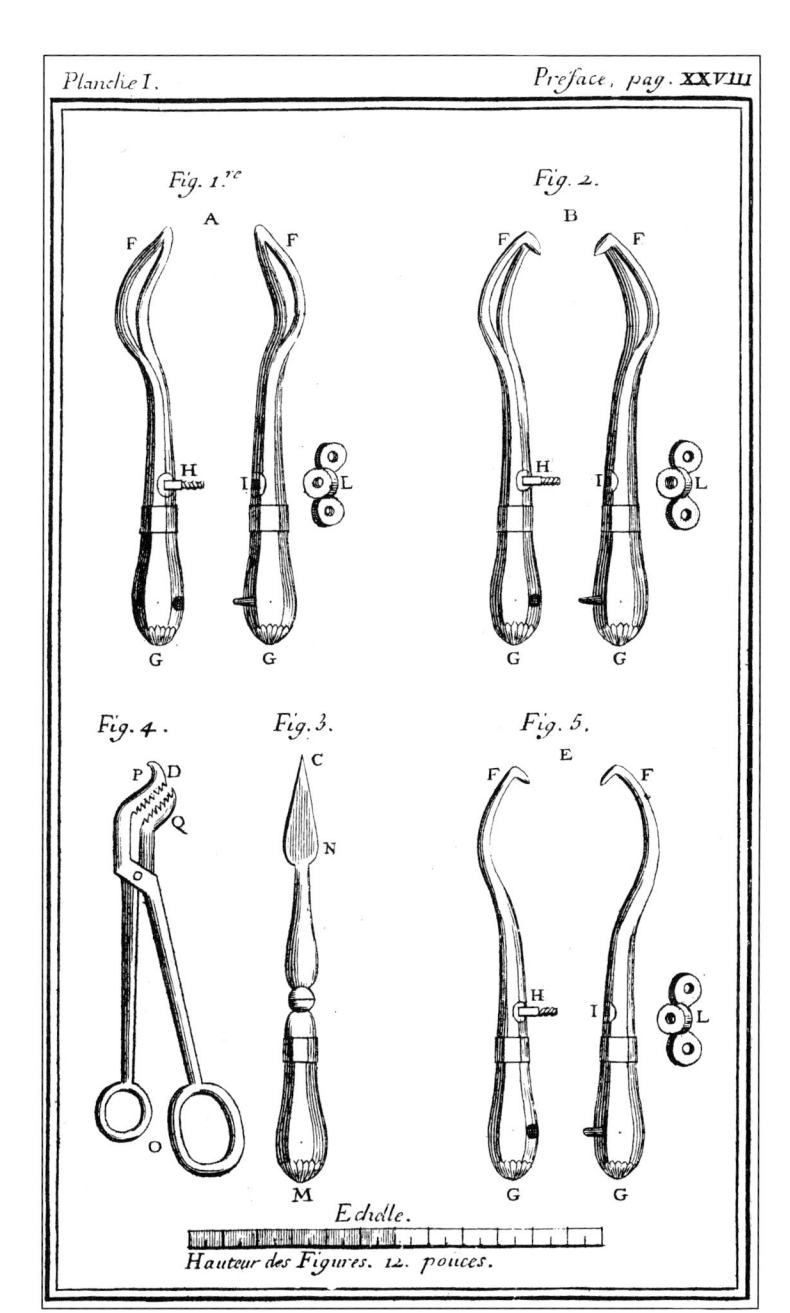

FIGURE 10.1.
Mesnard's instruments. The set comprises: Figure 1. *tenette en cuiller* (forceps). Figure 2. *tenette à crochet* (essentially the forceps with teeth). Figure 3. *perce-crâne*. Figure 4. *tenette à conducteur* (craniotomy forceps). Figure 5. Double crochet. (Mesnard, 1753).

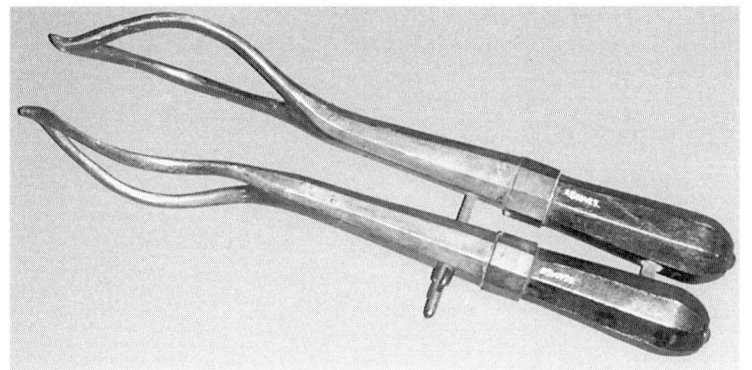

FIGURE 10.2.
Mesnard's *tenette en cuiller* (model). (Science Museum, London)

NONCROSSED, OR PARALLEL, FORCEPS 137

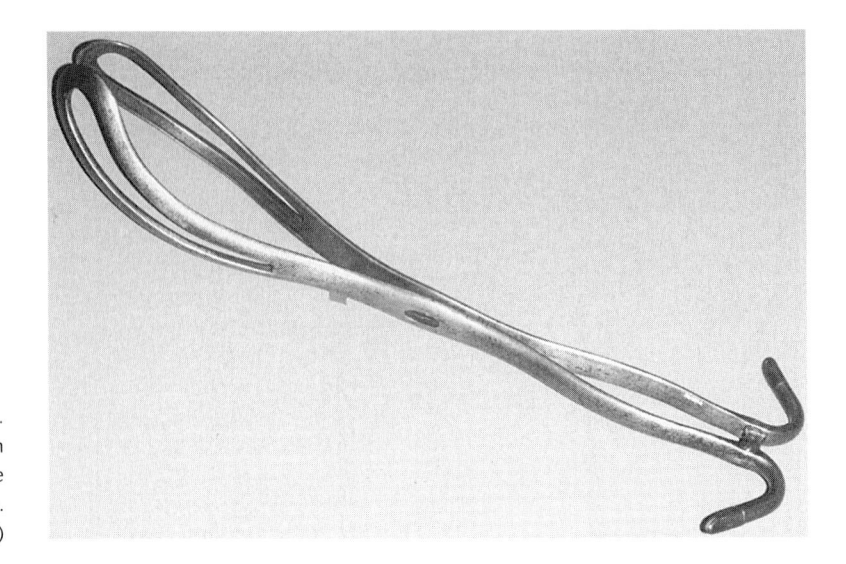

FIGURE 10.3.
Thenance's forceps. There is a loose articulation with a pin at the end of the handle. The perforations were to accommodate a napkin. (Science Museum, London)

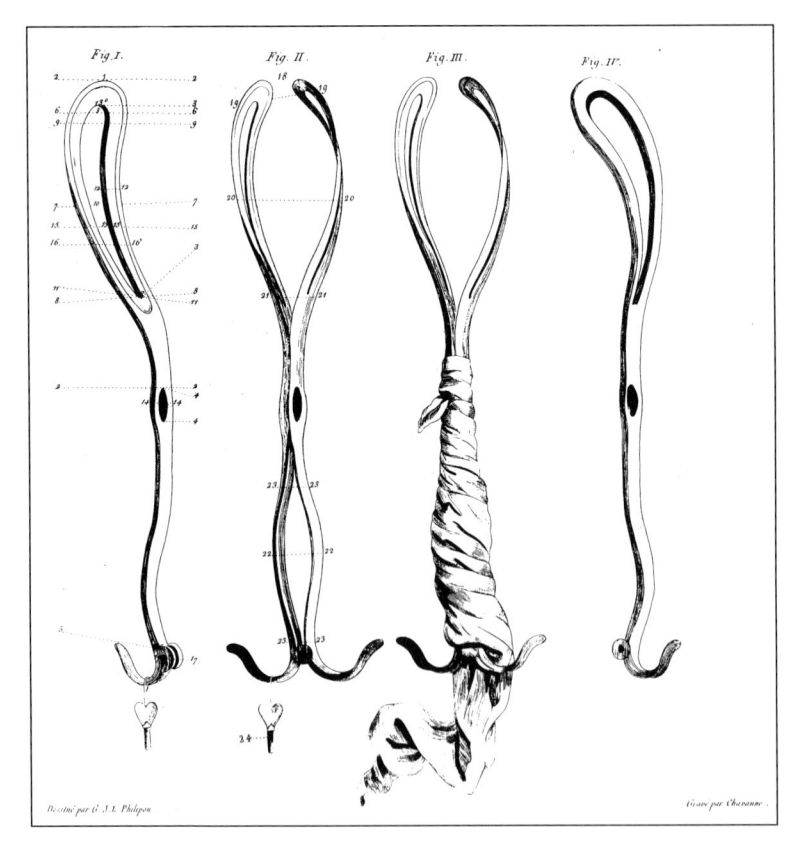

FIGURE 10.4.
Thenance's forceps. The components and method of assembly are shown. (Thenance, 1802)

138 CHAPTER 10

FIGURE 10.5 (TOP).
Valette's forceps. A revival of Thenance's forceps but of lighter construction. The blades are detachable. (Science Museum, London)

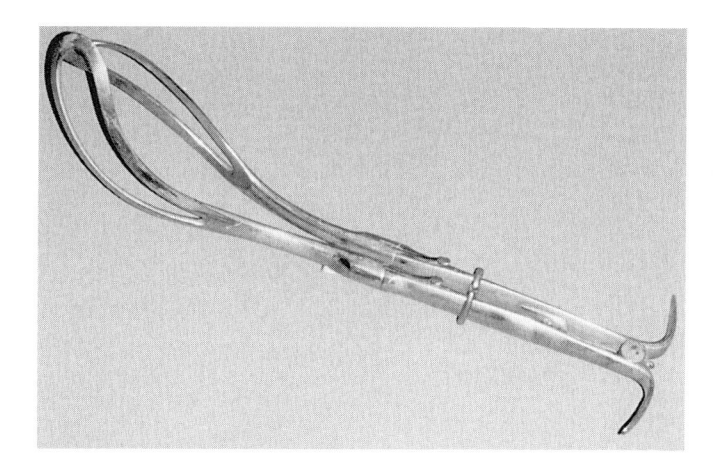

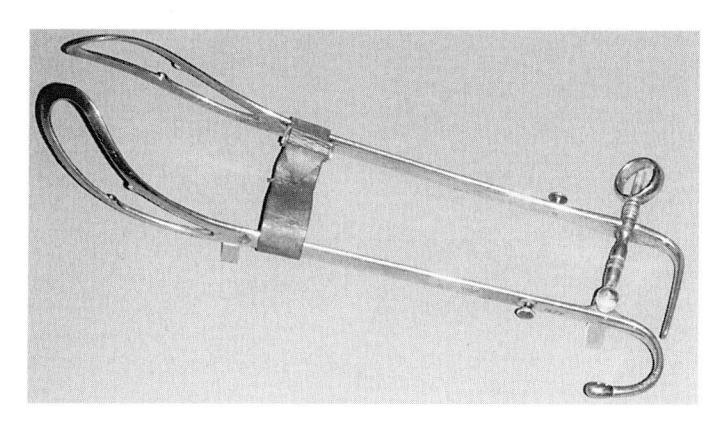

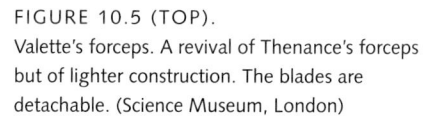

FIGURE 10.7 (BOTTOM).
Chassagny's early parallel forceps. There were several variants. A cap on one handle conceals a sharp crotchet. Note the hooks on the inside margins of the blades for attaching lacs or tapes. (Science Museum, London)

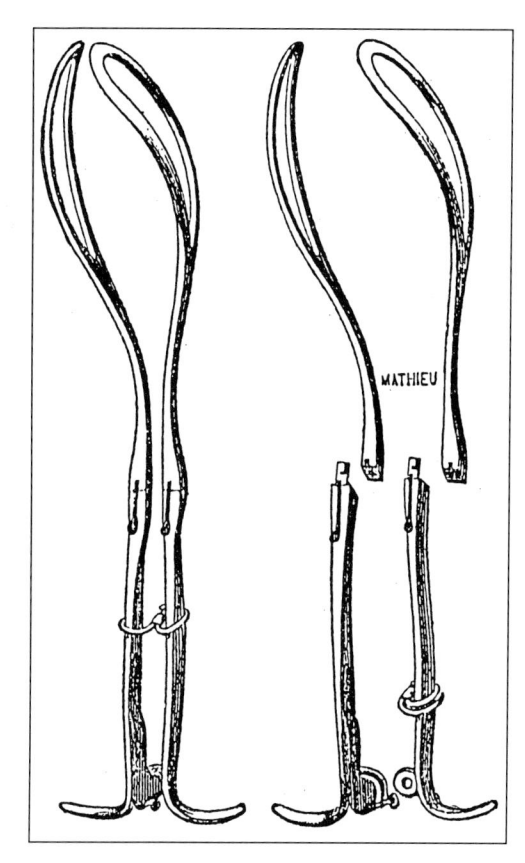

FIGURE 10.6.
Valette's forceps. Showing the separate blades and the ring for attaching a napkin. (Valette, 1857)

Chassagny's rotating forceps (Figure 10.8) incorporated the same principles but were of lighter steel construction. A pivot at the end of the handle enabled the blades to be folded one inside the other for portability and there were two hinged finger rings.

The more commonly known later models of Lyons forceps from around 1885 were double curved and elliptical in shape, with the shanks contiguous and the ends of the handles joined by adjustable hinged plates, which were held together by either a screw or a sliding collar (Figures 10.9, 10.10). Chassagny claimed, as did so many other designers of parallel forceps, that they adapted perfectly to all heads with a minimum amount of compression force.

J. Poullet, who was a younger contemporary of Chassagny, made many attempts to reduce trauma to the fetal head, starting with his *sericeps* and soon followed by his *forceps souple à tractions indépendantes* (Chapter 11), his antero-posterior *forceps général* (Chapter 9), and axis-traction forceps (Chapter 12). Ultimately he returned to a parallel forceps design, which he combined with traction tapes. In 1883 and 1884 he published lengthy critiques of landmarks in forceps development and the weaknesses of earlier designs. He then described his new parallel forceps that he claimed both overcame all the problems he had enumerated and fulfilled his essential criteria, which included a good cephalic grip without undue compression, a pelvic curve, axis traction,

NONCROSSED, OR PARALLEL, FORCEPS 139

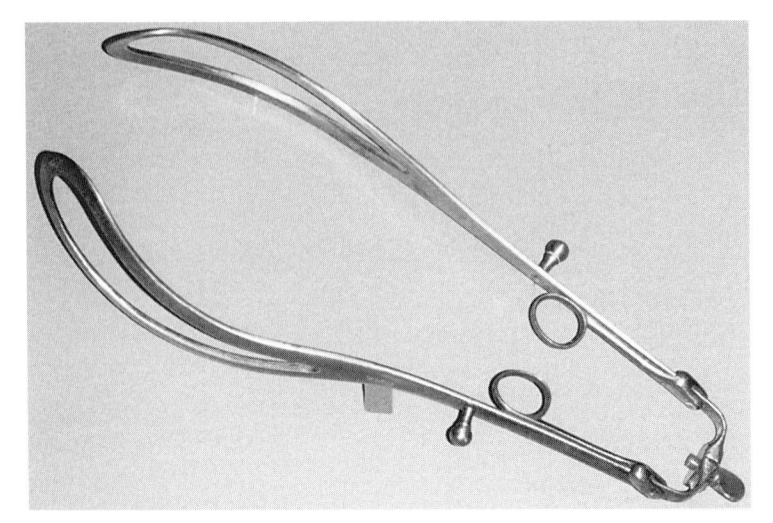

FIGURE 10.8.
Chassagny's rotating forceps. They are of lighter construction. The finger rings are hinged. (Science Museum, London)

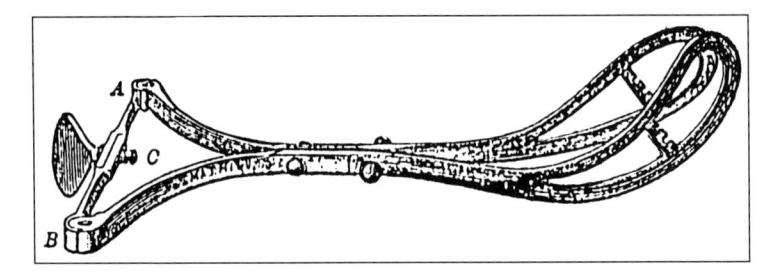

FIGURES 10.9, 10.10.
Two versions of Chassagny's later forceps. They both have a pelvic curve and devices for attaching lacs. The articulations and the adjustable plates joining the ends of the handles differ, although they are of a similar principle. (Chassagny, 1891)

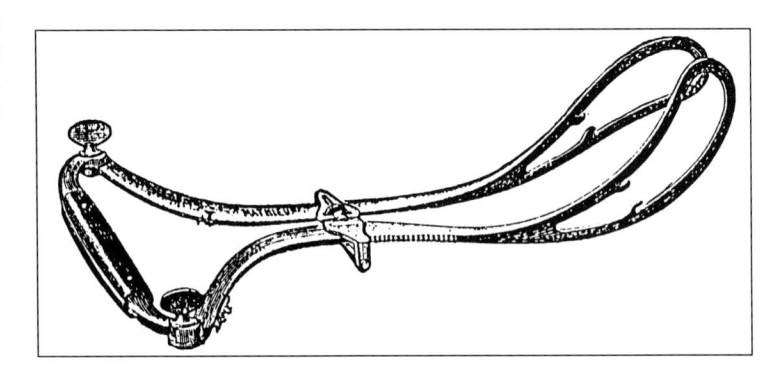

FIGURE 10.11.
Poullet's later parallel forceps. The double crossbars give stability. They both have screws so that the angles and distance between the blades is adjustable. (E. Hubert, 1884)

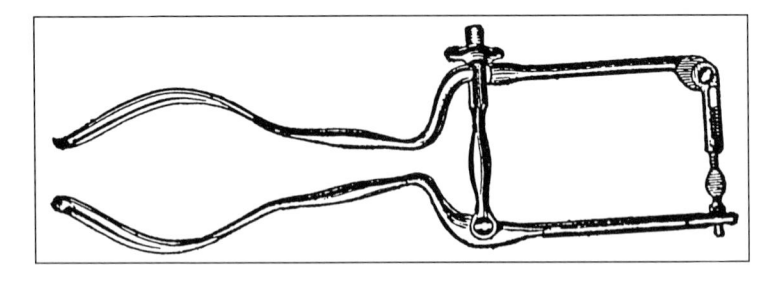

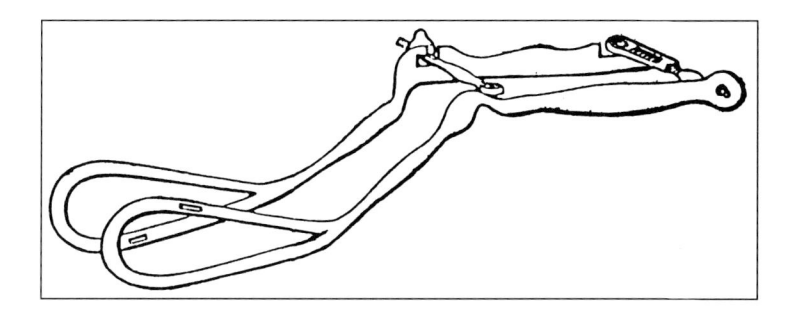

FIGURE 10.12.
Poullet's parallel forceps with perineal step. The crossbar design has been simplified compared with Figure 10.10. (Poullet, 1884)

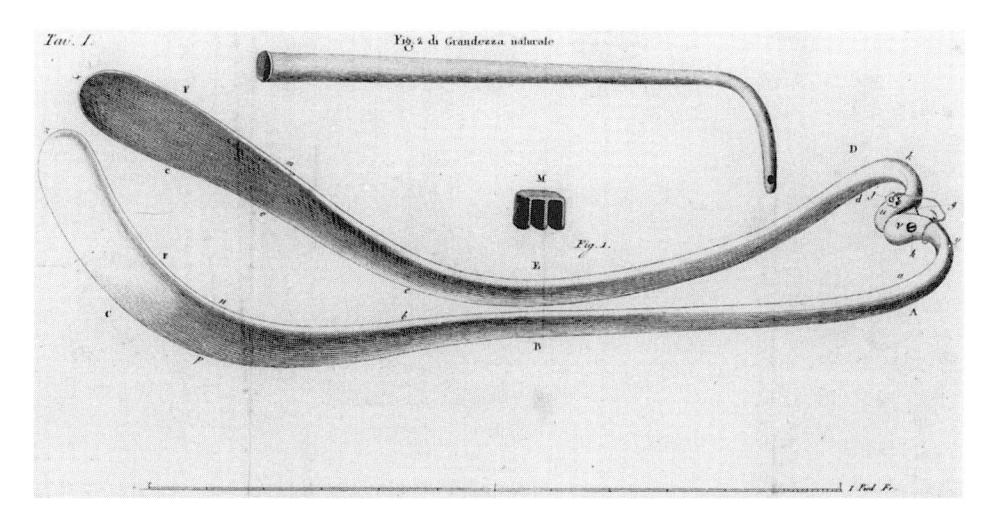

FIGURE 10.13.
Assalini's original design. The solid blades have a pelvic curve. The handles are joined by a mortise and tenon and can be locked with a pin. There is a separate E-shaped clip to hold the shanks together. A catheter is also shown.(Assalini, 1811)

freedom of movement, and relationship of the shape of the blades to the shape of the head. In particular they reputedly overcame the weaknesses of the popular forceps of his contemporaries, Chassagny and Tarnier. The instruments (Figure 10.11), of which there were a number of minor variants including detachable blades, had handles with two detachable crossbars forming a hinged parallelogram. This construction allowed a certain degree of movement of the blades and variation in the distance between them without disturbing the relationship of the cephalic curve to the head, thereby avoiding inappropriate compression. The shank was set at an angle of 150 degrees to form a perineal step (Figure 10.12). Axis traction could be achieved by a combination of tapes strung through holes in the blades and a metal rod with a transverse handle(see also Chapter 12).

Other European Developments

Although the Lyons school made the most sustained and scientific developments in parallel forceps design, the principle was explored by a number of other practitioners. Preeminent among these was Paolo Assalini.

Paolo Assalini's (1759–1840) parallel forceps (1811) were of simple design (Figure 10.13) and found immediate popularity in Europe, continuing to be manufactured and used well into the twentieth century. They were made entirely of metal and the handles were incurved and linked by a loose mortise and tenon joint. The original models were straight, with spoon-shaped, solid blades, but Assalini later incorporated a fenestrated blade. Subsequent copies embraced a range of variations in length, with blades that were both solid and fenestrated, straight and with a pelvic curve (Figure 10.14). An optional extra was an E-shaped clip to hold the blades together at about their midpoint for more stability.

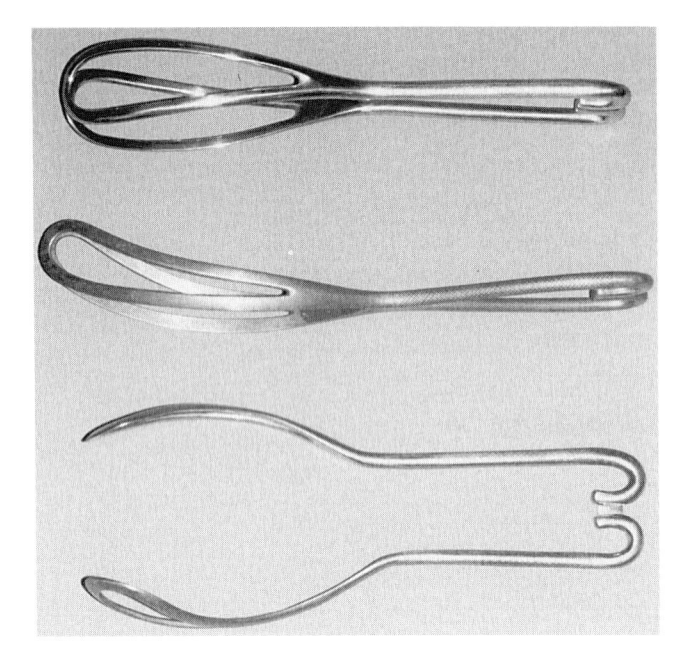

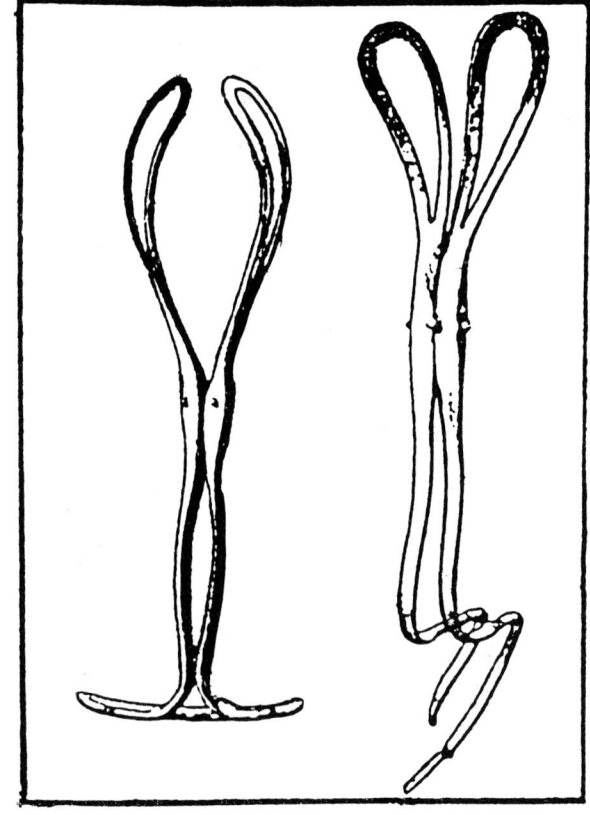

FIGURE 10.14 (ABOVE).
Assalini's forceps. Later straight and curved variants with fenestrated blades. The locking pin and E clip have been abandoned. (RCOG)

FIGURE 10.15 (ABOVE RIGHT).
Bernard's forceps. The shanks are joined by a chain and the handles, bent to a right angle, have a locking mechanism. (Bernard, 1636)

FIGURE 10.16.
Mattei's leniceps ("to hold softly"). The transverse handle is in two parts, with a three-position mortise joint. (Science Museum, London)

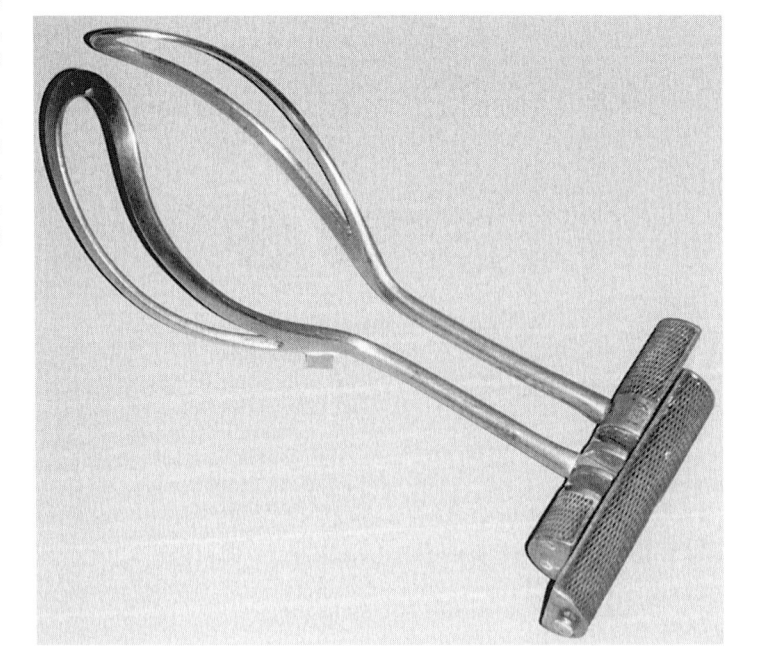

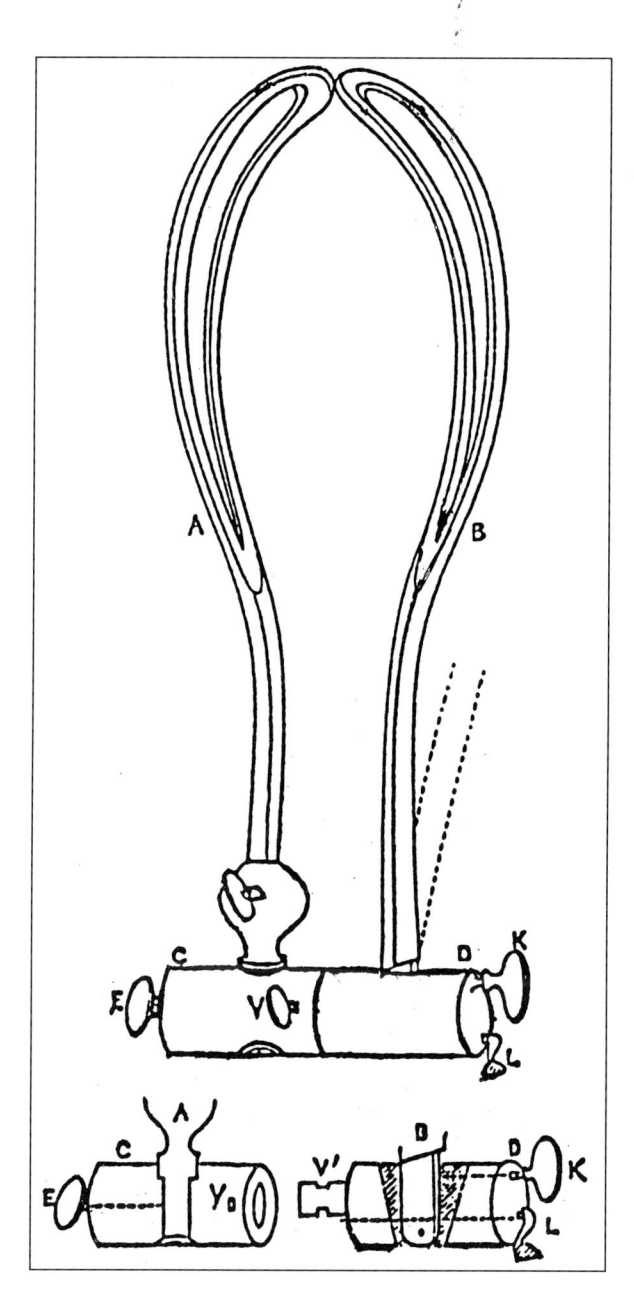

FIGURE 10.17.
Mondotte's forceps. This is a more complex development of the leniceps. In addition to the width adjustment one blade is hinged and the other pivoted. (Meadows, 1867)

The *forceps assemblé* (1836, 1853) of C. Bernard from Apt, comprised two branches joined by a chain (Figure 10.15). The blades were introduced superimposed on each other and finally positioned on the head by "wandering." This practice was not uncommon but some claimed that it caused trauma to mother and child.

A. Mattei had a novel design of parallel forceps (1859), which he termed *leniceps* ("to hold softly") (Figure 10.16). They were short and light in construction, with no pelvic curve. The straight shanks were united by a mortise-type joint to a detachable transverse handle that was in two parts, with perforations at varying distances so that the space between the blades could be varied. Mattei claimed that they could be applied at a lesser cervical dilatation, that they were easy to carry in the pocket, and that their application was gentle and easy. Indeed, so easy was their use that they could be applied without the woman being aware of it! (see also Chapter 8, Draper)

Mondotte's forceps (circa 1864), exhibited at the 1866 Obstetrical Society *Conversazione* (Meadows, 1867), were of a similar design to the leniceps and the distance between the blades was similarly adjustable (Figure 10.17). The only es-

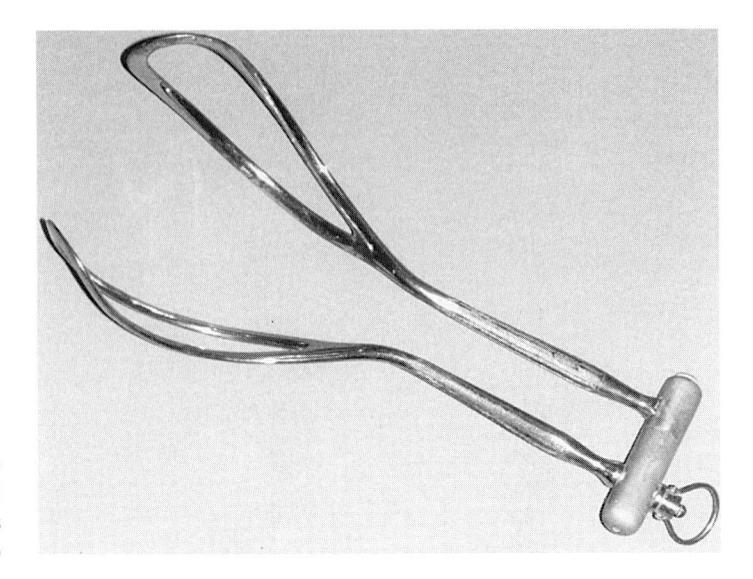

FIGURE 10.18.
Hamon's retroceps. Another development of the leniceps. The left blade has a sliding joint and the right blade is pivoted, as in Mondotte's forceps. (Science Museum, London)

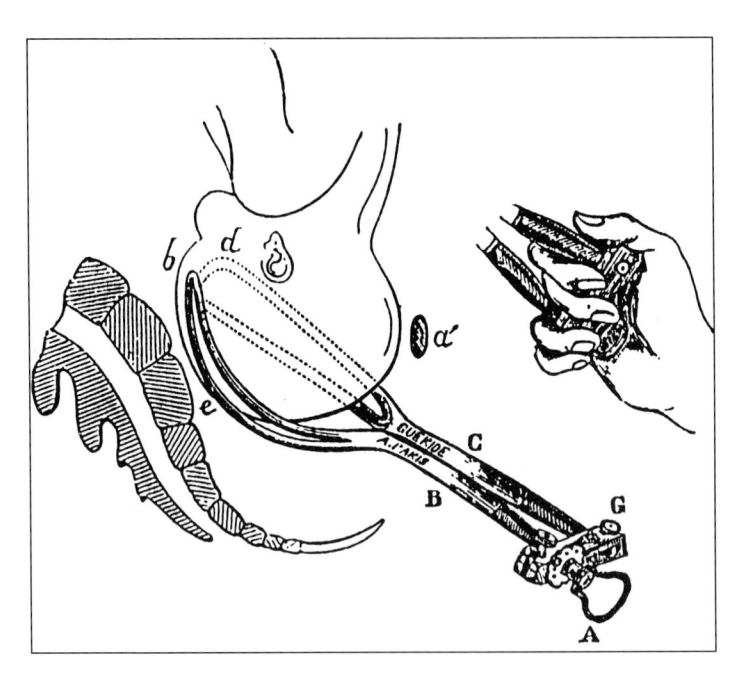

FIGURE 10.19.
Hamon's retroceps. Showing the method of application and traction. (Charpentier, 1883)

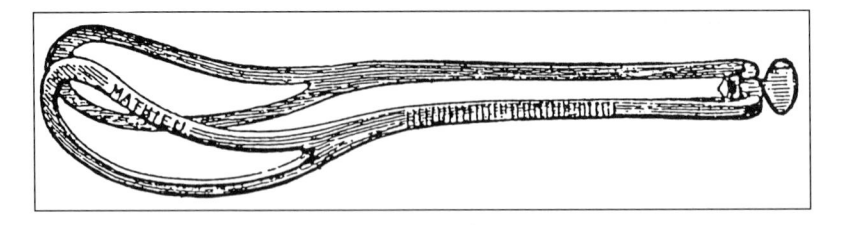

FIGURE 10.20.
Trelat's forceps. The design is based on Chassagny's rotating forceps. The blades are flexible. (Witkowski, 1887)

144 CHAPTER 10

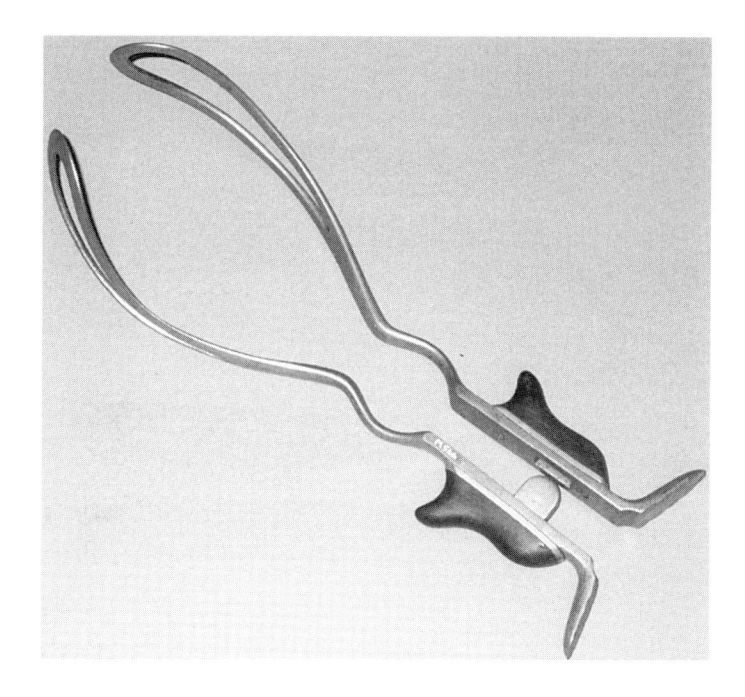

FIGURE 10.21.
Lazarewitch's parallel forceps. One of his designs for parallel forceps that differ only in detail. He had versions with straight and curved blades. (RCOG)

sential difference was in the design of the handles and articulation, which was much more complicated and unstable than that of the leniceps, even though the principle was similar. The handle was in two parts, joined by a mortise and tenon. One blade was hinged on the handle and the other pivoted.

L. Hamon of Fresnay described an instrument (1864a, 1864b), the *retroceps* ("to hold behind"), which is usually regarded as a parallel forceps and has many points of similarity with Mattei's leniceps, with the blades jointed to a common transverse handle. The left blade, which could move from side to side in a mortise slot on the handle, was fixed with a nut, while the right blade had a circular mortise joint so that it could rotate in its long axis (Figures 10.18, 10.19). However, the mode of use of the instrument was more akin to that of a double-bladed lever than forceps, as the blades were inserted posteriorly and did not directly face each other; thus they did not grasp the baby's head. Without regard for the inefficiency of the instrument for traction Hamon subsequently added features for attaching tapes and a traction assembly (Chapter 11).

Ulysse Trelat, Jr. (1828–1890), a professor of surgery at Necker, invented forceps that were also shown in 1866 at the Obstetric Society *Conversazione* (Figure 10.20) (Meadows, 1867). They were similar to Chassagny's rotating forceps (Figure 10.8). Because of their flexibility and elasticity they were dubbed "sugar pincers." It is unlikely that they gave a very effective grip on the head and the absence of any listing in major instrument makers' catalogues suggest that they were a misconception.

J. Lazarewitch (b. 1829) of the University of Kharkoff was another prolific designer of instruments, which he presented at various international meetings (1868b, 1869b, 1877b, 1881a), and in consequence numerous, often inaccurate, copies emerged, to which he drew attention at the International Medical Congress of 1881. His curved parallel forceps were first shown at the Obstetrical Society of London in 1866 at the *Conversazione* (Meadows, 1867). They had no outstanding original features apart from having the lock in the handle (Figure 10.21). He thereafter changed the design several times. In a model he exhibited in 1881, and in subsequent models, he dispensed with the pelvic curve, probably because they were short forceps. The lock was stronger than his previous version and constructed of a mortise and tenon in the handle and a screw passing right through, which enabled the blades to be kept parallel or diverged at an angle. He also added additional crossbars at the base of the shank that permitted considerable traction force, especially if a tape was attached. He claimed that placing the tape round the proximal finger rests avoided any compression force on the head, whereas if the tape was placed distally compression was achieved.

Toward the end of the nineteenth century, a number of other noncrossing forceps were developed in Europe but they were primarily axis-traction forceps and are described in Chapters 12–14. Carof's jointed forceps are described in Chapter 8.

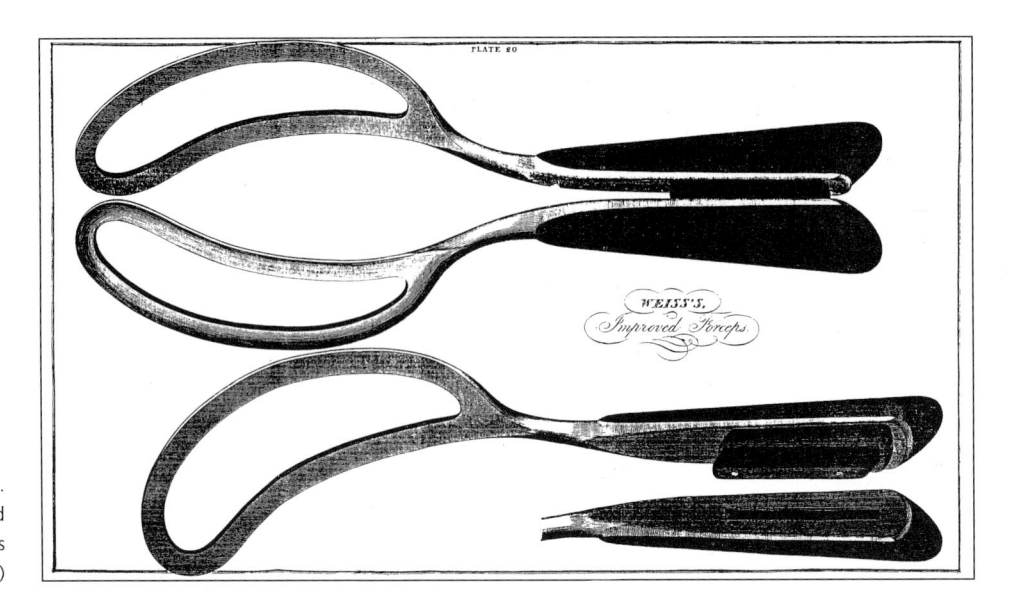

FIGURE 10.22.
Weiss's parallel forceps. The mortise and tenon joint predates Lazarewitch's design. (Weiss, 1831)

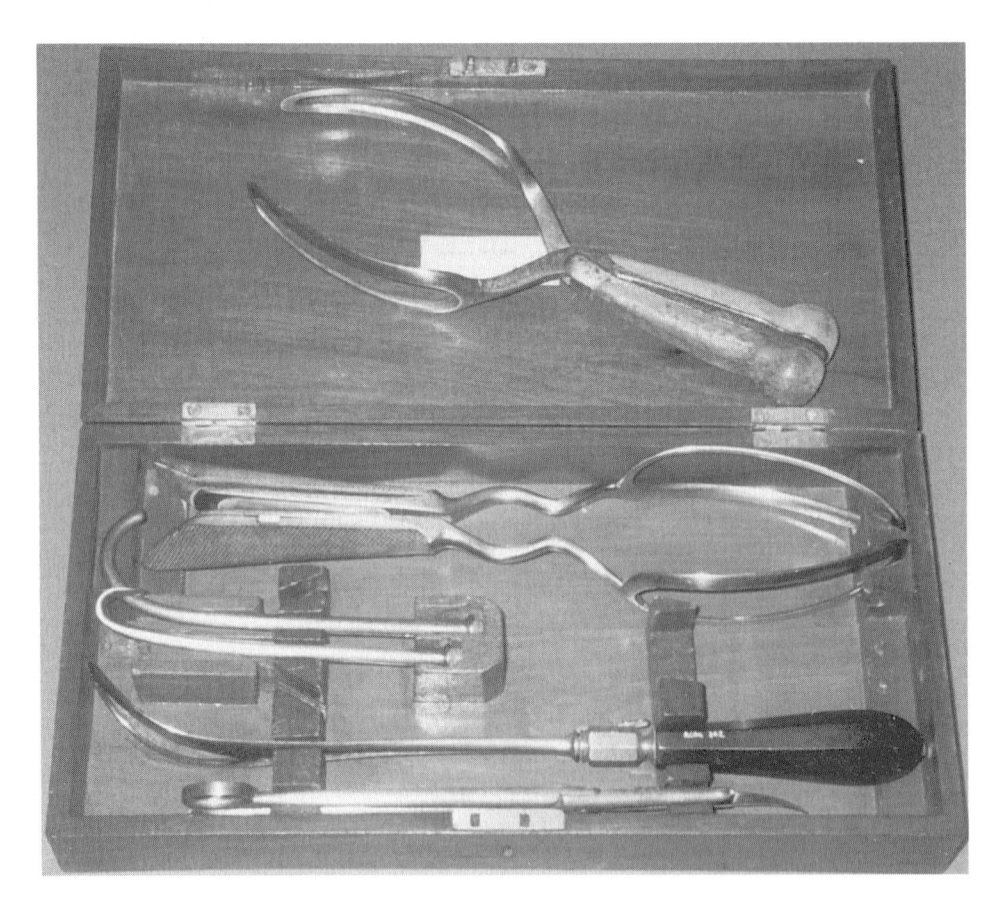

FIGURE 10.23.
Weiss general practitioners instrument set (mid-nineteenth century). The set comprises short straight forceps; parallel forceps; hook, crotchet, and lever with interchangeable handle; Denman's perforator. (RCOG)

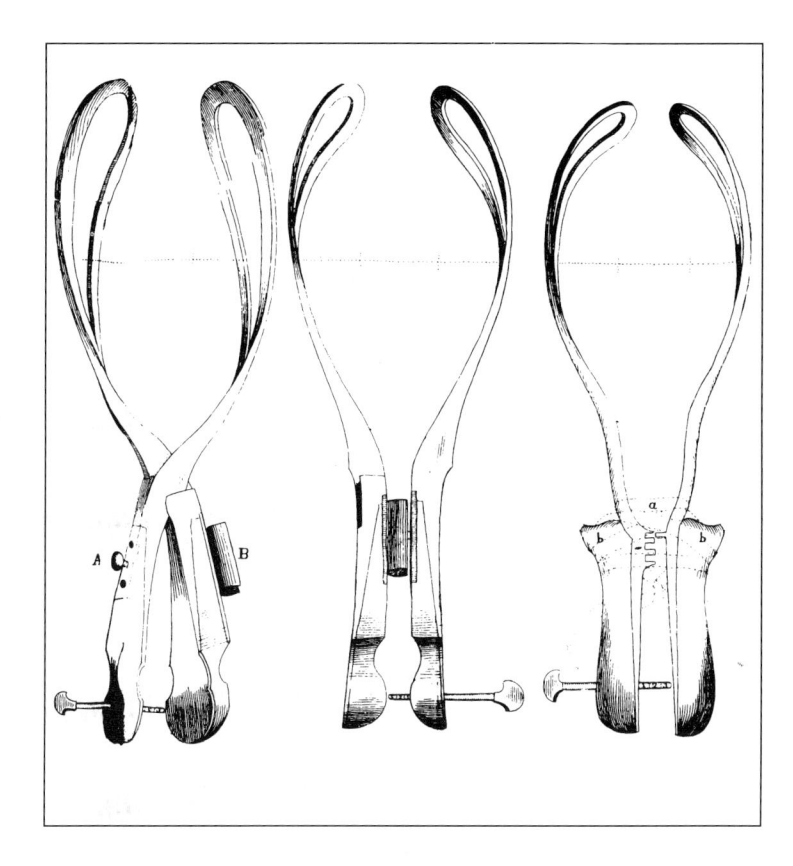

FIGURE 10.24.
Aitken's parallel forceps. In the first model (left and center), which can be used either crossed or uncrossed and asymmetrically, a ball-headed pin A articulates with an open-sided cannula B on the other handle. In the right-hand version a pin on one handle fits a three-position slotted joint on the other. Note also the "cephalometer" in the handle. (Aitken, 1786)

Britain and America

Noncrossing forceps never achieved significant notice outside Continental Europe and, for example, in Britain the catalogues of the major instrument makers of the nineteenth century such as Arnold, Down, and Maw offered only Assalini's curved forceps. However, the concept was not unknown in Britain. The innovative instrument maker John Weiss described and illustrated an "improved forceps" in 1831, which he claimed were based on Assalini's concept but with a better joint. They were short, curved, parallel forceps with a long mortise and tenon joint in the handle (Figure 10.22) and a similar instrument was in a set of obstetric instruments made by Weiss in the second half of the century (Figure 10.23). In fact, these instruments bear little resemblance to Assalini's, the only similarity being that these and Assalini's were parallel forceps.

Also toward the end of the eighteenth century and contemporaneous with Thenance, John Aitken (d. 1790) of Edinburgh described and illustrated two different parallel forceps in his *Principles of Midwifery* (1786; Plate NN, figures 4–6) (Figure 10.24). In the first pair, based on Smellie's forceps and with a crossover joint, he added a ball-headed pin on the outside of one handle and an open-sided cannula on the outside of the other handle to admit the ballhead. Thus the instrument could be used as a conventional forceps or as a parallel forceps, which would also allow for a degree of asymmetry, and was applicable when the blades could not be locked conventionally as in the crossover forceps articulations. The second pair had a simple lug and three-position slot joint, and stability was achieved by tying the blades together with a tape. In addition the handles incorporated finger rests and the roots of the blades were separated to allow a finger to go between them. Another interesting feature was that both pairs had a pressure-regulating screw that he termed a *cephalometer* (see also Chapter 5, "Pressure-Regulating Devices and Labimeters").

Bowers's forceps (circa 1885) were made by Arnold but are neither mentioned nor illustrated in their catalogues. They are listed but not illustrated in Weiss's catalogue. The pair

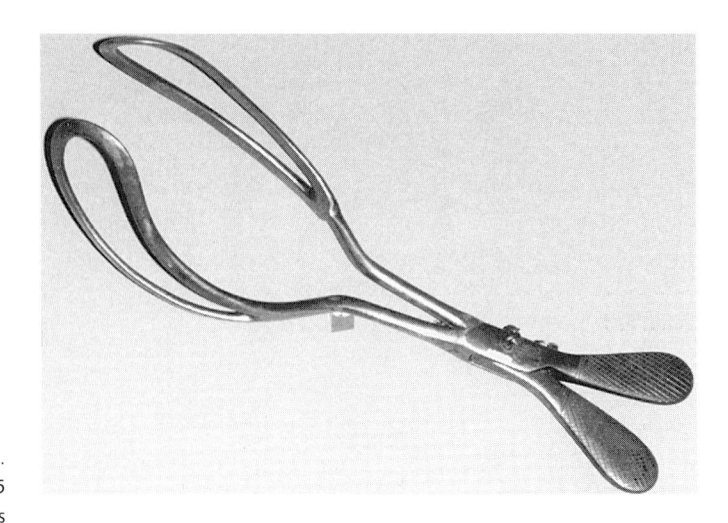

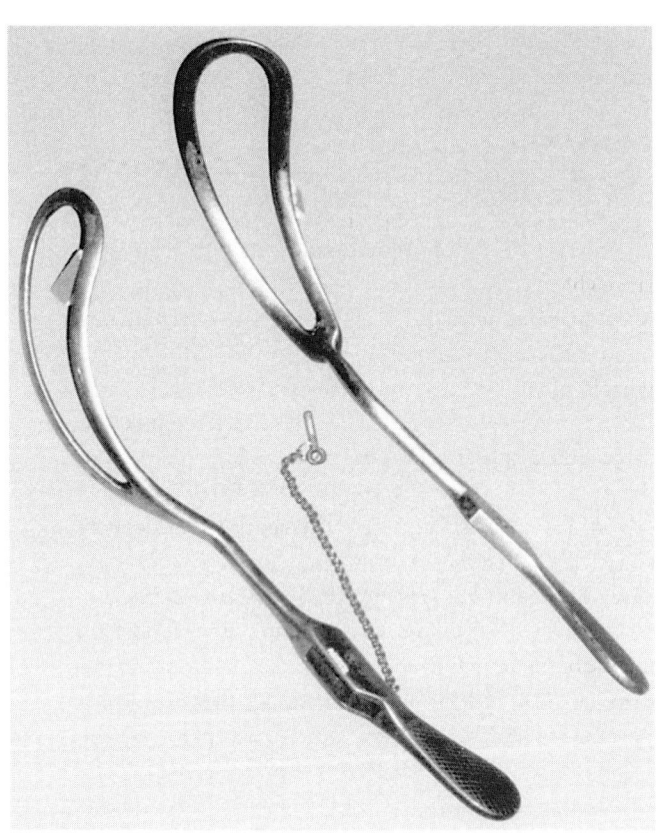

FIGURES 10.25, 10.26.
Bowers's forceps. They date from about 1885 but no written account is available. The joint is secured by a chain and pin. (Science Museum, London)

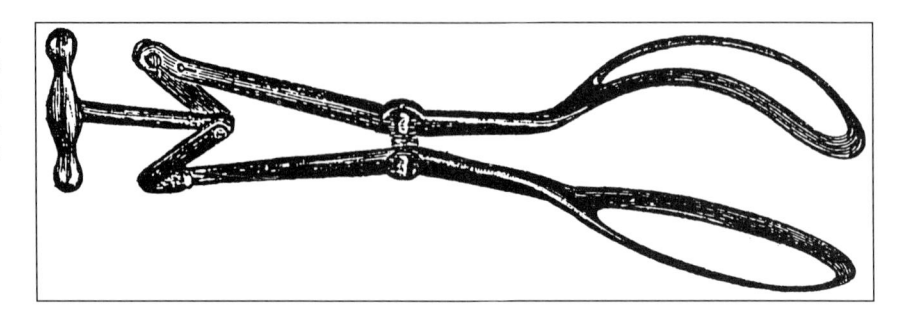

FIGURE 10.27.
Stewart's forceps. The ingenious coupling of the traction handle results in increased traction increasing the degree of head compression. (Stewart, 1889)

illustrated in this book is in the Wellcome collection (Figures 10.25, 10.26). The curved blades are of the Simpson type and the blades are secured at the shank by a chain and pin.

No parallel forceps featured in Tiemann's (New York) comprehensive catalogue of 1889 although there was at least one original American design, a novel and ingenious instrument described by W. S. Stewart, Professor of Obstetrics and Clinical Gynecology at the Medico-Chirurugical College of Philadelphia. Because of difficulties he experienced in locking crossover blades he designed a noncrossing pair of forceps with a loose joint at the shank (1887, 1889). He also addressed the problem of the degree of compression force to be used and was concerned about the use of a compression screw. His device to vary the compression force in relation to the traction force is shown in Figure 10.27. The traction handle was coupled to the handles of the forceps by a double-hinged lever system so that when traction was applied the ends of the handles were forced apart and the blades were brought together.

. . .

The sporadic designs for uncrossed forceps in the mid- to late eighteenth century were possibly attempts to improve on Palfyn's instruments. In France a major interest, centered on the influential school of Lyons, did not reawaken until the mid-nineteenth century. In the mechanical mood of the times these designs became more and more complex and most of them appear to have had a limited life, judging from the instrument makers' catalogues of the time.

The one enduring design, that of Assalini, came from Italy and antedated the prolific inventors of Lyons. With no more than minor and unimportant modifications, they continued to be used in several European centers until at least the middle of the twentieth century. This was no doubt due to their simplicity of design and functionality, contrasting with the complexities of the mid-nineteenth century instruments.

AIDS TO TRACTION (*TRACTIONS MÉCANIQUES*) AND DYNAMOMETERS

11

In Britain and most of Europe any desire to increase traction force was generally met by relatively simple means. The more conservative practitioners usually used no more extra force than that achieved by tapes passed through the fenestra, often attaching them to a blunt hook. Purpose-designed hooks were also used or adapted to give maximum traction force. Alexander Duke (d. 1915), of the Rotunda Hospital in Dublin, devised an attachment that he used with a modified pair of Morgan's traction rods. (Morgan's hooks, and others intended primarily for axis traction, are discussed in Chapter 14). Duke's graphic description reads:

> Having seen more than once an experienced accoucheur fail with all his force to deliver till at length, assisted by another grasping him round the waist, he was enabled to do so (with no detriment to either mother or child), I had often thought if some means could be devised which, in a difficult case, would give the required power without the necessity of calling an assistant (even if one were always at hand). When additional traction is required, as in cases of convulsions, haemorrhage, etc., where time is very important, I slip the rings of my tractors into an ordinary swivel attached by metal band to a strap which I have previously buckled round my waist, and can thus make any amount of traction *consistent with safety*, with the greatest of ease to myself, and without fatigue, or perspiring profusely, as I often did and many do still. (1879) (Figure 11.1)

In addition, Duke attached cricket spikes to the soles of his shoes to keep his feet from slipping (1880).

In France during the third quarter of the nineteenth century many practitioners, in keeping with their tendency to use heavier instruments and greater force, felt a need to augment the traction force that could normally be achieved with forceps. This desire led to the development of various devices (*tractions mécaniques*) that had considerable mechanical advantage and could be used to apply sustained traction rather than the commonly employed intermittent traction, a policy advocated over many years by Chassagny in particular. This traction was often mediated through tapes or hooks with handles passed through the fenestra, thus, unwittingly in most cases, applying to some degree the principles of axis traction. However, much of the traction force was uselessly expended on pulling the head against the pubes, with the attendant risks of trauma to the baby and the birth canal. Apart from any arguments concerning the relative merits of intermittent or sustained traction these aids suffered many disadvantages, such as complexity and difficulty in application and, in particular for many devices, the difficulty in altering the direction of traction. The considerable degree of force that could be exerted was also a major hazard, although the introduction of the dynamometer to measure the traction force mitigated this to some degree. Possibly the concept of a dynamometer had arisen from devices used in Japan earlier in the century, such as that illustrated by Witkowski (1887) (Figure 11.2).

In Britain the mechanically ingenious but dangerous European machines discussed in this chapter did not find favor and also became less popular in France following the appreciation of the components of the forces involved in delivery, and the introduction of true axis-traction forceps by Tarnier in 1877 (Chapter 13).

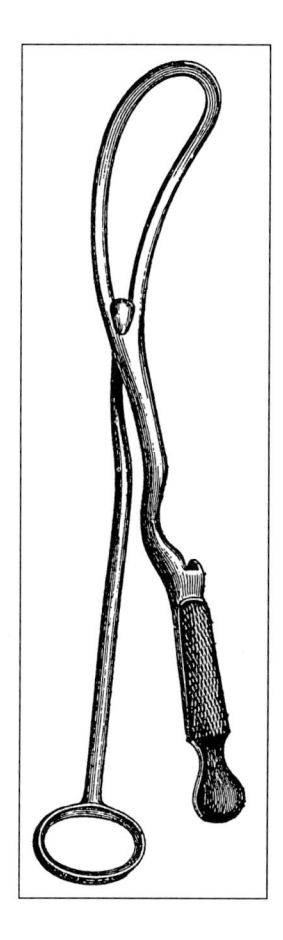

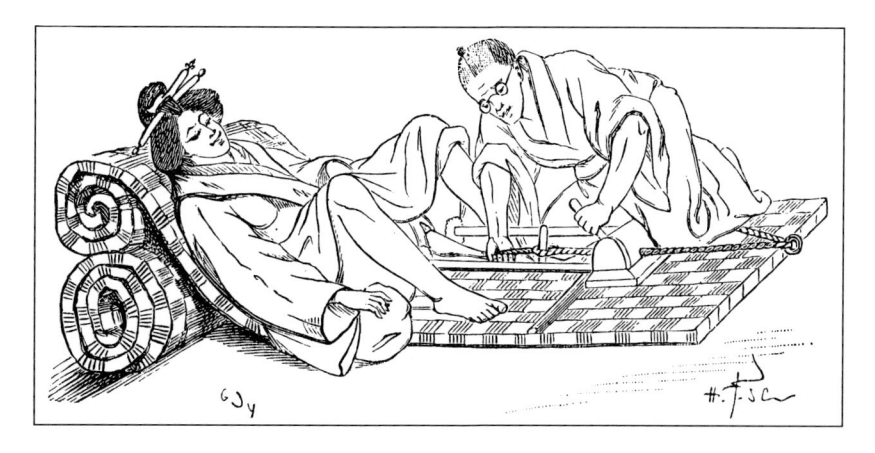

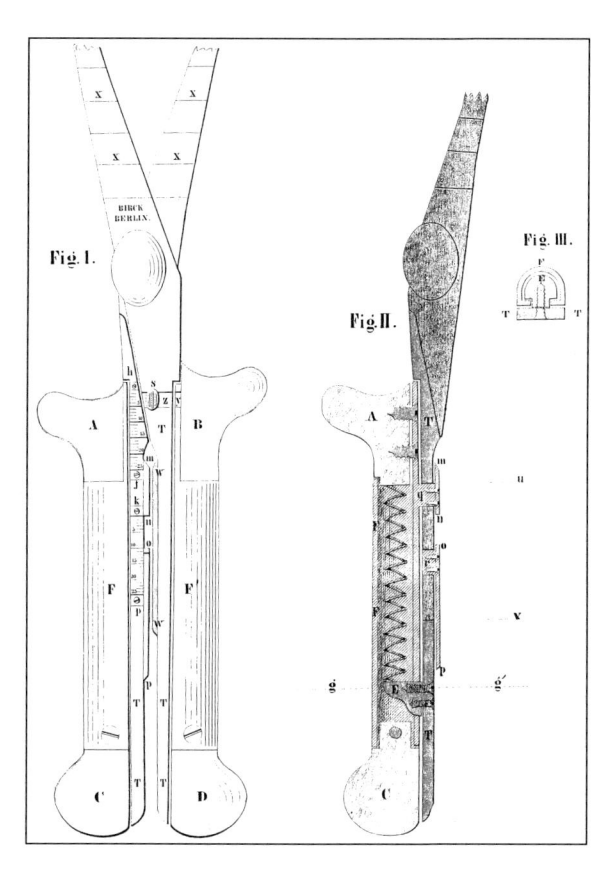

FIGURE 11.1.
Duke's tractors. They could be used with any fenestrated forceps. (Duke, 1879)

FIGURE 11.2.
Japanese tractor. The device was in use early in the eighteenth century. (Witkowski, 1887)

FIGURE 11.3.
Kristeller's forceps. A strong spring pressure gauge is built into each handle, the scales being on the upper surface of the handles. The handles slide on the shank but can be fixed with a pin if desired. (Kristeller, 1861)

Dynamometers

Concern with the potential traction force led to the incorporation of dynamometers in several traction systems in order to measure the force exerted. These were usually of a standard type based on a double elliptical spring and dial that measured the compression of the springs, which was equivalent to the traction force. Examples in relation to the tractors of Joulin, Xavier Delore (b. 1828) of Lyons, G. Pros of La Rochelle, and Poullet are illustrated below.

Samuel Kristeller (1820–1900) of Berlin, presented a complicated but ingenious forceps to the Berlin Obstetrical Society in 1860, which he illustrated in his 1861 article. The instrument was described in detail by Doran (1921). The forceps incorporated a spring measuring gauge in the handle (Figure 11.3). In each handle was a brass cylinder that could slide along the extension of the shank of the forceps and contained a strong spring that was compressed when traction was applied through the finger lugs. The traction force was read on a brass scale. Each handle also had a slide catch to enable it to be fixed to the shank if the dynamometer was not required.

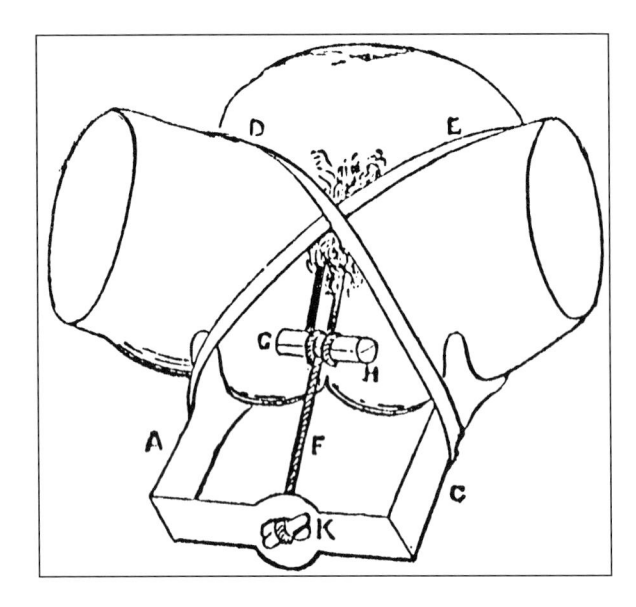

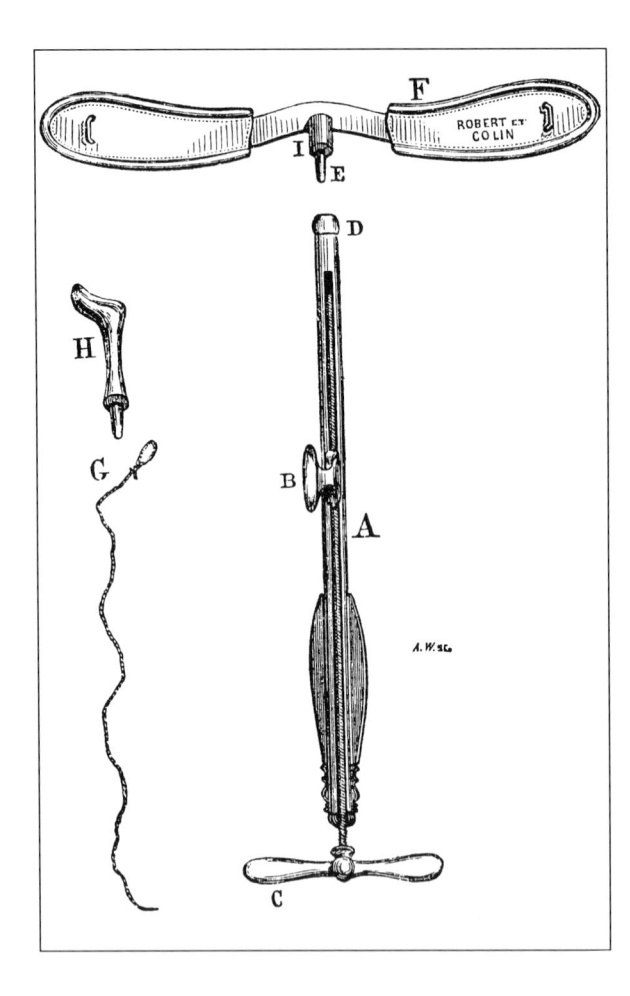

Tractions Soutenues

A. Mattei, who invented the leniceps (Chapter 10), was one of the first surgeons to construct an apparatus that could be used to provide prolonged and forcible traction. He eventually demonstrated this new instrument at the 1866 Obstetrical Society *Conversazione* (Meadows, 1867) (Figure 11.4). It comprised a U-shaped steel framework with a concave termination to the limbs to receive the patient's thighs. It was held in position by diagonal straps that crossed the front of the pubes and wrapped around the thighs. A rope was attached to the handle of the leniceps and to a screw in the U-frame. Sustained forcible traction was achieved by rotating the screw.

Joulin's *aide-forceps* (1867) was described by Charpentier (1883) but it was poorly designed and relatively ineffective, principally because the transverse bar that was applied to the ischial tuberosities was designed to lie in front of the forceps and was therefore obstructive, limiting the direction and control of traction. Attached to this plate was a steel tube within which was a threaded rod with a distal handle (Figure 11.5). A cord was passed through the fenestra of the blades and hooked on to the threaded rod. Traction was applied by turning the handle so that the threaded rod was drawn up the tube. In addition the apparatus could be fitted with a chain saw to function as an écraseur.

Joulin's *aide-forceps* was important because he was the first to interpose a dynamometer between the cord and the hook on the screw (Figure 11.6). The force deployed varied between 20 and 60 kilograms (44 and 132 pounds). Joulin claimed that with sustained traction delivery was effected in 10 to 30 minutes. A similar apparatus was described by Roussel of Geneva in about 1874 and is illustrated by Witkowski (1892) (Figure 11.7). The crossbar was perforated to sit more readily over the ischial tuberosities than did the flat bar of Joulin and the tapes were attached directly to a drum with a worm screw and thumb-wheel mechanism.

Also in 1867 Xavier Delore (b. 1828) of Lyons devised a traction system involving pulleys. A plank of wood with a screw ring was bolted to the floor or a pillar and a double pulley was connected to the forceps with an interposed dynamometer (Figure 11.8). Although the direction of traction

FIGURE 11.4.
Mattei's steel frame for sustained traction. It is held in position by diagonal straps C,D. (Meadows, 1867)

FIGURE 11.5.
Joulin's *aide-forceps*. A cord passed through the fenestra of the forceps is attached to the hook *B* on the worm screw *A* and sustained traction is increased by turning the handle. Also shown is a chain saw *G* and attachment *H*. (Charpentier, 1883)

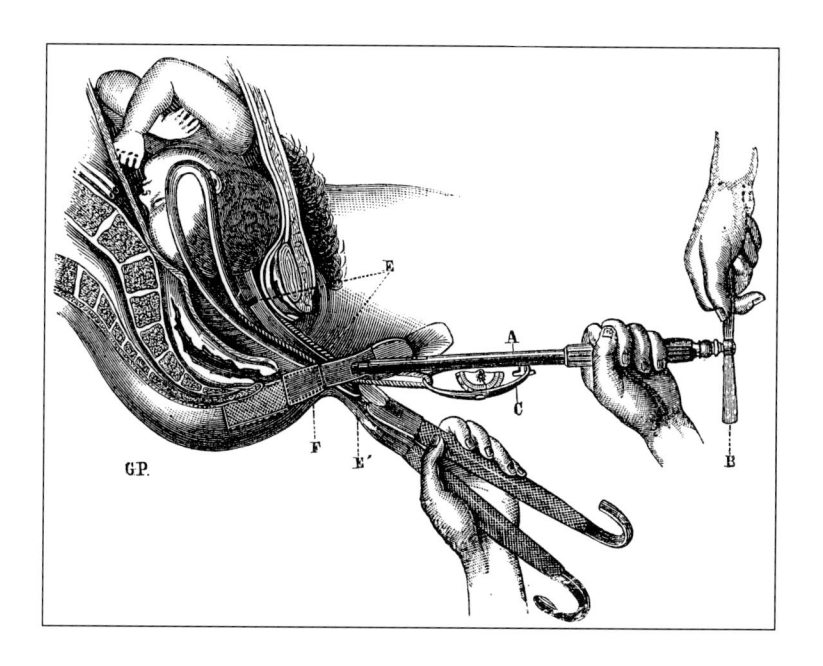

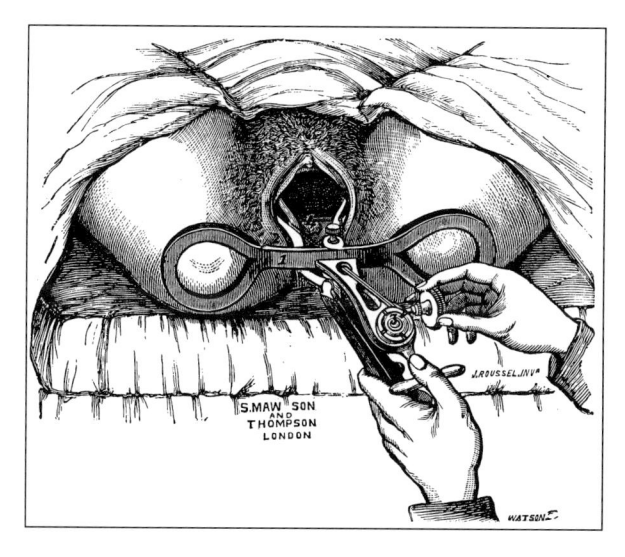

FIGURE 11.6.
Joulin's *aide-forceps*. The apparatus in use. A dynamometer *(C)* to measure the traction force has been added. (Charpentier, 1883)

FIGURE 11.7.
Roussel's *aide-forceps*. Similar in principle to Joulin's apparatus but with a wheel mechanism to apply traction. (Witkowski, 1887)

FIGURE 11.8.
Delore's cord and pulley tractor. A dynamometer is interposed in the pulley system. (Charpentier, 1883)

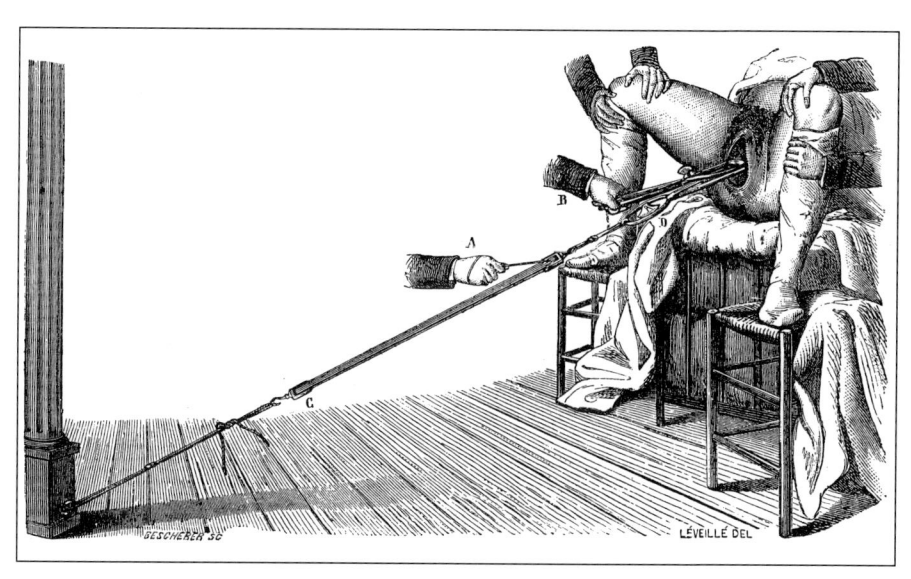

AIDS TO TRACTION AND DYNAMOMETERS   153

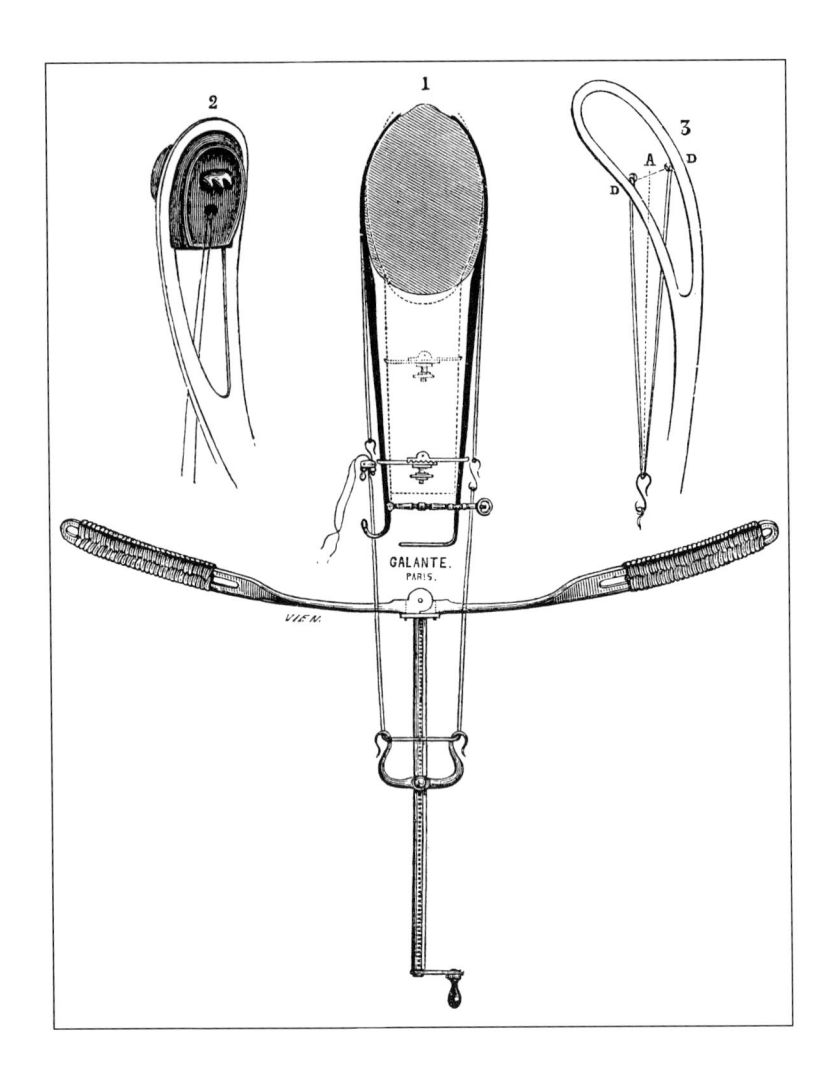

FIGURES 11.9–11.11. Chassagny's *forceps à tractions soutenues*. 11.9: In this version two methods of attaching the cords are shown. Figure 2 utilizes a special attachment with teeth that fits inside the fenestra. Figure 3 shows hooks inside the fenestra. A worm screw is used for traction (Charpentier, 1883.) 11.10: This has a cog wheel and chain mechanism (Charpentier, 1883). 11.11: Another version of Figure 11.9 with padded buttock rests. (Hubert, 1889)

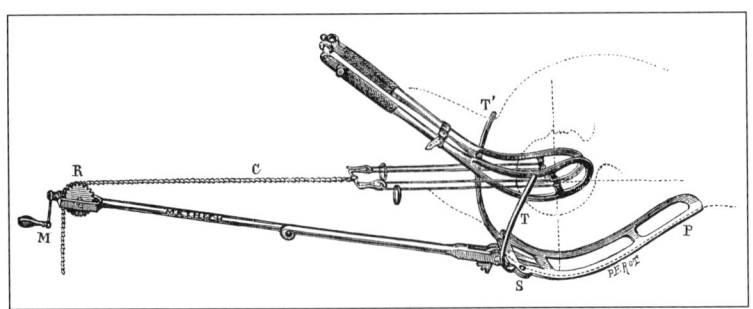

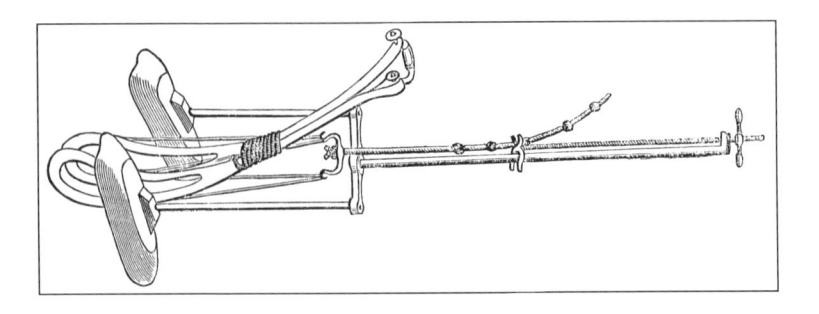

154   CHAPTER 11

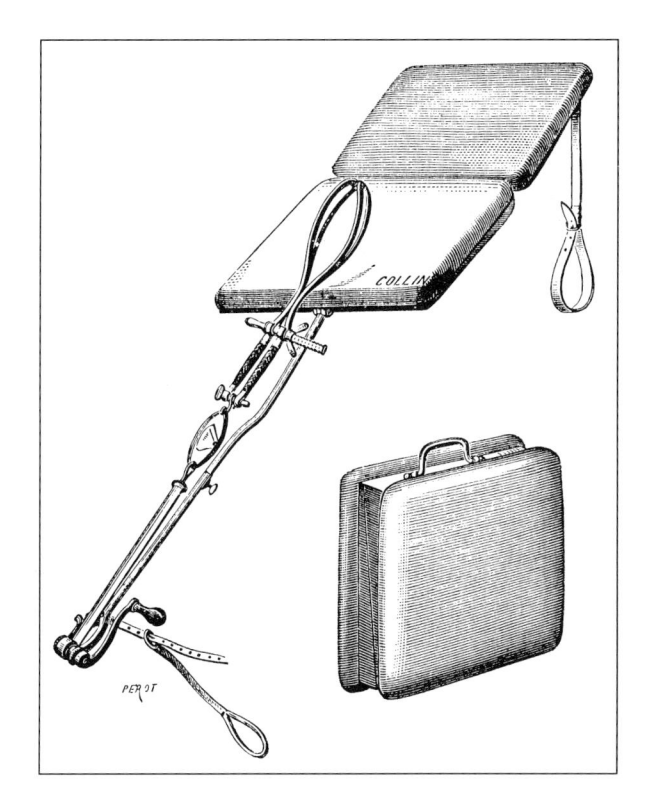

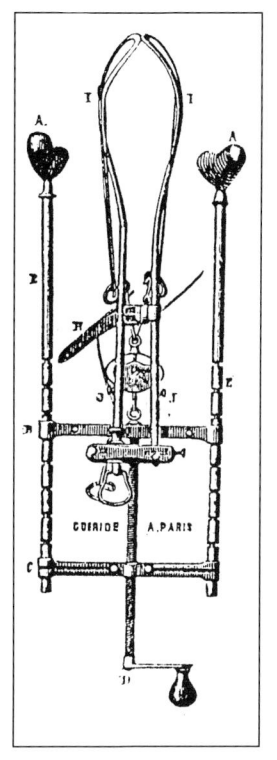

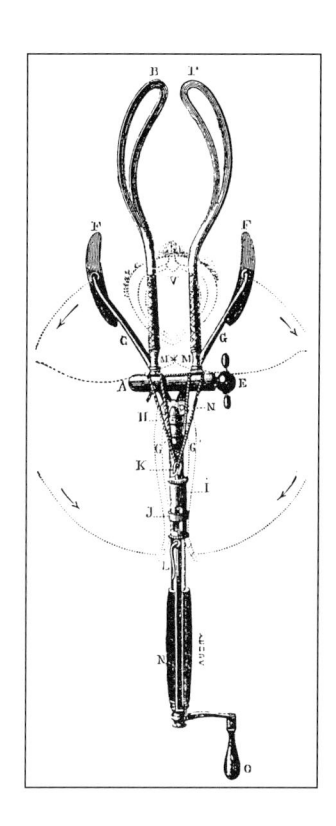

FIGURE 11.12.
Pros's portable tractor. This is one of several versions. The hinged rod allows for variation in the direction of traction. (Witkowski, 1887)

FIGURES 11.13, 11.14.
Hamon's mechanical tractors. 11.13: early model. 11.14: late model. (Witkowski, 1887)

was fixed the angle of the blades to the birth canal could be controlled manually. The only limit to the traction force that could be applied was the amount of counter force that the assistants holding the patient could exert.

Although M. Chassagny of Lyons, who designed many types of parallel forceps (Chapter 10), was one of the first to experiment with mechanical traction, a technique already known to veterinary surgeons (Chassagny, 1860–1861, 1863, 1871), he did not publicize his mechanical tractor, or *forceps à tractions soutenues,* for "continued traction and progressive pressure" until 1875. This was an apparatus with perineal rests, initially made of wood but later steel. Although the traction apparatus could be used with conventional forceps, Chassagny used purpose-designed, long parallel forceps with flexible blades and cords connecting the blades to a long screw, with a cranked handle attached at right angles to the perineal plate (Figures 11.9–11.11).

Chassagny was one of the few surgeons who persisted with the philosophy of continuous traction and described at least three modifications, not significant, of his original apparatus, two of which were illustrated by Charpentier (1883) and one by Hubert (1889). As late as 1891 Chassagny was still promoting the principle in his text, *Fonctions du forceps.*

In 1874 G. Pros of La Rochelle constructed a tractor on the Chassagny principle and claimed priority over Chassagny (1875, 1876, 1877) (Figure 11.12). The apparatus, which is illustrated with various modifications, essentially consisted of a wooden frame covered with cloth that was placed under the buttocks. Leather straps anchored the woman to the frame. An adjustable rod was attached to the board in the midline by a hinge. At the end of the rod was a winding handle and strap, the latter being attached to the forceps by a transverse bar, with an intervening dynamometer. Because the rod was hinged the direction of traction was easily and accurately adjustable. Pros mentions a traction force of between 60 and 80 kilograms (132 and 176 pounds), rather more than that employed by Joulin.

In 1877, L. Hamon, also from La Rochelle, constructed a mechanical tractor for use with his retroceps (Chapter 10). This was rather surprising since he extolled the gentleness of his retroceps that were, in any case, not a very efficient tractor. The general concept was similar to that of Chassagny's earlier model, with two crutches that rested in the genitocrural fold and a long screw with a cranked handle (Figure 11.13). He later designed another, more complicated, model (Figure 11.14). Both of these were illustrated in

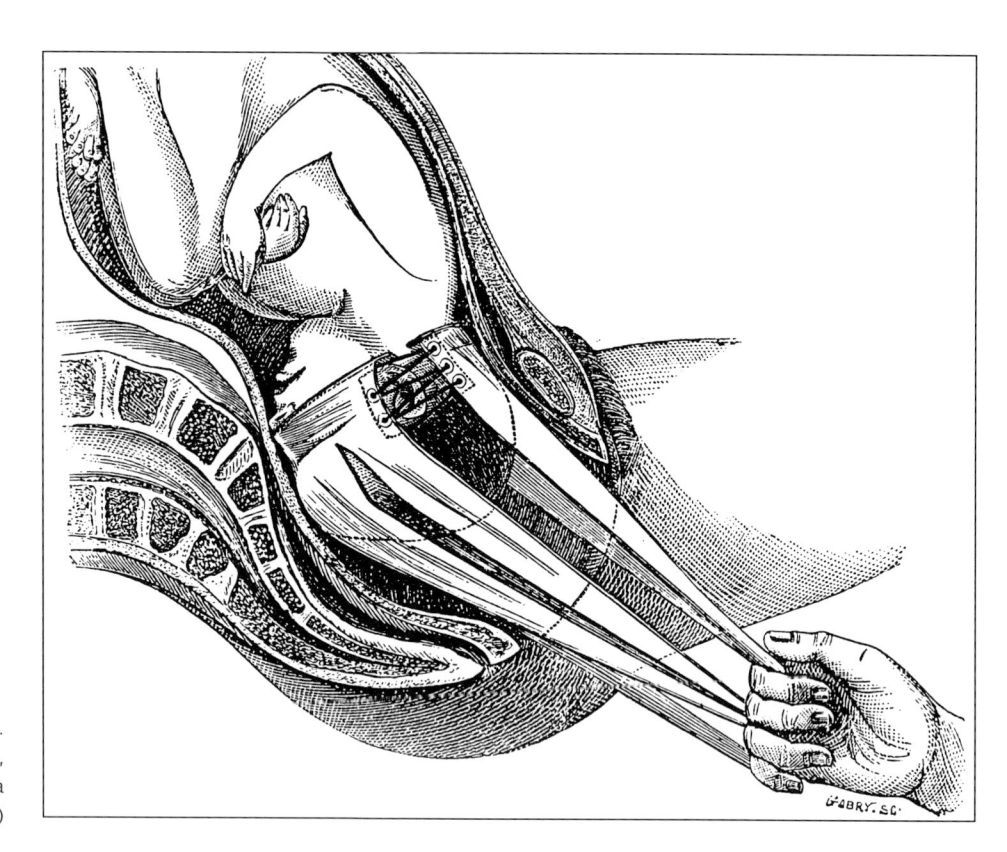

FIGURE 11.15.
Poullet's original sericeps. This device, based on a Japanese concept, was not a success. (Poullet, 1875)

Witkowski's *Histoire des accouchements chez tous les peuples* (1887).

J. Poullet of Lyons (Chapter 9), who was a thoughtful innovator, gave a critical appraisal of the various mechanical tractors then available in his *Diverses Espèces de forceps* of 1883 and described his own contrivances and apparatus, which, he claimed, overcame the disadvantages of his predecessors. In 1875 Poullet had presented to the Imperial Academy of Medicine with John Anne Henri Depaul (1811–1883), his new traction device, the *sericeps* (1875a) (Figure 11.15). This instrument was based on an earlier Japanese idea and was constructed of fabric in the manner of a pair of laced corsets to encompass the head, with four prolongations of the material to form the hand grip. A steel forceps was used to introduce the sericeps. In spite of the apparent advantage of using a soft material rather than metal, the sericeps proved to be dangerous to the fetus and Poullet encountered such problems with neonatal apnea that he renounced the equipment after using it in ten cases.

Also in 1875 Poullet published a description of his *tracteur pour appliquer la force mécanique* (1875b) (Figure 11.16). He described it as having three components: a pelvic arc in two pieces (*ABCD* in Figure 11.16), the ends of which were lozenge shaped and covered with rubber, to fit against the ischial tuberosities; and a rod (*EF*) attached to the arc at one end and to the third component, the cannula, at the other. The rod and cannula were set at an angle to each other; the cannula (*FG*) enclosed a long screw with a threaded hook (*H*) attached. Rotation of the screw moved the hook along the cannula, thus providing the traction force. The traction chains were inserted in holes in the blades of the forceps at one end and to the hook at the other, with an interposed dynamometer. The angle of the tractor could be altered, as is shown in Figure 11.17, thus allowing for axis traction. Poullet also illustrated the apparatus in use with his *sericeps* (Figure 11.18), although he probably never used this combination.

Poullet continued to experiment with variations on his mechanical novelties and in 1881 introduced his *forceps souple à tractions indépendantes* (Figure 11.19). This instrument was also designed to encompass the head firmly and allow strong traction but it was clearly difficult to apply and had the potential for damage to the face and head, as is evidence by the illustration.

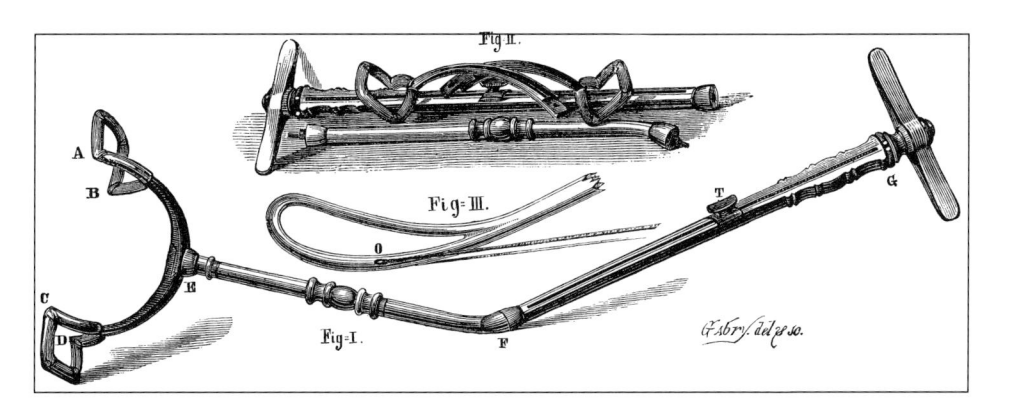

FIGURE 11.16.
Poullet's *tracteur pour appliquer la force mécanique.* The individual components are shown. (Charpentier, 1883)

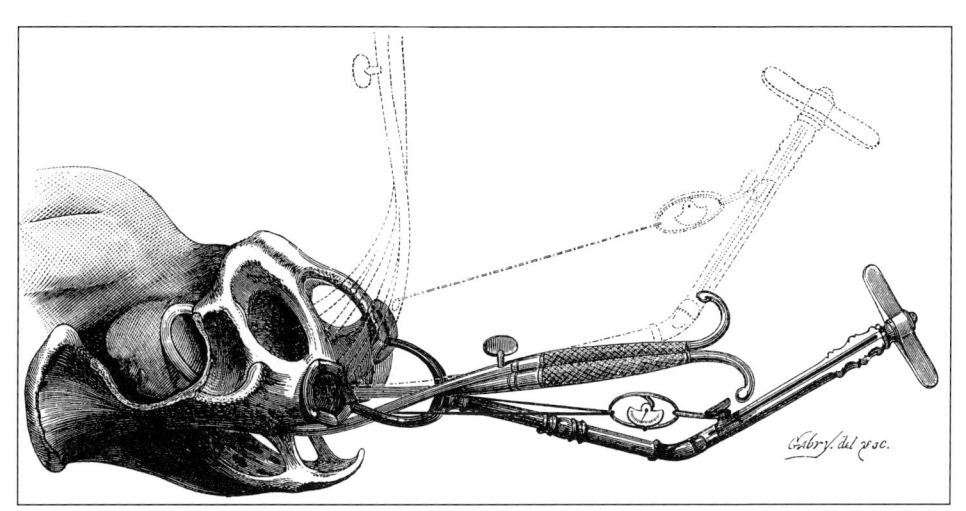

FIGURE 11.17.
Poullet's tractor. In use with forceps. Note the adjustable angle on the rod and the interposed dynamometer. (Poullet, 1875)

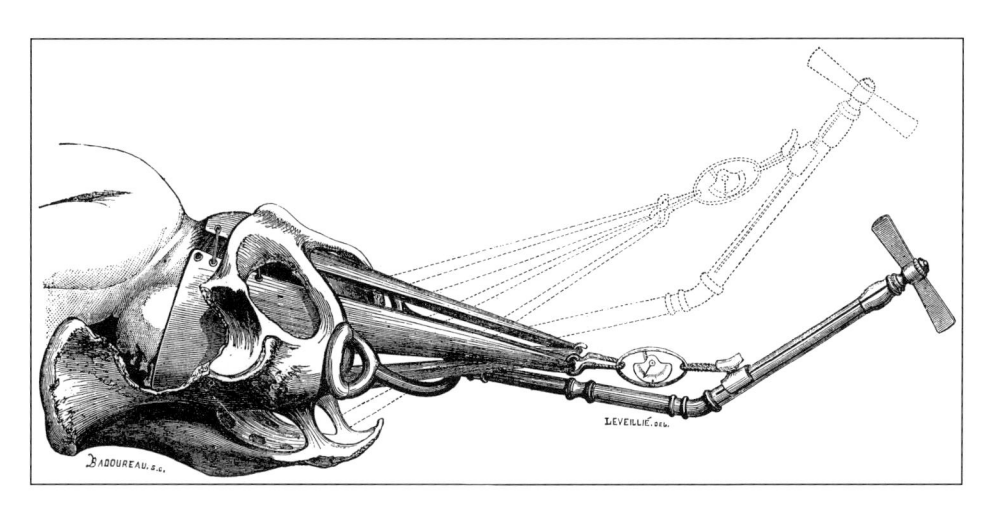

FIGURE 11.18.
Poullet's tractor. In use with the sericeps. (Poullet, 1875)

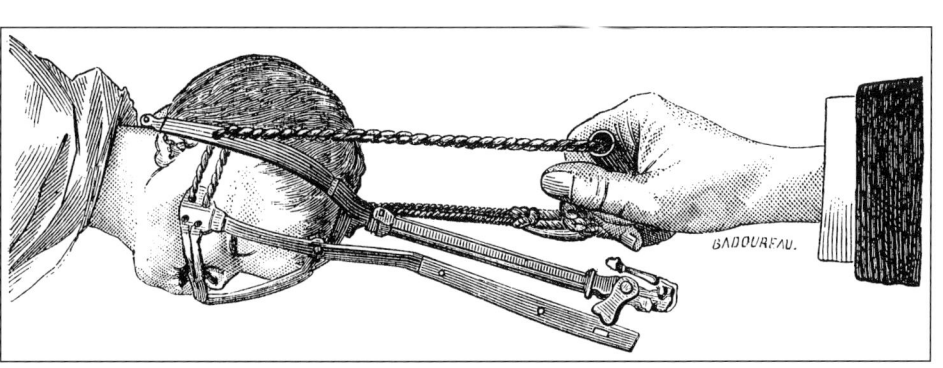

FIGURE 11.19.
Poullet's *forceps souple à tractions indépendantes.* One of his later novel designs, termed *nouveau sericeps* by Charpentier. (Charpentier, 1883)

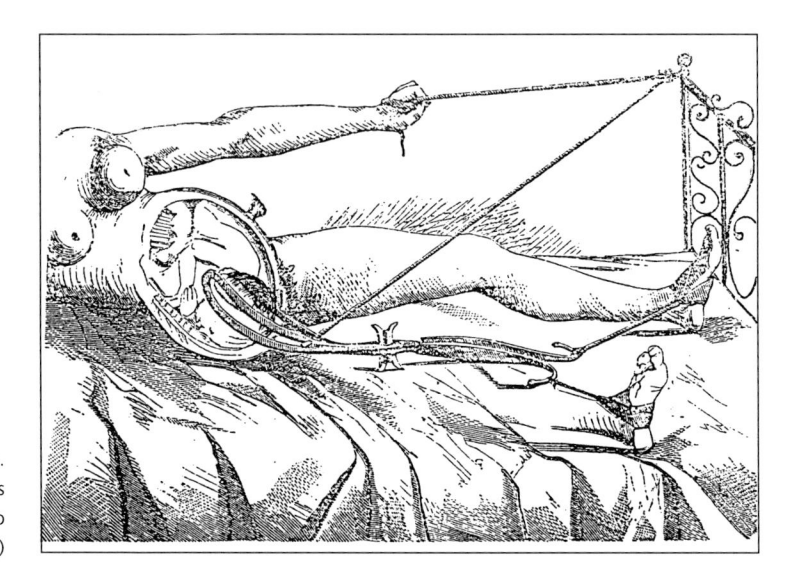

FIGURE 11.20.
Giordano's *forcipe a staffe briglie*. The patient is applying traction via a rope and pulley, and also by foot stirrups. (Giordano, 1865)

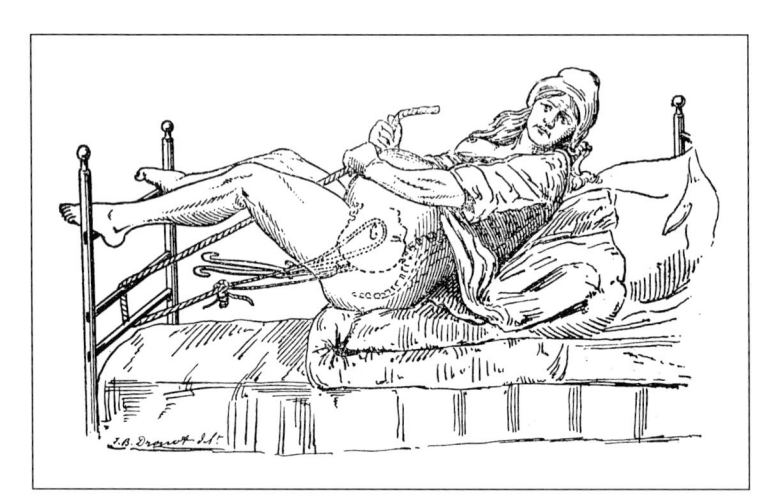

FIGURE 11.21.
Roussel's *ex tempore* use of patient traction. (Witkowski, 1892)

"Auto-Traction"

A curious diversion was the use of arrangements for the patient herself to apply traction, an action that could be referred to as "auto traction."

Scipione Giordano of Turin described his *forcipe a staffe briglie* in 1865, using a traction cord held by the mother passing through a pulley on the foot of the bed and attached to the fenestra of the forceps. In addition stirrups in which the mother's feet were inserted were attached by cords to the handles of the forceps (Figure 11.20).

Another situation in which a similar contraption was used, reported by Roussel of Geneva, developed by chance and is chronicled by Witkowski (1892) (Figure 11.21). The obstetrician, being on holiday and with an injured arm, went to the aid of a woman with obstructed labor who had not responded to the midwife's administration of ergot. He applied forceps, with ropes through the fenestra and, because of his injury, instructed the husband to pull. The husband fainted and disappeared so he put the cord around the cross bar at the foot of the bed and enlisted the help of the mother. She instinctively pulled during contractions and delivered herself in seven or eight minutes.

. . .

The aids to traction described in this chapter had a limited vogue of no more than thirty years and would probably have fallen into oblivion but for their interest as items of curiosity and the fact that they were present in some widely read and enduring publications such as Witkowski's *Histoire* and Meadows's *Catalogue and Report*. The need for sustained traction was not widely accepted and the opportunity for abuse with such powerful tools is self-evident. In addition, little consideration was given to the mechanics of parturition, although by this time the more scientific approach leading to the concept of axis traction was becoming well established.

EARLY AXIS-TRACTION FORCEPS AND THEIR PRECURSORS

12

In the eighteenth and early nineteenth centuries there was increasing understanding of the shape of the birth canal and the mechanism of delivery. In particular, the forward curve of the canal caused problems with maintaining a good grip of the fetal head with the forceps as it descended, and hence the introduction of the pelvic curve by Smellie and Levret. In addition the concept of episiotomy had not yet developed and trauma to the perineum was to be avoided whenever possible because of the high risk of infection. Improvements introduced by the Edinburgh school of Johnson, Young, and Hamilton (Chapter 4) included modifying the shape of the tip of the blades and altering the angle at which the blade was set to the handle by a reflex perineal curve (Figure 12.1). The main purpose for these modifications was to reduce perineal trauma while applying traction when the head was high in the birth canal.

"Axis traction" refers to the principle of applying traction to the head in the axis of the birth canal at the level at which the head is situated, so that the direction of traction varies as the head descends. When the head is at the level of the pelvic brim the axis of traction would lie through the anus and coccyx and the progressive maneuvers and designs of forceps to overcome this problem are discussed in this and the following two chapters. The stages in the development of axis traction in the eighteenth and nineteenth centuries were reviewed in 1881 by A. H. Smith at the American Gynecological Society and were summarized diagrammatically (1882) (Figure 12.2).

A common and long-standing procedure to improve the mechanics of traction force was what came to be known generally as Pajot's maneuver (Pajot, 1877) (Figure 12.3), although it had been described nearly a century previously by Osiander (1796). (Figure 12.2, A) and by Saxtorph and Scheel (1804) and subsequently modified by Smith (Figure 12.2, L,M). Pajot's maneuver consisted of applying downward pressure to the shank of the forceps during normal traction, the resultant of the two forces, if judged correctly, being a traction force in the pelvic axis. Naegele achieved the same effect by looping a fillet over the shank (Figure 12.2, B). This procedure was only possible with long forceps having a deep pelvic curve such as those of the Levret type and, although not widely advocated in Britain, was popularized in America by H. L. Hodge (1864), who preferred the European type of long forceps.

The Osiander/Pajot maneuver continued to be widely used in America but Richard Cleeman of Philadelphia, who was in the practice of using the popular Hodge forceps, was concerned that they frequently slipped off the head when applied above the pelvic brim and combined with the Pajot maneuver (1878). He ascribed this problem to having to apply traction in the wrong direction (not in the pelvic axis) and modified the Hodge forceps by bending the shank to an angle of 120 degrees (Figure 12.4). The extracting force was obtained by perpendicular pressure on the handles, rather than by traction, and hence the slender handles without finger grips. As soon as the head had entered the pelvis the instrument was replaced by conventional forceps.

Tapes (or Lacs)

Saxtorph and others had suggested putting traction tapes through the fenestra of the blades, which primarily facilitated traction, but Saxtorph also claimed that it improved the direction of the traction forces, which was partly true. However this was apparently forgotten, to be reintroduced

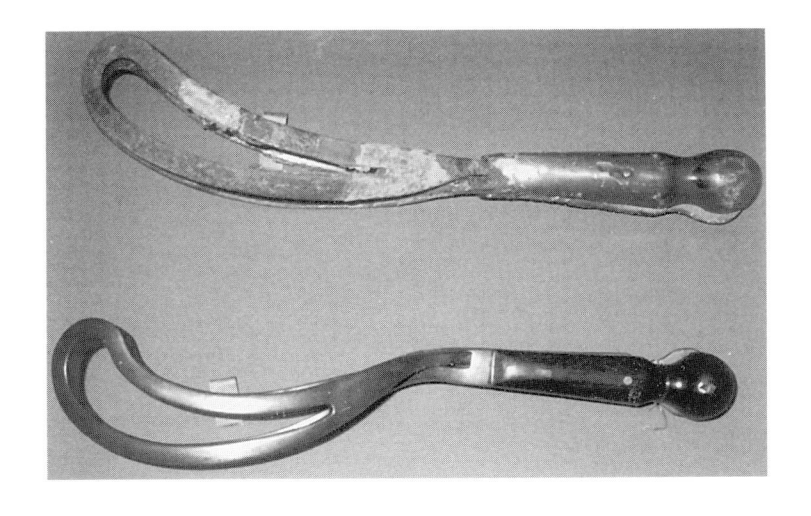

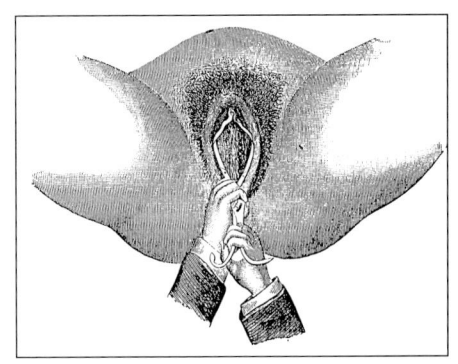

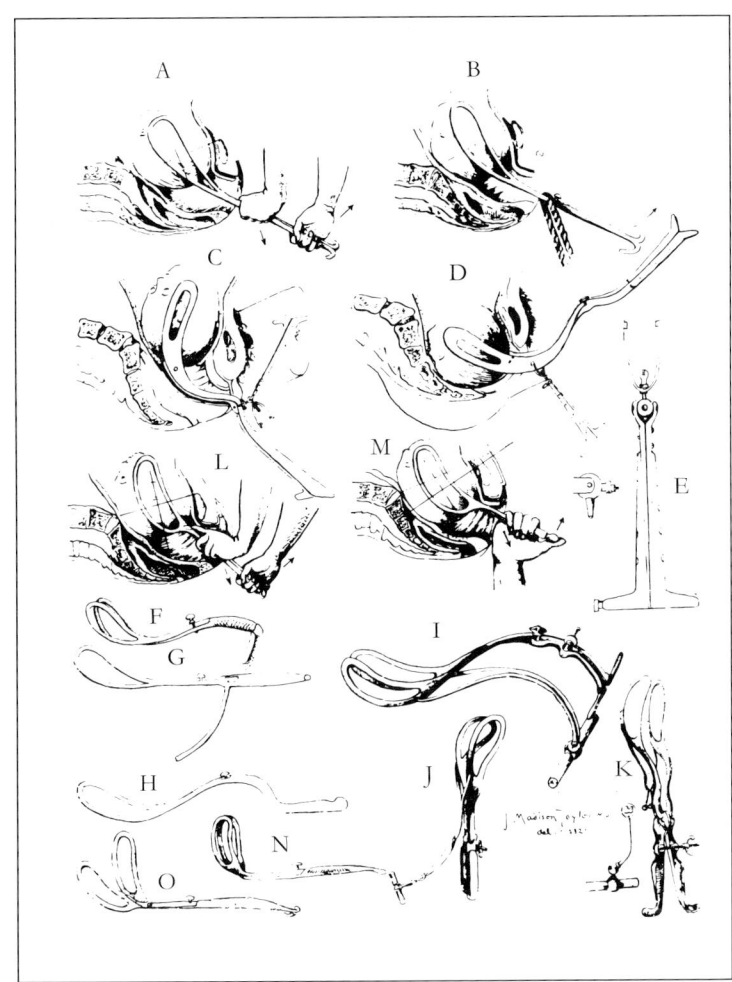

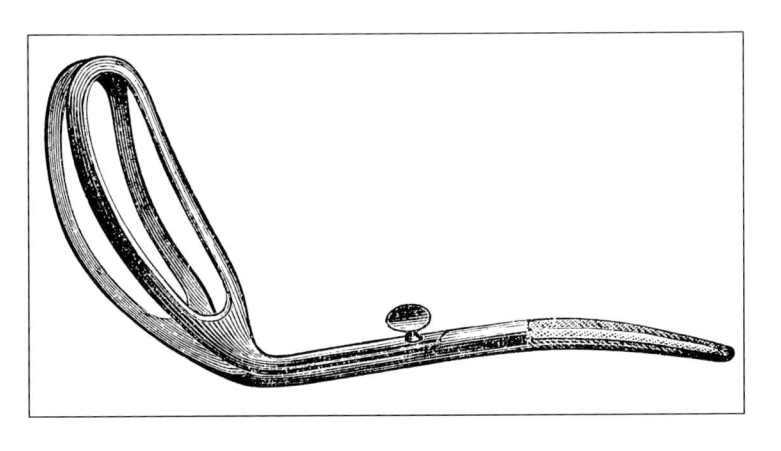

FIGURE 12.1 (ABOVE LEFT).
Smellie's and Johnson's forceps compared. In the Smellie instrument (top) the pelvic curve is almost in the axis of the handle. The Johnson blades are of similar size but have modified tips and are set back on the handle. (RCOG)

FIGURE 12.2 (LEFT).
Smith's illustrations of the development of axis traction (1882). A: Osiander's maneuver (1799). B: Naegele's fillet over the lock (1843). C,D,E: Hermann's adjunct, used above the lock for downward pressure, or below for downward traction (1844). F,G: Hubert's forceps (1869). H: Moralés's forceps (1871). I: Tarnier's first model (1877). J: A. R. Simpson's first model (1879). K: Lusk's modification of Tarnier's forceps (1880). N: Cleeman's forceps (1879). O: McFerran's forceps (1879). L,M: Smith's modifications of the Osiander/Pajot maneuver for use with Davis's forceps.

FIGURE 12.3 (ABOVE RIGHT).
Pajot's maneuver. The left hand is pulling the shank toward the perineum while traction is maintained by the right hand. (Pinard, 1879)

FIGURE 12.4 (BOTTOM LEFT).
Cleeman's forceps. A modification of Hodge forceps with the blades set at an angle of 120°. They were intended as an alternative to Pajot's maneuver. (Cleeman, 1878)

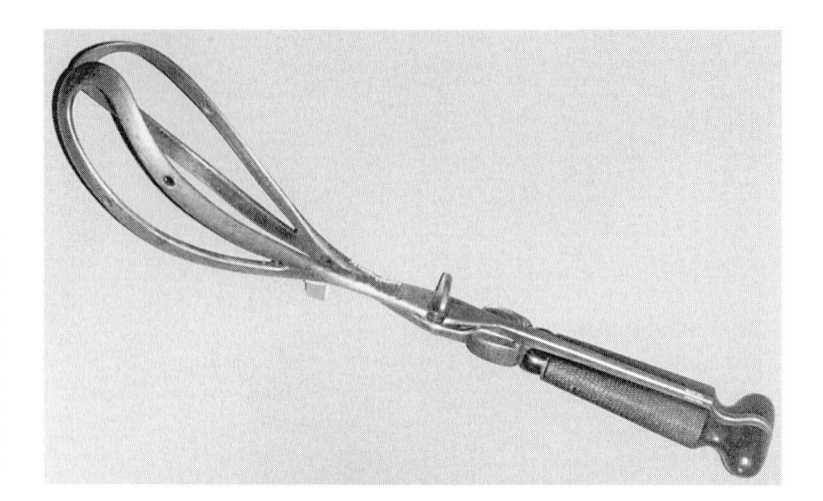

FIGURE 12.5.
Laroyenne's forceps. The upper and lower limbs of the blades are perforated to accommodate tapes. Although tapes had been used earlier by passing them through the fenestra, this had been mainly to increase the traction force, whereas this design was specifically to improve the axis of traction. Note also the folding finger lugs. (Science Museum, London)

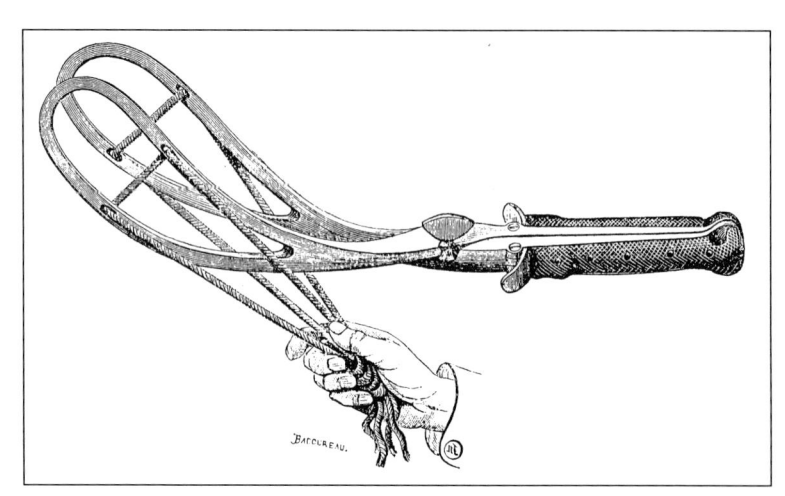

FIGURE 12.6.
Laroyenne's forceps, showing the method of use. (Laroyenne, 1875))

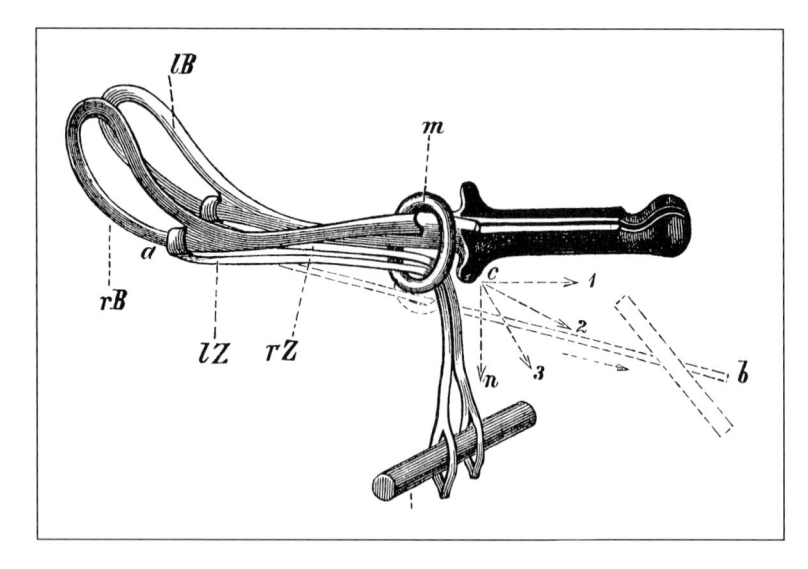

FIGURE 12.7.
Sänger's forceps. The tapes are held close to the shank by a loose ring m. The angle of traction can be varied by repositioning the ring. (Sänger, 1881)

on the Continent late in the nineteenth century by, among others, Lucien Pierre Laroyenne (1831–1902) (Figures 12.5, 12.6) (1875) and Poullet (1884). They sought to achieve traction more specifically in the pelvic axis by passing the traction tapes through slots in the limbs of the blades.

Max Sänger of Leipzig (1853–1903), used tapes with a

162 CHAPTER 12

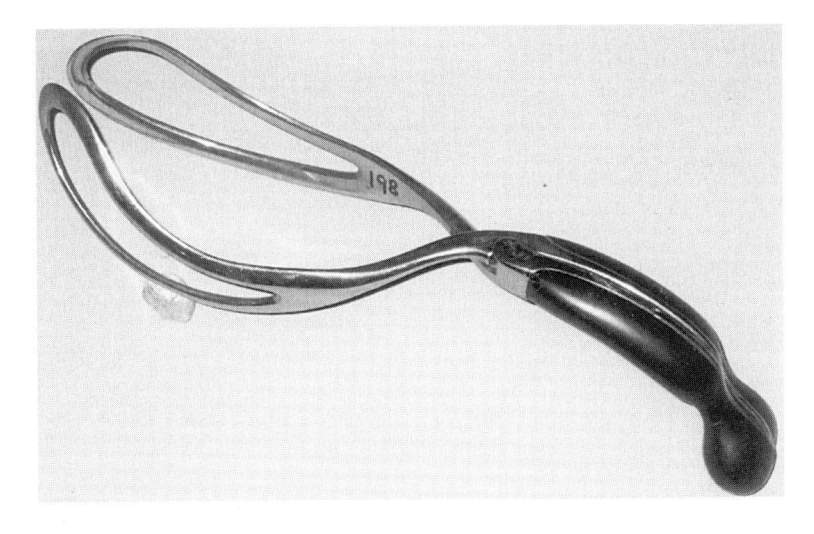

FIGURE 12.8.
Aveling's forceps. The curve of the shank and handle was intended to facilitate both insertion and traction. (RCOG)

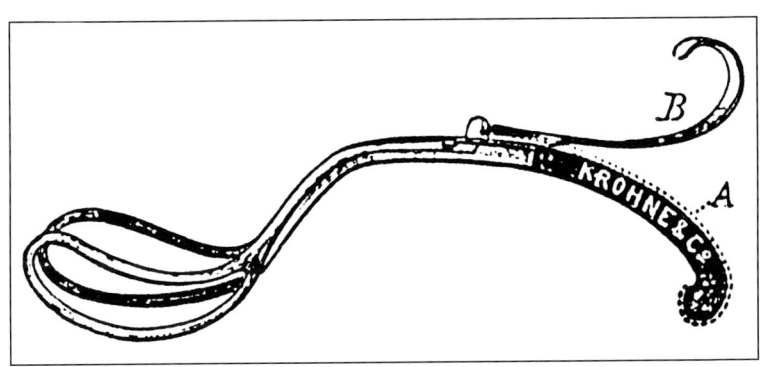

FIGURE 12.9.
Holland's forceps. An attempt to improve the function of Aveling's forceps. The supplementary handle B is fixed to the shank of Aveling-type forceps A by a ball-and-socket joint. It is not clear how it would have facilitated axis traction. (Holland, 1886)

crosshandle and kept them close to the shank with a rubber ring (1881) (Figure 12.7).

Perineal Steps and Curved Handles

Forceps incorporating perineal steps in the shanks and/or curved handles altered the angle of traction but were not true axis-traction forceps at all planes in the pelvis. It might be thought that the major mechanical developments already beginning to appear in the middle of the nineteenth century, and which are discussed subsequently in this and following chapters, would have soon made the stepped designs obsolete, but the more complex designs were often met with distrust and new designs of stepped forceps continued to appear until the end of the century.

Great Britain

Although in the 1870s revolutionary changes in forceps design were beginning to occur in Europe, in Britain the next evolutionary steps were major redesigns of the shank and handle by Aveling (1870, 1879), Galabin (1877b), and later Wagstaff (circa 1890) and others. The concept of incorporating a perineal step in the forceps design to minimize trauma by modifying the direction of traction developed from Young's alteration of the set of the blades' angle.

James Aveling (1828–1892), who founded both the Jessop Hospital, Sheffield, and the Chelsea Hospital for Women, London, was a prolific writer and innovator, particularly on the obstetric forceps and their use. He and some of his contemporaries recognized the impossibility of achieving a correctly directed traction force with forceps having curved blades and a straight handle. He described the use of curved handles in 1870, a pair of which he had demonstrated previously at the Obstetrical Society of London (of which he was a founding member) in 1868 (Figure 12.8). The backward curve of the handles was intended to facilitate insertion and traction but, though the idea was a good one and a step forward in forceps design, it unfortunately did not work satisfactorily.

Edmund Holland tried to improve Aveling's instrument by a curved traction rod attached on the upper surface by a ball-and-socket joint (Figure 12.9). Holland stated that the supplementary handle acted "as a lever of the first kind, as

FIGURE 12.10.
Galabin's forceps. Although of the same principle as Aveling's forceps, these are heavier and have serrated handles and finger lugs, allowing greater traction force. (RCOG)

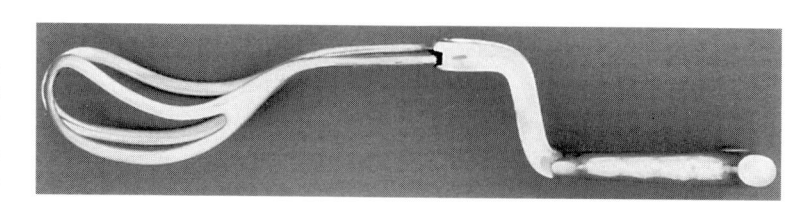

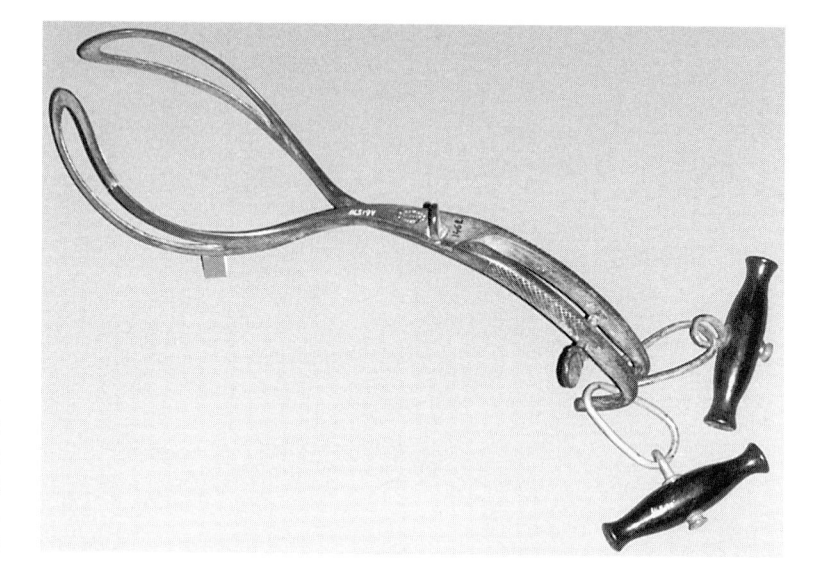

FIGURE 12.11.
Christie's forceps. Another sigmoid design with the addition of hooked handles to which traction rods could be attached. There is also a pressure-regulating screw in the handles. (Science Museum, London)

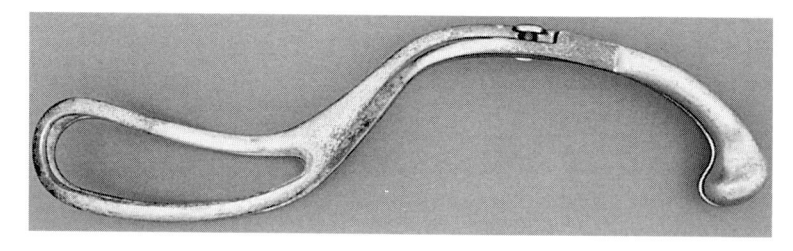

FIGURE 12.12.
Wagstaff's forceps. A sigmoid design with a Brunninghausen-type lock. (RCOG)

well as a tractor, and by its means a greater axial control over the instrument [was] effected than by any other mechanism with which I am acquainted" (1886). However, this glowing testimonial did not seem to lead to any widespread enthusiasm for its use.

Alfred Galabin (1843–1914) was an obstetric physician and a lecturer at Guy's Hospital and was one of the first obstetricians to carry out gynecological operations, at that time firmly in the province of the general surgeons. Galabin first demonstrated his forceps to the Obstetrical Society of London in 1877. This was a meeting at which Tarnier's early axis-traction forceps had been demonstrated and debated (see below). Galabin's forceps were a modification of Aveling's (Figure 12.10). They had cranked shafts, which reduced perineal trauma and allowed traction to be applied in the axis of the pelvis, depending on the level of the head. The serrated handles and finger lugs at both ends of the handles allowed a powerful degree of traction, unlike the handles of Aveling's forceps, which were specially designed with a smooth finish to avoid excessive traction force.

David Christie (d. 1917) of Donegal used the sigmoid shape, as did Aveling, with the curve of the handles mirroring the pelvic curve of the blades (1878). The handles terminated in a blunt hook to which a traction handle was attached by a large ring (Figure 12.11). The ring was so shaped that traction tended to bring the two handles together. The joint was a slot and screw and a compression screw in the handle could be used to regulate the degree of apposition of the blades.

Although British designs of forceps based on Tarnier's (see below) principles started to appear in the early 1880s, modifications of the Aveling/Galabin type, that is, forceps with a sigmoid shape based on the concept of a perineal step or curve, continued over the next fifteen years. Wagstaff (circa 1890) (Figure 12.12) and Wales (1895) described similar for-

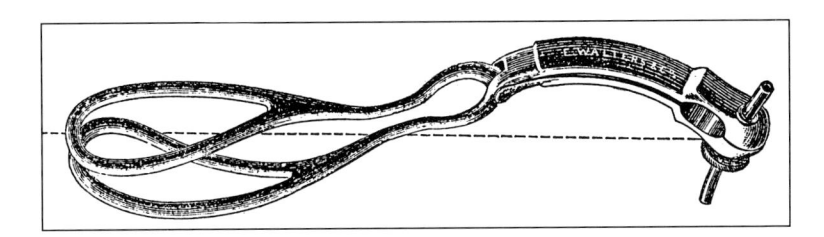

FIGURE 12.13.
Taylor's forceps. Two finger rings and a transverse traction bar at the end of the handle facilitate axis traction. (G. Taylor, 1892)

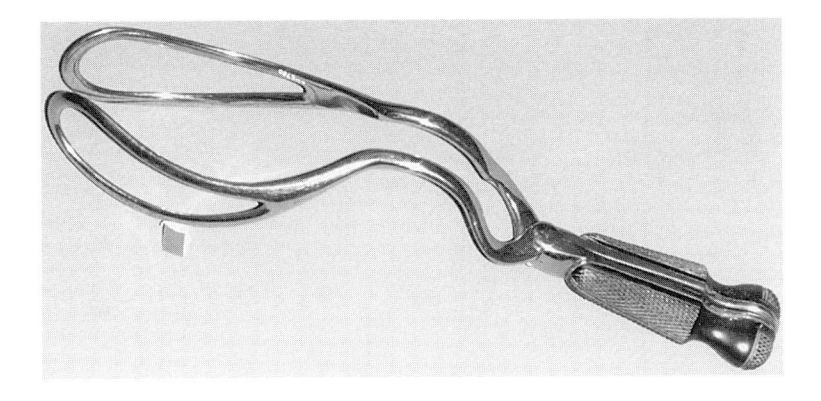

FIGURE 12.14.
Pearse's forceps. The straight handle makes it less mechanically efficient than those with curved handles. (Science Museum, London)

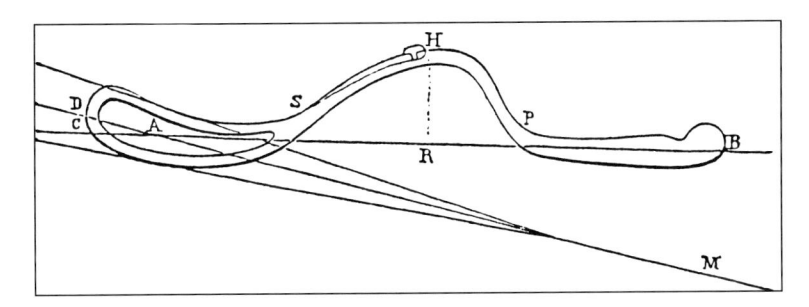

FIGURE 12.15.
Moralès's forceps. The cranked shaft also appeared in Continental designs but they were superseded by the popularity of Tarnier's instruments. (Moralès, 1871)

ceps but the former had a pivot and notch joint of the Brunninghausen type (Chapter 5).

G. Taylor (1892) also used a sigmoid design with the addition of a Barnes's finger ring and a second finger hole at the end of the handle. A transverse bar and thumb screw secured the handles distally (Figure 12.13). In 1890 T. F. Pearse, who had designed a hinged forceps in 1887, introduced a forceps with a marked reflex perineal curve but with a straight handle of the Barnes type (Figure 12.14; see also Figure 6.25).

Europe

The cranked shaft also appeared in Continental designs of the period, such as those of Moralès, which he called *forceps à trois courbures* (1871), and one of Poullet's models (1884) (see below). Tarnier was critical of Moralès's design in that while Moralès claimed that the line of traction was AB,

Tarnier contended that it should be DM, which was well below the axis of the forceps (see Figure 12.15).

Poullet designed a number of forceps of varying complexity that are described elsewhere (Chapters 9, 10). His axis-traction forceps (1881) were a more practical proposition in which he tried to combine the good qualities of the freedom of movement allowed by tape tractors with those of the rigid stems of Tarnier. The forceps were of the conventional French pattern (see Chapter 5) but with perforations in the blades to accommodate the tapes or, in a variation, with a perforated bar across the fenestra (Figure 12.16). The tapes were threaded onto a rigid, curved traction rod. The same principle was used by Herff of Basel (1892).

However, Poullet subsequently returned to the concept of parallel forceps, which were popular in his native Lyons. He modified the parallel forceps described in Chapter 10 (Figures 10.10, 10.11) by adding a rather unnecessarily compli-

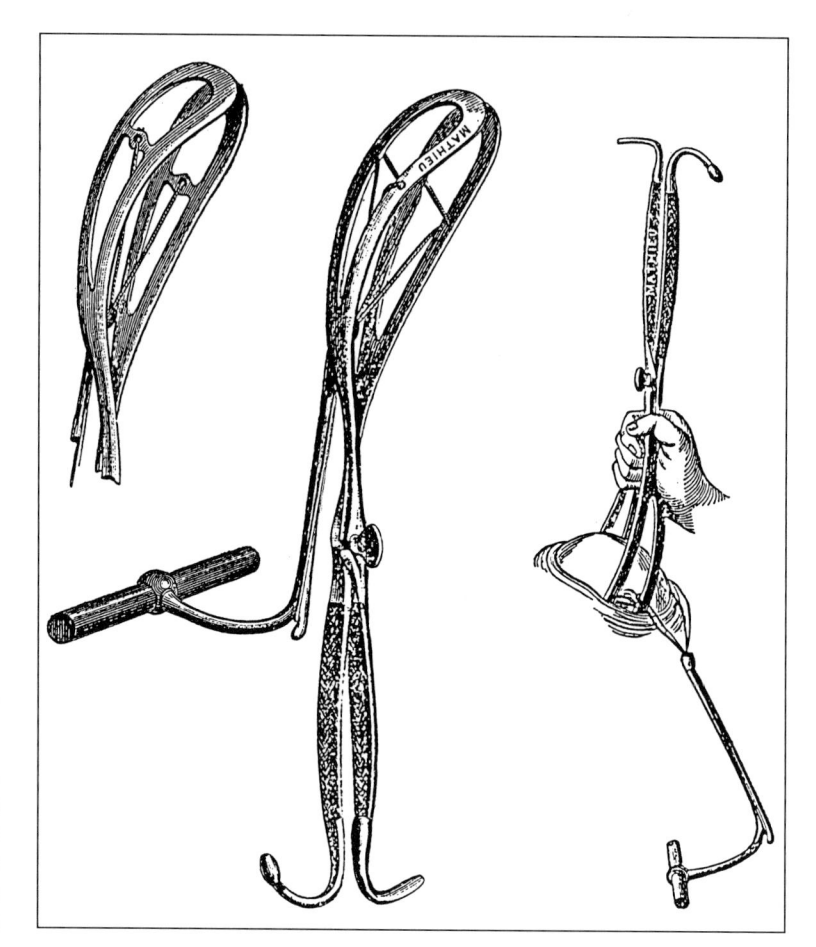

FIGURE 12.16.
Poullet's axis-traction forceps. Tapes are attached to the blades either by perforations in the limbs of the blades (left) or to a crossbar (center). Distally they are tied to a rigid rod with a crossbar handle. (E. Hubert, 1884)

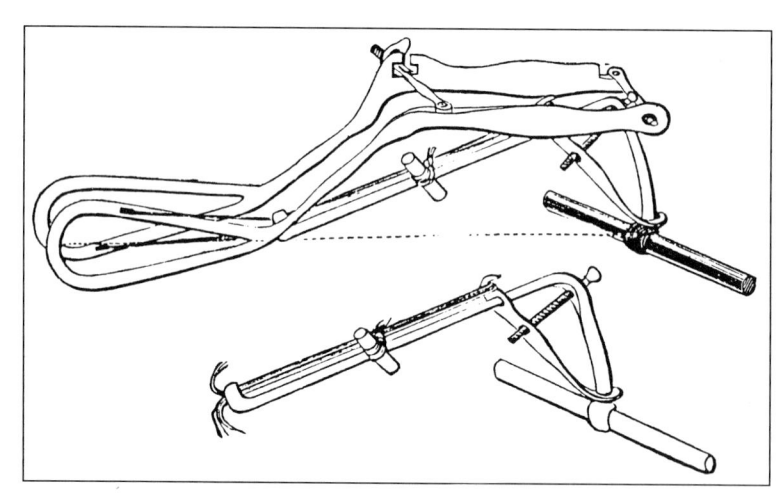

FIGURE 12.17.
Poullet's axis-traction attachment for his stepped parallel forceps. A development of one of his original designs (Figure 12.12). The attachment comprises tapes passing through holes in the blades and attached to a bar and traction rod with a screw tensioner. (Poullet, 1884)

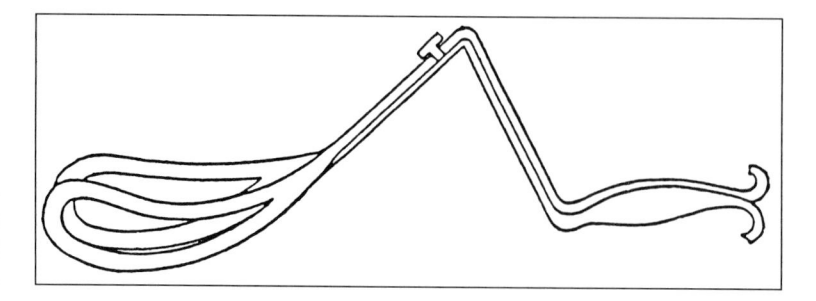

FIGURE 12.18.
Dewees's early forceps. A simple response to Tarnier's complicated designs. However, it did not endure. (Dewees, 1892)

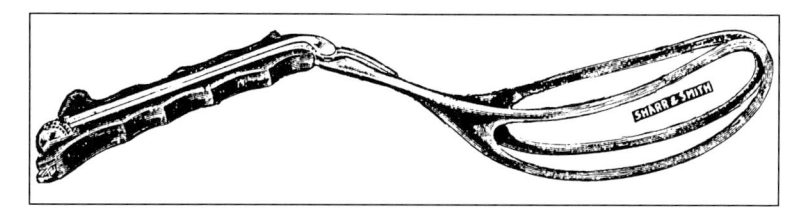

FIGURE 12.19.
Knox's forceps. An American step design with a compression screw in the handle. (Parvin, 1890)

cated tape and traction-rod attachment (Figure 12.17). The tapes were passed through perforations in the blades and were then attached to an angled rod with a crossbar handle. A rod with a screw adjustment allowed the tension on the tape to be varied. Poullet claimed that, apart from obtaining traction in the long axis of the blades, the design allowed a good fit both to the fetal head and in relation to the birth canal, while the independent movement of the two blades made the instrument ideal in cases of asynclitism.

America

The concept of axis traction did not develop until later in America, after the advent of Tarnier's forceps and the various derivatives thereof. W. B Dewees of Kansas, whose philosophy was that "real wisdom is always simple," predicted that the day would dawn when instrumental delivery would only be done by axis traction and presented, with considerable self-confidence, a simple, stepped forceps (Figure 12.18), (1892, 1894, 1895) which he was to replace, with even greater self-confidence, with a more advanced design only three years later (Figure 14.15). A little later an instrument by J. S. Knox of Rush Medical College was described by Parvin in 1890. It was similar to the Dewees instrument but had a J. Y. Simpson-type handle with finger lugs (Figure 12.19; see also Chapter 6).

Application of Geometric Principles to Axis-Traction Problems

In 1840 Hermann of Berne introduced a forceps that incorporated a perineal step in the shank and a second pair of straight handles (the "adjunct") attached by a link joint to the blade (Figure 12.20). The first written description of these forceps did not appear until 1844 in his son's treatise, together with a diagram of the parallelogram of traction forces associated with his forceps (Hermann, T., 1844). The adjunct could be attached above the shank for downward pressure when the head was at the brim, thus providing a mechanical means of implementing Pajot's maneuver. In addition the adjunct could be attached to holes in the blades

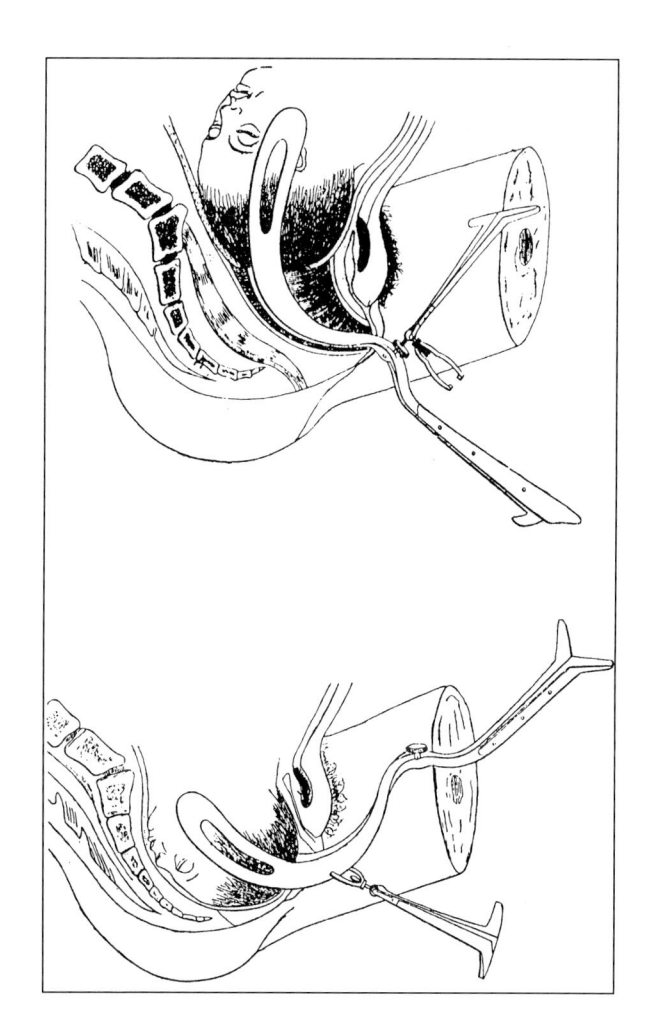

FIGURE 12.20.
Hermann's forceps. The additional rod, or *adjunct,* could be used (top) for downward pressure on the shank, mimicking Pajot's maneuver; or attached to the root of the blades to achieve a close approximation to axis traction (bottom). (Pinard, 1879)

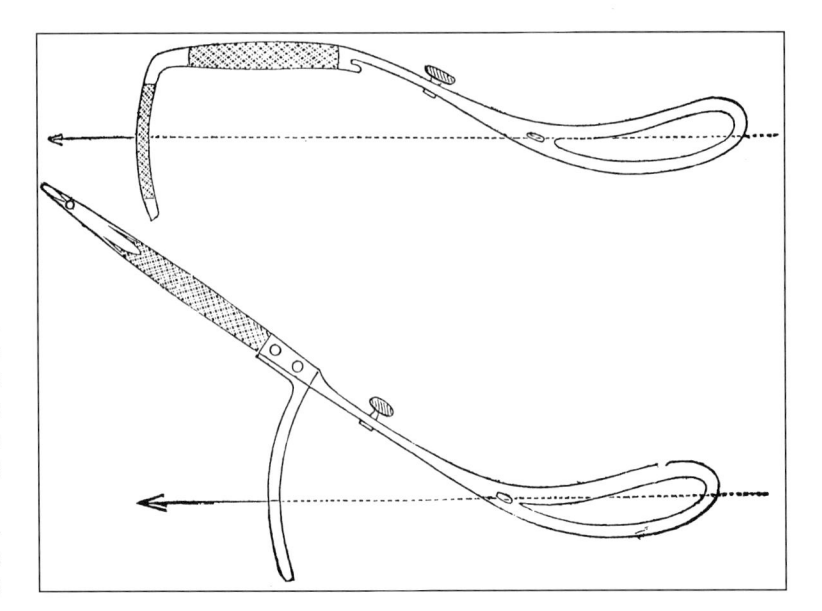

FIGURE 12.21.
L. J. Hubert's forceps. Early and late models. The fixed bar at the root of the handle made it difficult to apply to a high head. Both models have holes for traction tapes at the roots of the blades. (E. Hubert, 1884)

FIGURE 12.22.
L. J. Hubert's forceps versus Pajot's maneuver. Comparison of the forces. (E. Hubert, 1877)

to assist traction, thus antedating by more than thirty years Tarnier's idea of attaching hinged traction rods to the blades of the forceps.

Greater consideration of the mechanics of delivery resulted in the development of truer axis traction and Louis Joseph Hubert (*père*) (1810–1876), Professor of Obstetrics at the Catholic University of Louvain, was the first person to show, by geometric demonstration, that the pelvic curve of the forceps made it impossible to pull the head in the right direction and that the traction force could be considered as two components at right angles to each other, one producing advancement of the head but the other serving only to compress the maternal soft tissues (1860b). For example, a traction force of 50 kilograms (110 pounds) applied with conventional forceps at an angle of 45 degrees to the axis of the birth canal would result in a useless pressure of 35 kilograms (77 pounds) being expended against the pubis. He emphasized the adverse effects of the compressive force caused by traction in the wrong direction and stated what was to become an established principle: "The direction of traction must coincide with the line which constitutes the axis of the blades of the forceps."

E. Hubert (*fils*) described the development of his father's forceps in his 1884 article. L. J. Hubert tried the use of crotchets hooked into the forceps blades to create a double-lever system but subsequently designed two novel instruments (Figures 12.21, 12.22). In the first model the handle was extended and bent over in an arc, an arrangement that seemed to be suitable for axis traction at the level of the pelvic brim but not at the lower planes. In the later model a rigid bar was attached at right angles to the handle close to the shank and traction was applied at the point in the arc of the at-

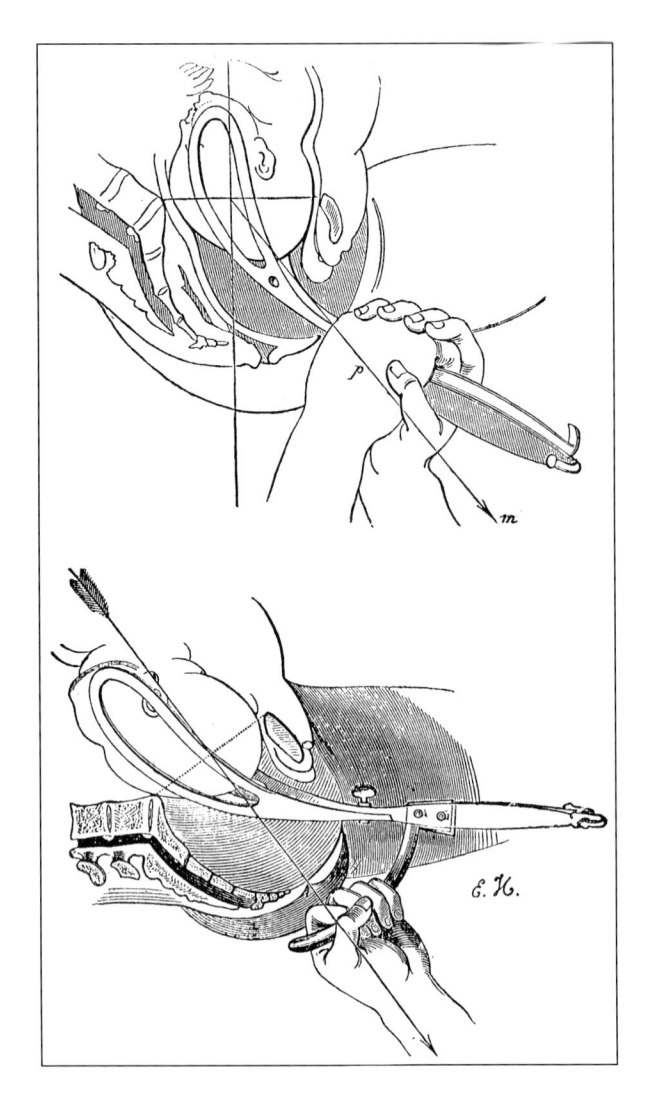

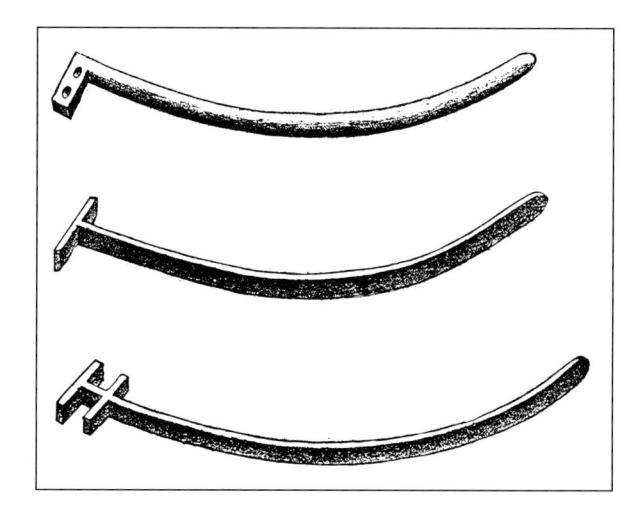

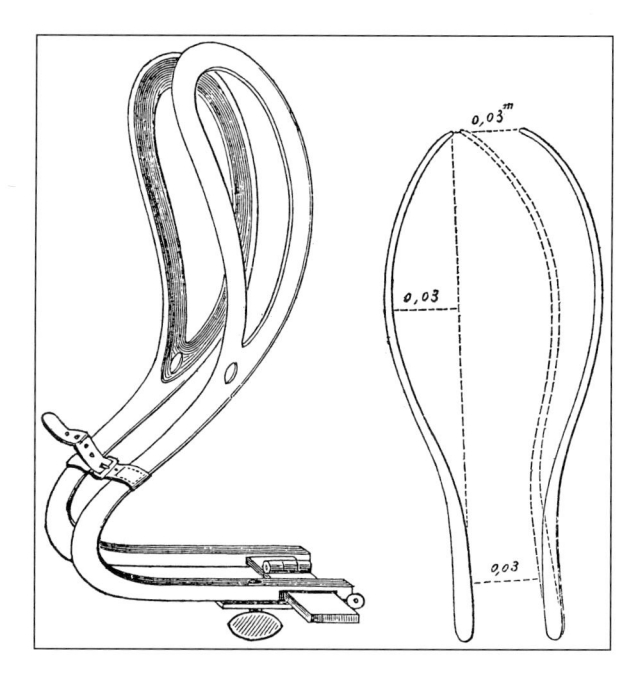

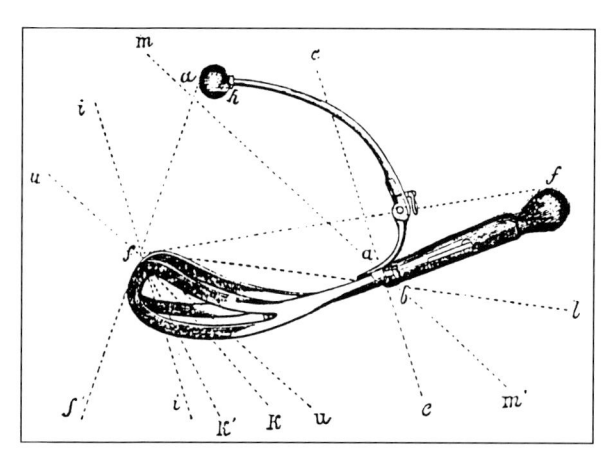

FIGURE 12.23 (TOP LEFT).
Traction rods for L. J. Hubert's forceps. Top: L. J. Hubert's original design. Center: Lanteneer's modification. Below: Van Ermengem's modification. (E. Hubert, 1884)

FIGURE 12.24 (LEFT).
E. Hubert's forceps. Hubert applied his father's sigmoid shape to parallel forceps in the Lyons tradition, with a sliding lock at the end of the handle and a strap at the shank. (E. Hubert, 1877)

FIGURE 12.25 (ABOVE).
Hartmann's forceps. This was another attempt to mimic Pajot's maneuver. Pressure on the rod *ad* in the axis *ee* gives a resultant force in the axis *fl*. (Charpentier, 1883)

tachment that was in the line of the axis of the blades. Both designs had perforations at the root of the blades to take traction tapes. Lanteneer and Emile P. Van Ermengem made simple modifications to the traction rod to make it easily detachable (see Hubert, E., 1884; Figure 12.23).

E. Hubert (1877), while adhering to his father's principles and retaining the sigmoid shape, radically changed the design. Following the example of the Lyons school (Chapter 10), he favored parallel blades. He also eliminated the conventional element of the handles as being useless and dangerous and turned the residual handles at an angle of 120 degrees to the shank (Figure 12.24). The shanks were joined by a strap and the handles by a transverse sliding bar and screw pivot so that the distance between the blades could be adjusted. He also put holes at the base of the blades so that tapes could be used for traction if desired. However, this could be interpreted as lack of faith in the efficacy of his own design.

R. Hartmann (1870) addressed the same geometric problems as Hubert, but with rather less clarity, and designed a forceps with the traction rod *above* the lock (Figure 12.25). In normal use it was intended to replace Pajot's maneuver but Hartmann discussed various parallelograms of forces showing the purported effects of pressure at different points and in different directions. There is no indication of how much his hypotheses were put to the test in practice, nor what was the outcome.

• • •

The worthy attempts to solve the problem of axis traction described in this chapter represented significant advances, particularly the objective scientific analysis of L. J. Hubert. However, all the proposed solutions had deficiencies and it required the major changes in logical thought and design initiated by E. S. Tarnier in 1877 to make any further significant advances in this field.

TARNIER AXIS-TRACTION FORCEPS AND THEIR MODIFICATIONS

13

The credit for further developing an understanding of the detailed geometry and for designing the first forceps that truly allowed efficient traction through the curving axis of the birth canal goes to Etienne Tarnier. In Tarnier's time the Levret type of forceps was in general use in France but the principles that Tarnier established were for the most part regarded as sound and his new designs soon became widely adopted. True axis-traction forceps appeared in profusion in the last two decades of the nineteenth century and even into the twentieth century. Das (1929) listed nineteen new axis-traction forceps described between 1900 and 1910.

Tarnier's Designs

Etienne Stéphane Tarnier (1828–1897), *chef de clinique*, Paris Maternité, and Professor of Obstetrics at the University of Paris, first described his revolutionary concept for axis traction in 1877, a project in which he was assisted by an artillery colonel and a craftsman. Tarnier described his early models in a monograph, *Description de deux nouveaux forceps* (1877a) and illustrations of many of his prototypes, including versions using lacs, may be seen therein. In this paper he first showed the fallacies of the Levret design, demonstrating that when the head is at or above the pelvic brim it is impossible to pull in the correct axis (that is, at right angles to the plane of the brim). Following L. J. Hubert's example and analyzing parallelograms of forces, he also showed that with any long, curved forceps used for high application, a dangerous degree of pressure could be exerted against the symphysis pubis. For example, he estimated the components of a resultant of 40 kilograms (88 pounds) comprised 30 kilograms (66 pounds) of downward force and 26 kilograms (57 pounds) against the pubis.

Tarnier's main tenet was that for the forceps to be used at all levels of the pelvis they must be in two parts, one fixed and one mobile. For the first time the additional rods were used exclusively for traction, the conventional fixed handles being used only for application of the blades. The stated purposes of the design were to (1) allow constant and easy transition along the axis of the pelvic planes, (2) allow freedom of movement of the head, as in normal labor, and (3) provide an indicator to show the direction of traction.

Tarnier's early models were relatively simple, with a sigmoid shape based on the designs of L. J. Hubert (1860b) and Moralès (1871). He added traction rods attached by hinges to the lower limbs of the blades, with the curve following closely the line of the shank and handle so that the whole assembly comprising each blade could be introduced easily (Figures 13.1, 13.2). A large, swiveling, transverse wooden handle on the traction rods permitted a two-handed grip and the potential for considerable traction force, while the fixed handles terminated in hinged crossbars that could also be used for traction in the lower strait.

Thereafter Tarnier made numerous modifications, over thirty during the next four years according to William Wright Jaggard (1857–1896) of Chicago (1886). In later developments the traction rods were jointed as well as being hinged on the blades, the traction handle was fully articulated with the rods, and a needle indicator was incorporated to indicate the direction of traction. Tarnier also dispensed with the sigmoid shape. The ultimate result, which was intended to replace the simple but long and heavy Levret/Dubois instruments (Chapters 3, 5) for high forceps delivery, was a very complex

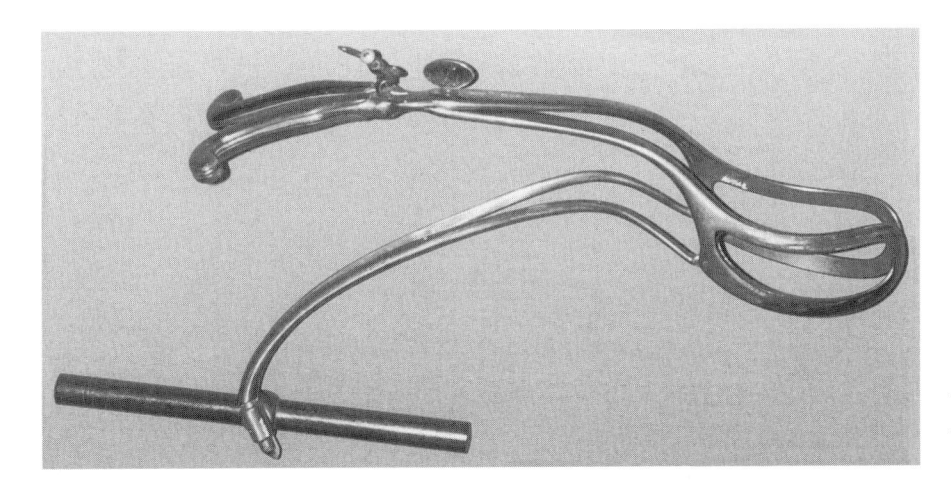

FIGURE 13.1.
Tarnier's forceps. An early sigmoid pattern with the curve of the rods following the curve of the shank and handle. (Science Museum, London)

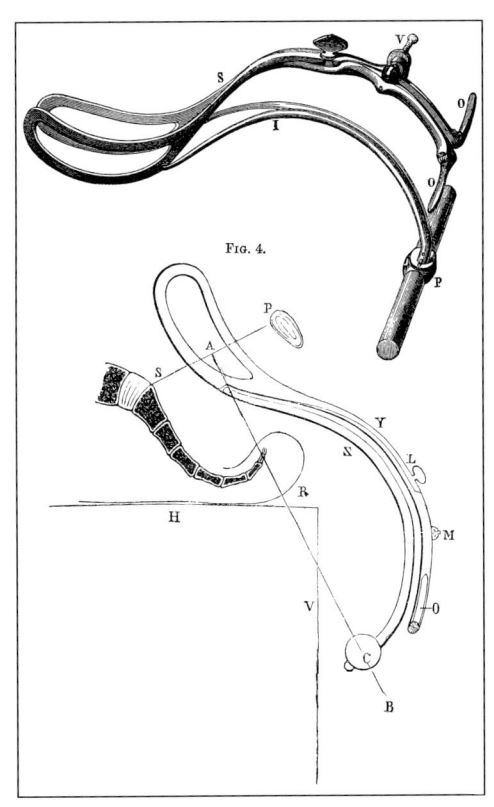

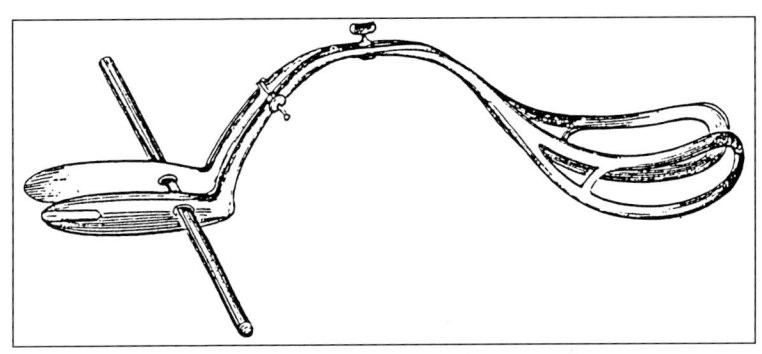

FIGURE 13.2 (ABOVE).
Tarnier's forceps. Another early design as demonstrated by Wiltshire to the Obstetric Society of London. (Wiltshire, 1877)

FIGURE 13.3 (ABOVE RIGHT).
Tarnier's *forceps à branches croisées et à manches immobiles*. Traction was provided by a transverse bar passing through perforations in the handle. (Tarnier, 1877)

instrument that was rather unwieldy and unduly expensive to manufacture.

Among the many models that Tarnier described, one had a longer shank and hinged handles that could be locked in a transverse position or brought together under the arch of the shank and thus lying in the axis of the blades, thereby acting as an indicator for the direction of traction to be followed as the head descended. The fenestra were divided by a bar through which lacs could be passed. Axis traction could be provided either by the tapes or by attaching a rod and handle to the ends of the handles when they were in the folded position.

In a further modification of lighter construction (Figure 13.3), a fixed handle was perforated to take a transverse-traction handle, while lacs were passed through the fenestra. Subsequently perforations in the lower limbs of the blades were provided to accommodate the lacs.

Tarnier's other move, in about 1878, was to devise a traction rod that fit onto the articulation of the ordinary long

TARNIER AXIS-TRACTION FORCEPS **171**

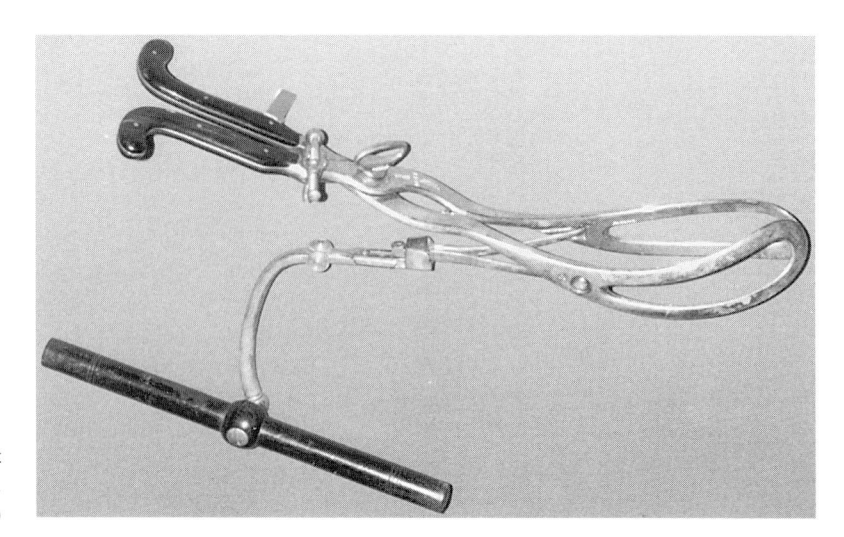

FIGURE 13.4.
Tarnier's forceps. A late model (circa 1878) that became widely used. (Science Museum, London)

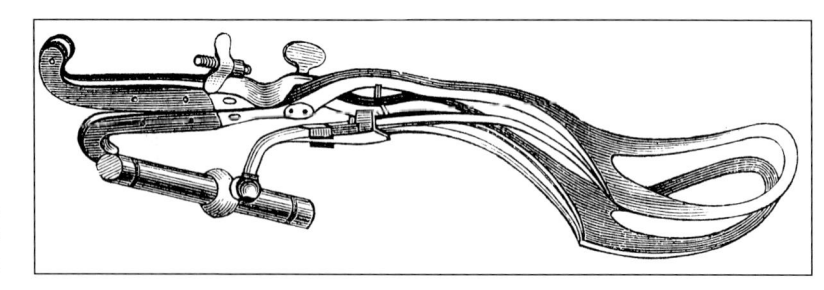

FIGURE 13.5.
Tarnier's forceps. A variant of Figure 13.4 demonstrated by Breus. (Breus, 1885)

FIGURE 13.6.
Tarnier's late forceps in use. (Charpentier, 1883)

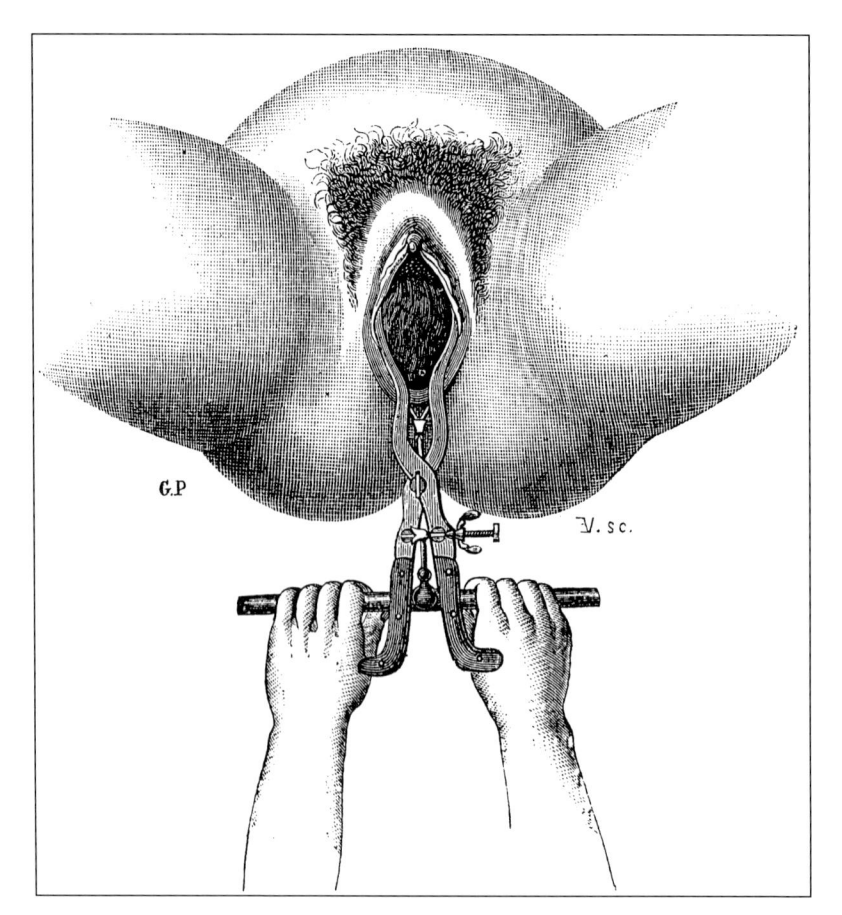

curved forceps of the Levret type (Figures 13.4–13.6). In a paper given at the International Medical Congress in 1881 he stated that he had abandoned the perineal curve because it made direct application more difficult and in oblique applications contact with the pubic ramus caused deviation of the handle of the instrument. In an expanded version of this paper published the following year he illustrated long curved forceps with straight handles and traction rods attached to the blades with a multijointed handle. It is versions of this instrument that became most widely available commercially. Word of the new instruments spread rapidly but initially they did not find favor with a number of influential obstetricians, partly as a result of vested interests.

The British Response

By May 1877 Tarnier's forceps were commended for study in the *British Medical Journal*, while in November of that year Alfred Wiltshire (1839–1886), Lecturer in Midwifery and Assistant Physician-Accoucheur at St. Mary's Hospital, London, demonstrated them to the Obstetrical Society of London (1877) (Figure 13.2). In general the reception of Wiltshire's demonstration was unfavorable and reactionary. Lack of practical experience with the instrument did not inhibit pontification and rejection. In the discussion following the demonstration J. Braxton Hicks (1823–1897, Obstetric Physician to Guy's and St. Mary's Hospitals, London, was not impressed with Tarnier's forceps, though he had no practical experience with them, and favored Pajot's maneuver, an entrenched view typical of the time. James Mathews Duncan (1826–1890), Physician-Accoucheur at St. Bartholomew's Hospital, London, agreed with Hicks but accepted that the forceps were "a model of scientific ingenuity." Later, in 1887, he stated that a scientifically constructed instrument was not necessarily better than a scientifically imperfect instrument that had been well tested and improved in practice. Galabin was critical and anxious to promote his own new design of forceps, which he showed later in the meeting, and Aveling confined himself to agreeing with the perineal and handle curves. In 1878 Aveling said that Tarnier's forceps were "undoubtedly theoretically excellent but practically far too complicated to come into general use" (1879). In Britain more general acceptance had to await the modified designs of A. R. Simpson (see Chapter 14).

The European Response

In Europe Pajot saw the Tarnier forceps as displacing his own maneuver, but when Tarnier replaced him as Professor of Obstetrics at the University of Paris, Pajot's influence waned. Gustav Augustus Braun (1829–1911), the head of the Vienna Maternity Clinic and an influential figure of the day, used the forceps in twelve cases and concluded that there were decided advantages, particularly that less forcible traction was required (1880). However, the introduction of the forceps was more difficult and great experience was required. He recommended them for high operations by the experienced surgeon but dissuaded the beginner or less experienced surgeon from using them.

The American Response

In America, by October of 1877, Fordyce Barker (1877, 1878) was championing the Tarnier cause at the New York Academy of Medicine. However, in the ensuing discussion James Platt White (1811–1881), a professor of obstetrics in Buffalo, was unable to see the utility of the instrument and believed it to be a substitute of mechanical device for skill, predicting that within twenty years it would be among the obstetric curiosities. He also disliked the concept of an occipitofacial application because of the damage it could cause to the fetus. At the time Professors Thomas Lusk (see below) and G. Taylor both preferred the long straight forceps. However Lusk changed his opinion and subsequently favored Tarnier's forceps, which he modified (1880a,b) and which are described later in this chapter (page 183). Lusk claimed that "the most important contribution made in the last ten years to the obstetric armamentarium is unquestionably the Tarnier forceps" (1880b) and wrote in the fourth edition of his textbook *The Science and Art of Midwifery*, "To one accustomed only to the familiar forceps, the facility with which delivery can be accomplished by Tarnier's instrument would seem hardly credible" (1892).

As stated in Chapter 12, Albert H. Smith gave a lengthy critique of axis traction at the American Gynecological Society and claimed that the idea of axis traction sent obstetricians "into a state of effervescence" on recognition of the true mechanics of labor and the bad practices of the past (1882). He objected to the Tarnier instruments, without any basis of personal experience, on the grounds of complicated design, difficulty in disinfection, the use of a compression screw, and cost, especially as Tarnier seemed to produce a new, improved model every six months! Smith gave a full description of Osiander's technique, which had been abandoned because it included either a pendulum action or rotary movement, both of which had been widely discredited. Nevertheless, Smith strenuously supported the modified Osiander or Pajot-type maneuver (although he did not refer to Pajot by name) in the belief that simple manual dexterity rendered mechanical axis traction superfluous. The lengthy discussion, led by such luminaries as Lusk, Barker,

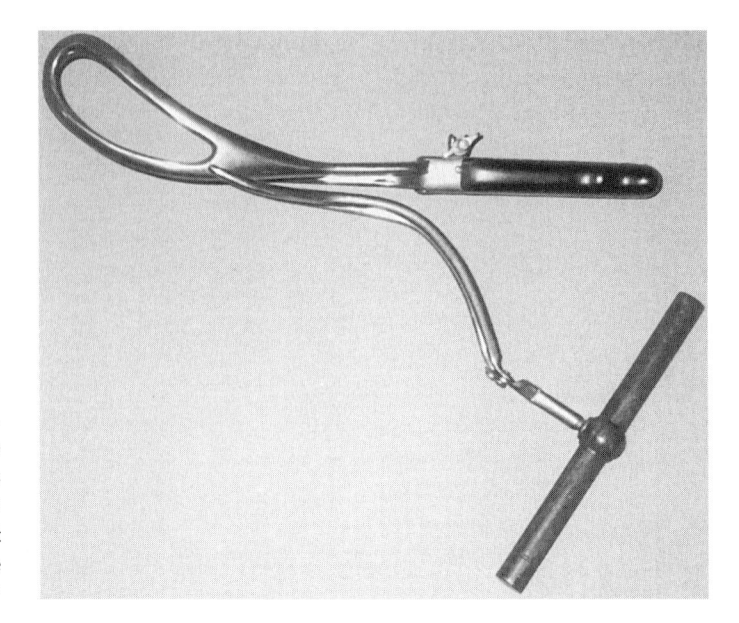

FIGURES 13.7–13.9.
A. R. Simpson's forceps (RCOG). 13.7: The traction rods have a fixed hinge. Earlier designs had detachable rods. The handle is large enough for a two-handed grip. 13.8: Detail of the joint on the traction handle. 13.9: Inscription on the inner face of the handle: "LEFT LOWER FIRST."

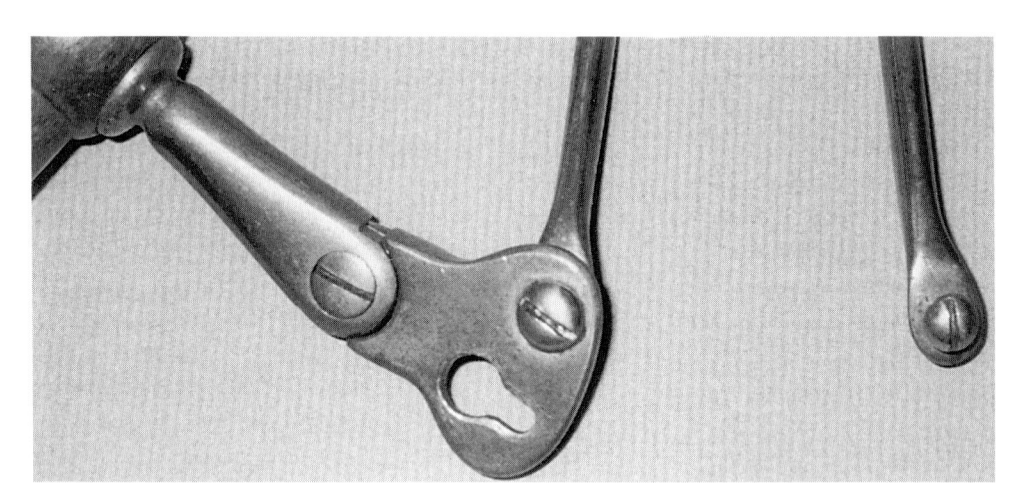

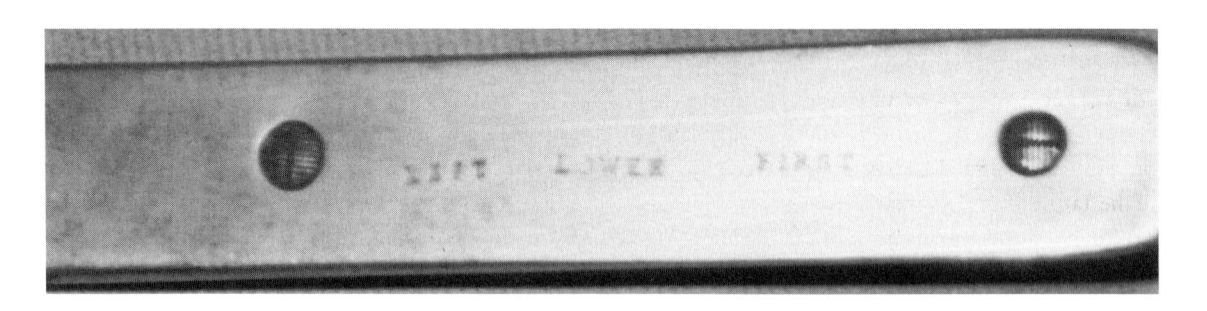

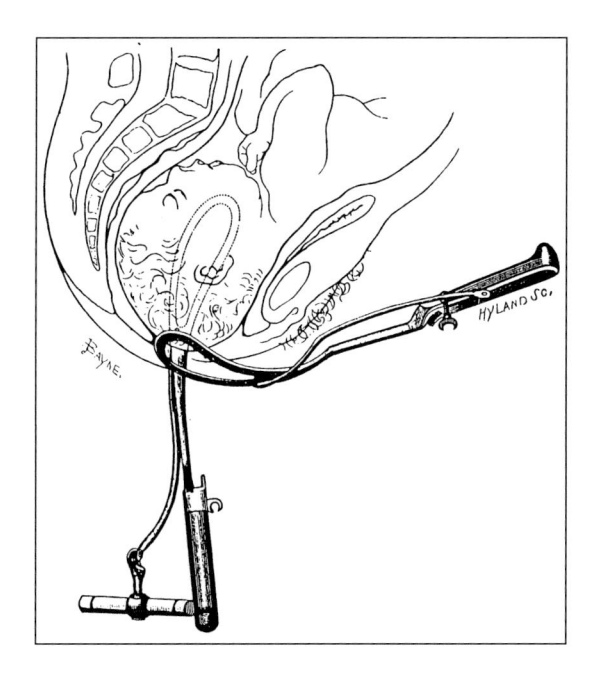

FIGURE 13.10.
A. R. Simpson's illustration of his forceps application. Note the rod pushed above the shank. (A. R. Simpson, 1881)

and Howard, that followed his paper was generally unsympathetic to his cause. Although by 1888 T. Opie of Baltimore claimed that only traction-rod forceps should be used for high operations, enthusiasm for axis traction in America continued to be muted. In a survey conducted by H. D. Fry of Washington (1889a) only thirty of eighty-two (37 percent) obstetricians said that they recognized the value of axis traction.

Modifications of Tarnier's Forceps

British Developments

In Britain Robert Barnes made some minor modifications to Tarnier's design (1878), but the most important development came from A. R. Simpson. Simpson wrote excellent critiques of Tarnier's forceps (1881, 1883) and gave graphic descriptions of the considerable force used, often inappropriately, by some practitioners. He summarized the benefits of the Tarnier-type forceps as follows:

> The attachment of rods to the blades allows of direct traction on the head in their embrace. The backward compensation curve (perineal curve, it is sometimes called) of the rods allows of the traction by a curved instrument through a curved canal without loss of power, and without misdirection of force. The jointing of the rods allows the advancing head to move the application handles in the constantly-changing direction along which it is travelling; and the direction of application handles thus furnishes the operator with an unerring index to the proper line of traction. (1883)

Simpson modified and simplified Tarnier's traction rods and adapted them to his uncle's (J. Y. Simpson) long forceps (Figures 13.7–13.10). He first demonstrated them in 1879 at the Obstetric Society of Edinburgh and gave a detailed description in 1880 (1880–1881). The handles of the J. Y. Simpson forceps were made smooth and the finger lugs were removed. As an *aide-mémoire* "LEFT LOWER FIRST" was stamped on the inside of the handle of the left blade (a device later used on some of Milne Murray's forceps) (Figure 13.9). A bar and screw were attached to the handles so that they could be held together firmly, thus maintaining a grip on the fetal head. However, Simpson emphasized that this attachment should not be used for compressing the head. The blades were of the original J. Y. Simpson design (Chapter 6) and the traction rods were articulated to the roots of the blades. The traction rods in A. R. Simpson's early design were detachable but he soon became convinced that the long forceps should never be used without axis traction and so attached the rods with permanent hinges. The form of the rods followed closely the line of the forceps blade and shank, and the handle was permanently fixed to the distal end of the left rod, while the right rod had a pin that passed through a keyhole slot on the handle plate (Doran, 1921). After further experience Simpson made a number of technical modifications that included lengthening the forceps and altering the attachment of the traction handle to make it stronger and easier to apply.

Charles Cullingworth (1892) had been a pupil of A. R. Simpson and was experienced in the use of his forceps but saw room for some minor improvements, mainly by increasing the strength of the components. They were of firmer construction, made entirely of metal, and with stronger

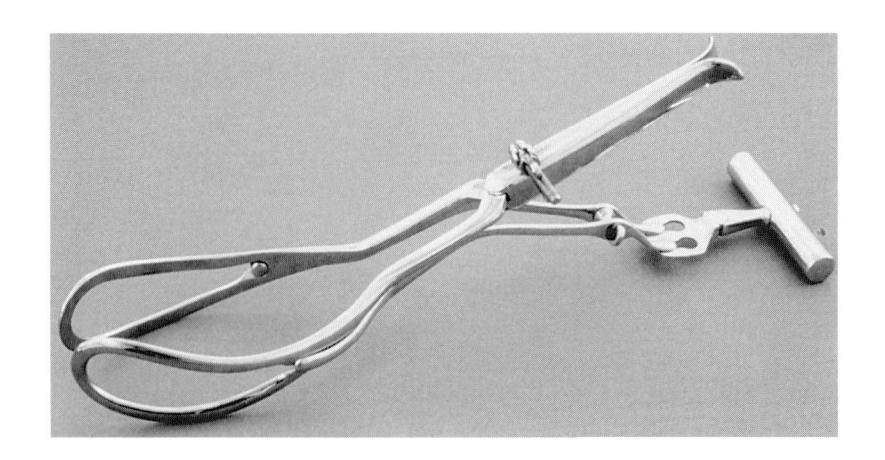

FIGURES 13.11–13.13.
Milne Murray's forceps (RCOG). 13.11: Later
version with detachable traction rods. 13.12:
Detail of handle lock. 13.13: Detail of fixed and
detachable rods.

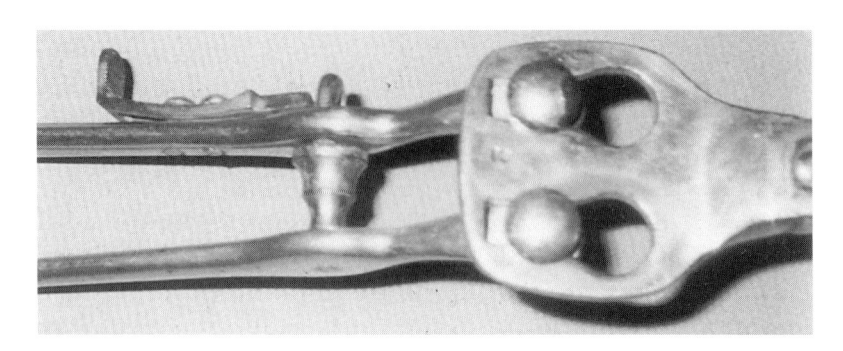

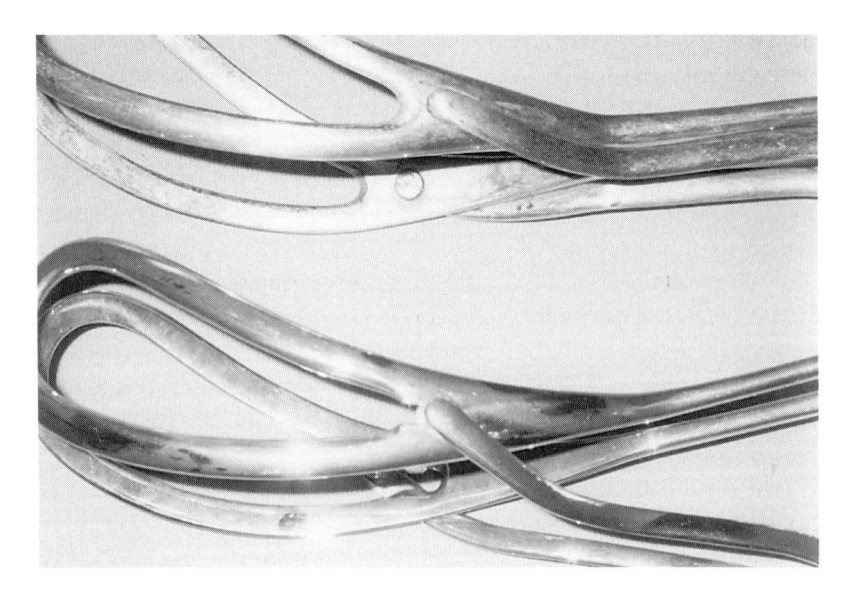

screws and studs. The blades were narrowed near the shanks to reduce the degree of perineal distension.

Robert Milne Murray (1855–1904) was a physician at the Royal Maternity and the Simpson Memorial Pavilion in Edinburgh. He had a highly scientific, analytical mind and considerable mathematical ability that he applied to the mechanics of forceps delivery. His work is worthy of close study even today. From a mathematical point of view, he readdressed the problems of a design to achieve true axis traction without risk of perineal trauma, analyzed the mechanics of the earlier axis-traction forceps, and made his own designs, which became very popular in Britain. In his paper to the Edinburgh Obstetrical Society in 1891 he stated the problem simply as being "to draw the foetal head through the birth canal with the least expenditure of force. Any force expended above that needed to overcome the resistance of the birth canal is likely to cause injury."

Milne Murray identified two major factors that made the solution complex: (1) the pelvic canal is curved and (2) the fetal head is not a sphere but an irregular ovoid or asymmetrical wedge. He observed that the immediate effect of traction with straight forceps was to encourage deflexion of the head and therefore increase the dimensions of the presenting diameter. With the curved forceps the grasp of the head was symmetrical to its mass, so that the contour of the head determined its presentation. However, this was offset by the faulty direction of traction with the curved forceps, a long-recognized problem partially corrected by Pajot's maneuver or by design modifications mentioned previously in Chapter 12.

Having critically analyzed the geometry of other forceps Milne Murray constructed his own instruments (Figures 13.11–13.13). He emphasized that the traction-rod hinge must be attached to the blade as near to the center of it as the fenestra permitted and he reduced the size of the fenestra to allow for this. The line of the traction rods was as close as possible to the outside of the shanks and handle to reduce the space that they occupied and the rods were fixed to the blades so that only antero-posterior movement was possible. The distal ends of the rods curved backward so that with the rods lying close to the shanks, the traction bar and pivot formed a tangent to the middle point of the arc of the curve of the blades. The rods were attached to the traction handle by studs fitting into keyhole apertures on the plate of the handle. Lightness in design was emphasized and the handles, no longer required for traction, were made smooth and light.

Milne Murray, while retaining the basic principles of the Tarnier and A. R. Simpson forceps, devised various improvements, including all steel construction, detachable traction rods, a detachable traction handle with a simple double keyhole and stud joint to the rods (Figure 13.12), and a traction-rod lock comprising a pin on one rod engaging with a mortise on the other and held by a simple bolt. These were all described in a seminal paper that Milne Murray gave to the Edinburgh Medical Society in 1891. He subsequently made the rods detachable, which facilitated cleaning but made them more unsteady in use (Figure 13.13). This was the reverse of A. R. Simpson's method, who started with detachable rods and changed to permanent hinges. The widespread popularity of both the Simpson and, later, the Milne Murray forceps led to most manufacturers taking up the designs and adding their own minor modifications in construction. Many of the instruments were Simpson/Milne Murray hybrids. Some of the more significant variations introduced by later obstetricians are described later in this chapter.

However, Milne Murray's most novel development was an adjustable axis-traction forceps (1896), which he regarded as desirable for abnormally shaped pelves, such as the flat pelvis and that with a low angle of brim inclination. The forceps itself was identical with the original model described above but the traction rods were radically altered. The distal segments of the rods turned at a right angle and had a graduated scale. The traction handle was fixed to the rods by a perforated block and adjacent to the hinge of the handle a sector scale indicated the appropriate angle of traction for the position of the handle on the rods (Figures 13.14, 13.15). In addition Milne Murray had a similar pair of forceps but with a reduced pelvic curve for use in occipito-posterior cases; he argued that the pelvic curve gave a better grip and helped to promote flexion of the head.

A similar design was subsequently adopted by George Porter Mathew (1898), who virtually eliminated the handles (Figure 13.16). The blades were smaller and narrower than conventional British blades, which, he claimed, made them easier to introduce and less likely to damage the head, especially when the head was lying transversely at a flattened pelvic brim. The principle of adjustable traction rods was subsequently revived in the twentieth century by Victor Bonney (1872–1953) of Middlesex Hospital, London. However, the benefits of adjustable rods were more theoretical than practical and their use was eventually abandoned.

Soon after A. R. Simpson introduced his forceps J. G. Lyon of Glasgow described his "remarkable Axis-Traction rods for midwifery forceps" (1881) (Figure 13.17), which could be attached to any curved forceps by a minor modification of soldering a small bridge across the base of the fenestra to make a socket into which his hooked rods would fit. Instead of using a compression screw he used a strong rubber ring to hold the handles together. The left rod had a swivel-jointed handle attached to it. The right rod was in two halves, one

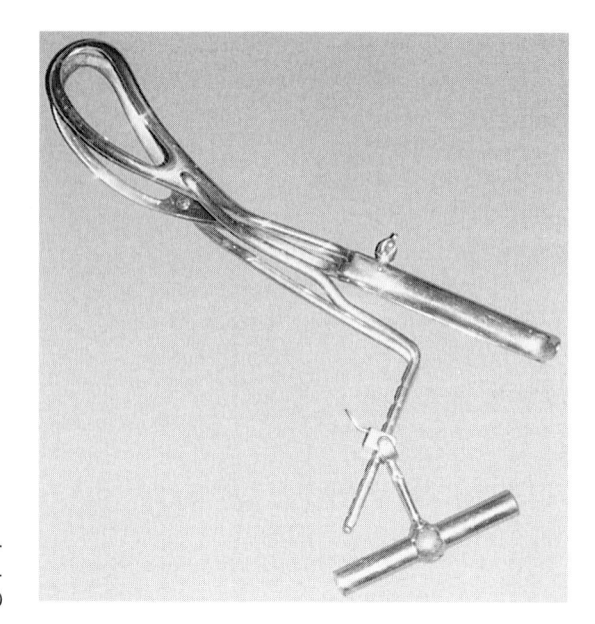

FIGURE 13.14.
Milne Murray's adjustable axis-traction forceps.
(Science Museum, London)

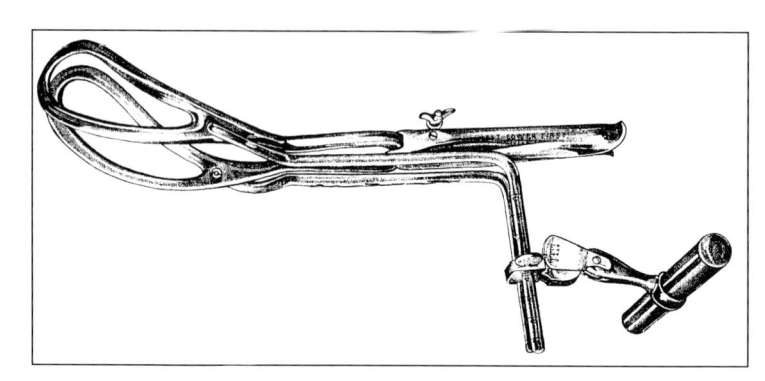

FIGURE 13.15.
Milne Murray's adjustable forceps. Showing the fixed hinge joints, the scales on the traction rod arm and the handle attachment. (Milne Murray, 1896)

FIGURE 13.16.
Porter Mathew's adjustable forceps. A development of Milne Murray's forceps, with truncated handles. (RCOG)

end being attached to the handle and fitted with a wedge lock to join it to the proximal (hooked) half.

David William Aitken (1893) claimed to improve the Milne Murray type of axis-traction rods by placing them exactly in the line of traction. However, the notable features of his forceps were that they were parallel and fixed together with a plate and screw where the joint would normally be. In addition the handles were detachable, sliding off slender rods that were left to act as pointers (Figure 13.18). In spite of his claim, Aitken's contribution was not significant to the practicalities of axis traction.

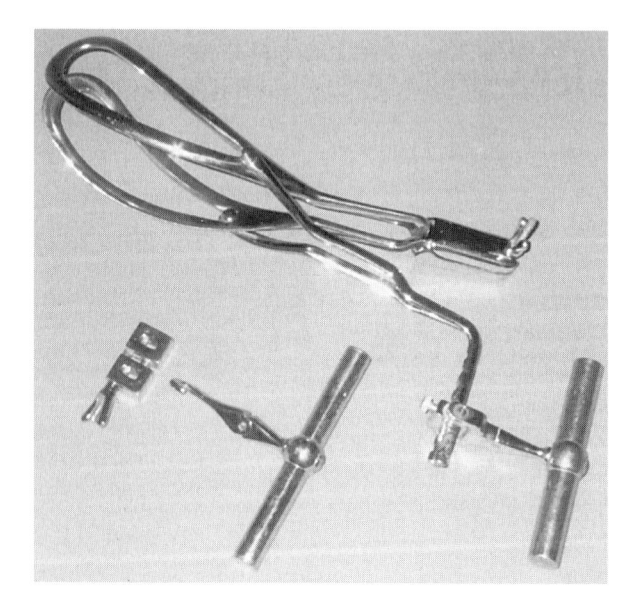

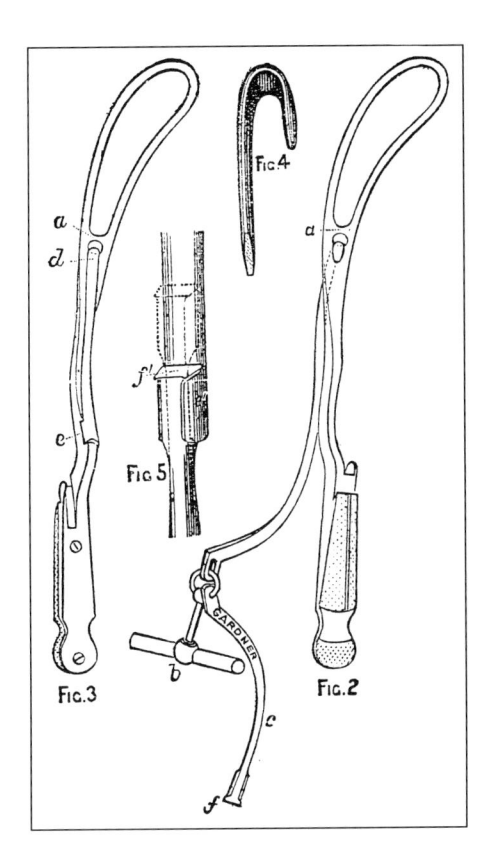

FIGURE 13.17.
Lyon's forceps. The traction handle *b* is attached by a swivel handle to the left blade and the lower half of the right rod *c*. The other half of the right blade is clipped to the shank *e* during insertion. The two parts of the right rod are joined by a wedge lock. (Lyon, 1881)

FIGURE 13.18.
Aitken's forceps. A solid block and screw replace the normal joint. The handles are detachable, leaving rods that act as pointers. (Aitken, 1893)

FIGURE 13.19.
Mackness's forceps. Another modification of Milne Murray's forceps, with a short handle. Figure I is the original version with button attachment of the traction handle. Figure II shows the later design with keyholes replacing the buttons. (Mackness, 1896)

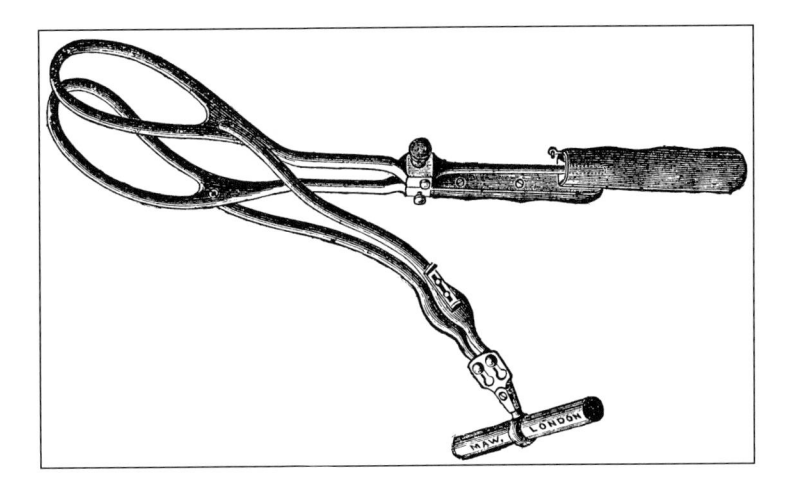

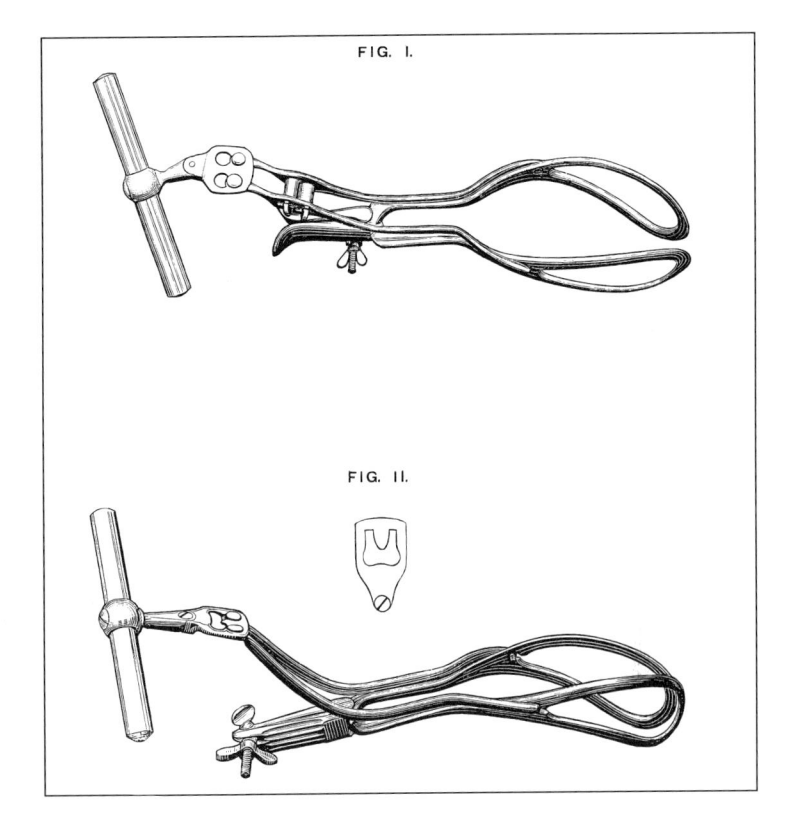

George Owen Carr Mackness of Forfarshire's designs were based on Milne Murray's, with detachable traction rods (1896) (Figure 13.19). He shortened the handles to 76 millimeters (3 inches), which, he claimed, made for ease of application, particularly with occipito-posterior positions. In his early model (Figure 13.19, Figure I), the traction handle was attached by buttons that were difficult to remove, so he reverted to the keyhole design (Figure 13.19, Figure II). He also moved the locking screw from the proximal to the distal end of the handle.

TARNIER AXIS-TRACTION FORCEPS 179

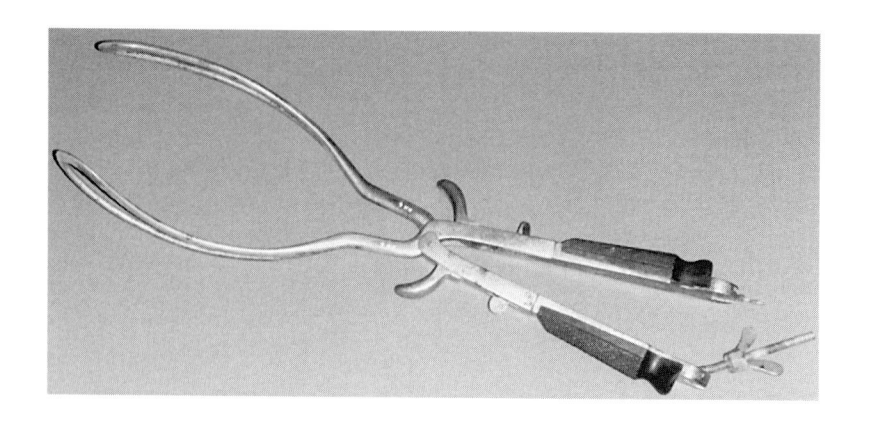

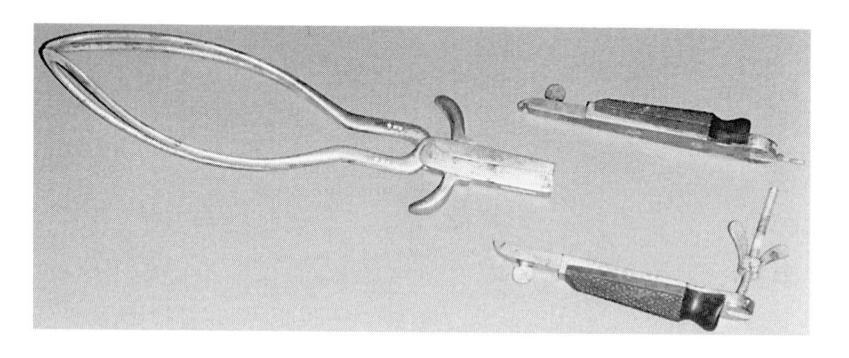

FIGURES 13.20, 13.21.
More Madden's compression forceps (RCOG).
13.20: These heavy forceps could be used for crushing. 13.21: The long compressing handles are detachable, allowing the instrument to be used as a short forceps (traction rods not shown).

FIGURE 13.22.
More Madden's compression forceps with traction rods attached. (More Madden, 1888a,b)

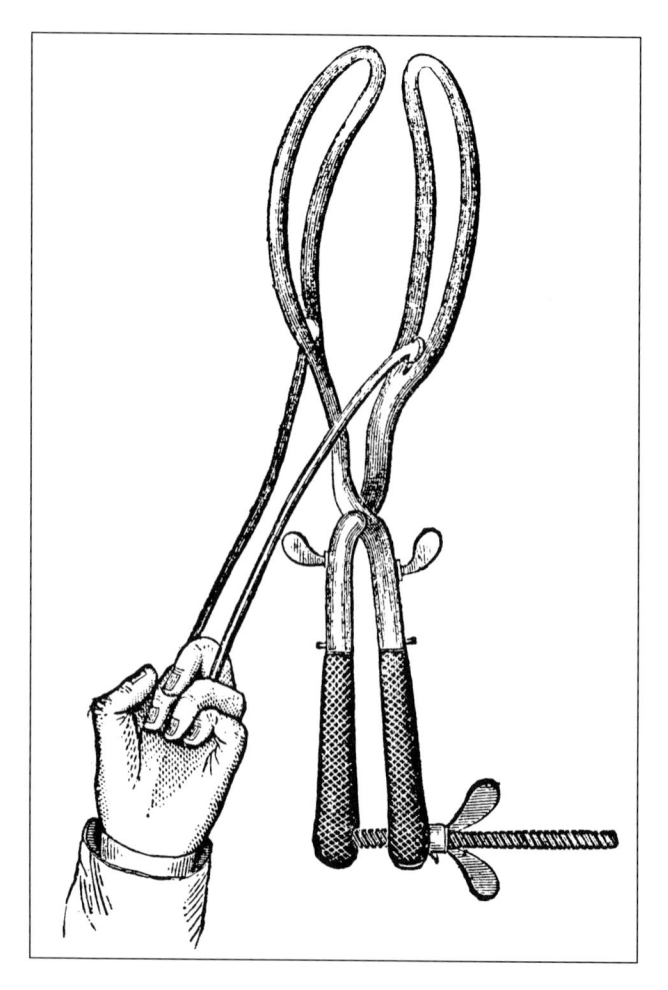

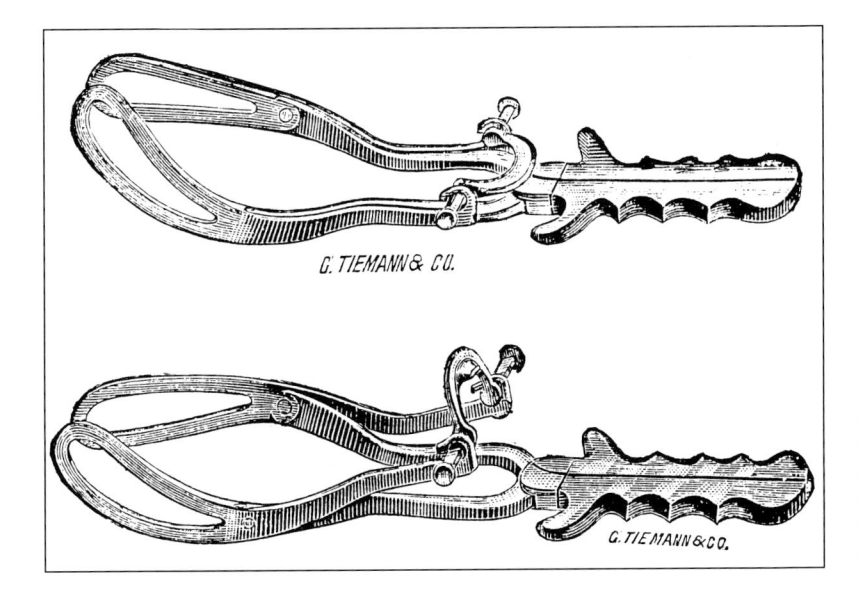

FIGURE 13.23.
Braun's *forceps trimorpha*. The handles are articulated to the root of the blades, which are extended backward. They are illustrated with the crossbar above the handles but they could be used with the crossbar below, thereby increasing the pelvic curve. (Braun, 1886)

Thomas More Madden, Obstetric Physician to the Mater Misericordiae Hospital, Dublin, seemed to be influenced by Continental practice when he described his "compressing double forceps" (1874b, 1888a,b) (Figures 13.20–13.22), intended for cases of difficulty and pelvic flattening. He described the forceps as being "of considerable length and strength, approximated by a powerful screw... I need hardly add that such an instrument requires caution and skill in its use, and should be employed chiefly as a substitute for embryotomic implements"(1888a). The traction rods, which appear to have been almost an afterthought with no obvious designed slot or other articulating device, hooked into the fenestra to give even greater traction force. They were designed so that they could be used on any fenestrated forceps. The main handles could be removed to provide a short forceps with finger grips.

European Developments
Germany Max Sänger (1853–1903) of Leipzig initially used Brunninghausen-type forceps (Chapter 5), to which he attached straps and a buckle of leather (1880). He later substituted a ring pessary instead of the buckle. He also described an instrument based on the Tarnier/Simpson designs, which he called the "German axis traction forceps." This was essentially a pair of Busch forceps (Chapter 9) without a fixation screw, with traction rods that were similar to A. R. Simpson's and were permanently attached by hinges to the blades, although the locking plate was removable.

Austria Carl Braun of Vienna (1823–1891) devised and modified various instruments as well as introducing some innovations of his own. According to Jaggard (1886), A. R. Simpson had sent a pair of his own forceps to Braun in 1880 and Braun immediately adopted them for use in his clinic. He subsequently modified them and, in 1886, used them as a basis for his *forceps trimorpha*, the instrument for which he is best known. The essential feature of the Braun forceps was an extension of the blades backward as spurs to form traction rods that turned upward at an angle. They were joined by a detachable stirrup-shaped crossbar that hooked into notches on the rods (Figure 13.23). The handles were hinged by an articulation at the base of the blade. When used with the handles below the blades the axis of the forceps was straightened, facilitating insertion. The pelvic curve could be increased by linking the fenestra handles under the lock. As with other hinged forceps, they were not very successful in meeting practical requirements (Chapter 8) and, according to A. R. Simpson, the only function of the extension of the blades was to provide an indication for the correct direction of traction.

Carl Breus (1852–1914) was assistant to Braun at the Vienna Maternity Clinic. Before Braun's article appeared, Breus had described a pair of forceps similar to Braun's, which he called "pelvic entrance forceps"(1882, 1885). They were of lighter construction and had a simple transverse pin to join the rods (Figure 13.24).

T. Felsenreich, also of Vienna, endeavored to improve on the Simpson's instrument with some minor modifications, including a buttonhole hinge for the traction rods, a removable compression thumbscrew at the end of the handles, and a hard rubber handle for the traction rods (1886) (Figure 13.25).

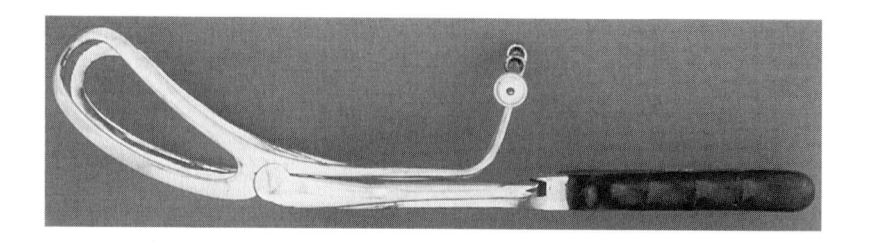

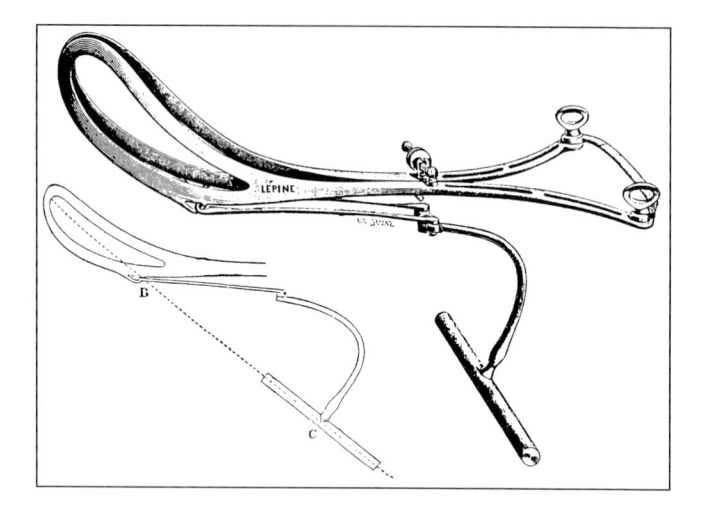

FIGURE 13.24 (TOP).
Breus's "pelvic entrance" forceps. These are lighter than those of his chief, Braun, and have a simple rod connection. (RCOG)

FIGURE 13.25 (RIGHT).
Felsenreich's forceps. These forceps are a modified A. R. Simpson-type with a compression screw. They were introduced as an alternative to the Braun/Breus instruments. (Felsenreich, 1886)

FIGURE 13.26 (ABOVE).
Demelin's forceps. The curved traction rod is hooked into rings on the lower surface of the blades. Parallel forceps were chosen to reduce the compression force. (Demelin, 1899)

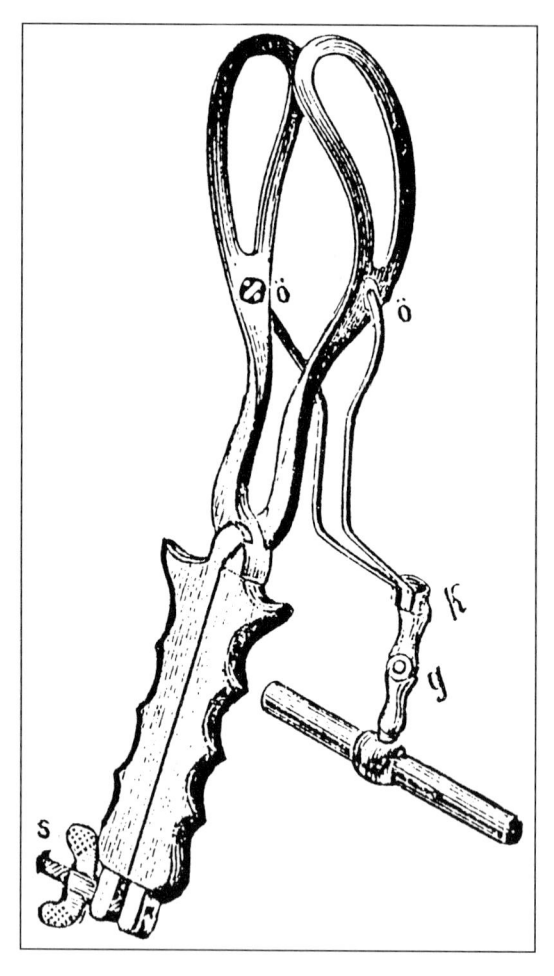

France Tarnier's forceps became so widely used that there was little competition, the only significant development coming from Poullet, referred to earlier. Poullet used, among other designs, a curved traction rod attached to tapes that passed through perforations in the blades (Chapter 12).

At the end of the century L. Demelin described a novel parallel axis-traction forceps (1899) (Figure 13.26). After application of the blades they were kept in place by screws and bolts at either end of the handle. Traction rods hooked into holes on the lower edges of the blades. Following manometric experiments he claimed that the compression force was several times less than that which occurred with Tarnier's forceps.

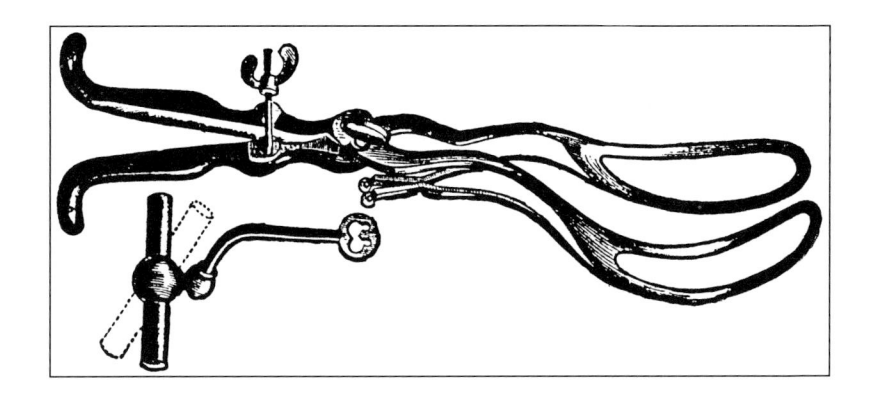

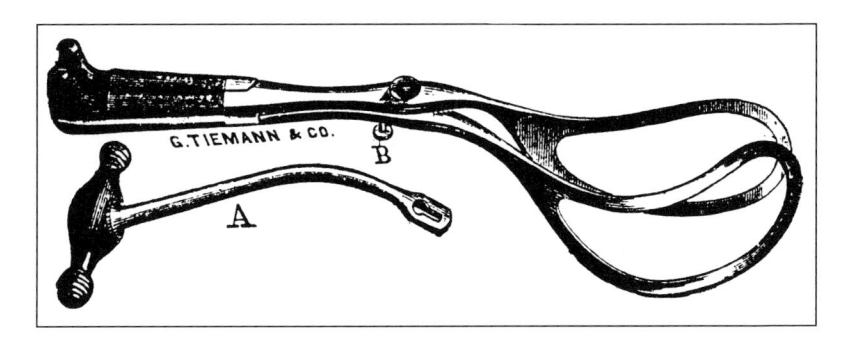

FIGURES 13.27, 13.28.
Lusk's axis-traction forceps. 13.27: His original modification of Tarnier's forceps. 13.28: The later simplified traction mechanism with a single noninvasive rod. (Lusk, 1880b, 1892)

American Developments

J. Bartlett of Chicago introduced a forceps similar to those of L. J. Hubert, of which he claimed to be unaware at the time (1880), but instruments based on the Tarnier principle were reputedly introduced in America by W. T. Howard of North Carolina. However, there is no written description of his forceps and their date is uncertain (Simpson, 1883).

The revolutionary designs of Tarnier were soon adopted in America and seem to have taken precedence over British axis-traction forceps, such as those of A. R. Simpson. For example, at the end of the century the illustrious and influential John Whitridge Williams (1866–1931), a professor of obstetrics at Johns Hopkins and author of the most enduring textbook on obstetrics, favored J. Y. Simpson's forceps for general use when axis traction was not required and the later versions of Tarnier's axis-traction forceps, which could be used either with or without the traction rods.

The first authenticated record of a new American design based on Tarnier's instruments is that of Thomas Lusk (1838–1897), who spent seven years (interrupted by returning to America to fight in the Civil War) studying in various European centers. He became a professor at Bellevue Medical College in New York and wrote one of the most successful American textbooks of midwifery. He modified and simplified the Tarnier design by making a lighter instrument (1880b) (Figure 13.27) based on Wallace's forceps (Chapter 7), which were at that time in widespread use in America. In a later model (Figure 13.28) he used a simple, single rod with a key attachment to the shank of the forceps rather than the clumsy socket joint, which was more difficult to assemble, to attach the handle to the rods. In the fourth edition of his *Science and Art of Midwifery* (1892), he had come to regard A. R. Simpson's forceps as "a most valuable addition" to his equipment for use when the head was in the pelvic cavity, when it "answer[ed] every indication." However, for high operations he "sometimes found it convenient to lay it aside for a longer forceps with a backward curve."

L. E. Neale, Chief of the obstetric clinic at the University of Maryland, added detachable traction rods and a compression screw at the end of the handle to J. Y. Simpson's forceps and acknowledged that he took the idea from Felsenreich, whom he had visited in Vienna (1885) (Figure 13.29). The forceps of E. Reynolds of Boston and of William S. Gardner of Baltimore (1892) were modifications of Simpson's style. Reynolds later simplified the basic Simpson design, utilizing curved traction rods with a hook at either end, one of which fit into the angle of the fenestrum and the other into a transverse, swivel-traction bar (1888). A separate clamp was used to fasten the forceps together.

Later, in 1895, Charles Jewett (1839–1910), a professor of obstetrics and gynecology at Long Island Hospital, modified Milne Murray's forceps, the main differences being a slotted Brunninghausen-type lock and reduced mobility of the traction bar (Figure 13.30).

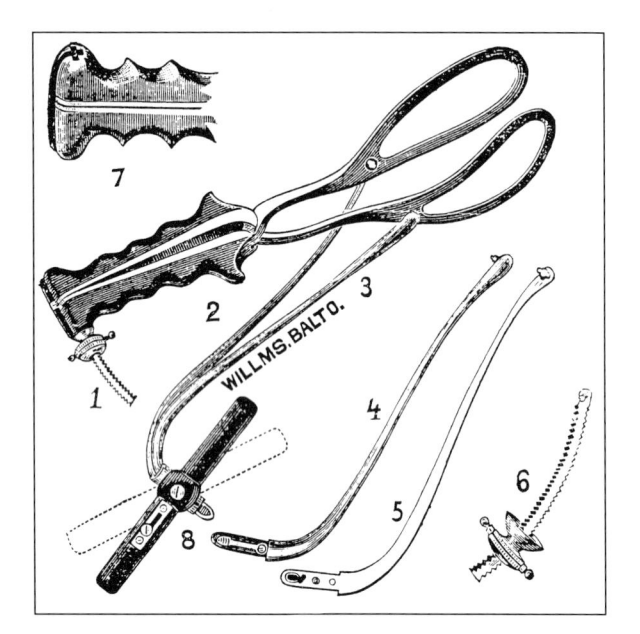

. . .

The philosophical principles and designs of Tarnier took the obstetric world by storm but the application of scientific principles had led to increasing complexity of design and practical difficulties in use. Soon more thought was being given to simplification and Mathews Duncan's view, as expressed earlier, that a scientifically imperfect instrument proved in practice might be better than a more scientifically designed instrument, became more prevalent.

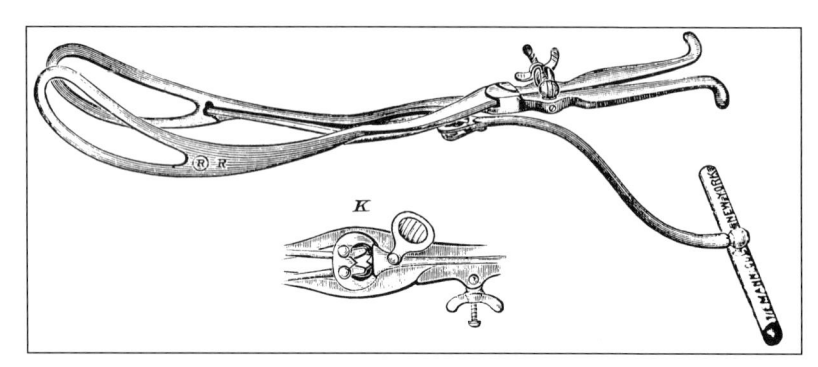

FIGURE 13.29.
Neale's forceps. An American adaptation of Felsenreich's forceps. (Neale, 1885)

FIGURE 13.30.
Jewett's axis-traction forceps. The insert shows the detail of the lock for attaching the traction handle to the rods. (Jewett, 1895)

OTHER AXIS-TRACTION FORCEPS AND ATTACHMENTS

In the latter part of the nineteenth century a lingering unhappiness remained among practitioners with the practical aspects of the designs based on the Tarnier and A. R. Simpson patterns. These designs had resulted in instruments that, although mechanically efficient and based on sound principles, were difficult to use, especially for the occasional operator. They also suffered from complexity of design, manufacture, and reproducibility, and thus were very expensive. From the operators' and patients' points of view, they were difficult to apply and the loose ironmongery within the birth canal could cause trauma to the maternal soft tissues. In consequence there was a particular desire to avoid the use of intravaginal traction rods. The quest for simplification resulted in the appearance of many unsatisfactory instruments but the credit for achieving simplification without undue sacrifice of the mechanical benefits is largely due to William Neville of Dublin (see below).

Robert Harvey Hilliard of Edinburgh reported a forceps designed by his brother F. Hilliard, an instrument maker who also lived in Edinburgh, which comprised a simple double-hinged traction rod that fit by means of pins into slots added to the end of the handles of J. Y. Simpson's forceps (1880) (Figure 14.1). However it did not seem to find favor, probably because A. R. Simpson's axis-traction forceps were by then receiving an enthusiastic reception.

James Foulis (1846–1901) of Edinburgh used forceps similar to those of A. R. Simpson, but with a clamping screw on the end of the handle and an optional traction rod that could be fixed to the shank (1887, 1900) (Figure 14.2). He claimed that this facilitated downward and backward pressure to produce an appropriate compound force. The disadvantages were that the recurved handle was too close to the buttocks and the rigid handle was inferior to Neville's hinged handle.

A major and enduring contribution to simplification of the axis-traction forceps was made in 1886 by William Neville (d. 1904), who practiced obstetrics at the Coombe Lying-Hospital in Dublin but retired from active practice because of ill health. In 1904 he was appointed to the Rotunda Hospital as a pathologist but he died soon after. Although he designed his own forceps (Figure 14.3), his simple traction apparatus (Figure 14.4) could be adapted to any conventional long forceps. This apparatus was most commonly seen as an addition to the Barnes or Anderson forceps (Chapter 6) and these continued in widespread and regular use well into the mid-twentieth century (Figure 14.5). The device comprised an angled rod with a cross handle attached by a double pivot, allowing movement of the handle on the rod both vertically and horizontally. The rod was attached to the shank of the forceps by a pin that fit into a socket in the shank and was secured by a screw and a wing nut that fit into a slot on the shank of the other blade.

The advantages of simplicity, having the traction rod entirely outside the birth canal, and being able to fit it after the forceps had been applied, more than compensated for some small loss of geometric and mechanical advantage. Moreover, if desired, the forceps could be used conventionally without the traction rod if required.

In America, William Harrison Studley (1827–1892) of New York was critical of the hinges in the Tarnier-type traction system and believed that greater rigidity was required for effective control of the descent of the head (1882). His forceps had deeply concave blades, a strong shank, a perineal curve, and a rigid traction rod with a transverse handle that was attached to the shank by a thumb screw (Figure 14.6).

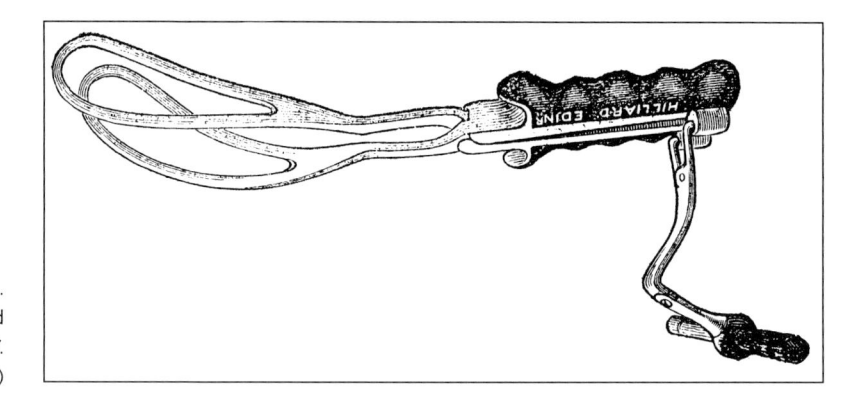

FIGURE 14.1.
Hilliard's forceps. The detachable traction rod fits into slots at the end of the handle of J. Y. Simpson's long forceps. (Hilliard, 1880)

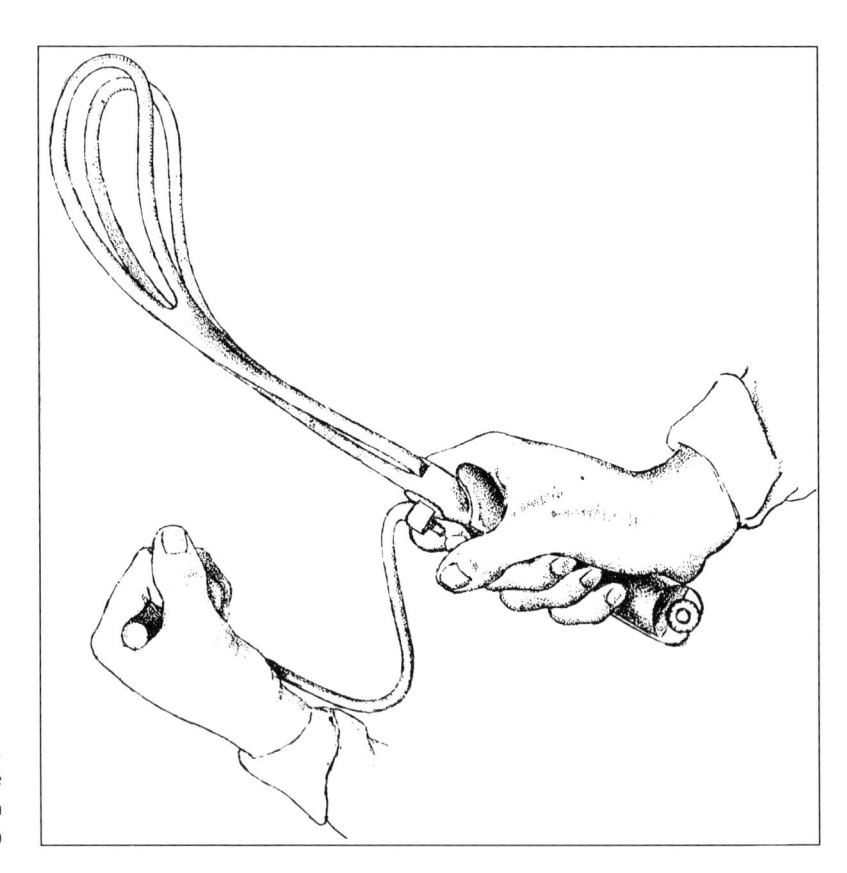

FIGURE 14.2.
Foulis's forceps. Another unsound design. The traction handle was too rigid and impinged on the buttocks. (Foulis, 1887)

FIGURE 14.3.
Neville's forceps. Original design, showing the double-jointed traction handle. (Neville, 1886)

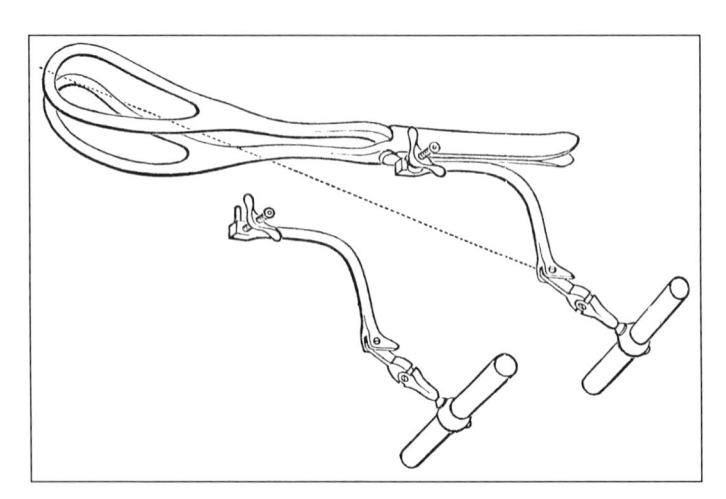

186   CHAPTER 14

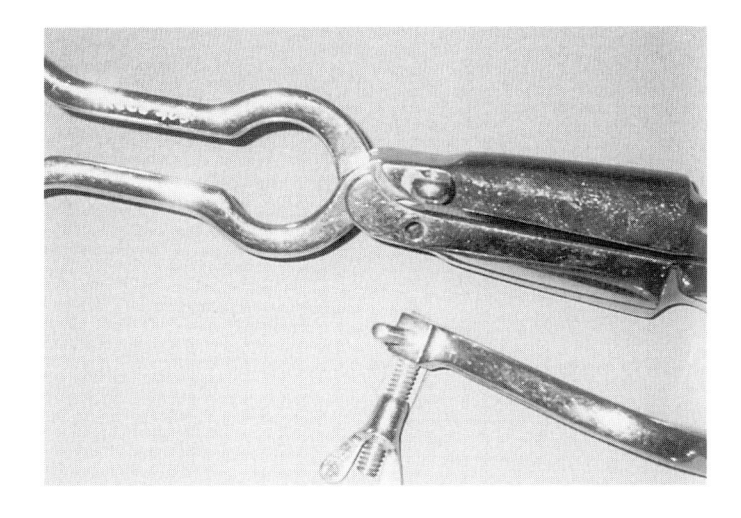

FIGURE 14.4.
Neville's traction rod. Detail of the attachment to the shank of the forceps. (RCOG)

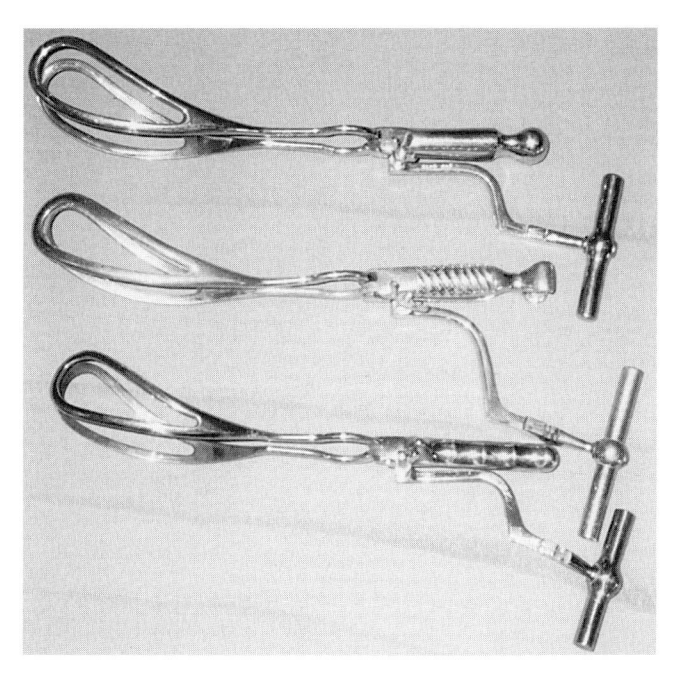

FIGURE 14.5.
Forceps adapted to take the Neville traction rod. Top to bottom: Barnes, Greville, Anderson. (RCOG)

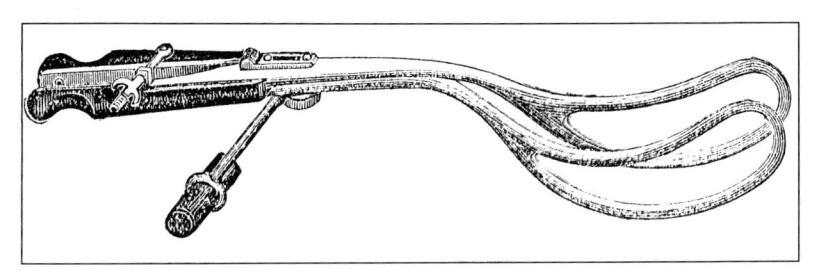

FIGURE 14.6.
Studley's forceps. The aim was greater rigidity, which was achieved by heavy shanks, a compression screw, and a rigid traction rod screwed to the shank. (Studley, 1882)

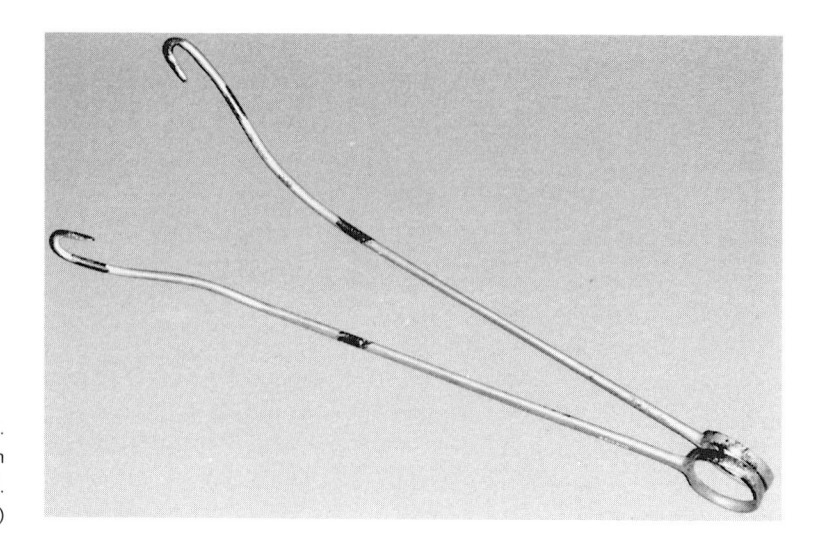

FIGURE 14.7.
Morgan's tractors. These simple hooks with finger rings are held together by a rubber band. (Science Museum, London)

FIGURE 14.8.
Le Page's tractor. Two versions that were widely advertised. The claws hook into the root of the blades. (Science Museum, London)

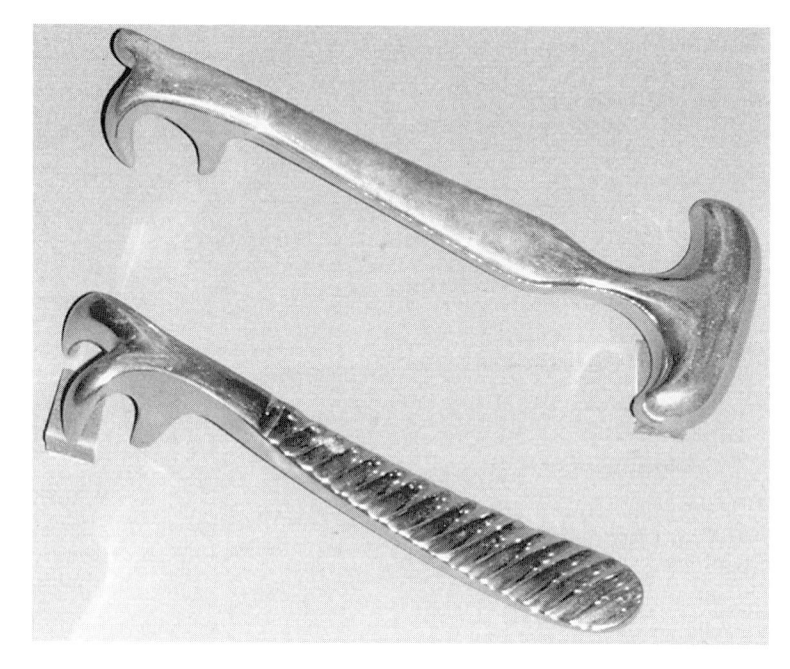

FIGURE 14.9.
Stephenson's tractor. Stephenson emphasized the desirability of maintaining a grip on the handle of the forceps, unlike Tarnier and others. (Stephenson, 1886)

FIGURE 14.10.
McLaurin's forceps. Parallel forceps with a sliding lock. The separate traction handle is also attached to the end of the handle. (McLaurin, 1886)

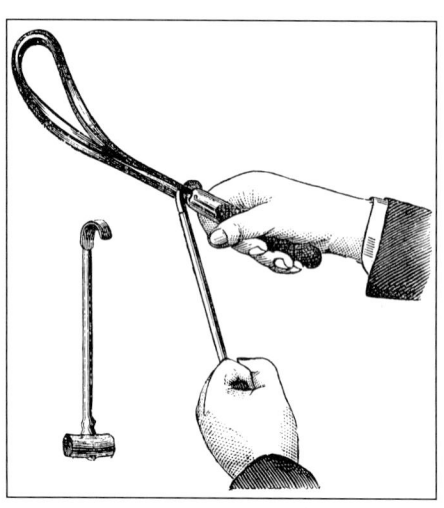

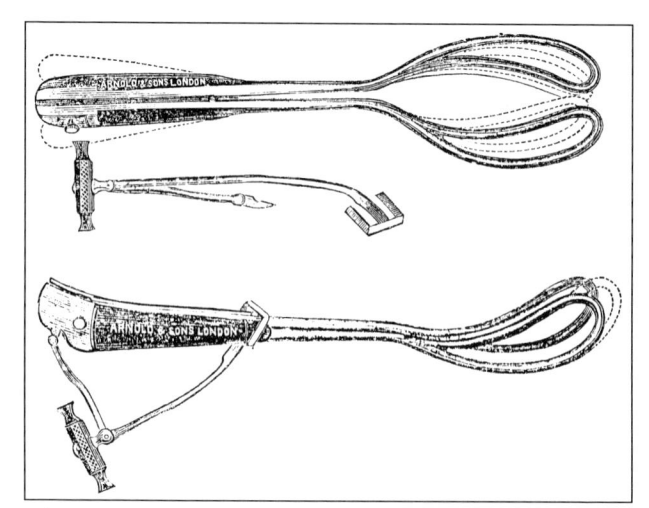

188 CHAPTER 14

Having a nonhinged traction rod did not necessarily increase the strength of compression but did alter the way traction was applied, which, in Studley's eyes, was an improvement.

Separate Traction Devices

Separate tractors to attach to conventional long forceps without adaptation being required became common in Britain and America and stemmed from the desire for simplicity and lower expenditure on equipment and forceps. The forceps could then be used conventionally when axis traction was not required. Some of these instruments were intended to hook into the fenestra while others were attached to the shank or handle to avoid invading the birth canal.

Europe

Some of the simple traction hooks were intended mainly to allow for greater traction and are described in Chapter 11. However, increasingly practitioners recognized their benefit in influencing the direction of traction.

Herbert Morgan of Lichfield summarized the situation relating to the practicalities of using the Tarnier forceps and looked for a simpler solution:

> When I had once thoroughly examined the ingenious new midwifery forceps of M. Tarnier I saw immediately that his principle gave to those who used the instrument a new power, in a new direction, I set to work to try if the best part of his principle could be arranged in an effective portable and cheap form so as to be applied to the different patterns of existing long curved forceps.... (1878)

Morgan's tractors (Figure 14.7) were a simple pair of hooks that slipped into the angles of the fenestra of the blades after they had been applied. The handles were held together with a rubber band. With this arrangement the direction of traction could be almost exactly in the pelvic axis. However, there was a risk of trauma as well as encroachment on the perineum.

Alexander Duke, who designed his tractor to give extra force rather than considering the direction of traction vis-à-vis any scientific principles, such as the parallelograms of forces (1879), has been discussed in Chapter 11. Duke found difficulty in attaching Morgan's rods after the forceps had been applied and modified them so that they could be introduced with the blades. Alexander Keiller (1811–1892), a physician at the Edinburgh Maternity Hospital and a lecturer at the Royal College of Surgeons in Edinburgh, claimed to have invented a similar device (1879).

J. F. Le Page of Paris's tractor was a very simple claw-like device that hooked onto the articulation (1883). It was easy to use and became very popular, even though its method of attachment was crude and it was not mechanically very sound (Figure 14.8). This type of attachment continued to be used for some time and, in the third decade of the twentieth century, the Holborn Surgical Instrument Company still marketed Le Page's tractor, their own variation of it, and another similar device by Penrose Williams.

William Stephenson (1837–1908), Professor of Midwifery at the University of Aberdeen, was one of the first to use an attachment that did not invade the birth canal (1886). Initially he used a crotchet hooked into the shank, the blunt hook at the other end serving as a handle, but later had a purpose-made instrument with a crosshandle (Figure 14.9).

William McLaurin (1846–1899), a surgeon at the Royal Maternity Charity in London, observed that when forceps were applied over the face and occiput the blades often were not level. He thus designed parallel forceps with a sliding lock to compensate for this unevenness (1886) (Figure 14.10). The axis tractor was a simple T-shaped rod that hooked over the shank and had a hinged extension near the traction handle that fit into the end of the main handle.

America

A. B. Lyman of Baltimore also designed a hook to fit into the shank of any forceps but this was of more complicated design than other separate traction rods (1891) (Figure 14.11), as it was intended to be used in the same manner as adjustable axis-traction forceps (see Chapter 13, Milne Murray, Porter Mathew). The terminal part of the rod was hinged to turn at a right angle and was threaded so that the handle could be fixed at any position from the rod according to the axis of the head in the birth canal.

D. Benjamin of New Jersey combined Simpson's blades with Hodge's handles and had a separate axis traction rod which could be used as required with any type of forceps (1898).

Robert W. Fisher of Salt Lake City utilized a simple iron bar with a slot to fit over the shank of the forceps, effectively converting the instrument to a modified Hubert's forceps (1895) (Figure 14.12). However, Benjamin's and Fisher's instruments were unremarkable and did not provide any significant benefits.

A more complicated independent device originated from Brooks H. Wells (d. 1917) of New York (1886) (Figure 14.13). The traction rod had a notched hook that fit between the shanks at the articulation and was provided with a transverse handle. In addition, an adjustable arm attached to the rod had a screw clamp that fit around the handles. Thus it

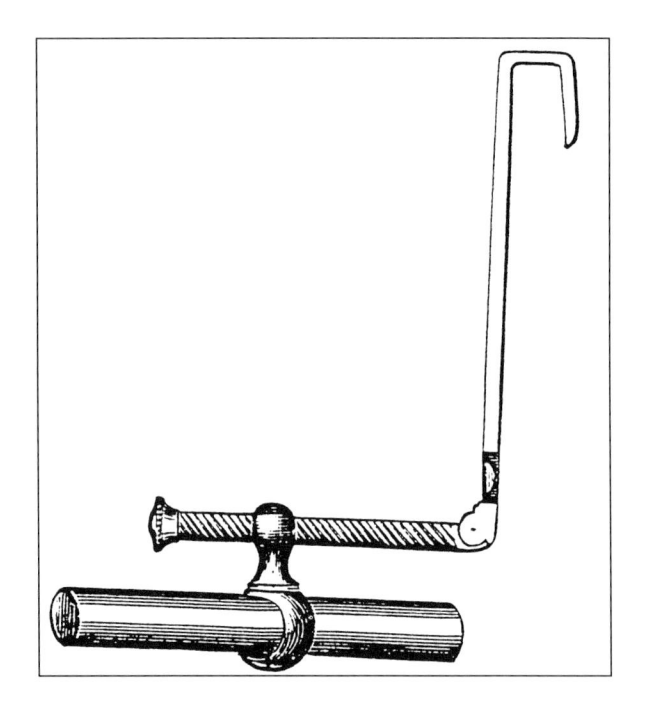

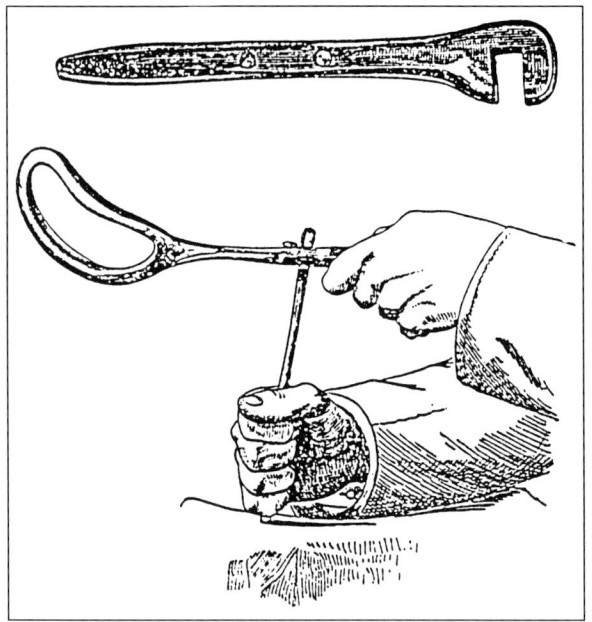

FIGURE 14.11.
Lyman's tractor. A separate hook-type traction rod with the handle adjustable on a screw shank to alter the traction angle. (Lyman, 1891)

FIGURE 14.12.
Fisher's tractor. A notched bar fits the shank firmly, intended to mimic Hubert's forceps. (Fisher, 1895)

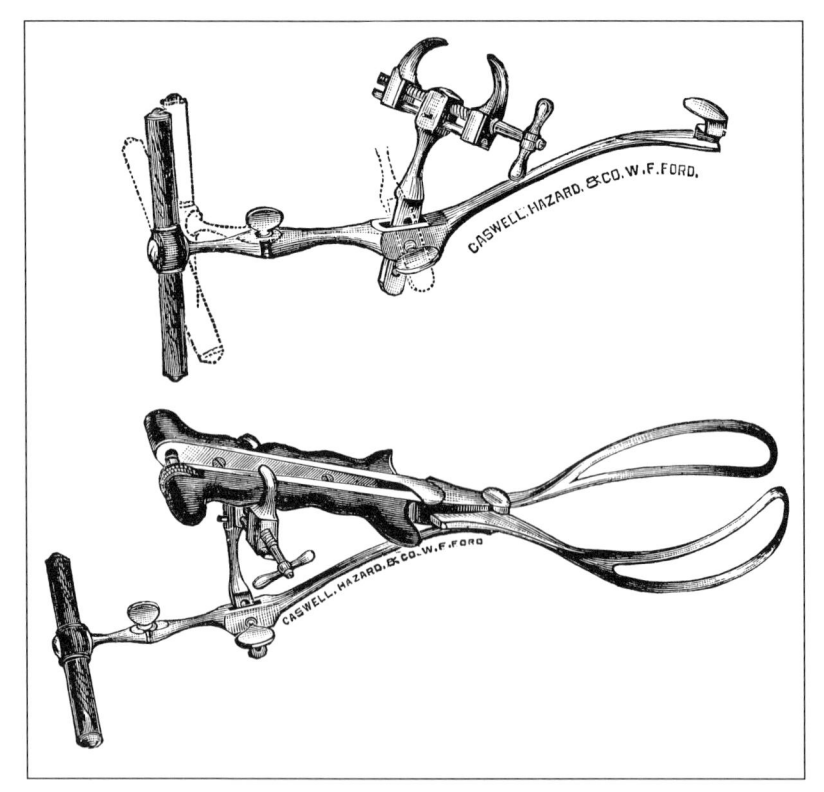

FIGURE 14.13.
Wells's forceps. The jointed tractor hooks into the root of the blades. The angle can be fixed by an adjustable arm that clamps on to the handle of the forceps. (Wells, 1886)

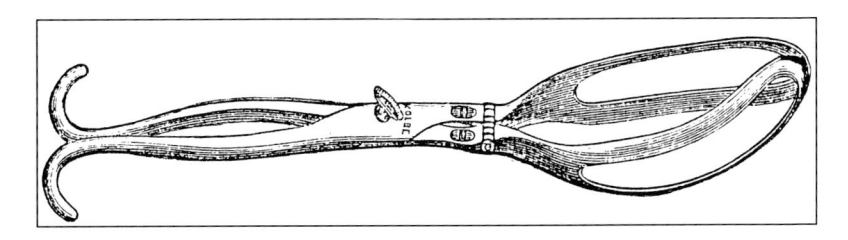

FIGURE 14.14.
McFerran's forceps. The vertical hinge in the shank gives little benefit and does not contribute to axis traction. (McFerran, 1877)

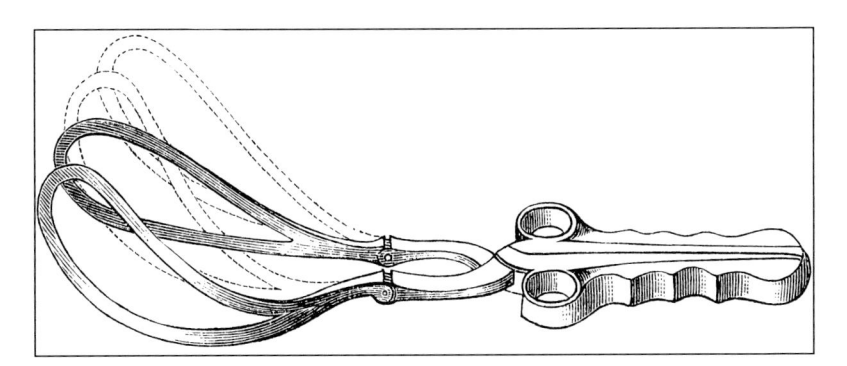

FIGURE 14.15.
Vedder's forceps. The model illustrated is a later all-steel instrument, the original having wooden handles (Vedder, 1878). Although the construction of this forceps is similar to Vedder's original instrument, it is based on J. Y. Simpson's rather than a European-type forceps.

was possible to fix the angle of the traction rod appropriate to the angle of the forceps being used and to adjust the angle according to the line of traction.

Hinged Shanks and Handles

Another alteration that had limited passing interest was to hinge the blade on the shank in a vertical plane, thus effectively altering the pelvic curve, unlike the hinges in the shanks allowing lateral folding, which have been mentioned previously (Chapter 8) in relation to portability and facility of application with the woman in the lateral position. Although it was often claimed that these instruments hinged in the vertical plane fulfilled the principles of axis traction, many of them clearly did not even approach this objective and did no more than overcome some of the difficulties of high forceps application. Early in the nineteenth century David Davis devised a pair of such forceps and these were found at University College Hospital (see Chapter 5; Figure 6.6) but as he did not describe them in any of his writings, including his *Atlas*, they were presumably a failure.

In the last quarter of the nineteenth century the hinged shank was again explored by a number of people, the first being Americans. Joseph A. McFerran of Philadelphia introduced a simple hinged forceps (Figure 14.14) based on the European pattern, with long, hooked, metal handles and a screw-and-slot articulation (1877, 1884). Hinges were interposed between the shanks and the fenestra. This design only allowed at best the same forces and direction of traction of older instruments with a perineal curve. It was clearly inferior to the sophisticated axis-traction instruments then available.

Maus R. Vedder of New York, whose forceps were a modified J. Y. Simpson instrument with a similar vertical hinge (Figure 14.15), claimed that his forceps were very nearly perfect (1878). In spite of this alleged perfection he suggested that Tarnier-type traction rods could be attached if more traction force was desired.

A number of attempts were made to design a functional hinged handle that would rotate up to 90 degrees from the shank, thus producing instruments functionally reminiscent of Hubert's and other stepped forceps and avoiding the need for intravaginal rods. One of the earliest of these was that of A. D. Macdonald of Liverpool, whose forceps blades were almost straight (1882) (Figure 14.16). The elongated handles were hinged vertically at their midpoint. The ends could be rotated up to 90 degrees and were perforated to take a transverse traction handle. The binding screw was graduated so that the size of the head could be measured and the degree of compression judged.

N. Grattan modified the Anderson-type forceps (Chapter 6) by fitting a spring catch in each of the handles so that they could be fixed at any angle up to 90 degrees, thus providing, in effect, a perineal curve serving the same function as the Aveling forceps (1888) (Figures 14.17, 14.18). J. F. Le Page's forceps were made on a similar principle to that of

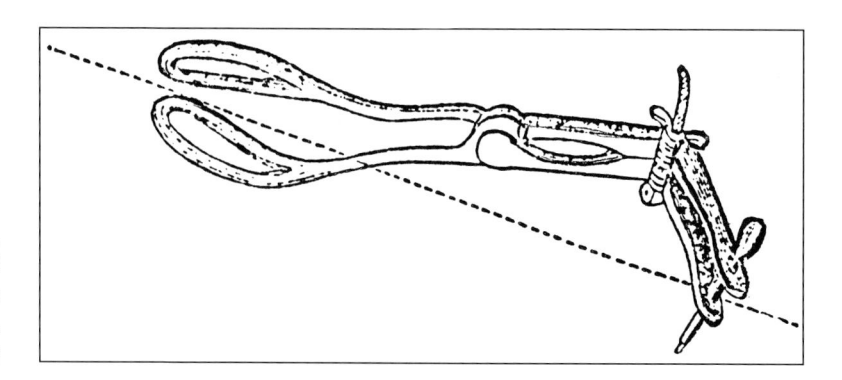

FIGURE 14.16.
A. D. Macdonald's forceps. The elongated handles can be rotated up to 90°. The screw connecting the handles is graduated. (Macdonald, 1882)

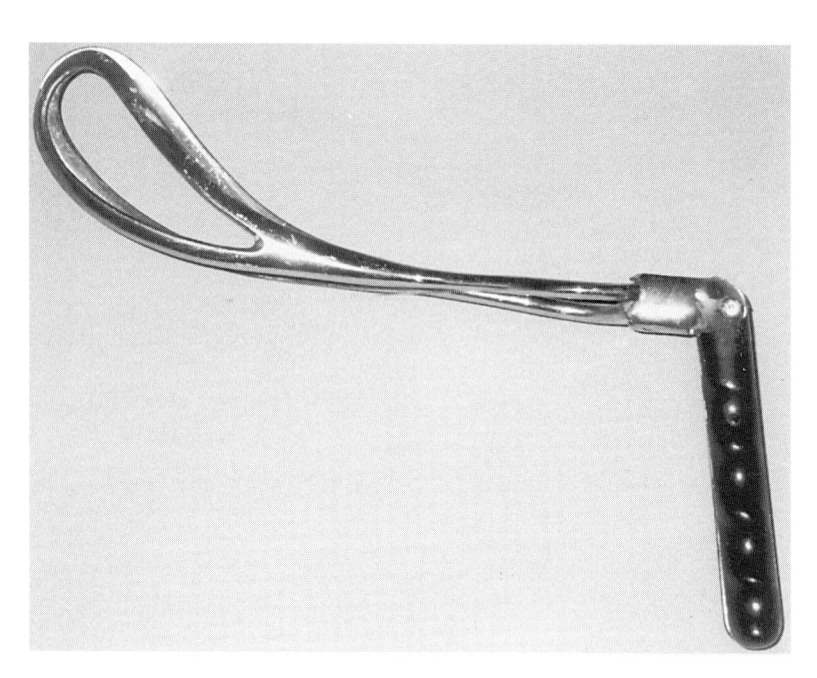

FIGURES 14.17, 14.18.
Grattan's forceps. The hinged handles can be fixed at any angle up to 90°. (Grattan, 1888)

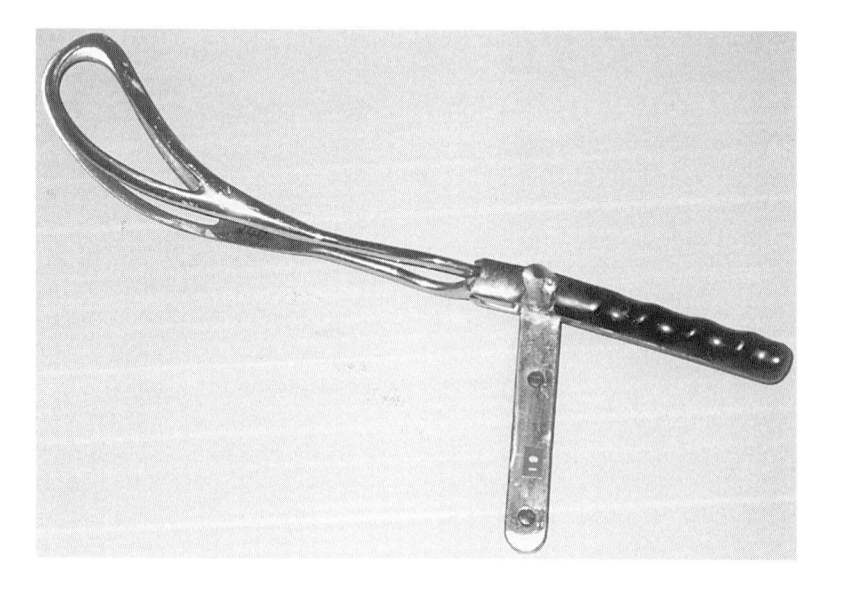

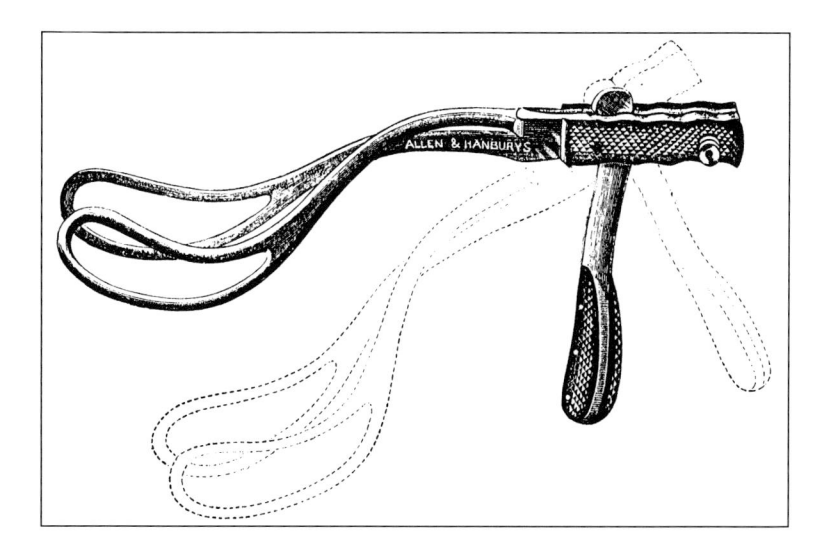

FIGURE 14.19.
Le Page's forceps. The hinged extension between the handles rotates up to 90° and is clamped by a fixing screw joining the handles. (Le Page, 1883)

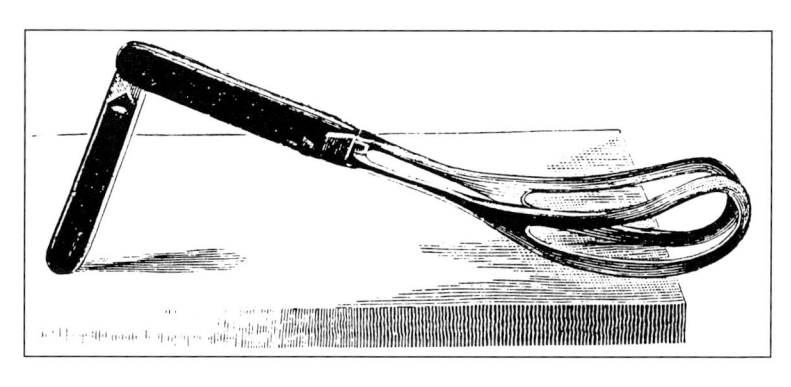

FIGURE 14.20.
McGillicuddy's forceps. An American version of the extended hinged handle. (McGillicuddy, 1889)

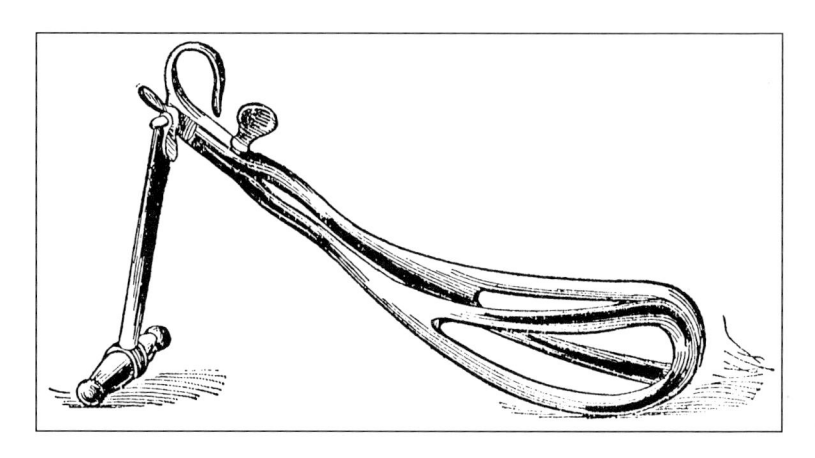

FIGURE 14.21.
Dewees's "axis-traction and anti-craniotomy" forceps. The conventional handle is replaced by the hinged traction handle. (Dewees, 1895)

Grattan, the only difference being a hinged extension to the handle (1883) (Figure 14.19).

In America, Timothy J. McGillicuddy (1857–1899) of New York added folding handles to the Simpson-type forceps (1889, 1891). These shorter additional handles were folded on the conventional handles when not required but could be rotated up to 90 degrees to provide axis traction (Figure 14.20).

Dewees, who in 1892 had described a simple stepped forceps, later discarded the conventional handles and fixed a hinged traction handle onto the shank just distal to the joint with a compression screw, an instrument he described as an "axis traction and anti-craniotomy forceps" (1895) (Figure 14.21). He thought he had achieved the most perfect instrument yet devised as the result of his riper experience and more extended study. His claim that it was an "aseptic, eco-

OTHER AXIS-TRACTION FORCEPS 193

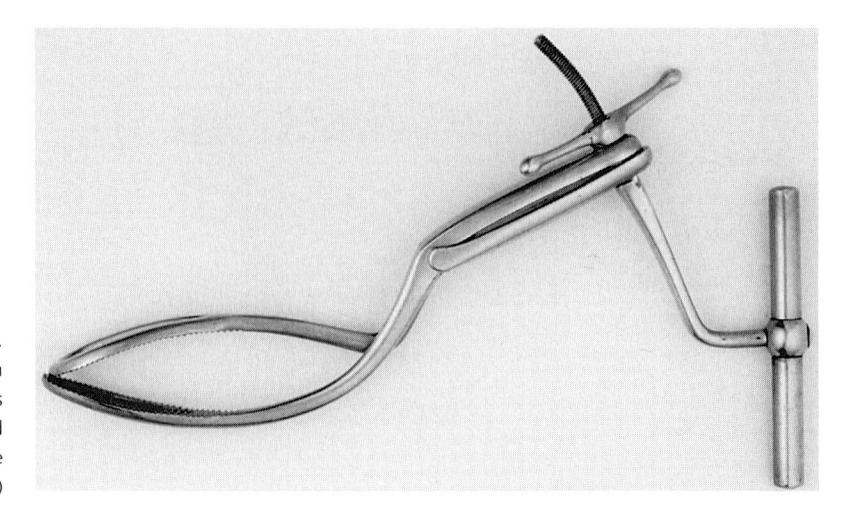

FIGURE 14.22.
Cameron's antero-posterior axis-traction forceps. One blade passes through the other, as in Ziegler's forceps. The handles are clamped together by a screw and wing nut on the traction rod. (RCOG)

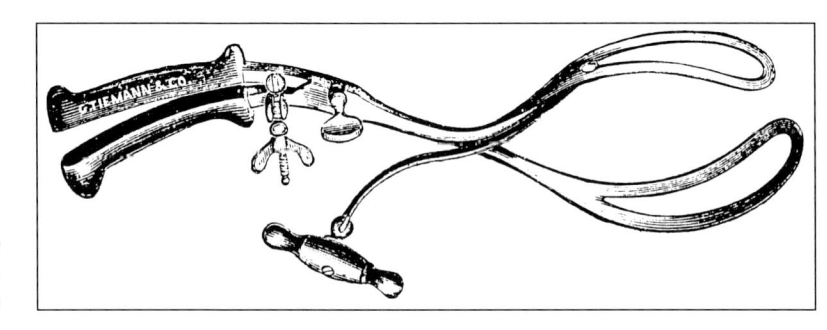

FIGURE 14.23.
Fry's antero-posterior forceps. The single traction rod hooks into the anterior blade. (Fry, 1889b)

nomic, safe, efficient and uncomplicated instrument" might equally well be applied to many other designs of the time and his did not seem to have widespread appeal.

Axis Traction with Antero-Posterior Forceps

One of the major difficulties with the Tarnier/Simpson forceps was that they could not be applied in correct cephalic application when the head was in the transverse position. Several instruments were devised to try to overcome this problem. McLaurin's forceps (1886) were intended to increase the adaptability of the blades to the head and have already been described.

Murdoch Cameron (1846–1930), Regius Professor of Midwifery, University of Glasgow, created antero-posterior forceps around 1893 that were specifically intended for use in cases of major pelvic contraction, with a true conjugate of as little as 76 millimeters (3 inches), which was not uncommon in the Glasgow slums at that time. The posterior blade had an elongated fenestrum through which the anterior blade was passed. Traction was provided through a simple rod and crossbar that screwed onto the end of the handle and also served to hold the blades together (Figure 14.22).

Fry reviewed the reasons for failure of earlier antero-posterior forceps (Chapter 9). His instrument was specifically designed for application before anterior rotation of the head had occurred. It had a pelvic curve on the flat and the blades were of unequal length, the anterior being shorter. The traction rod fit into the angle of the fenestra of the anterior blade only (Figure 14.23). The blades were applied by a "wandering" technique and the traction rod was attached after positioning of the blades (1889b).

. . .

The innovations described in this chapter showed ingenuity and, in most cases, attempts to simplify designs while retaining the principle of axis traction. However, most of them achieved little more than local popularity. The notable exception was the Neville traction rod, which sacrificed little in geometric terms while providing simplicity of design and use, the ability to be used on almost any long forceps with only minor modification, and more safety because of its noninvasive rod.

VACUUM EXTRACTORS

The first functional instrument utilizing suction to aid delivery is generally attributed to J. Y. Simpson but the principle has a much longer history. In the seventeenth century a number of surgeons advocated suction devices to raise depressed skull fractures in children. These included Fabricius Hildanus (1643) (Jones, 1960), who used a leather sucker, and Ambroise Paré (1614), who favored a cupping glass, or *ventouse* (Figure 15.1). In 1706 James Yonge reported to the Royal Society of London on an unsuccessful attempt to deliver a child by attaching a cupping glass to the scalp with an air pump.

Neil Arnott (1788–1874) of London described a children's game of the time in which a piece of wet leather with a string attached could be used to lift a smooth stone by its suction force, the theoretical load being up to 15 pounds per square inch (4.98 Nm^{-2}, that is, atmospheric pressure). Based on these measurements he proposed a "pneumatic tractor" consisting of a circular piece of leather that was kept extended by solid rings, or "radii" (1829). He estimated that with a 76-millimeter (3-inch) diameter disk, a traction force of 45.5 kilograms (100 pounds) was possible. Initially he considered its value in surgery but subsequently suggested that it could be used as a substitute for obstetric forceps "in the hands of men who are deficient in manual dexterity, whether from inexperience or natural aptitude." Such a recommendation was hardly likely to endear the instrument to obstetricians who were proud of their skills and there is no record of Arnott or any other contemporary obstetrician actually using the device.

The evolution of vacuum extractors has been well reviewed by Chalmers in his work *The Ventouse* (1971). J. Y. Simpson, after some years of experimentation, described a suction tractor at the Edinburgh Obstetric Society in 1848 (Simpson, 1849a). He likened the action to that of a cuttlefish's adhesion and paid tribute to Arnott, whom he quoted at length, for the original idea. His prototype instrument comprised a tubular, metal vaginal speculum fitted with a piston. The end was covered with leather and smeared with lard. He was successful in delivering a baby with this device, although two or three reapplications were necessary. He described the instrument as "rude and imperfect" and indicated various possibilities for improvement, including experiments with a dynamometer.

Within a short time Simpson (1849b) described in detail his preferred model of suction tractor, which comprised a short brass pump with a double-valved piston, similar to a breast pump of the period (Figures 15.2, 15.3). The detail of the instrument was illustrated by Scanzoni (1853) (Figure 15.4). The piston was attached to an inner metal cup 38 millimeters (1.5 inches) in diameter and 13 millimeters (.5 inches) in depth and to a deeper outer cup of vulcanized rubber. Within the inner cup was brass wire gauze covered with flannel to protect the scalp from damage. In his experiments he found that this would lift a weight of 13.6 to 18.2 kilograms (30 to 40 pounds), while a 76-millimeter (3-inch) cup would lift from 27.3 to 36.4 kilograms (60 to 80 pounds). He used this version in several cases but saw room for further improvement. However soon after this, in a letter to a patient (Duns, 1873), he expressed the belief that the instrument was now nearly perfect and sent two instruments for her father's use. In the same letter he described the reception his instrument had received, including a demonstration he gave to

FIGURE 15.1.
Paré's *ventouses*. (Paré, 1655)

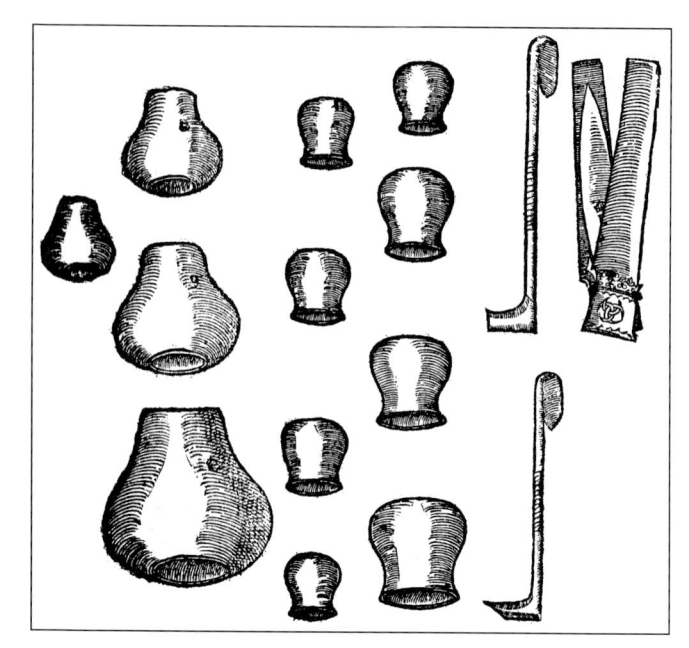

FIGURES 15.2, 15.3.
Simpson's air tractor. The brass double-valved syringe is attached to a metal cup covered with vulcanized rubber. (University of Edinburgh)

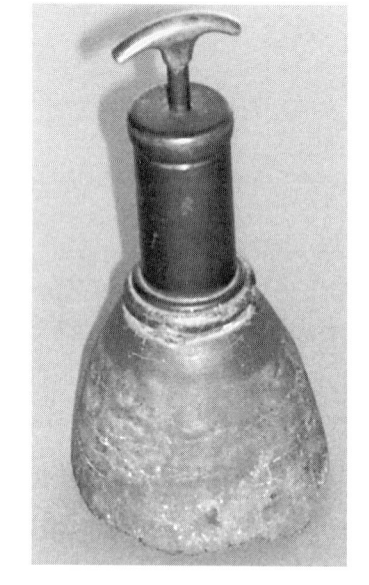

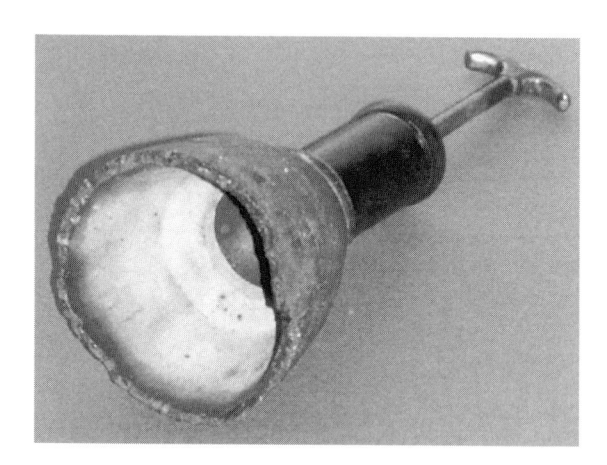

Dr. Marginles, a physician at the St. Petersburg Court. He reported that "[t]he Russian danced with joy, crying, 'C'est superbe, superbe; c'est immortalité à vous.'"

Simpson envisaged that the main use of the suction tractor would be to bring down the high head into the pelvic cavity, the circumstances in which he had used his prototype and a particularly hazardous procedure with the forceps. He also thought it could be used for rotating the head and possibly applied to the breech as well. When the head was low in the birth canal and uterine action was poor it could be used to augment contractions and would be safer than pharmacological uterine stimulants such as ergot of rye.

Unfortunately, over the next few months some vigorous, even vitriolic, correspondence followed in the *London Medical Gazette* (not an uncommon occurrence at that time) concerning Simpson's vacuum extractor. F. H. James of Exeter claimed to have designed a similar instrument independently but his device was very rudimentary and there is no evidence that he ever used it (1849). A former pupil of Simpson, James Mitchell of Nottingham, in three letters to the *Gazette* (which had to be edited and were rejected by other journals because they were considered libelous) accused him of plagiarism and claimed to have designed a similar instrument that he had described in an examination paper while he was in Edinburgh from 1847 to 1848. (1849). Simpson and

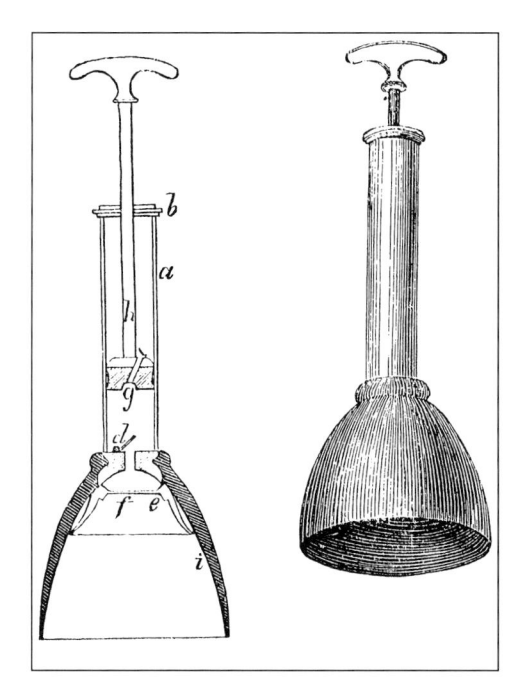

FIGURE 15.4.
Scanzoni's representation of Simpson's *aërotractor*. *d,g*: the two valves; *e*: inner brass cup; *f*: wire lattice; *i*: outer protecting bell.
(Scanzoni, 1853)

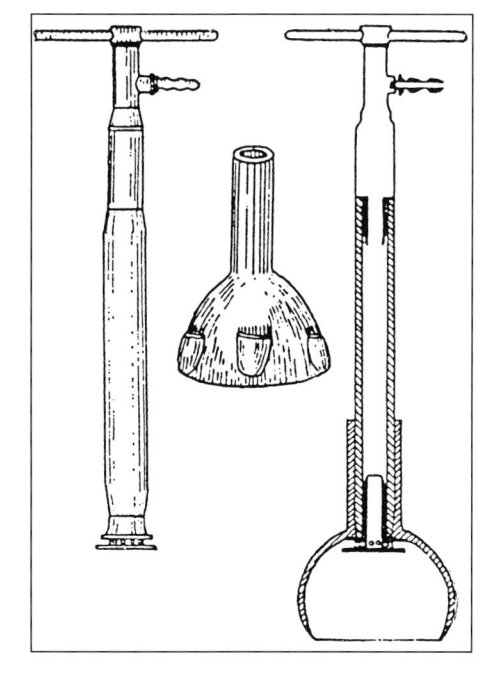

FIGURE 15.5.
Saleh's vacuum extractor. The cup, which has finger pockets to aid insertion, and possibly rotation, can be separated from the pump.
(Witkowski, 1887)

Mathews Duncan (1849), at that time an assistant to Simpson and the person who had marked the examination papers, both denied Mitchell's claim. The correspondence was finally closed by the editor, who reiterated Mathews Duncan's judgement of "He alone discovers who proves," a fair comment on Simpson as an achiever that could be applied to many of his other ideas that, while not original, he brought to practical fruition, most notably the use of chloroform.

In spite of his initial enthusiasm and a number of successful deliveries, Simpson appears to have dropped the suction tractor in favor of his new forceps design, which he described in the same year (Chapter 6). The failure of the tractor to be more widely adopted appears to be mainly because of the difficulty with its application. Simpson suggested a folding version, like an umbrella, to overcome this problem but never made one (1849a). W. H. Priestley and H. R. Storer reported in 1855 that subsequent to his presentations in 1849 Simpson used the tractor to raise depressed fractures, in the manner of Paré, and also used it successfully in breech delivery.

Simpson did not pursue the further development of his tractor, but concentrated on his long forceps. No other obstetrician took up the idea so that in Britain, the concept received little or no attention for nearly a century. Cazeaux of Paris said that Simpson's instrument deserved mention, if only on the score of its originality, but doubted that it would ever come into general use (1850). Scanzoni gave a detailed description and explanation but recorded some unsuccessful experiments in Würzburg, the failure due to the fact that he could not induce sufficient suction force (1853). However, the novelty of the concept continued to attract some attention in Europe and in America in the last quarter of the century. Soubhy Saleh of Paris devised an instrument that he used to deliver the head and also to aspirate the cranial contents after perforation (1886) (Figure 15.5). The rubber cup had finger grips around its perimeter; these could be used for both traction and rotation. The vacuum pump was separate from the cup, unlike the previous devices of Simpson and Scanzoni.

In America, Herbert L. Stillman patented a device in 1875, described as merely a surgical instrument, that served as a cervical dilator as well as a vacuum extractor (Figure 15.6). An oval cup was surrounded by a ring of dilators that could be expanded after introduction of the instrument, with an elastic band encircling their distal ends. This is the only mention in the nineteenth-century literature of the appli-

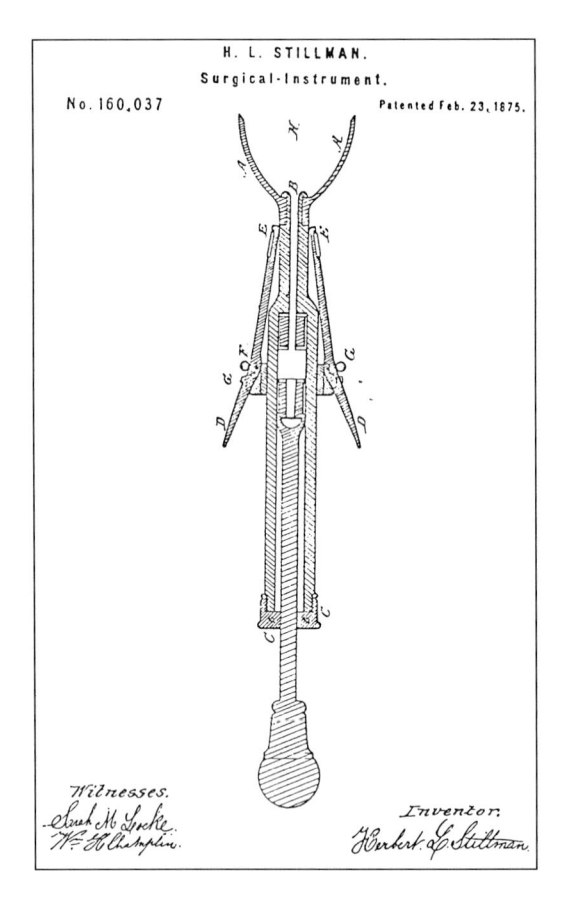

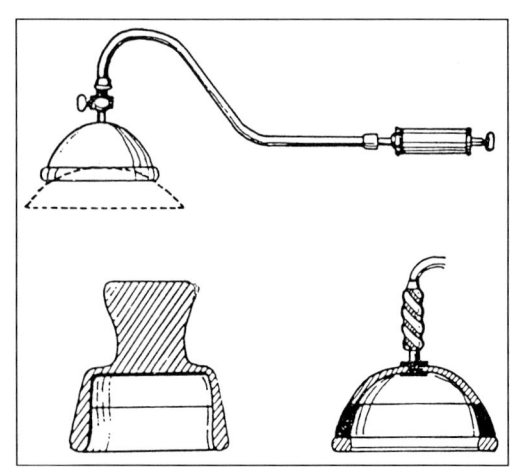

FIGURE 15.6 (LEFT).
Stillman's dilator and extractor. After insertion of the cup *AA* through a partially dilated cervix the cervix could be stretched by a series of levers *DGF*, using a rubber band over the arms *DD*. (From Chalmers, *The Ventouse—The Obstetric Vacuum Extractor* [London: Arnold, 1971])

FIGURE 15.7 (ABOVE).
McCahey's atmospheric tractor. Various cups of metal and soft rubber were made. The pump is separate. (From Chalmers, *The Ventouse—The Obstetric Vacuum Extractor* [London: Arnold, 1971])

cation of a vacuum extractor before full dilatation of the cervix. Chalmers (1971) was unable to find any record of its use in practice.

Peter McCahey of Philadelphia made several variations of his "Atmospheric Tractor" (Figure 15.7). The important innovation was that he separated the suction pump from the cup, thus facilitating the application of the latter (1890). After experimenting with metal cups of different shapes, McCahey settled for a soft rubber cup, which he recorded as having used successfully in five cases. This instrument was the nearest forerunner of the twentieth-century instruments, but it was not until 1912 that a pressure gauge was incorporated by Kuntzsch of Potsdam. His *Vakuumhelm* had a rubber cup reinforced with metal that was attached by a flexible rubber tube to a pump with a pressure gauge. Kuntzsch considered that negative pressures of greater than 1 kilogram per square centimeter resulted in considerable risk of scalp trauma.

. . .

Interest in the concept of vacuum extraction did not revive until the middle of the twentieth century, when a number of new designs appeared, of which the Malmström instruments and their modifications led the field. It was only then, a century after Simpson's experiments, that the prophesy of Priestley and Storer was fulfilled, that there was "Hope that, at some future time [the device] be so far improved, as to be easily applied and used" (1855).

FILLETS, LEVERS, AND OTHER NONDESTRUCTIVE EXTRACTORS

Fillets

Fillets (also known as loops or lacs) have an important place in the history of obstetric instruments, as they are probably the first devices used to assist delivery with minimal trauma and the possibility of saving the child. They had been in use from the time of Hippocrates, at least, and were initially of simple construction, utilizing materials such as cotton, silk, and leather. Over the years fillets became more refined and were made of cane, whalebone, horsehair, and wire or steel strips, usually in wood or metal mounts. Because of the nature of the materials the early soft fillets made of fabric or leather tended not to survive but those in the Chamberlen instrument set are well preserved (Figure 16.1).

Fillets of this type seem to have been in world-wide use, for Charpentier illustrated variants in use in Japan during the early years of the nineteenth century (1883) (Figure 16.2), but little is known of their manner of use or popularity. Lazarewitch described a later Japanese fillet that came into his possession (1881a) (Figure 16.3). This fillet comprised a polished, wooden blade with holes in it through which was passed a strong cord to form a loop.

The concept of the fillet was seductive, especially in times when other extractors were regarded with fear. It was claimed that fillets were easy to apply, whatever the position of the head, and even when the head was too high for the safe application of forceps. They also were supposed to allow sufficient traction force to be applied for extraction and to present minimal hazard to the mother and baby. However, such expectations were not realized. Fillets of soft material were difficult to introduce, particularly when they were used around the groin in breech presentations, although many had a cane or whalebone insert to facilitate introduction. They were also very likely to slip and tended to alter the position of the head adversely, creating new difficulties. The expectation of minimizing trauma was also reduced by the ability to use considerable traction force, which nullified the benefits of the soft materials used.

J. L. Baudelocque (1790) saw little benefit from using the fillet. He did not use it on the head, confining its application to the foot, groin, hand, or axilla. Thus he applied the fillet to parts of the already delivered child, such as a leg, while exploring for the other leg. He also used the fillet to apply traction to parts that could not be easily secured with the hand or hook.

By the mid-eighteenth century disapproval was being voiced by Smellie and by Pugh. Both Alexander Hamilton (1775) and Merriman in London (1826) recounted stories of inadvertent decapitation by the fillet, the latter giving a particularly lurid account of the proceedings in a case attended by his uncle. In the latter part of the century, in the time of Bland and Denman, fillets had been largely abandoned in Britain.

One nineteenth-century British proponent of the use of the soft fillet in certain circumstances was Joseph Griffiths Swayne (1819–1902), Consulting Physician, Bristol General Hospital, who reverted from using a blunt hook for groin traction to a tape or bandage sling with a modified blunt hook as an introducer (1876) (Figure 16.4). The sling comprised a strong silk cord with a loop at each end, padded in the center and covered with India rubber. He used this specifically for delivery of the impacted breech. The handle of the hook was detachable and was placed through the loops of the sling to apply traction.

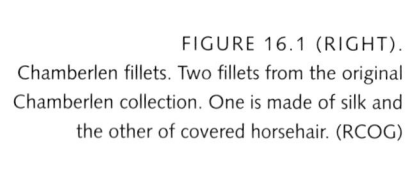

FIGURE 16.1 (RIGHT).
Chamberlen fillets. Two fillets from the original Chamberlen collection. One is made of silk and the other of covered horsehair. (RCOG)

FIGURE 16.2 (BELOW LEFT).
Japanese fillets and introducers. Fillets of different materials are being used for extraction and for extraction. The introducers are also in various forms.(Charpentier, 1883)

FIGURE 16.3 (BELOW RIGHT).
Japanese fillet as shown by Lazarewitch (1881a).

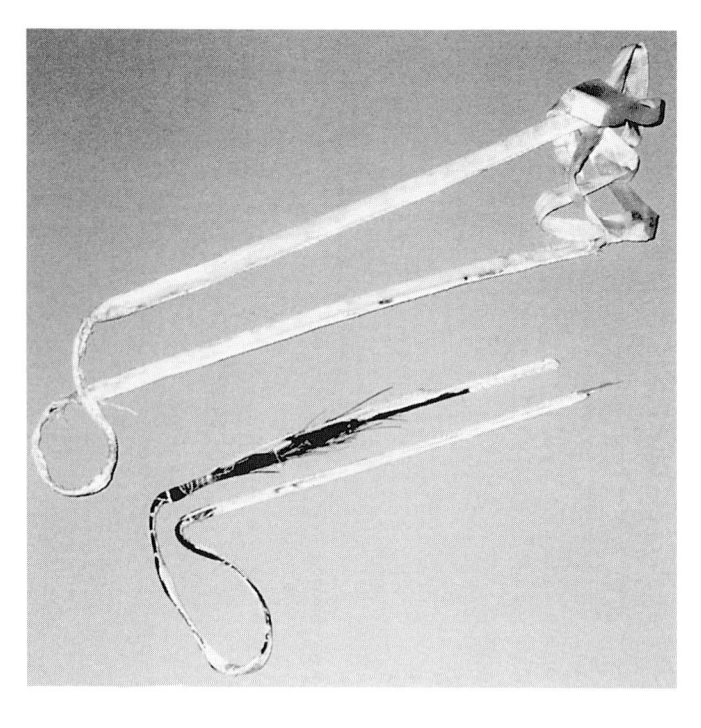

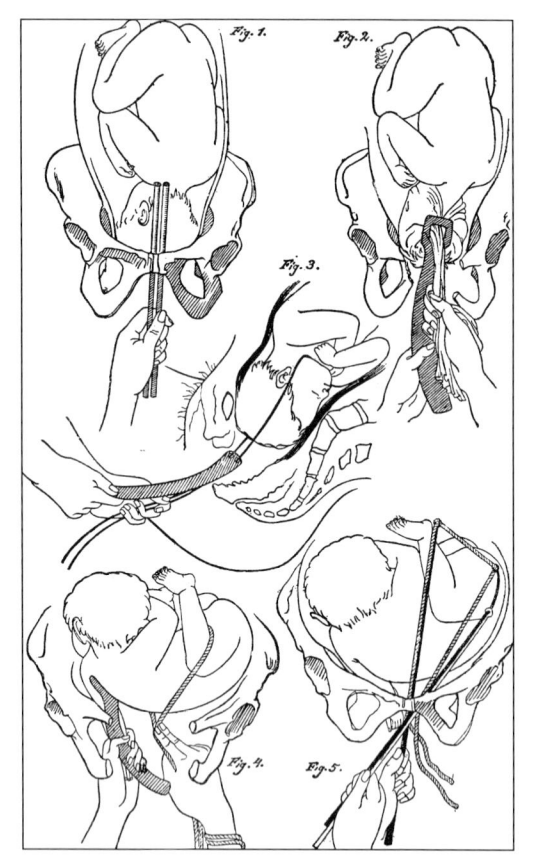

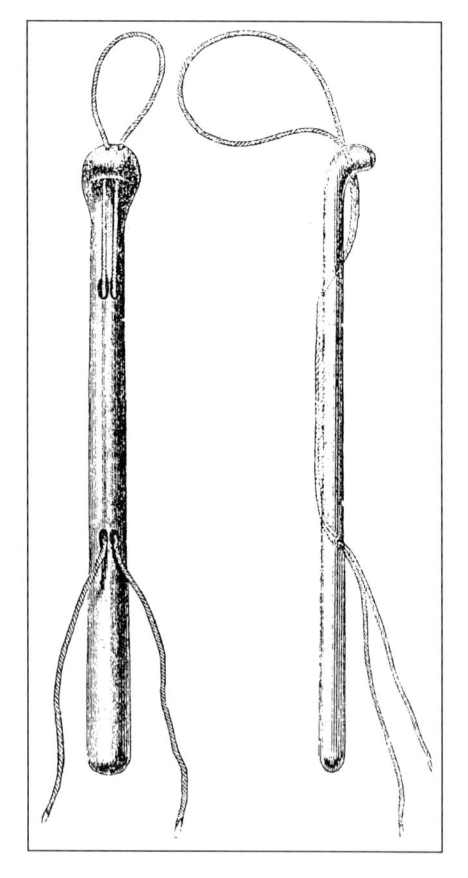

200 CHAPTER 16

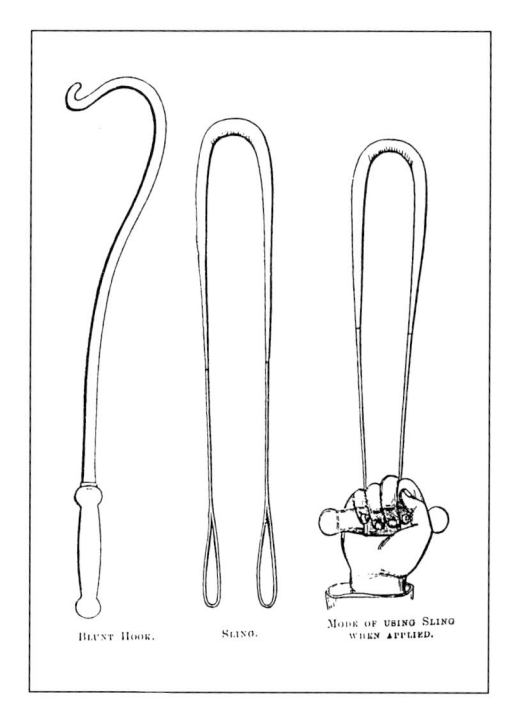

FIGURE 16.4 (ABOVE).
Swayne's blunt hook and sling introducer.
(Swayne, 1876)

FIGURE 16.5 (ABOVE RIGHT).
Hubert's *porte fillet*. The tip is turned at a right angle and is perforated, with another perforation 50mm (2ins) below. (Science Museum, London)

FIGURE 16.6 (RIGHT).
Lazarewitch's *porte fillet*. (Science Museum, London)

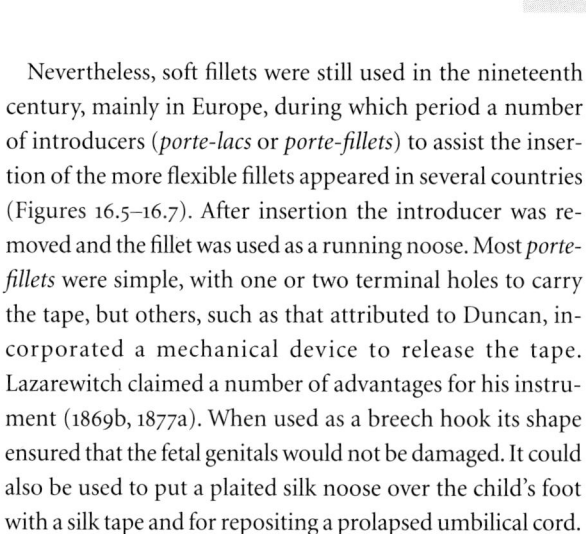

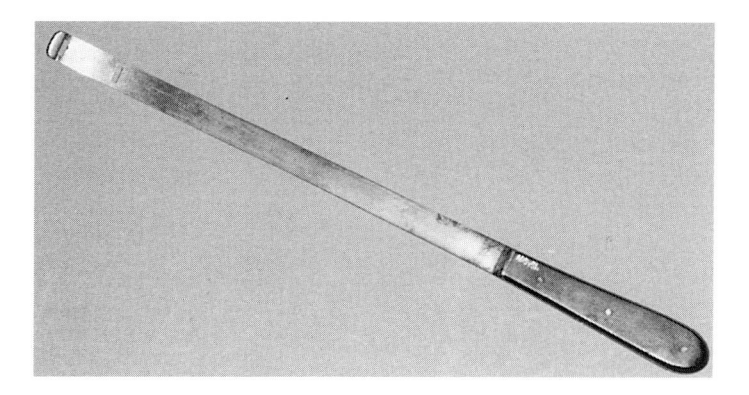

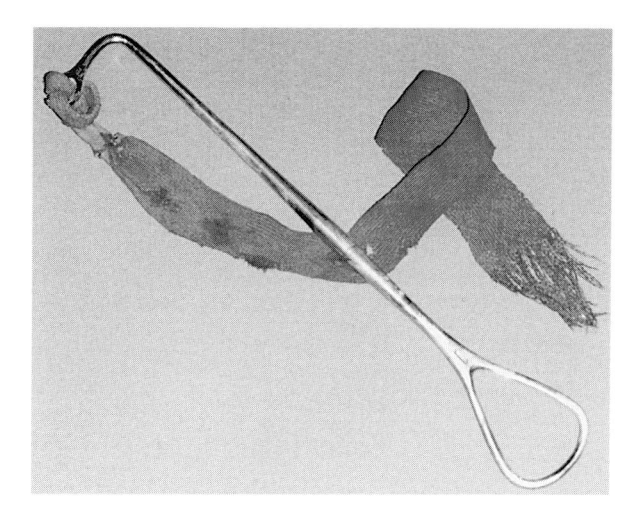

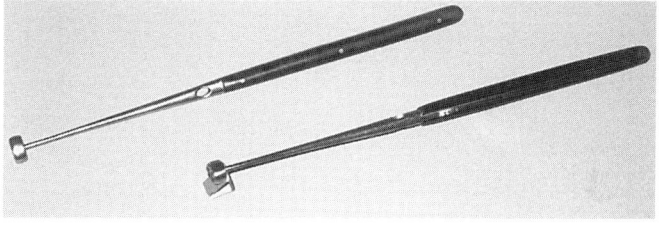

FIGURE 16.7.
Unidentified *portes fillets*. Both the tip and the shaft are perforated. (RCOG)

Nevertheless, soft fillets were still used in the nineteenth century, mainly in Europe, during which period a number of introducers (*porte-lacs* or *porte-fillets*) to assist the insertion of the more flexible fillets appeared in several countries (Figures 16.5–16.7). After insertion the introducer was removed and the fillet was used as a running noose. Most *porte-fillets* were simple, with one or two terminal holes to carry the tape, but others, such as that attributed to Duncan, incorporated a mechanical device to release the tape. Lazarewitch claimed a number of advantages for his instrument (1869b, 1877a). When used as a breech hook its shape ensured that the fetal genitals would not be damaged. It could also be used to put a plaited silk noose over the child's foot with a silk tape and for repositing a prolapsed umbilical cord.

FILLETS, LEVERS, AND OTHER NONDESTRUCTIVE EXTRACTORS 201

FIGURE 16.8 (RIGHT).
Turning rods. These were used to help manipulation of the fetal lie. (RCOG)

FIGURE 16.9 (BELOW).
Simple rigid fillets. (Science Museum, London)

FIGURE 16.10 (BOTTOM LEFT).
Sheraton's folding steel fillet (RCOG). Left: folded for insertion. Right: open for use.

FIGURE 16.11 (BOTTOM RIGHT).
Whalebone fillets (Science Museum, London). Left: Unidentified. The handles are not detachable. Center: Westmacott. This a later version with a longer handle than originally described. The fillet is held on the handle by screws. Right: Eardley-Wilmot. An improvement on Westmacott's fillet with a slit in the handle to facilitate manipulation.

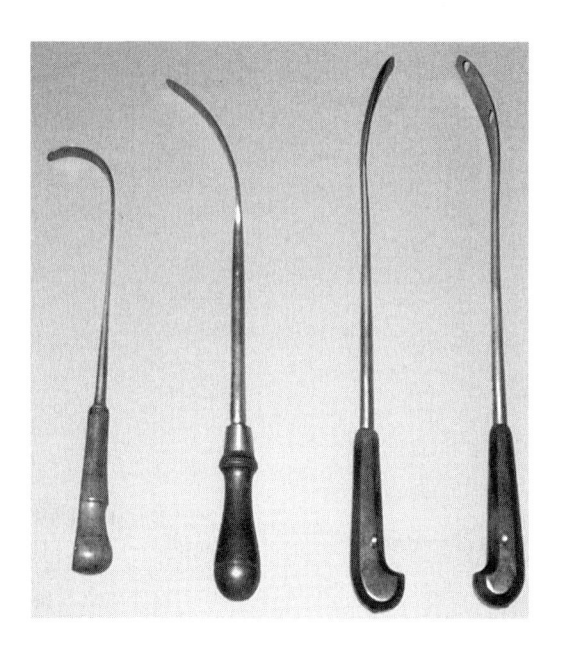

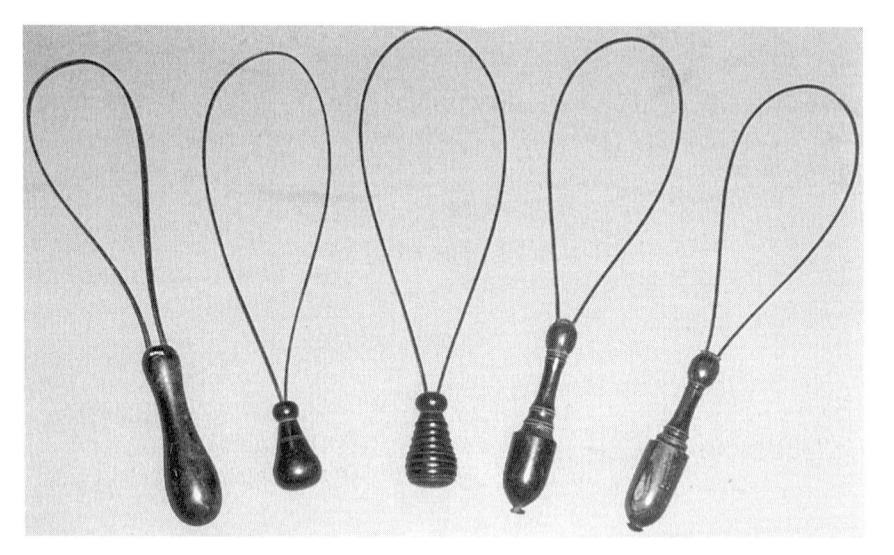

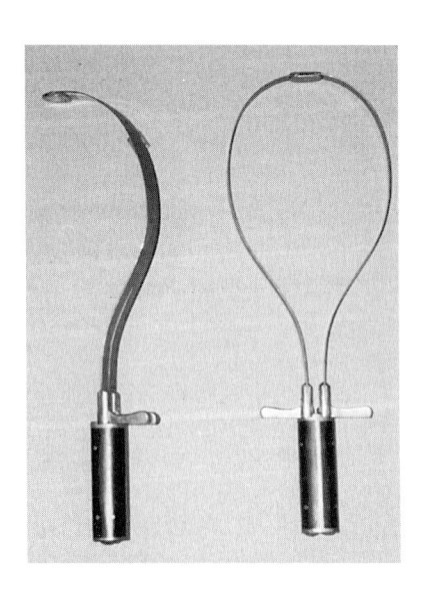

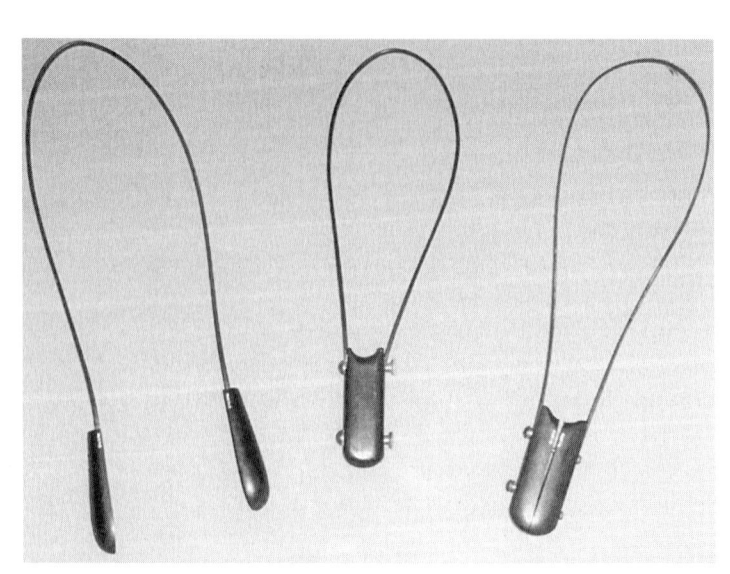

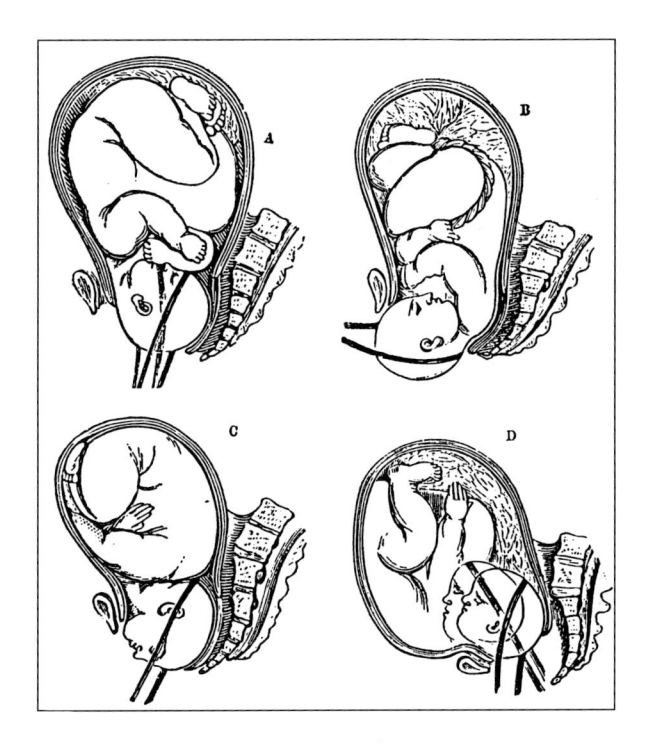

FIGURE 16.12.
Illustrations from Westmacott showing various cephalic presentations. (Westmacott, 1869)

Turning Rods

Fillet introducers were sometimes designed to be used also as blunt hooks or as aids to manipulating the position of the fetus. However turning rods designed for the specific purpose were also made (Figure 16.8).

Late Nineteenth-Century Renaissance of the Fillet

In spite of the earlier setbacks the fillet, now modified, more sophisticated, and made from more rigid materials, staged a comeback in Britain later in the nineteenth century, possibly as a reaction to the heavy destructive instruments that were coming into vogue (Figure 16.9). However, difficulties in application remained until jointed and detachable handles were introduced.

E. R. Sheraton of Durham obtained a patent for his "New or Improved Instrument to be used in cases of Difficult Parturition" (1867) (Figure 16.10). His stated intention was that it would supersede the forceps and vectis. The flexible steel blades were united distally by a pin and were attached proximally to a two-part hinged handle. Thus they could be folded, forming a half hoop to facilitate insertion over either the occiput or the chin, and then opened to encompass the fetal head. Judging by the appearance of this instrument in manufacturers' catalogues for several decades and the number of instruments still extant, the device must have achieved a significant degree of popularity.

John G. Westmacott, who was the senior medical officer at the Paddington Provident Dispensary in London, presented another novel version of the fillet to the Obstetrical Society of London in 1869 and said that he seldom attended a labor case without it in his pocket (Figure 16.11, center). The loop was of whalebone with the ends fixed in brass sockets that were attached to the handle by two knurled screws. Westmacott regarded the fillet as a good alternative to the forceps when the patient was exhausted and contractions had ceased, or when there was "partial obstruction." In his illustrations he tried to show the versatility of the instrument in various cephalic malpresentations (Figure 16.12). In the discussion that followed his paper it was evident that the fillet was quite widely used in some areas but some notable obstetricians, such as Robert Barnes, Graily Hewitt, and W. S. Playfair, continued to discount it, questioning its mode of action and claiming, correctly, that it was no substitute for the forceps.

Robert Eardley-Wilmot of London continued to champion the fillet in preference to the low forceps operation so long as no serious obstacle requiring much force existed. He simplified application of the fillet by dividing the handle of Westmacott's instrument longitudinally and providing a twin pin-and-socket joint (1874) (Figure 16.11, right). An

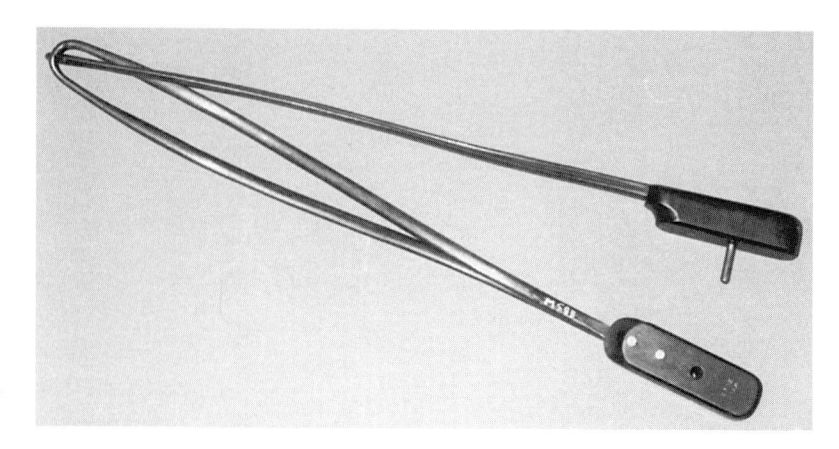

FIGURE 16.13.
Debenham's double fillet. The two whalebone fillets are interlocked. (RCOG)

FIGURE 16.14.
Japanese adjustable whalebone fillet. The longitudinal handle slides up the fillet, acting as a snare. (Science Museum, London)

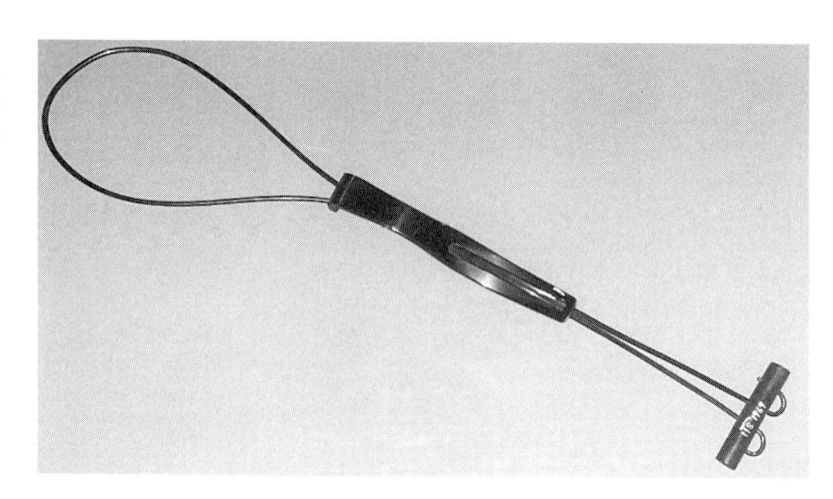

additional benefit, not noted by earlier writers, was that chloroform, which was becoming commonplace for forceps delivery, was not required for application of the fillet. However, when he presented his paper to the Obstetrical Society of London, condemnation by eminent practitioners of the day far outweighed support.

Another attempt to facilitate ease of use and adaptability was made by R. K. Debenham (1867-1868) with his interlocking double whalebone fillet (Figure 16.13). Although there are a number of examples of Debenham's fillet in existence it was not promoted in the texts of the time and had no obvious advantages.

More advanced fillets were also in use in Japan (Figure 16.14), Europe, and America (Olivier, 1883; Lusk, 1892). William Lusk also used it for breech extraction when the legs were extended. However, the fillet tended to slip onto the thigh and cause extension of the leg. Adolf Victor Olivier (b. 1853) of Paris claimed that this could be overcome by pressure from a finger in the rectum.

Europe did not follow the design developments that had been occurring in Britain, probably because of the greater commitment to forceps. However, soft fillets, or lacs, continued to be used in France and Germany, and the *porte-lacs* referred to previously were used for their introduction. A more refined device that found favor was that of Olivier (1883). His *porte-lac* was a hollowed-out, blunt hook with an olive-shaped end. A long strip of whalebone ran through the tube. There was a metallic eye at one end to which a loop could be attached and a button at the other end. A screw just above the handle enabled the whalebone to be fixed at any desired position (Figure 16.15). The instrument was introduced around the groin or shoulder and the whalebone advanced until it could be withdrawn from the vulva and a fillet attached to the loop. The procedure was reversed to get the fillet into position. Any suitable material could be used for the fillet but Olivier recommended a lace covered with rubber tubing.

American attitudes to the fillet were, if anything, muted. Theophilus Parvin, Professor of Obstetrics at Jefferson Medical College, Philadelphia, in the quite extensive section on operative delivery in his *The Science and Art of Obstetrics* (1890), did not mention the fillet, even to discount it. Tho-

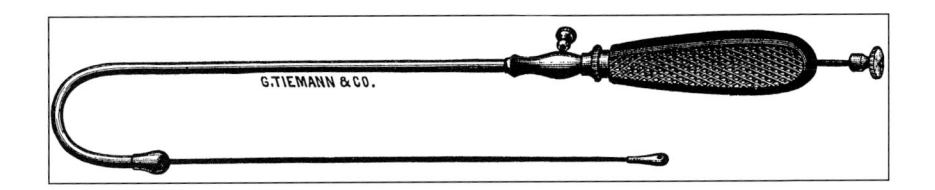

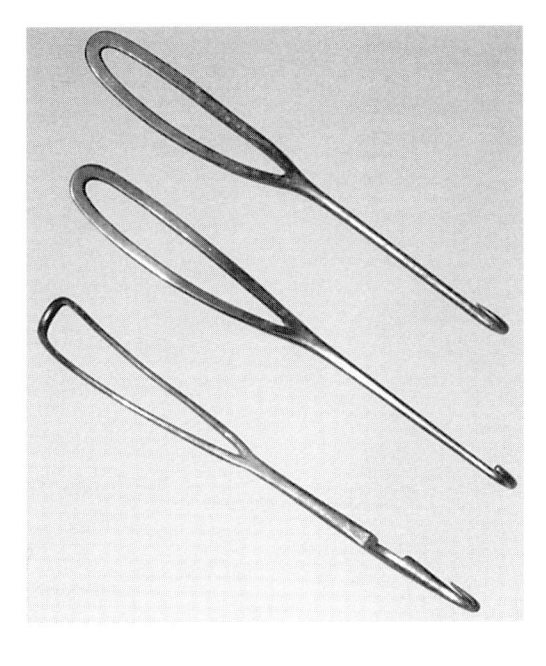

FIGURE 16.15.
Olivier's *porte-lac* as illustrated by Tiemann (Figure 3780).

FIGURE 16.16.
Chamberlen levers. The earliest fenestrated levers, with blades similar in shape to their forceps. (RCOG)

mas Lusk, in *The Science and Art of Midwifery* (1892) admitted to a limited place for the fillet in breech presentation if forceps delivery failed or was contraindicated because of nonengagement of the breech. His recommendations were based on results that he quoted from the Munich Lying-in Institution, where fillets were in more common use than elsewhere in Germany, and he noted that out of thirty breech deliveries using the fillet, twenty-three children were healthy and in all cases showing pressure marks from the fillet rapid healing occurred. One child had a fractured femur. Lusk also drew on the experience of Olivier and recommended his *porte-fillet* but only for breech presentations;. he made no reference to the recent (at that time) British designs. The Olivier instrument was the only fillet marketed by Tiemann (1889).

The Japanese use of soft fillets has been referred to earlier. They apparently continued to develop the principle as a Japanese whalebone fillet and introducer of late design, for which no details are available, is in the Wellcome Collection (Figure 16.14).

By the end of the nineteenth century little was being heard of fillets. In the discussion following Eardley-Wilmot's 1874 paper, W. S. Playfair summarized attitudes to the fillet. No fact in the history of obstetrics was more curious than the way in which the fillet would crop up again and again as an obstetric instrument. It seldom happened that many consecutive years passed without some one writing a paper to show its advantages; and invariably it again shortly fell into what he [Playfair] could not help thinking was a very well-merited oblivion. But the truth was, as Aveling had remarked, that the fillet was essentially an unscientific instrument.

Levers (Tractors or Vectis)

The common use of the lever dates from the time of the Chamberlens and Roonhuysens (Chapters 1, 2). As with the forceps, the history of levers in the sixteenth and seventeenth centuries is obscured by professional secrecy. It has been generally overlooked that the Chamberlen family also used levers, which were fenestrated and of design similar to their forceps, and that these dated from the same period (Figure 16.16). They only came to light with the discovery of the instruments at Woodham Mortimer in 1813.

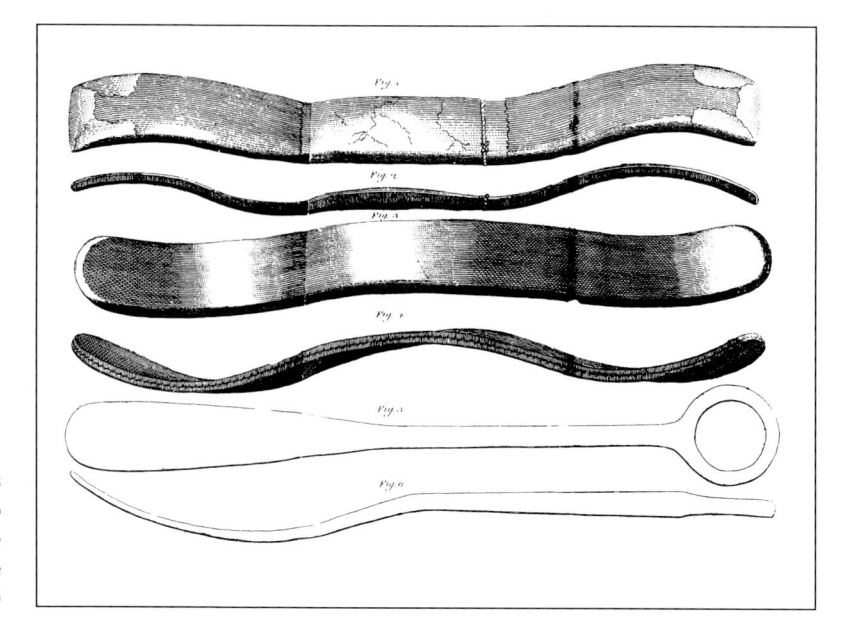

FIGURE 16.17.
The Roonhuysen lever. The steel version is covered with soft leather (Figures 1–4). Also illustrated is Aitken's spatula, which could be heated and curved to serve the same purpose (Figures 5–6). (Aitken, 1786)

The first levers of the Roonhuysen type were made of bone or ivory, but soon iron and, later, tempered steel were introduced. These levers were about 280 millimeters (11 inches) long, 25 millimeters (1 inch) wide, straight in the middle, and slightly curved at each end. The steel versions were covered with soft leather. This simple blade of Dutch origin developed into more complex forms that were fenestrated and approximated to the shape of a single forceps blade, usually with the handle hinged or detachable.

A lever could be used in three ways. The most common use occurred when there was arrest in the pelvis with an occipito-anterior position. In this situation it was used as a first-degree lever to ease the head out in the manner of a scoop, with the maternal pubic arch as a fulcrum. The lever could also be used as an antagonist to the left hand when placed on the contralateral side of the head, thus altering the position of the head. Finally, it could be used for direct traction, in which case the blade had to be curved to afford an adequate grip on the head. Eventually levers were used more to alter the position of the head rather than as true levers, but opinions differed widely as to their appropriate indications. By the mid-nineteenth century only the latter use was considered reasonably safe as a possible alternative to low forceps delivery.

Aitken illustrated levers in common use toward the end of the eighteenth century (1786) (Figure 16.17). The designs remained relatively simple and based on individual preferences but steel covered with leather became more common than the bone and wood that had been used previously. The French, notably Mauriceau (1668), adopted designs more akin to one blade of Palfyn's forceps, with a solid curved blade, straight shank, and wooden handle. However, after

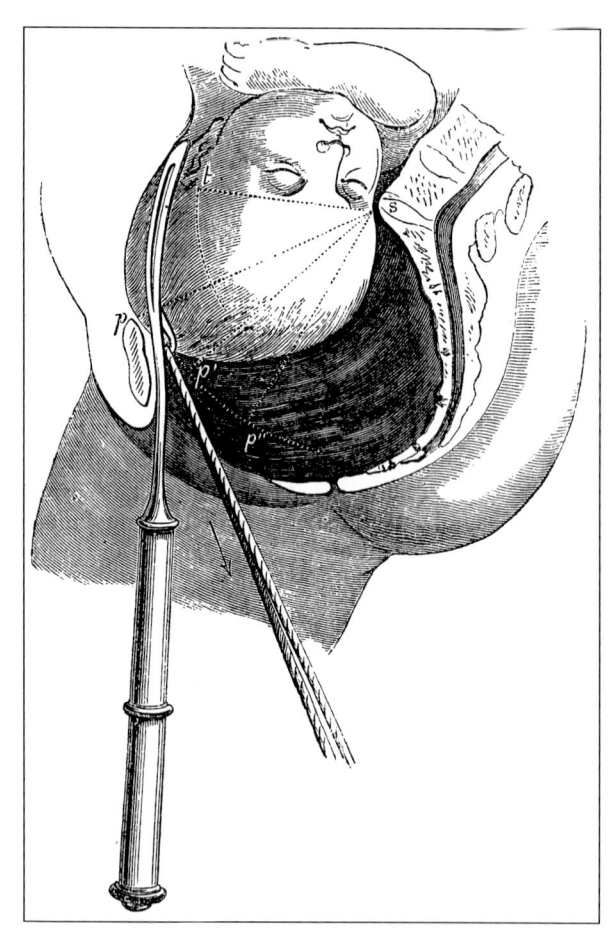

FIGURE 16.18.
L. J. Hubert's lever and lac. (Charpentier, 1883)

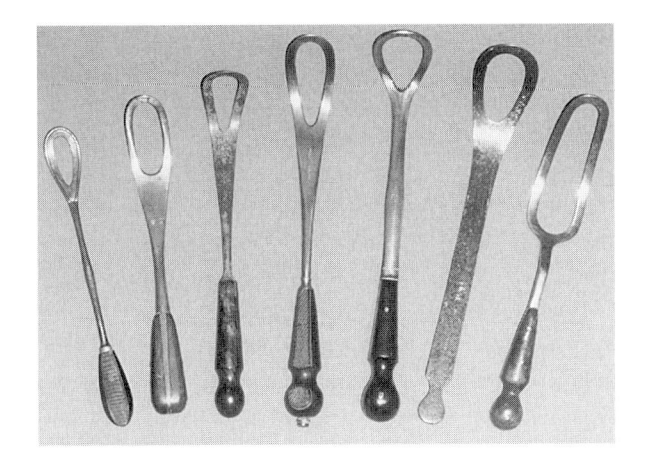

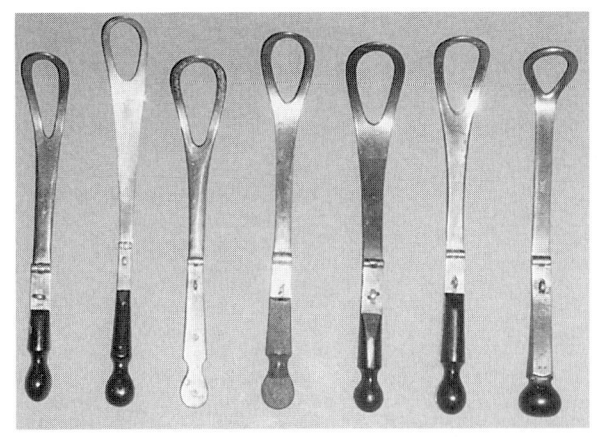

FIGURE 16.19.
A selection of simple levers from the eighteenth and nineteenth centuries. They all have curved fenestrated blades. (Science Museum, London)

FIGURE 16.20.
A selection of folding levers of the same period. (Science Museum, London)

FIGURE 16.21.
Detail of the hinges and locks of folding levers.

the advent of the forceps, levers never had any great popularity in France, where the forceps became the instrument of choice in most cases.

Considering the origins of the lever it is not surprising that it was widely used in the Low Countries and Joannes de Bruyn of Amsterdam (quoted by J. L. Baudelocque (1790), claimed to have used it in eight hundred cases over a period of forty-two years, a record that Baudelocque interpreted as being the result of de Bruyn's abuse of the instrument and his lack of skill. Generally, French authors gave little value to the vectis. Baudelocque devoted a large section of his book to criticism, sometimes vitriolic, of the techniques described by the various proponents of the lever, particularly M. G. Herbiniaux (b. 1740) of Brussels who had previously had the temerity to criticize Baudelocque's methods of using the forceps (1794). Baudelocque concluded that in most cases the use of the lever had been unnecessary and that possibly the most benefit had come from stimulating uterine contractions. He thought that it was rarely indispensable, that it should only be used in the manner of a blunt hook and not a lever, and that it should always be applied over the occiput and used to promote flexion.

At the end of the eighteenth century Baudelocque remarked that the form of the lever had been changed by every hand that touched it (1790), but he was referring primarily to levers with solid blades and more was yet to come. Fenestrated blades did not come into general use until the beginning of the nineteenth century and possibly originated in Germany. Kuhn and Tröhler (1987) illustrated designs of F. B. Osiander and A. E. von Siebold dating from about the turn of the century. The fenestrated blade was also adopted subsequently in Belgium, a notable design being that of L. J. Hubert (Figure 16.18). Hubert improved the potential of the instrument for traction by adding a small ring at the base of the blade through which a tape could be passed. His accompanying diagram showed its method of use.

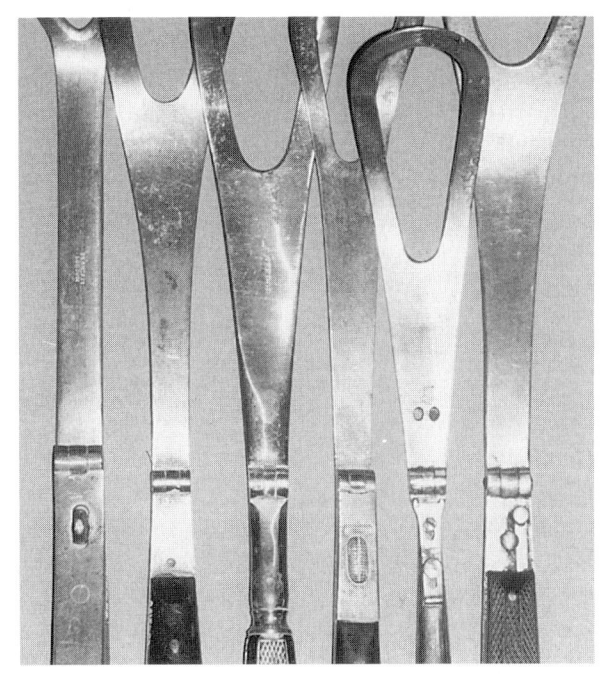

In Britain at the end of the eighteenth century and up to the mid-nineteenth century a wide range of levers emerged, characterized by having a small spoon-shaped fenestrated blade and a wooden handle, but with minor variations in length and size and curvature of the blades. (Figure 16.19). Many had folding handles to aid portability (Figures 16.20, 16.21). Others had detachable handles and these were usually part of an interchangeable set that might include a blunt hook, a crotchet, and/or a decapitator, such as that of Radford (Figure 16.30).

In the early nineteenth century Samuel Merriman made a balanced appraisal of the lever and forceps as used in Britain (1828). Among his conclusions were that "in general, the *forceps* effects the delivery better than the *lever;* but that, in a few rare instances, the *lever* may be beneficially employed to effect the delivery, before it is possible to use the *forceps.*" Because the lever, like the fillet, was easier to introduce, especially earlier in labor, it was more often used unnecessarily and with more hazard to the fetus and the mother. In company with others Merriman was concerned about the morality of using it secretly, which seems to have been a not uncommon practice. This concern was expressed repeatedly over the next half century.

The controversy over the respective merits of the lever and the forceps was exemplified by the disagreement between Denman and Osborn referred to previously (Chapter 4). The very conservative Denman was a proponent of the lever, which he came to prefer to forceps, while Osborn feared that the use of the lever could be mischievous and excessive. Hamilton favored Lowder's design, which had a hinged handle and a fenestrated blade with an arc of 97 degrees and a radius of 100 millimeters (4 inches), and a semicircular end. He would use it even if the head was not in the pelvis but particularly favored it for the correction and delivery of face presentations (1775).

W. Gaitskell advocated an instrument 330 millimeters (13 inches) long with a handle of rough wood to ensure a firm grip. The handle was made to be screwed on rather than hinged, which made introduction inconvenient (1823). For introduction all the fingers of one hand were to be inserted into the vagina and the blade "wandered" into position until it was over the occiput. Traction was then applied during uterine contractions until the head was on the perineum. The instrument was then removed and reinserted over the face to deliver the head by extension. Gaitskell gave a graphic and horrendous account of trauma following abuse of the vectis and listed all the abuses that might result in trauma. In the case that he reported the accoucheur had applied the vectis with such force that the mother had to be held down for three hours with only short intervals of rest. He eventually delivered the head, on which were many lacerations but the shoulders were impacted so he applied a strong traction with a towel tied round the neck of the baby. As the baby was delivered the mother had a gush of urine and sustained severe trauma involving the rectum, bladder, and cervix. Gaitskell's list of abuses illustrated by this case included applying the lever before full dilatation, rupturing the uterus during introduction, introducing the vectis outside the uterus, ignoring the position of the fetal head in the birth canal, failing to wait for natural contraction, and continuing pressure between contractions.

Blundell commended the lever to his pupils on the grounds of safety, portability, and ease of application (1840). He also favored the blade design of Lowder and advised having available two instruments with differing degrees of curvature. A bold curve retained its position better and was therefore more effective but a straighter blade was more easily introduced. Blundell described in detail the use of the lever for the commonest mechanical problem of the time: arrest of the head at the brim. He emphasized that the instrument should be used as a tractor, not a lever, with the blade over the occiput. When the head was arrested at the pelvic brim he advocated the principles of the technique described by Gaitskell, with modifications, applying traction only during contractions. Thus the head was not only brought down but encouraged to flex. Once the head was in the pelvis spontaneous delivery could be anticipated but if further assistance was required the lever was reapplied over the face and chin of the fetus but then "wandered" to the side of the head, as in a forceps application. Two fingers were then inserted over the other side and the head grasped between the fingers and the lever. Even if the lever had not been used to bring the head down Blundell still preferred it to the forceps for delivery of the head already in the pelvis.

David Davis's lever had the inner surface covered with short, pin-sized teeth and it was specifically designed for changing the position of the head in face presentations prior to forceps application (1825) (Figure 16.22). However, his successor at University College Hospital in London, Murphy, used the lever much more extensively. He used it as an extractor for assisting poor uterine action, for correcting malpositions of the head, and to overcome undue resistance of the perineum (1862). He considered it to have little power and not to be regarded as a substitute for the forceps and certainly not, as advocated by Blundell, when the head was arrested at the brim. Thus he promoted its use only when the head was low in the pelvis and contractions had waned. While he accepted its use to correct malpositions of the head he considered that one blade of the forceps was equally useful.

Later in the century A. B. Steele, Physician to the Liverpool Lying-In Hospital, reviewed the history and the then current role of the lever in his article "The Vectis As an Obstetric Instrument" (1875), with extracts from some of the most eminent writers including Blundell (1840), a very conservative obstetrician, who said that it was "an instrument excellent and of great effect in dextrous hands. If skill and

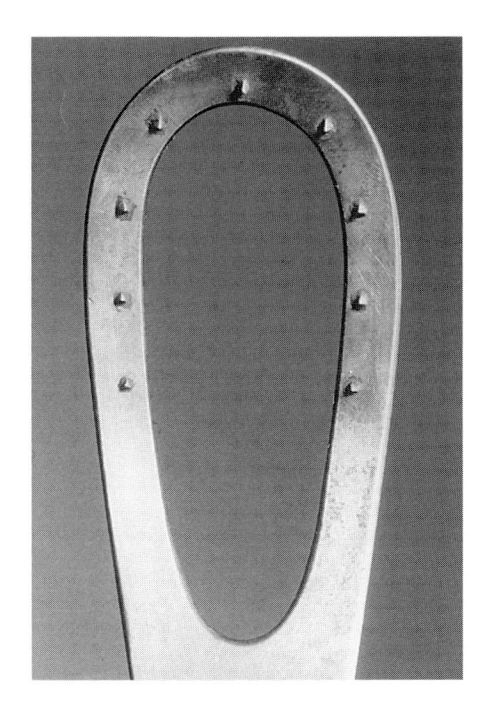

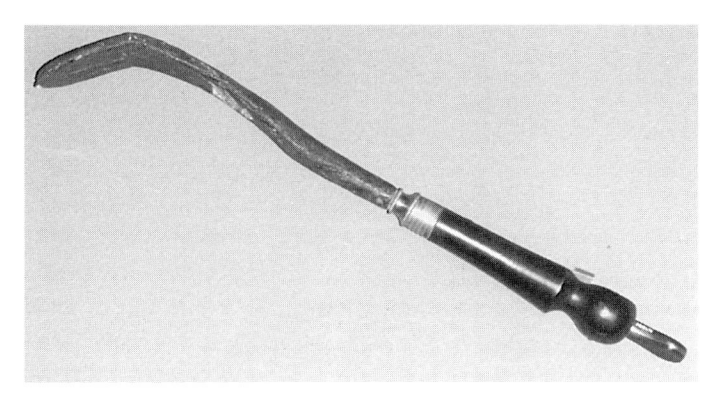

FIGURE 16.23 (ABOVE).
Aitken's "living lever." The hinged blade is bent by a screw mechanism in the handle, which shortens flexible steel strips attached to the tip of the blade. The instrument is leather-covered. (Science Museum, London)

FIGURE 16.22.
Davis's lever. Close-up view to show the fine teeth on the inner surface of the blade. It was specifically intended for use in face presentation prior to forceps application. (RCOG)

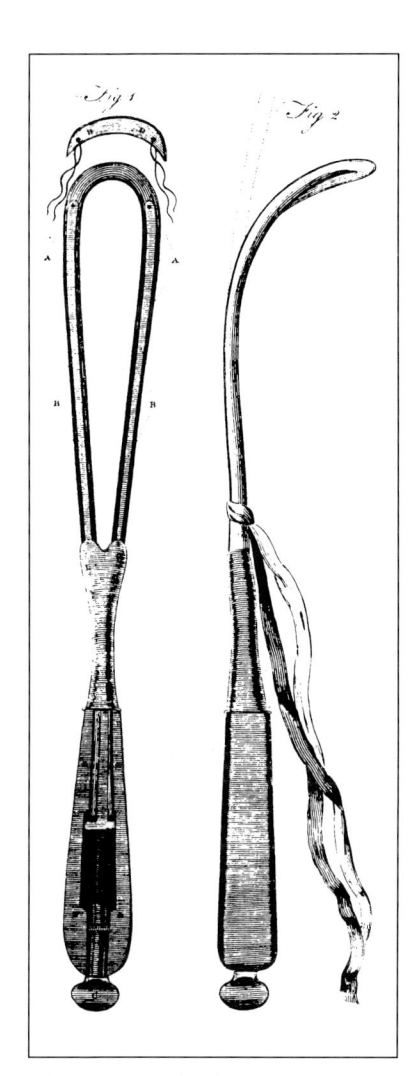

FIGURE 16.24.
Aitken's "living lever." Detail of the construction. A grooved attachment is also shown, intended for reposition of a prolapsed umbilical cord. (Aitken, 1786)

judgement are wanting, even the tractor (vectis) may inflict dreadful injuries, but in such hands still greater mischief may be expected for the long forceps"; and a quote from Conquest (1837), a more advanced thinker, who believed that "[w]hilst under some circumstances the lever is doubtless preferable to the forceps, the latter is now very generally admitted to be in the majority of cases by far the most useful instrument." Steele believed that in the first half of the nineteenth century the dangers of instrumental delivery were exaggerated. However, attitudes eventually changed with better knowledge of the physiology and mechanism of parturition. So it was that from the middle of the nineteenth century onward most teachers of repute relegated the lever at best to a limited role, to either correct malpositions or overcome minor impediments to delivery of the head.

Flexible Levers

Aitken devised a flexible "living lever," so named because the blade could be flexed and its motion resembled that of the fingers (1786) (Figures 16.23, 16.24). This ingenious but simple mechanism comprised two steel strips riveted to the tip of the blade and connected to a screw within the handle. Tightening the screw resulted in flexion of the blade to fit the contour of the fetal head, thereby diffusing the pressure

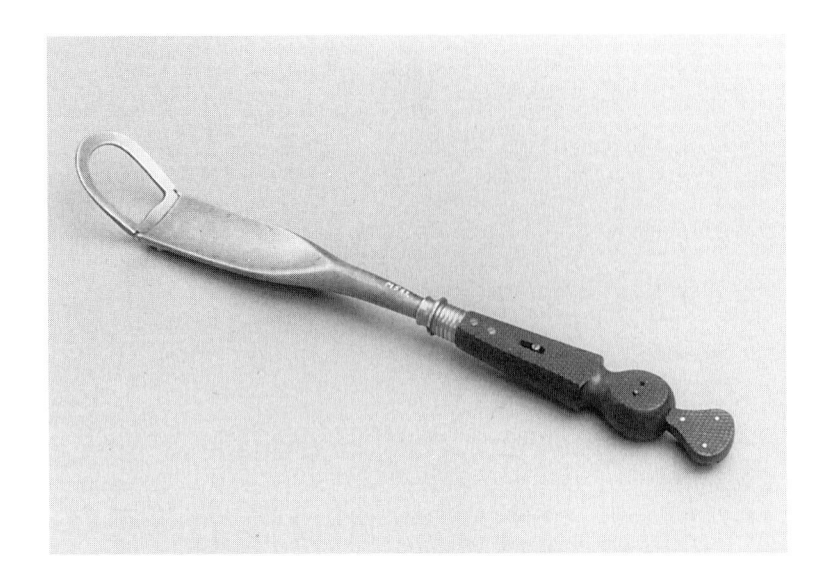

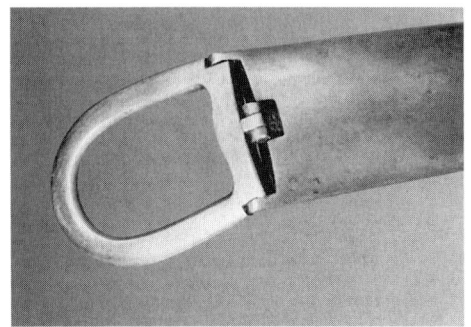

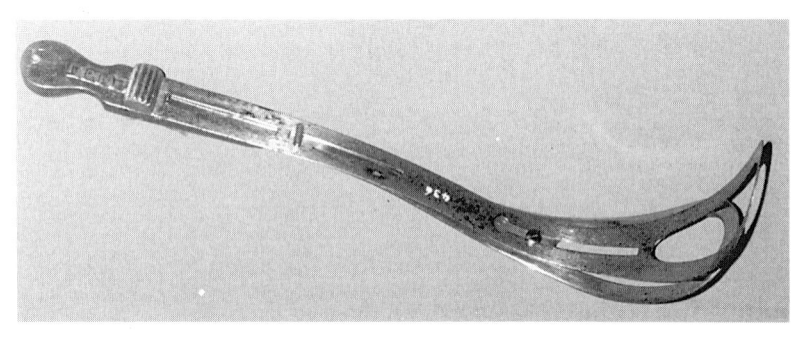

FIGURES 16.25 (TOP LEFT), 16.26 (TOP RIGHT).
Weiss's flexible lever. A more refined version of the Aitken principle. The actuating mechanism is concealed in the hollow blade. The detail of the end of the blade is shown in Figure 16.26. (RCOG)

FIGURE 16.27 (ABOVE).
Robertson's lever with flexible extendible sliding blade. (RCOG)

on the head. In addition Aitken created perforator and crotchet attachments to tie on to the tip of the blade. This concept was improved upon later by David Davis, who created a better design (1825), and by the instrument maker Weiss (1831) (Figures 16.25, 16.26).

Robertson adopted a different method for increasing the curvature by adding a flexible sliding blade to the inner face of a conventional lever (Figure 16.27).

In the face of more skilled obstetricians, better appreciation of the mechanics of delivery, and the ascendancy of the forceps, the days of the lever were numbered and some of Steele's conclusions make a fitting epitaph for an instrument that had a longer history than the forceps:

> To those who have recently recorded great results accomplished by the vectis I would accord a tribute to their exceptional dexterity and mechanical skill, but cannot admit that they have thereby proved the greater excellence of the suitability of the instrument they use... we would advise obstetricians not to sacrifice their time and labour in striving to acquire the supererogatory mechanical skill to qualify them to effect with an incomplete and one-handed instrument that which can be done more easily, more safely, and more effectually by the more perfect two-handed forceps. (1875)

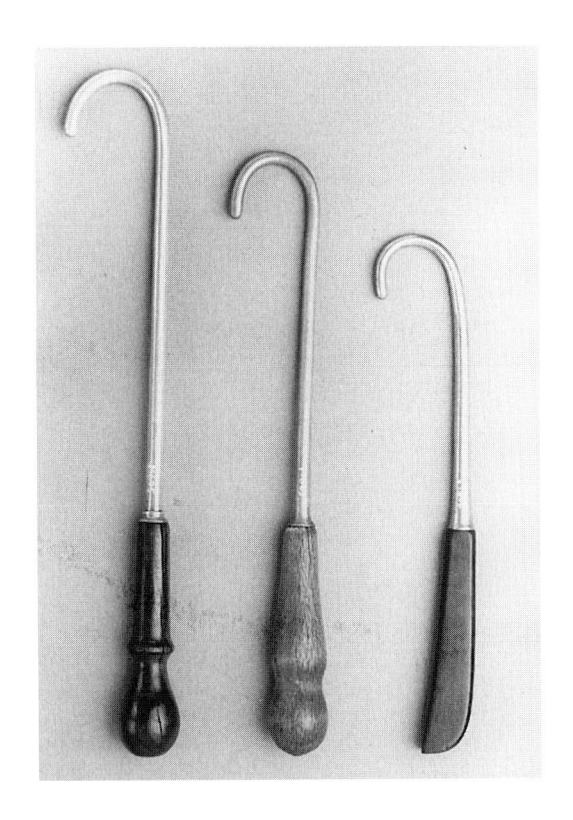

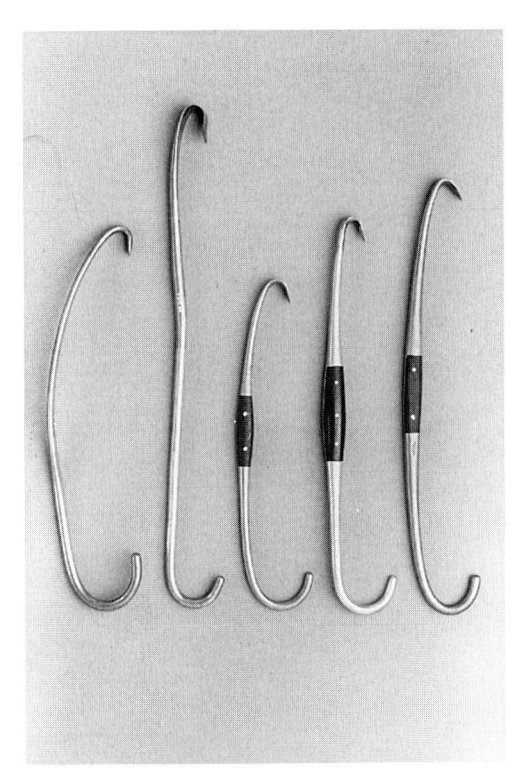

Blunt Hooks

Blunt hooks are among the oldest aids to delivery and until the end of the eighteenth century many were of crude construction. Although blunt hooks have been included under "nondestructive" instruments because by the nineteenth century they were used principally for hastening the passage of the breech or an arm, they were previously also used for altering the position of the fetus and for mutilation. They were commonly combined with crotchets as double-ended instruments and will be discussed again in Chapters 18 and 20. The use of hooks diminished with the introduction of the forceps but they continued in common use throughout the nineteenth century and appeared in instrument makers' catalogues well into the twentieth century. Because their use came to be limited to groin traction they were latterly known as "breech hooks."

Blunt hooks of the nineteenth century, although rarely worthy of individual mention, were of more thoughtful design (Figures 16.28, 16.29). More sophisticated instruments had detachable handles as part of a set (Figure 16.30).

Toward the end of the nineteenth century the days of the blunt hook, which had served obstetricians well for so long, when the well-being of the fetus was of little concern, were clearly numbered. Few obstetricians would use it on a living fetus other than for breech extraction and even on this indication there was concern about trauma to the legs, especially dislocation of the hip and fractures of the femur.

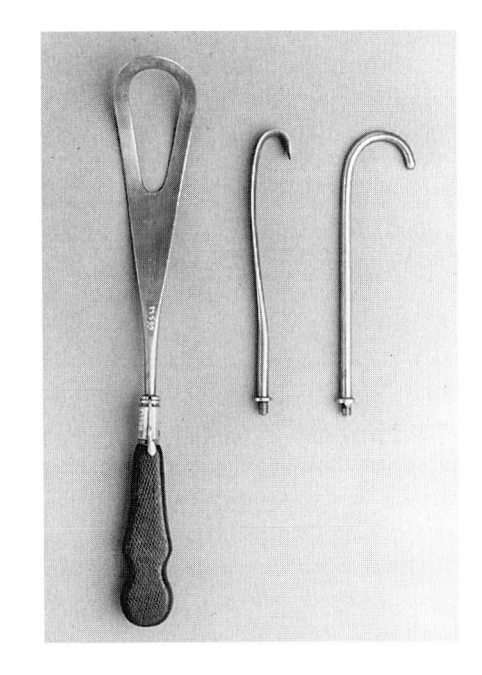

FIGURE 16.28 (TOP LEFT).
Nineteenth-century blunt hooks. (RCOG)

FIGURE 16.29 (TOP RIGHT).
Combined blunt hooks and crotchets. (RCOG)

FIGURE 16.30 (ABOVE).
Radford's interchangeable set. The handle has a bayonet fitting to accommodate a blunt hook, a crotchet and a vectis. (RCOG)

FILLETS, LEVERS, AND OTHER NONDESTRUCTIVE EXTRACTORS

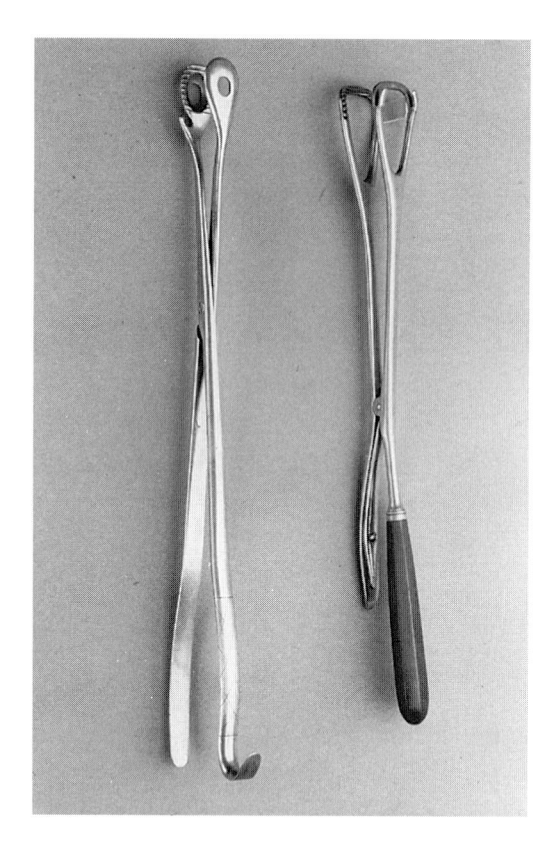

FIGURE 16.31.
Foot forceps made by Nyrop. Top: Grönning (1815). Bottom: Districtsloege (1853). The small hook on one blade was intended as a tape introducer. (RCOG)

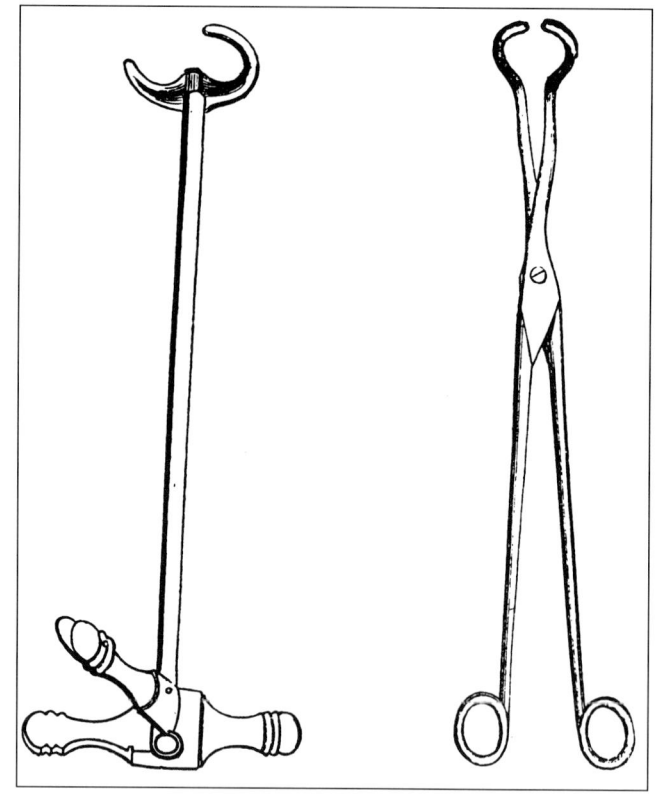

FIGURE 16.32.
Rizzoli's foot forceps. One pair has a simple scissors action, with the curved end at an acute angle. The lower pair has a slit handle and shaft so that closure is effected by rotation of the free portion of the handle. (Meadows, 1867)

Foot Forceps

Foot forceps were used, mainly on the Continent, for bringing down a leg but never came into general use. At the Obstetric Society *Conversazione* (Meadows, 1867) four designs were exhibited from Copenhagen, Russia, and Italy. Two were shown by Nyrop (instrument makers in Copenhagen) and were attributed to Drs. Grönning and Districtsloege. Examples of these in the museum of the Royal College of Obstetricians and Gynaecologists are shown in Figure 16.31. They were clearly potentially traumatic and likely to injure the foot and ankle bones as well as the soft tissues. In addition, on one blade there was a small hook for introducing a tape.

F. Rizzoli, Professor of Obstetrics at the University of Bologna was a prolific designer of instruments and exhibited two designs of foot forceps (1856) (Figure 16.32). The first was a simple scissors-action instrument with curved ends for embracing the ankle set at an acute angle to the shaft. The second was a more elegant hinged device in which the forceps could be opened and shut.

In spite of the publicity that foot forceps received at the Obstetric Society *Conversazione* in 1867, they never achieved popularity and had no mention in British or American texts of the late nineteenth century. It is unlikely that many obstetricians would see any need for them as, when necessary, a foot could usually be grasped and brought down manually and stabilized by a tape or loop.

METREURYNTERS AND CERVICAL DILATORS: INDUCTION AND AUGMENTATION OF LABOR

The concept of inducing the onset of labor prematurely is peculiarly British in origin and dates from the mid-eighteenth century. Robert Barnes comprehensively reviewed the history of the techniques for this procedure (1862), commenting that it stemmed from preeminently conservative English midwifery practice. He rather extravagantly claimed that it had probably been the means of saving more lives of mothers and children than any other operation. The common early indications were to avoid the birth of unduly large babies where there was potential cephalo-pelvic disproportion, severe antepartum hemorrhage, and eclamptic fits. Early simple methods of provoking labor, discussed below, were soon replaced or augmented by rupture of the membranes or devices to stretch the cervix, particularly hydrostatic bags, commonly called *metreurynters*, from the Greek words meaning "womb" and "to stretch." Toward the end of the nineteenth century more forceful mechanical dilators were introduced.

In the conservative climate of eighteenth- and nineteenth-century British obstetrics alternative strategies were being explored for minimizing the hazards of cephalo-pelvic disproportion, including suggestions that the size of the baby might be limited either by maternal starvation or by premature induction of labor (for which Barnes later coined the term *accouchement provoqué*). In France this was regarded as an immoral innovation and based on a philosophy quite contrary to the concepts of *accouchement forcé*, the forcible extraction of the unduly large fetus in cases of severe hemorrhage or obstructed labor. In 1827, The Academy of Medicine in Paris ruled induction of labor unjustifiable under any circumstances. In Germany induction of labor was not introduced on any scale until the mid-nineteenth century.

Lucas was an early proponent of restricted diet throughout pregnancy in cases of pelvic contraction, together with "occasional bleeding" and "moderate use of cooling aperients" (1794). When the problem was one of large babies rather than contracted pelvis he advised that the diet might only need to be restricted in the latter months of pregnancy. This advice tended to be copied by subsequent writers but, as with most such recommendations relating to diet, there was no objective evidence of benefit. Merriman thought that the benefits, if any, were minimal and thus the regime was only occasionally useful (1826). Also, Assalini, as quoted by Merriman, noted that women with hyperemesis throughout pregnancy, and therefore likely to be poorly nourished, nevertheless sometimes had large babies.

Denman reported a meeting of eminent men in London in 1756 at which the concept of premature induction of labor met with general approbation (1788). However, there were some misgivings about the moral rectitude of this practice because it had an inherent risk for the mother. Nevertheless, there was little doubt that at least some babies were saved from the death penalty of the perforator and the mother from the high risk of death from Caesarian section.

John Burns considered premature induction of labor as "defensible" if a destructive operation had been required in a previous pregnancy (1809), while Rigby the Younger went further in describing premature induction of labor as "perhaps the greatest improvement in operative midwifery since the invention and gradual improvement of the forceps" (1841). Robert Lee (1793–1877), Professor of Obstetrics, St. George's Hospital, London, declared the procedure safe, rendering Caesarian section totally unnecessary (1848). These overstatements were typical of nineteenth-century British

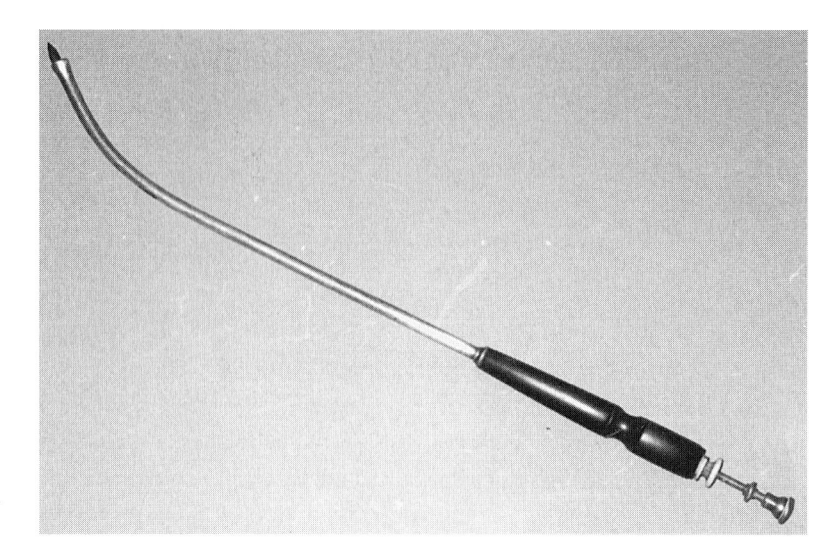

FIGURE 17.1.
Lee's membrane perforator. A triangular trocar is contained in a curved cannula with a bulbous end. The instrument is inserted with the trocar retracted. (RCOG)

attitudes to induction. Similar sentiments were expressed by Barnes at the Obstetric Society of London in 1862 and were reinforced by speakers in the subsequent discussion.

Methods of Inducing Labor

Methods of induction in use in the eighteenth and nineteenth centuries were reviewed by Barnes (1862), referred to above, and by Speert (1958). Many techniques, including Galvanism, irrigations with various fluids such as creosote water, carbon dioxide into the vagina, and stimulation of the breasts failed to stand the test of time. Lazarewitch (1868a) advised irrigation with warm water through a catheter. He reported twelve cases, the indications being vomiting, fits, and previous disproportion. The average induction-delivery interval was nineteen hours.

Artificial Rupture of the Membranes

The most commonly used method was rupture of the forewaters using a sharpened finger nail or a quill or other instrument such as a catheter or, later, a purpose designed instrument such as Lee's membrane perforator (1848) (Figure 17.1). However, there was concern that the loss of amniotic fluid might result in undue pressure on the fetus. To combat this Hamilton favored separation of the membranes for 51 to 76 millimeters (2–3 inches) around the os, while keeping them intact (1775). It was generally recognized that this was less effective than rupturing the membranes. In consequence forewater rupture continued although Hopkins advocated a compromise solution of rupturing the membranes remotely from the os and using a sound, with only partial release of the amniotic fluid (1816).

In Europe in the middle of the nineteenth century it was common practice to insert a bougie or flexible catheter between the uterine wall and the membranes and leave it *in situ* until shortly before the birth (see Barnes, 1862), a procedure for which Braun used 305-millimeter (12-inch) catgut bougies and that he described as "safe, painless and efficacious," with contractions commencing within six to twenty hours. The introduction of distensible bladders into the vagina were in vogue for a short time. These included Braun's *colpeurynter* (1851; see Barnes, 1862) and Gariel's air pessary (1852). Speert reported that Hüter and Busch had used animal bladders to reduce the hemorrhage from placenta previa.

Slow-stretching the cervix was also found to be efficacious in initiating labor and a favored technique was to insert a compressed sponge or a laminaria tent (the dried and compressed stalk of a sea-tangle [*laminaria digita*]) into the cervical canal. As water was absorbed the sponge or tent swelled and stretched the canal. Sponge tents rapidly became malodorous in spite of attempts to keep them free from infection by impregnating them with antiseptics, such as permanganate of potash. These were soon abandoned in favor of laminaria tents, which were cleaner in use though of limited effectiveness.

While membrane rupture, and to a lesser degree laminaria tents, stood the test of time, other methods proved relatively ineffective and in some cases potentially dangerous, with a high risk of air or fluid embolism, depending on the medium used in douches or bags, and a high stillbirth rate. However, the concept of stretching and stimulating the cervix, and of devices to tamponade the placental site in cases of hemorrhage from placenta previa, were logical and encouraged the development of better designs which, in turn, led to better results.

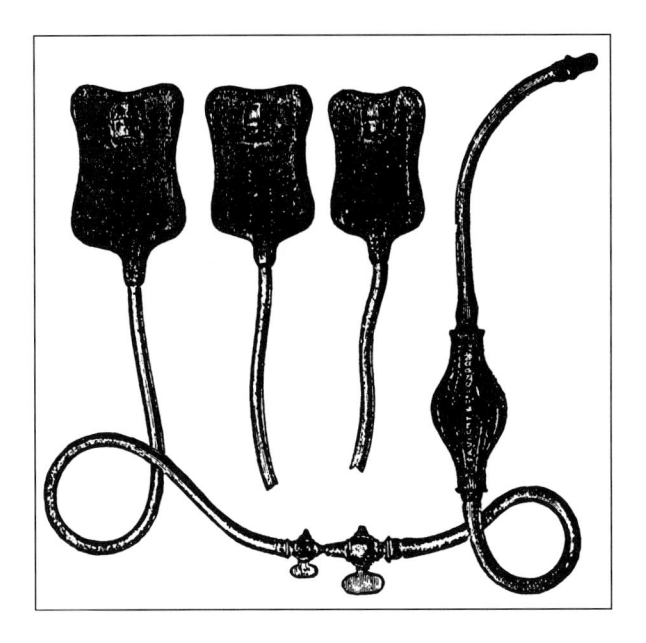

FIGURE 17.2.
Barnes's hydrostatic dilators. The fiddle-shaped bags fit in the cervical canal and are inflated with water using a Higginson's syringe. (Barnes, 1862)

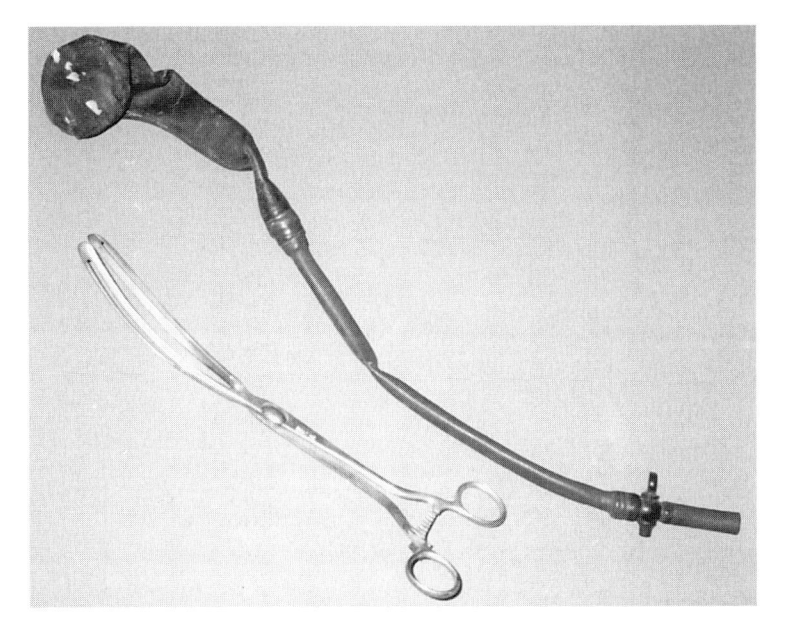

FIGURE 17.3.
De Ribe's hydrostatic bag and introducer. The collapsed rubber bag is grasped in the hollowed-out blades of the introducer. (RCOG)

Intracervical Rubber Balloons

More direct stimulation of the cervix took various forms. Brunninghausen (1820; see Barnes, 1862), Scholler (1842), and others introduced sponge tents into the cervix. However in the second half of the nineteenth century a number of distensible rubber balloons, or hydrostatic bags, of various designs for insertion into the cervix appeared.

In Britain Barnes was a strong protagonist of induction and acceleration of tardy labor but was critical of balloons placed in the vagina or uterus, the need being to stretch the cervical canal itself (1862). Barnes credited Jardine Murray (1859) as being the first person to use a bag inflated with air to plug and dilate the cervix; Murray used this bag in a case of placenta previa. Barnes devised fiddle-shaped bags of various sizes that were introduced into the cervix following overnight placement of an elastic bougie in the uterus (Figure 17.2). The bag was inflated until the cervix was dilated by 3 to 4 fingers and the membranes were then ruptured.

Playfair was concerned that the use of bags tended to dislodge the presenting part from the lower uterine segment and thereby encouraged malpresentation (1869). Barnes accepted this criticism but did not regard it as a major problem for he was prepared in such cases to undertake internal podalic version and bring down a leg.

The most well-known and enduring bag for cervical dilatation was that of Champetier de Ribes (Figures 17.3, 17.4), the director of obstetrics at the Hôtel-Dieu in Paris, which

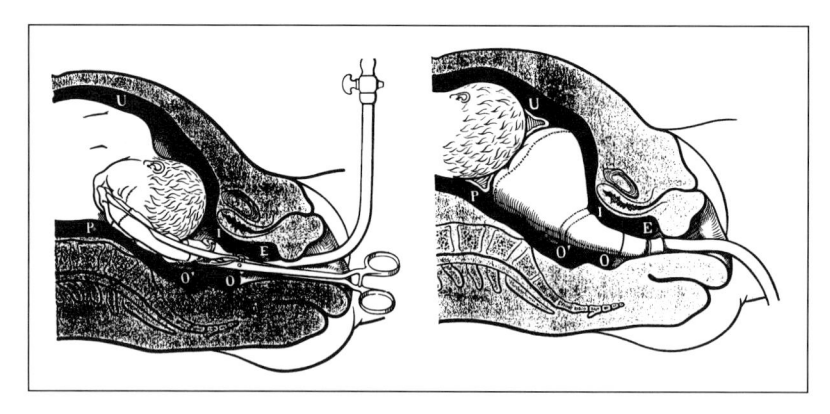

FIGURE 17.4.
Insertion of de Ribe's bag. The bag is inserted extra-amniotically (*PU*) until its neck is above the internal os (*O'I*). It is then filled by gravity via a funnel. (de Ribes, 1888)

FIGURE 17.5.
Voorhees's bags. These were improved versions of de Ribes's bags and were widely used in the USA. (Voorhees, 1900)

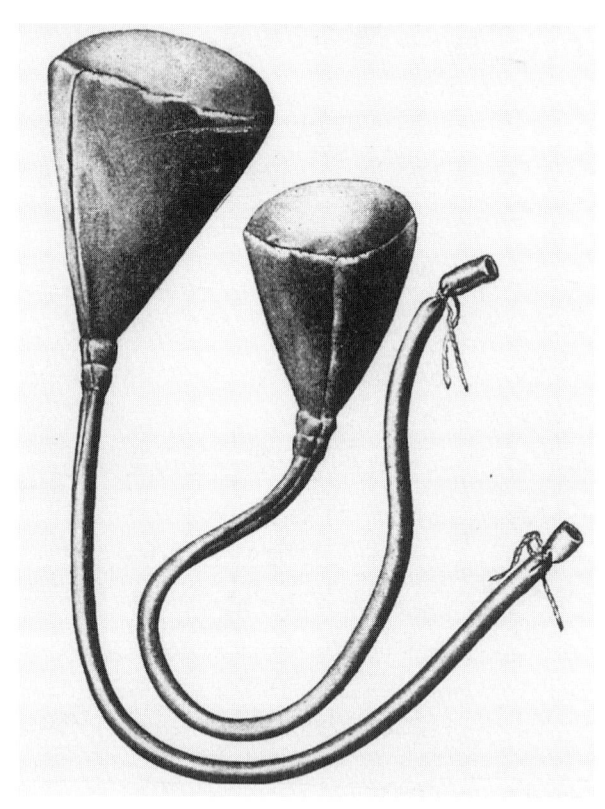

was used for induction and for stimulation of labor, particularly in placenta previa (1888). De Ribes claimed to have learned the idea from his former teacher, Tarnier, who had demonstrated a small, round balloon, his *ballon excitateur*, for induction of labor in 1878. The Tarnier *ballon* was a soft rubber bag the size of a hen's egg that was inserted through the cervix on the end of a catheter and was a refinement of the earlier techniques of using a pig's or dog's bladder inserted through the cervix to stem hemorrhage from placenta previa. De Ribes's bags were made of rubber-covered silk and were pyriform in shape. They were made in six sizes, ranging from 30 millimeters to 80 millimeters (1–3 inches) in diameter. The bag was folded and inserted using a special

introducing forceps and then filled with liquid, following which gentle traction was applied. In most of the eighteen cases reported by de Ribes the bag was expelled in less than twelve hours. De Ribes suggested that the bag could be used to induce labor in a variety of circumstances other than the control of hemorrhage from placenta previa. These included cases of polyhydramnios, severe albuminuria, shoulder presentation when version could not be achieved, and retained placenta with infection and a closed cervix.

In America the use of hydrostatic bags seems to have been variable. Lusk, in the fourth edition of his textbook (1892), recommended the use of Barnes's bags in a variety of circumstances to induce labor: placenta previa, eclampsia, hy-

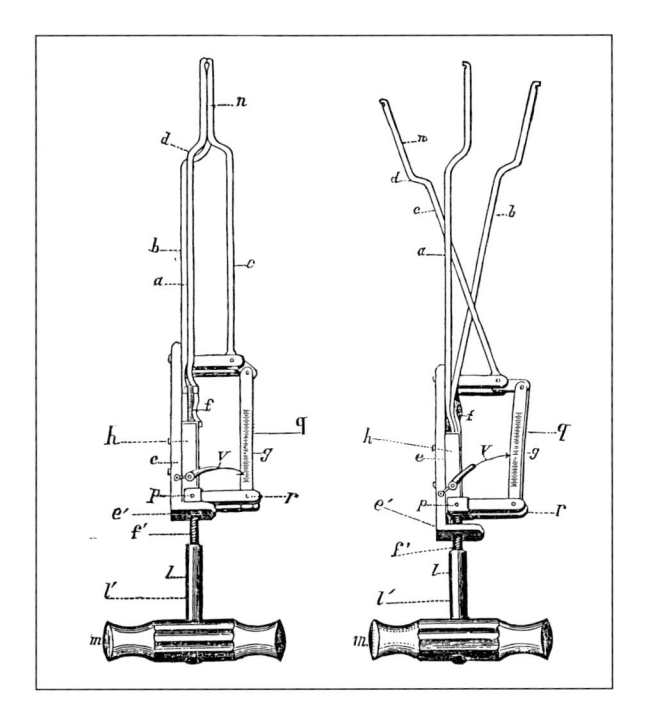

FIGURE 17.6.
Bossi's original cervical dilator. Three-bladed and of lightweight construction. The mechanical design is of interest. (Bossi, 1892)

datidiform mole, and in cases of tardy labor. However, McLane was less enthusiastic. He used modified Barnes's and de Ribes's bags but found them expensive and not durable (Voorhees, 1900). The resident obstetrician under McLane at the Sloane Maternity Hospital, James Ditmar Voorhees (1869–1929), was very critical of the Barnes's bags, particularly the bulkiness, which made introduction difficult, and the inappropriate shape and material led to early expulsion (1900). De Ribes's bags were difficult to obtain, expensive, and not robust. Voorhees described his own improved design based on de Ribes's bag, made of canvas covered with heavy rubber (Figure 17.5), and this rapidly replaced the de Ribes bag in America (Speert, 1958).

The appearance of several balloon designs over a relatively short space of time is probably related to the recent availability of vulcanized rubber, which replaced animal organs. The use of Barnes's, de Ribes's, and Voorhees's bags continued through the first half of the twentieth century. For example, Down Brothers, a major British instrument maker, still offered both Barnes's and de Ribes's bags in their 1929 and 1935 catalogues, together with a detailed description of the use of the de Ribes's bag in the 1929 edition.

Mechanical Dilatation of the Cervix

The techniques so far described were relatively gentle and encouraged natural but accelerated dilatation of the cervix while also helping to reduce blood loss in cases of placenta previa. Toward the end of the eighteenth century a more aggressive approach to achieving rapid delivery in cases of eclampsia and severe antepartum hemorrhage evolved. Instruments used included graduated bougies, expanding cutting blades, and blunt multibladed devices, which had considerable mechanical advantage and dilating force.

L. M. Bossi, a professor of obstetrics and gynecology at the University of Genoa, first described a mechanical cervical dilator in 1892 (Figure 17.6). Its main use was to hasten delivery in cases of eclampsia. The first model had three blades connected to a screw mechanism and handle. Although it was of relatively light construction, the leverage forces gave it considerable mechanical advantage.

In 1900 Bossi described his better-known and more robust four-bladed instrument (Figures 17.7, 17.8). The tapered, grooved blades had detachable lipped caps. A pivot and large turnscrew action were used to force the blades apart and a pointer indicated the degree of separation of the branches.

There were several variations of the Bossi dilator, two of which are illustrated in Figures 17.9 and 17.10. Preiss's instrument was very similar to Bossi's later model but was easier to assemble. Gustav Adolf Walcher (1856–1935), Director of the Würtenburg School for Midwives in Stuttgart, invented a dilator that worked on similar principles but had eight blades. Eight-bladed dilators were more complex in construction and therefore more difficult to clean and more expensive. The purpose of the extra blades was to distribute the stretching forces more evenly and therefore to reduce trauma but there is no evidence that this desired objective was ever achieved. Forceful mechanical dilatation of the cervix, an extension of *accouchement forcé* of earlier years, had a relatively short vogue, the resultant trauma often being more harmful than the condition that was being treated. On the other hand, artificial rupture of the membranes has continued in favor to this day, although the indications and technique have varied and have been influenced by the advent of antibiotics, oxytocic drugs, and the relative safety of Caesarian section.

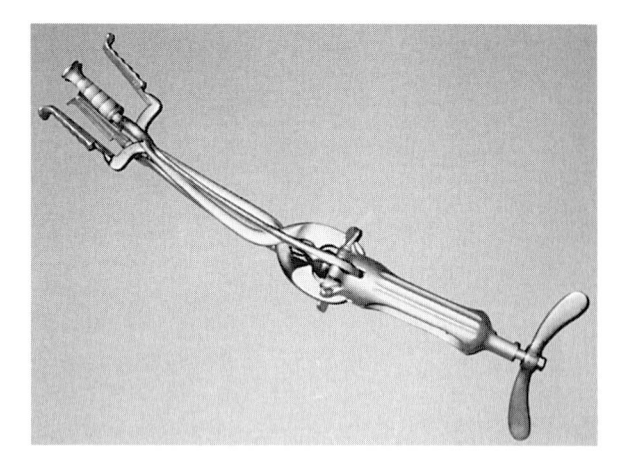

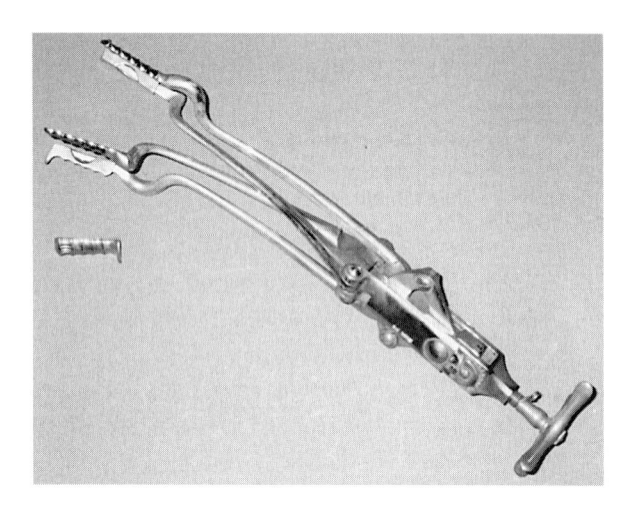

FIGURES 17.7, 17.8.
Bossi's later models. Refinements included a fourth blade, caps to go over the points to help retain the dilator in the cervical canal, improved mechanics, and simpler assembly to aid cleaning. (RCOG)

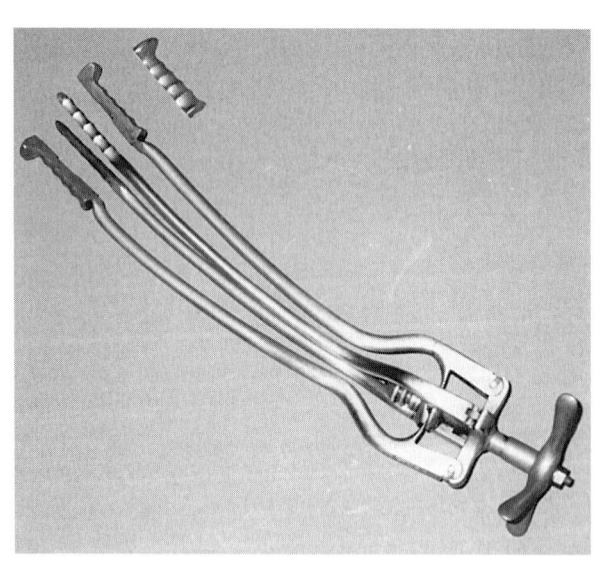

FIGURE 17.9.
Preiss's dilator. The construction is much simplified compared with Bossi's dilators. (RCOG)

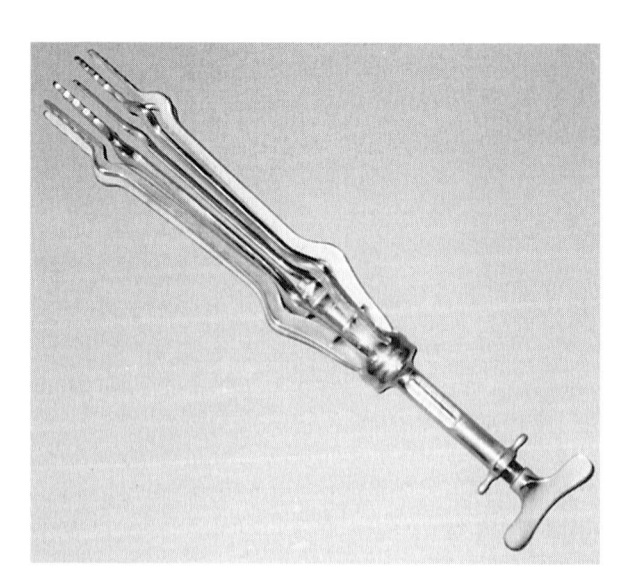

FIGURE 17.10.
Walcher's dilator. An eight-bladed version of Bossi's dilator. (RCOG)

PERFORATORS AND EXTRACTORS

In the eighteenth and nineteenth centuries most obstetricians (let alone the Church and the lay public) viewed destructive operations with fear and abhorrence, the more so if the fetus might still be alive. Destructive operations were only performed in extreme cases, usually after prolonged labors and various attempts at delivery by other means. Influential obstetricians in Britain still favored "turning" (podalic version) for obstructed labor whenever possible, even though some destructive procedure might still be necessary. In his lectures J. Y. Simpson, who had always been unhappy about destructive operations, especially on the living fetus, emphasized the benefits of turning as an alternative (Black, 1871). He also taught that the severity of maternal trauma was a function of time and that any intervention should be undertaken earlier rather than later, a criticism of the traditional conservatism that had ruled in Britain for so long.

Caesarian section was more freely used on the Continent, partly influenced by the Church in Rome and the teaching of St. Thomas Aquinas that the fetus could not be baptized in utero. In 1733 a panel of twelve doctors at the Sorbonne ruled that baptism in utero using a syringe was acceptable providing the holy water reached some part of the fetus. Bland claimed that this pronouncement reduced the Caesarian section rate (1794). To try to alleviate the problems of baptism in utero, a wide range of novel devices and procedures were introduced but few stood the test of time. Georges M. Herbiniaux of Brussels even devised a modified lever in which was incorporated a syringe for irrigations or possibly the introduction of holy water for intrauterine baptism (1794) (Figure 18.1).

One of the great quandaries of the time, therefore, was to determine whether or not the fetus was still alive. This was often in doubt as auscultation of the fetal heart was not introduced until the mid-nineteenth century. Obstetricians relied on a number of signs such as maternal rigors, a sense of coldness, fetid liquor amnii, and flaccid breasts with some discharge of milk, which all suggested that the baby was long since dead. R. W. Johnson would rely on three signs only: separation and looseness of the skull bones, peeling of the hairy scalp, and a cold, flaccid, nonpulsating umbilical cord that had been prolapsed for half an hour. Johnson claimed that "the practice of midwifery is now on such a footing ... as almost to explode the preposterous practice of extracting infants before they are known to be dead, by such instruments as cannot save them" (1769).

The rather basic types of instruments used for centuries for embryulcia and extraction of the dead fetus became more refined toward the end of the eighteenth century. Through the middle of the nineteenth century great efforts were made to be more scientific in the design of instruments, with an emphasis on safety for the mother (and for the obstetrician!). In the developmental process the equipment became larger and more complex, especially on the Continent, and this resulted in the introduction of new hazards. These efforts reached their heyday in the third quarter of the century and the range of apparatus was well reviewed by A. R. Simpson (1884b). He described three stages of embryulcia: perforation, comminution, and extraction. There were instruments designed primarily for each of the stages and every obstetrician was expected to have in his bag an instrument for each of these purposes. Although multipurpose instruments did evolve these required compromises in their design and many did not fulfill all their functions very efficiently.

Meanwhile Caesarian section was gradually gaining favor, with the consequential waning of the more horrendous of destructive procedures, such as piecemeal dismemberment.

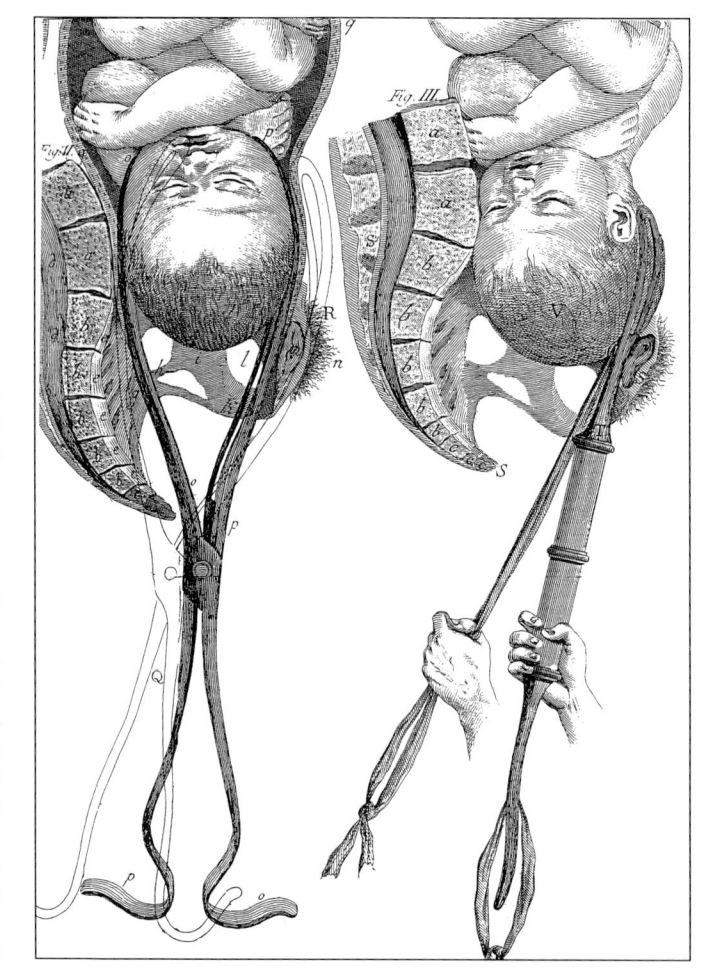

FIGURE 18.1 (RIGHT).
Herbiniaux's forceps and lever syringe. The left diagram shows a high forceps application and the oscillatory action advocated. The right diagram is the lever-syringe for irrigation. (Herbiniaux, 1794)

FIGURE 18.2 (OPPOSITE TOP).
Robertson's spear perforator. (RCOG)

FIGURE 18.3 (OPPOSITE LEFT).
Scissors-action perforators of the Smellie/Denman type. Earlier designs had straight blades but blades curved on the flat were soon adopted. The protective shoulder is the common feature. (RCOG)

FIGURE 18.4 (OPPOSITE RIGHT).
Cleveland's perforator. The addition of a screw in the handle facilitates separation of the blades. (Cleveland, 1868)

Merriman reported forty-six Caesarian sections with sixteen surviving children and no maternal mortality (1826). Also, the ever-recurring problem of accurate assessment of pelvic size led to some reservations so that Caesarian section tended to be restricted to women who had previously been delivered only after a destructive procedure.

By the 1860s Caesarian section was undoubtedly becoming safer and the "Caesarianists" were gaining ground, with such rational and balanced proponents as Thomas Radford (1869). Greenhalgh (1866) favored early Caesarian section in cases of extreme pelvic contraction, at least as a means of saving some babies if not their mothers. In particular he quoted the data of Keyser of Edinburgh based on 164 Caesarian sections. When the operation was performed within twenty-four hours of the onset of labor, forty mothers out of sixty died (67 percent) and forty-two of the babies were liveborn. Greenhalgh was "confident that the most skeptical must admit that the mortality to the mother is as great, if not greater, from craniotomy and crotchet operations in extreme distortion of the pelvis, as in the Caesarean section . . . nothing would induce me again . . . to attempt delivery by the crotchet where the conjugate (true) diameter of the brim does not measure fully two inches. . . ." In the ensuing discussion Barnes, not surprisingly, was more in favor of his own craniotomy forceps but Playfair quoted the results of Pihan-Dufeillay from France in which maternal mortality from Caesarian section in early labor was only 19 percent, compared with 81 percent in those cases where the mother was already suffering from exhaustion.

Perforators

Spear Perforators

Earlier perforators were of knife or spear form, sometimes protected by a sheath (Figures 18.2, 18.31). These very sharp

220 CHAPTER 18

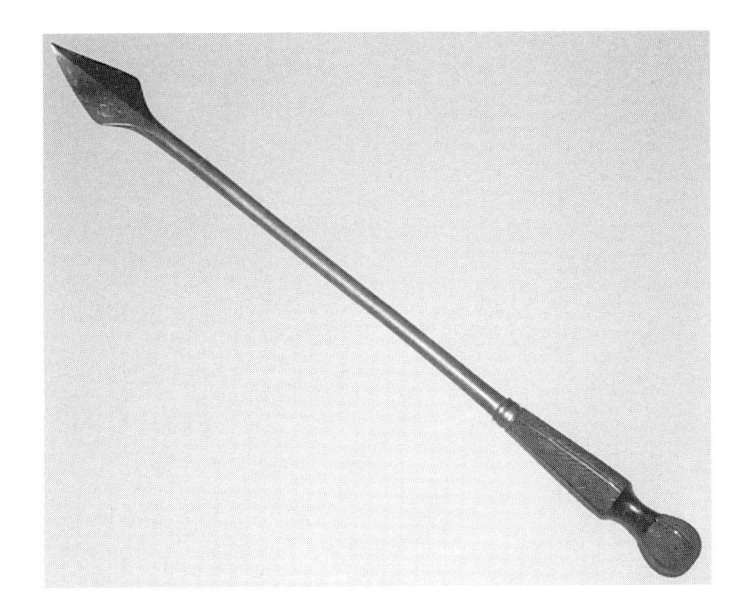

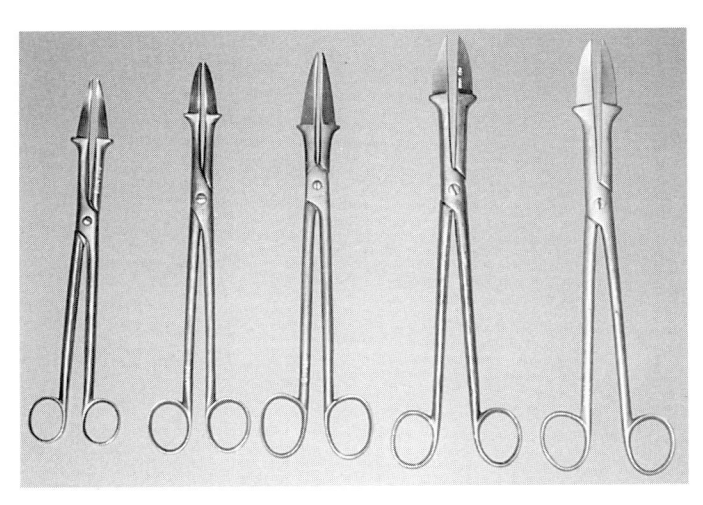

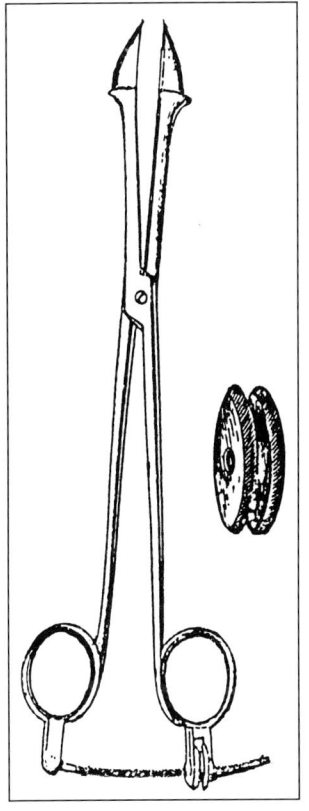

and relatively crude instruments were difficult to introduce and remove without damage to the birth canal, and possibly to the operator, and did not make an adequate opening in the skull. Their only possible advantages would have been cheapness and simplicity. Although they were soon superseded by the scissors type and other more sophisticated instruments, new designs of spear perforator continued to appear until at least 1871 in America (Garland, 1871). These were often part of a more complex instrument, incorporating a crotchet.

Jointed and Hinged Perforators
Wedge-scissors perforators were popularized by Smellie in the mid-eighteenth century. Some earlier instruments had both an inner and outer cutting edge but the inner cutting edge was soon dropped because it served no useful purpose.

Denman's perforator, which was of similar design but usually with curved blades, became the commonly used instrument (1788) (Figure 18.3). From the time of Smellie most scissors perforators had short pointed blades and a protective shoulder at the base of the blades.

The weakness in the design of these perforators was that they required the handles to be separated to cut or tear the tissues and thus required two hands. There were numerous modifications of the scissors design, such as that of William Frederick Cleveland, a surgeon at the Kilburn Hospital, London. He added a screw and wheel to the finger rings to force the blades apart (1868) (Figure 18.4).

A major improvement in the design of hinged perforators was a double crossover joint so that the blades were opened by squeezing the handles together, thus giving much greater mechanical advantage, as in the designs of Oldham

PERFORATORS AND EXTRACTORS **221**

FIGURE 18.5.
Oldham's and Holmes's perforators. The double crossover has the advantage that the blades are opened by closing the handles. In the Holmes perforator the point is on one blade only. (RCOG)

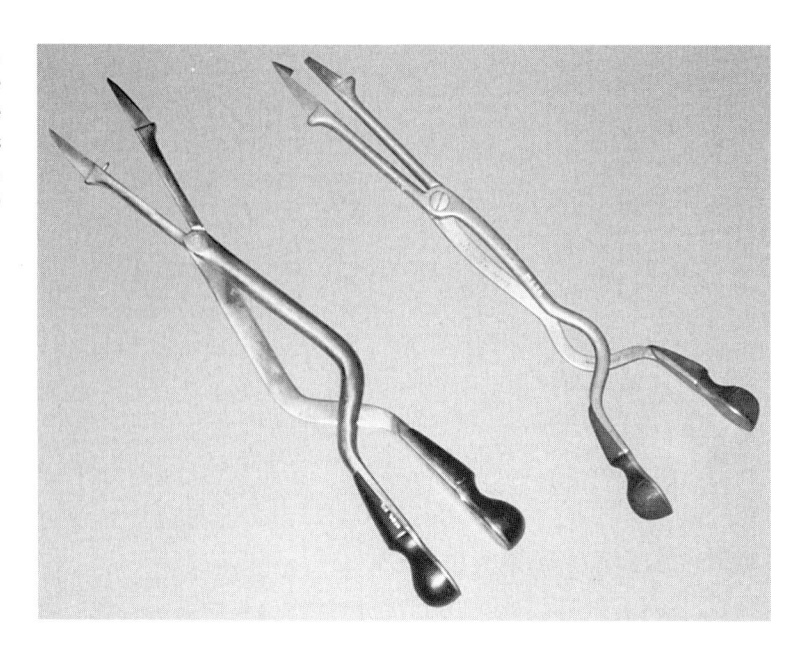

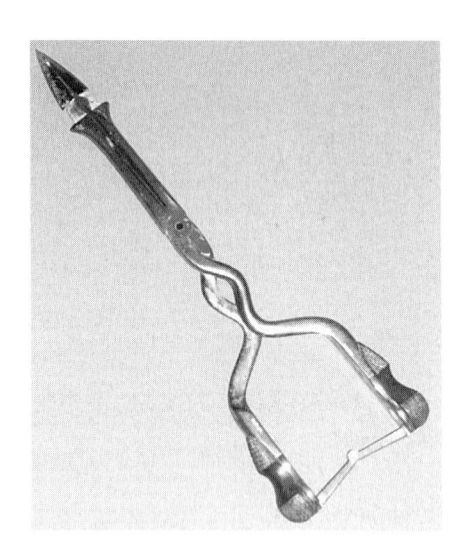

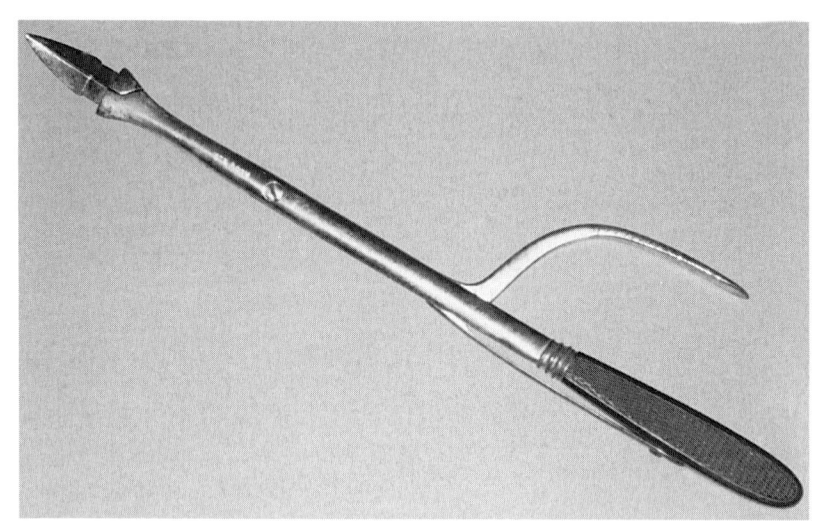

FIGURE 18.6 (ABOVE LEFT).
Greenhalgh's perforator. A double crossover similar to Oldham's and Holmes's with a locking bar between the handles. (Science Museum, London)

FIGURE 18.7 (ABOVE RIGHT).
Jones's perforator. A spring-loaded single-handed design. (RCOG)

FIGURE 18.8 (RIGHT).
J. Y. Simpson's spring-loaded perforator. (RCOG)

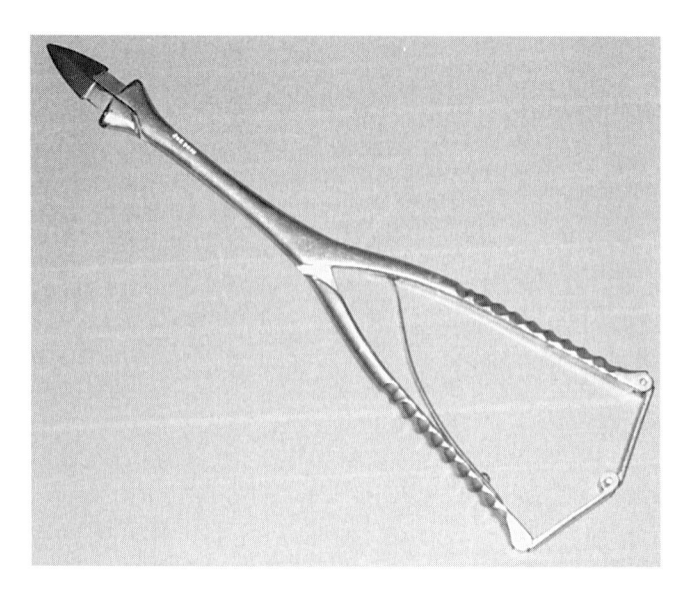

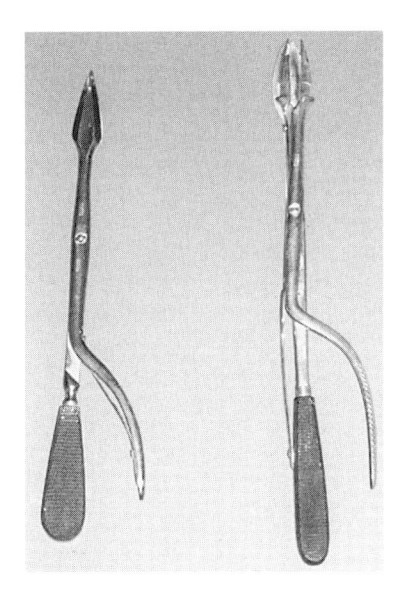

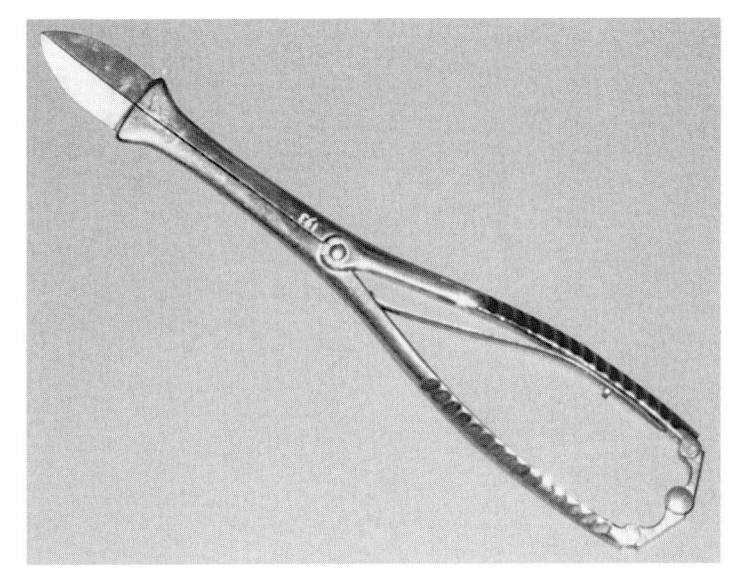

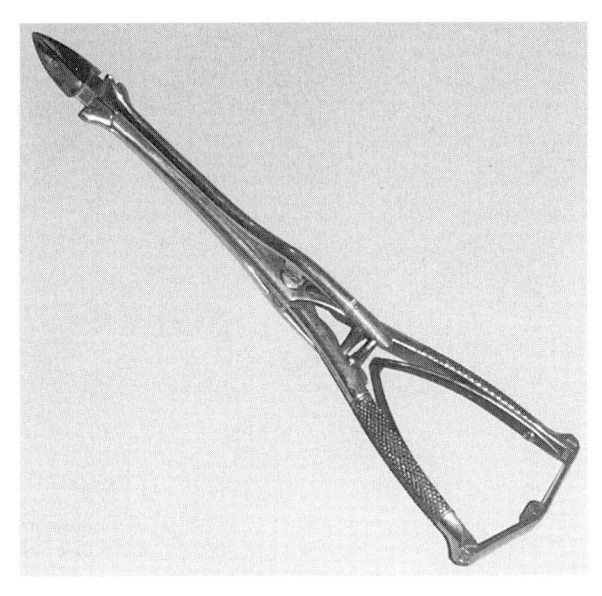

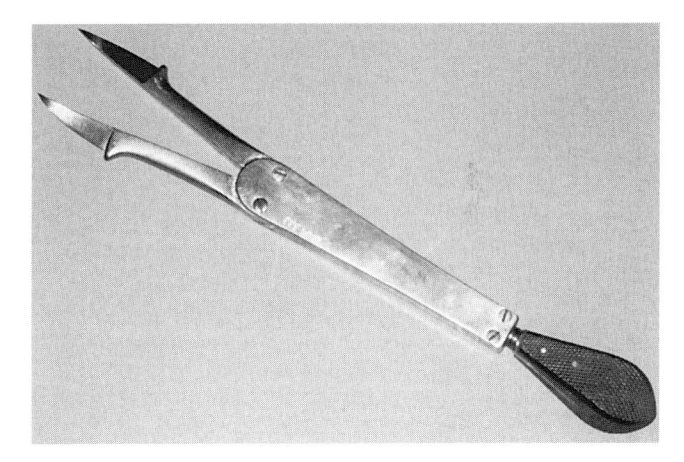

FIGURE 18.9 (TOP LEFT).
Blot's and Mathews Duncan's perforators. Both are of similar design to that of Jones. (Science Museum, London)

FIGURE 18.10 (TOP RIGHT).
Naegele's spring-loaded perforator. A modification of Simpson's design. (RCOG)

FIGURE 18.11 (ABOVE LEFT).
Godson's four-bladed spring-loaded perforator. (Science Museum, London)

FIGURE 18.12 (ABOVE RIGHT).
Weiss's screw-operated perforator. (RCOG)

and John Pocock Holmes (d. 1858) of London (see Blundell, 1834) (Figure 18.5). Holmes had the perforating point on one blade only, with the other blade truncated (1831). Greenhalgh added a hinged locking bar to the handle (1866) (Figure 18.6).

To further facilitate single-handed operation other designs were introduced, usually without a crossover joint but with a spring-loaded handle to keep the handles apart and the blades in apposition. These included Jones (Figure 18.7) and J. Y. Simpson's later model (1842; see Black, 1871) (Figure 18.8). Simpson had earlier used a simple scissors instrument of his own design. Other developments based on the Jones model included those of Hippolyte Blot (b. 1822) of Paris (1855a,b) and of Mathews Duncan (Figure 18.9), while Naegele (1830) modified Simpson's design (Figure 18.10) and Clement Godson, Consultant Physician at the City of London Lying-In Hospital, used a four-bladed perforator based on the same principle (circa 1880) (Figure 18.11).

Also, in keeping with the mechanical inventiveness of the time, more complex devices originated from the instrument makers, such as Weiss, which had a screw-operated handle to separate the blades (Figure 18.12).

PERFORATORS AND EXTRACTORS   223

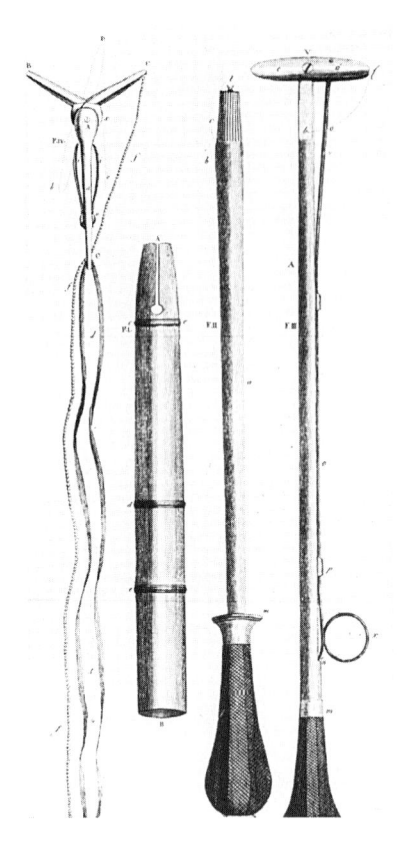

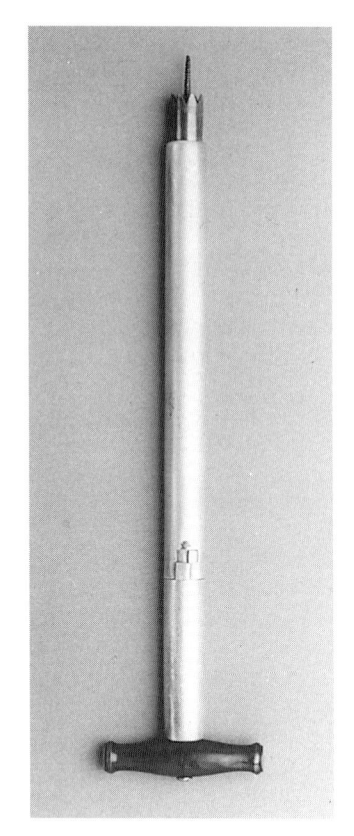

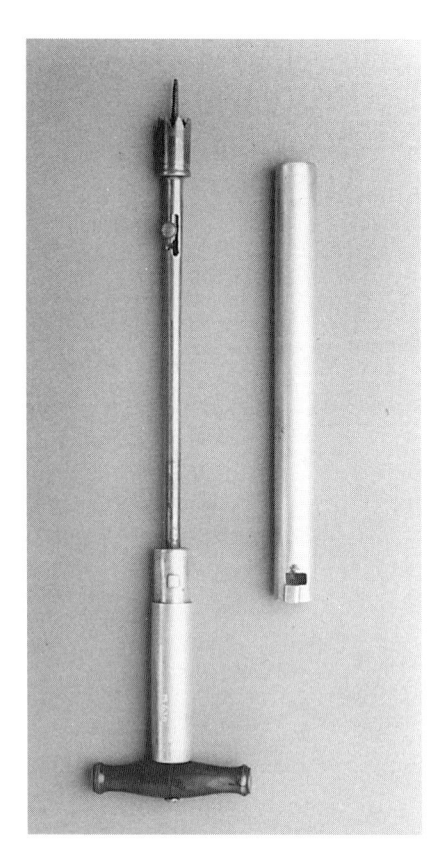

FIGURE 18.13 (ABOVE LEFT). Assalini's trephine perforator. The center illustrations show the components of the straight trephine. Left and right are the components of his hinged crotchets, which were inserted into the cranium and the wings then opened. (Assalini, 1811)

FIGURES 18.14 (ABOVE CENTER), 18.15 (ABOVE RIGHT). Mende's trephine perforator. 18.14: The assembled instrument. 18.15: The outer sheath removed, showing the components. (RCOG)

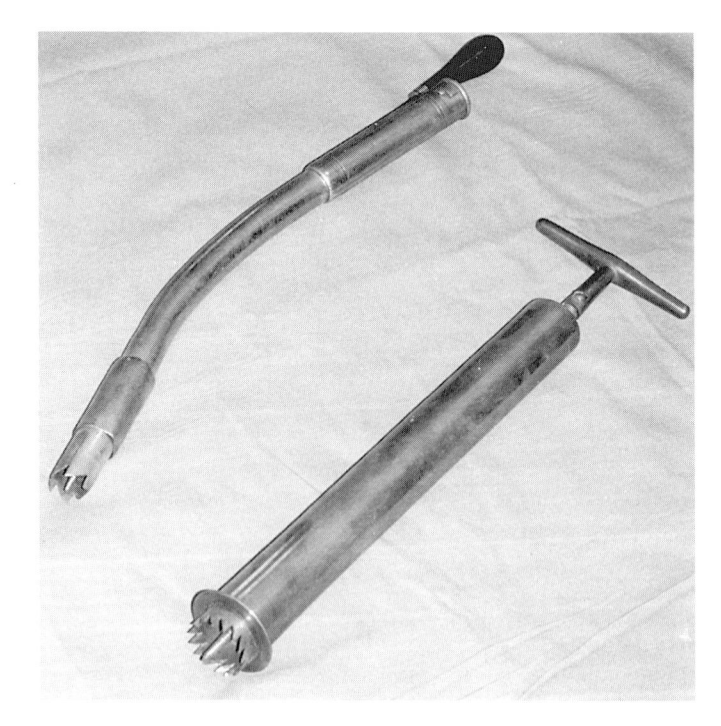

FIGURE 18.16. Trephine perforators. Top: Braun. Bottom: Jörg. (Charles University, Prague)

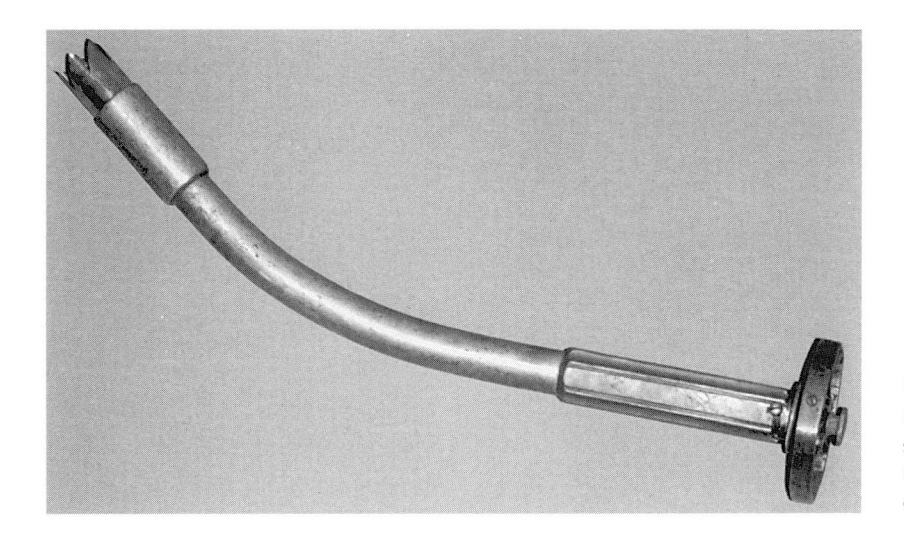

FIGURE 18.17.
Braun's trephine perforator. This model is of similar dimensions to that in Figure 18.16 but has a wheel screw instead of a crank. (Trinity Centre for Health Sciences, Dublin)

The method for using the perforator was fairly standard. The perforator was introduced with the tip guarded by the fingers. The skull was perforated preferably through the anterior fontanel but in cases of malpresentation through the most accessible point. The blades were then opened successively in two or more directions. However, there was no general agreement as to the timing or the best method of extraction after perforation. Although destructive operations were usually performed only after death of the fetus (if this could be determined), there were obstetricians who, in severe degrees of pelvic contraction, would perforate the head at the onset of labor. It was common practice, as advocated by, for example, Hamilton (1775) and Rigby the Younger (1841), to wait for several hours after perforation before attempting extraction in order that the head could soften and descend into the pelvic cavity and so the mother could rest. (Osborn advocated delaying up to thirty hours [1792].) However, a minority viewpoint, expressed by Burns (1809), among others, was that extraction with the crotchet should be done immediately after perforation unless there was gross pelvic contraction requiring complete breaking down of the skull.

According to Blundell the perforator was designed to be introduced with a boring action (1840). Because in many cases delivery might already have been attempted with the forceps he recommended leaving the forceps on the head and tying the handles tightly, thus stabilizing the head for the introduction of the perforator. He was prepared to use the perforator even if there was uncertainty as to whether the fetus was still alive and he emphasized the need for rapid and complete demolition of the brain to a pulp. Extraction could be performed either with the long forceps or with craniotomy forceps.

Osborn antagonized not only his former colleague Denman but also Alexander Hamilton over various matters of clinical management, inducing Hamilton to respond in a series of open letters in which he considered the relative merits of the crotchet (safe!) and Caesarian section (lethal) (1792). These letters continued the controversy over perforation, especially early perforation (that is, at the onset of labor) in cases where the true conjugate was less than 70 millimeters (2.75 inches), as advocated by Osborn, and particularly challenged the feasibility of making an accurate assessment of pelvic size clinically.

Trephine Perforators

In Paris the most popular perforator was that of Blot, according to A. R. Simpson, but trephine perforators, first used by Assalini (1811) in Italy (Figure 18.13), soon became popular in the rest of Europe, although they never became part of the British obstetricians armamentarium.

There were various modifications of the trephine perforator. The most widely used trephines were those of Mende of Göttingen (1825) (Chapter 5) and of Johan Christian Gottfried Jörg (1779–1856) (1807) (Figures 18.14–18.16, bottom). Both of these instruments were straight but Carl Braun modified the design by adding a pelvic curve (Figures 18.16, top; 18.17) (1859). Other trephines were of very strong construction, powerful enough to drill through the face if necessary. The trephines made a round hole in the head about 19 millimeters (.75 inches) in diameter and with clean edges, but their common failing, according to Rigby the Younger (1841), was that they did not make a big enough hole.

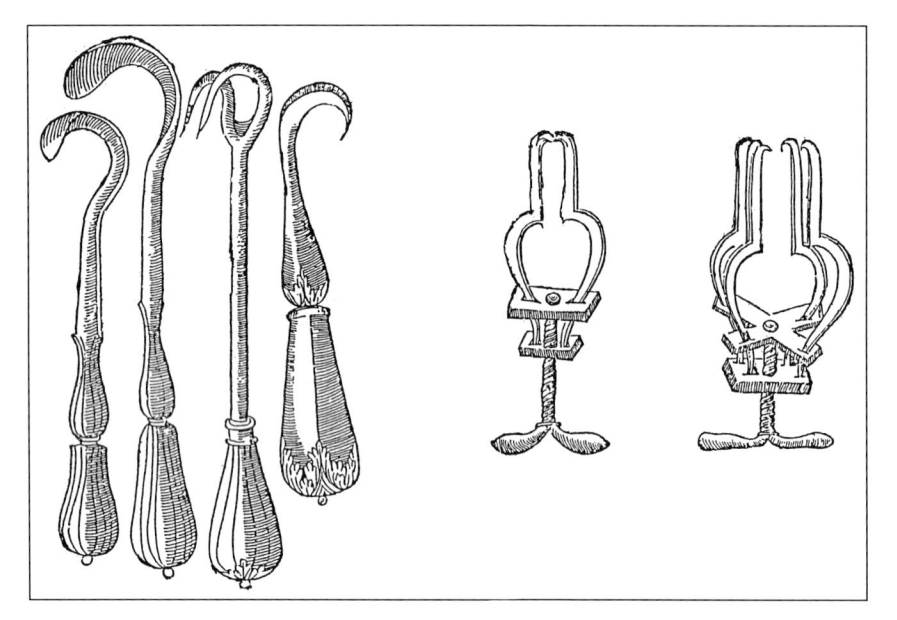

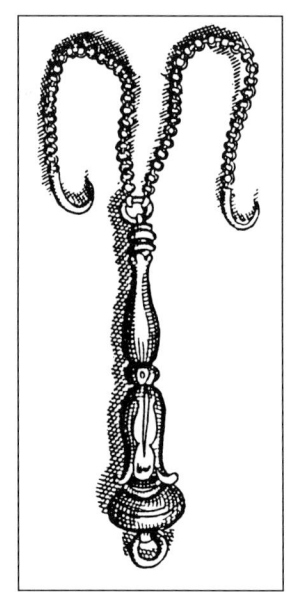

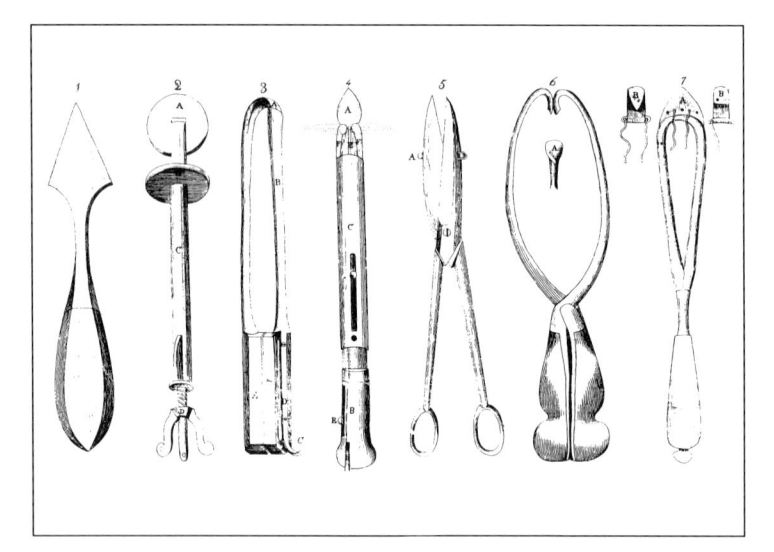

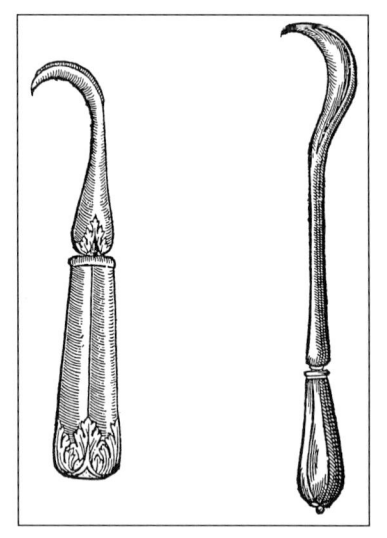

FIGURE 18.18 (TOP LEFT).
Paré's hooks and Gryphon's talons. (Paré, 1665)

FIGURE 18.19 (TOP RIGHT).
Scultetus's chains. (Paré, 1665)

FIGURE 18.20 (ABOVE LEFT).
Aitken's illustrations, Plate 4K. (Aitken, 1786) 1. Mauriceau's spear perforator; 2. Mauriceau's *tire-tête,* or extractor; 3. Levret's guarded crotchet (attributed to Mauriceau); 4. Ould's *terebra,* or perforator, modified by Burton by the addition of two folding wings for use also as an extractor; 5. scissors perforator; 6. Smellie's double crotchet; 7. Aitken's "living lever"

FIGURE 18.21 (ABOVE RIGHT).
Guillemeau's crotchet and curved knife. These are some of the earliest purpose-designed destructive instruments. (Guillemeau, 1612)

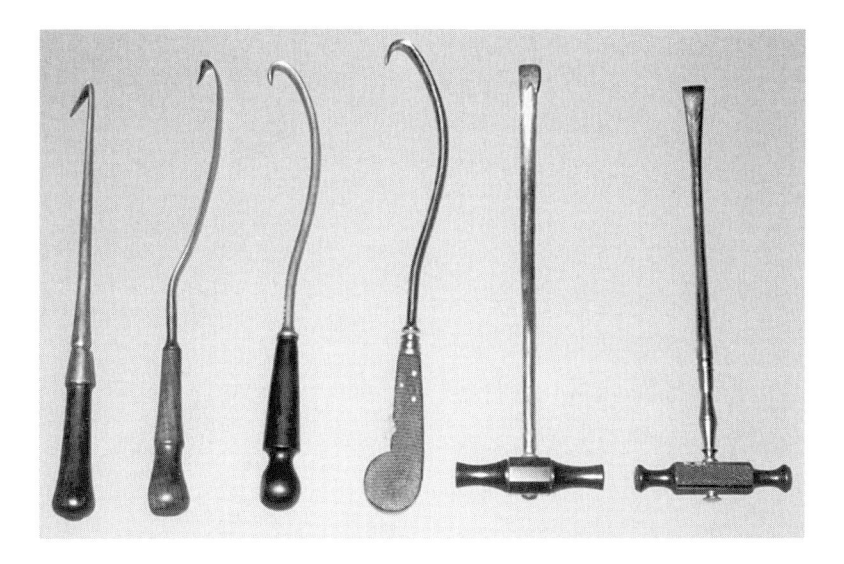

FIGURE 18.22.
A selection of crotchets. The three on the right all have detachable handles. (RCOG)

Extractors

Early extractors were in the form of talons and hooks, which could be either sharp or blunt, curved or straight, or on chains (Figures 18.18, 18.19) (Paré, 1665). The feature they had in common was that they were always dangerous, not only to the patient but also, as pointed out by Smellie (1751), to the operator.

In the seventeenth century Mauriceau devised a number of extraction instruments, some of which were later illustrated by Aitken (1786) (Figure 18.20). These included a simple spear perforator (1) and an extractor, or *tire-tête* (2), which comprised two circular plates, one fixed (*B*) and the other hinged (*A*) and attached by a threaded rod to a screw handle (*D*). The movable plate was introduced through the perforation in the skull and the skull was gripped between the plates by tightening the screw. His guarded crotchet (3) had a sliding cover extending from the handle to protect the tip. In the same plate Aitken showed the *terebra* (4), or perforator, of Fielding Ould (1742), which had an outer protective sheath and which was modified by Burton (1751) to function also as an extractor. This was achieved by two extendable wings (*EE*) at the distal end, operated by a button (*E*) on the handle. He also showed the scissors perforator, usually ascribed to Smellie, but with two button stops to limit penetration; the double crotchet (5), also usually ascribed to Smellie (see below); and Aitken's own "living lever" (6) (Chapter 16) converted into a perforator or a crotchet by tying on appropriate ends, a combination that Aitken described as "nearly sufficient for most cases of lingering birth."

Simple Crotchets

Simple crotchets or sharp hooks are among the oldest multipurpose destructive instruments, often adapted from instruments intended for other purposes. One of the early purpose-designed crotchets was described by Guillemeau (1609) (Figure 18.21), who believed it gave a safer and speedier solution than "turning" and breech extraction. If necessary a curved knife could be used to reduce the size of the fetus as, for example, in cases of hydrocephalus.

Both a crotchet and a blunt hook were essential items for the practicing obstetrician for nearly three centuries and, in spite of the advent of forceps, as late as 1875 Robert Lee, in his lectures at St. George's Hospital, London, taught that in cases of obstructed labor with a dead fetus extraction with a crotchet must be used, and not the forceps. At the other extreme, his contemporary Greenhalgh concluded that in cases of severe pelvic contraction nothing would induce him to use the crotchet again, his preferred solution being Caesarian section (1866).

Being of relatively simple construction early crotchets were commonly made to order locally and in consequence they are almost limitless in detail of construction (Figure 18.22). It became the usual practice to combine them in one double-ended instrument or as part of a set of instruments with an interchangeable handle; these have been illustrated earlier in Figures 16.25 and 16.26. Also, from the early days of forceps (late eighteenth century), a sharp, protected point had been included in one handle of several designs, especially on the Continent.

The turned-over, pointed end of the crotchet may have had one or more sharp teeth that would be used to hook into the head, orbit, clavicle, or any other accessible part. In some cases they were applied to the outside of the head, as advocated by Smellie, but could be inserted through the perforated head, as described by Alexander Hamilton (1775).

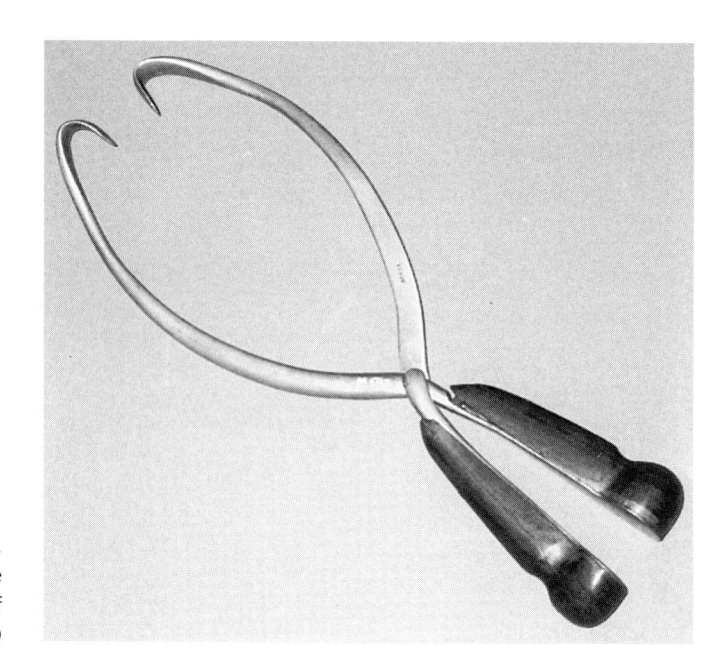

FIGURE 18.23.
Smellie's double crotchet. The blades could be used singly or in combination on the *outside* of the head. (RCOG)

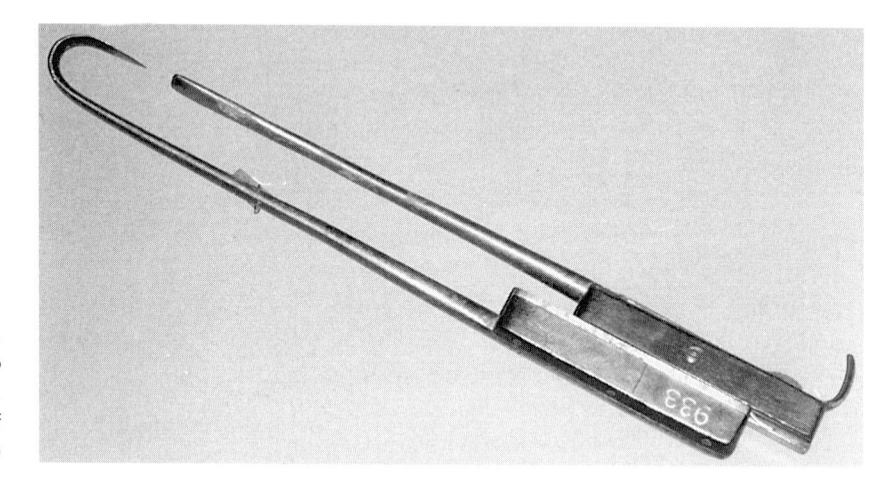

FIGURE 18.24.
Levret's guarded crotchet. The first design to facilitate insertion without maternal trauma. (*See also* Figure 18.20) (Middlesex School of Medicine)

Smellie also devised a double crotchet to be used singly or as a pair in the manner of forceps, but with teeth that embedded in the fetal head (Figures 18.23; 18.20[6]).

Guarded Crotchets

Crotchets were used not only for traction but also for piecemeal destruction of the fetus (*morcellement*) or for destruction of the fetus by such methods as ripping open the abdomen or thorax. In Chamberlen's translation of Mauriceau's textbook (1673), there is a graphic account of Mauriceau's encounter with a case of fetal hydrops in which his advice had been sought and rejected.

> He contented himself, without an exact Examination of the Case, to endeavour only the Extraction of it after his manner: And to effect it, he immediately pull'd and separated the Head wholly from the Body, which hung then but by a Skin, because the Midwives, as I said before, had pull'd it with so much Violence. Afterwards with his Crotchets he pull'd away both the Arms, and some of the Ribs, part of the Lungs and the Heart, one piece after another for above three Quarters of an Hour, that he was very wet with Sweat, altho' it were cold weather . . . After this he returns a second time with all his Strength to the Work, without effecting anymore because he had not yet open'd the lowr Belly, nor the *Diaphragma*, nor would not, as I had advised him every Moment, without which it was impossible to draw forth the rest of the Body.

Mauriceau eventually took over the delivery and, following perforation of the abdomen and release of dropsical fluid, extracted the trunk with ease.

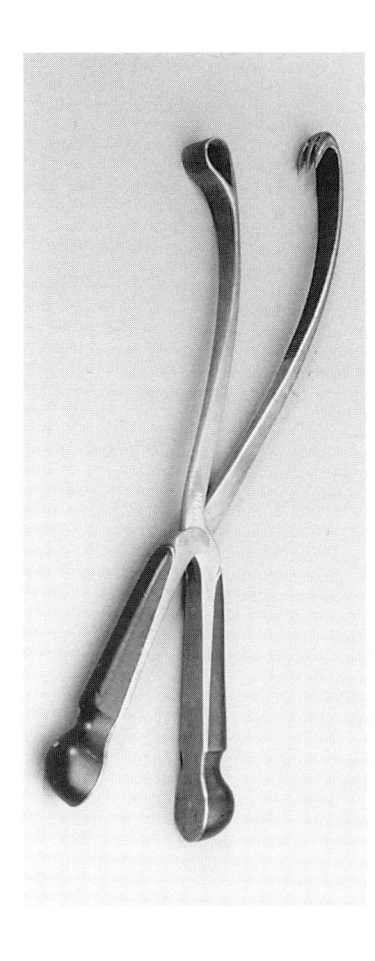

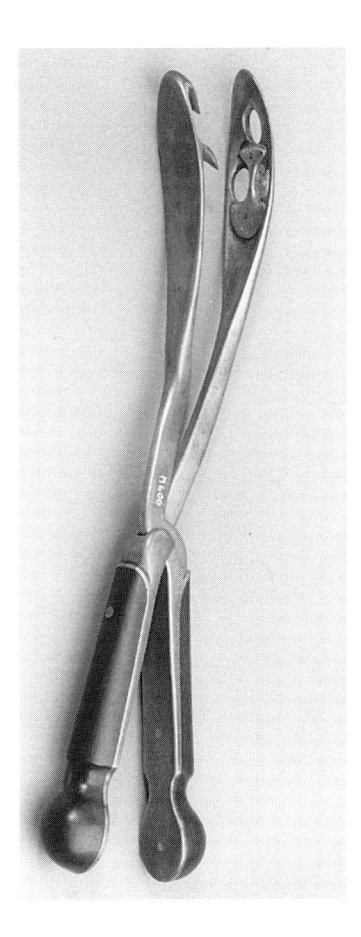

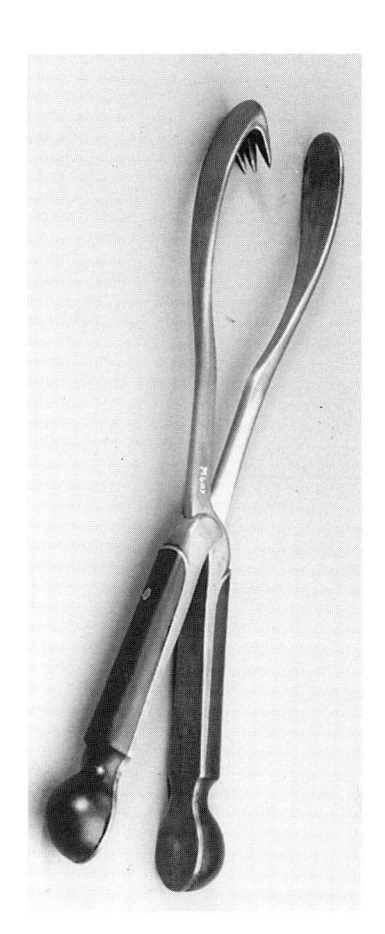

The potential for damage to the birth canal from the crotchet was obviously considerable and even from early times more refined versions had a guarded tip to facilitate atraumatic insertion. The first of these was described by Levret in 1762 (Figure 18.24) but Aitken (Figure 18.20) attributed an almost identical instrument to Mauriceau. The sharp, recurved tip was protected during introduction by an easily removable sheath on a sliding handle. However, in none of the illustrated editions of Mauriceau's book is there mention or illustration of a guarded crotchet.

David Davis favored immediate extraction after craniotomy and designed a number of hooks and forceps for what he termed *embryulcia* (1825) (Figures 18.25–18.30). His guarded crotchets were first described by him in 1817 and were designed for maternal safety as well as for obtaining a firm grasp of the head. The heavy crotchet had three sharp teeth and was applied to the outside of the cranium (Figures 18.25, 18.28). The guard blade was then passed into the cavity of the cranium. When the blades were locked the crotchet pierced the cranium and impinged on the guard. The blades could then be secured with a tape. As the more common practice of the time was to insert the crotchet into

FIGURES 18.25–18.27.
Davis's instruments for embryulcia (RCOG).
18.25: external head crotchet. 18.26: internal head crotchet. 18.27: body crotchet.

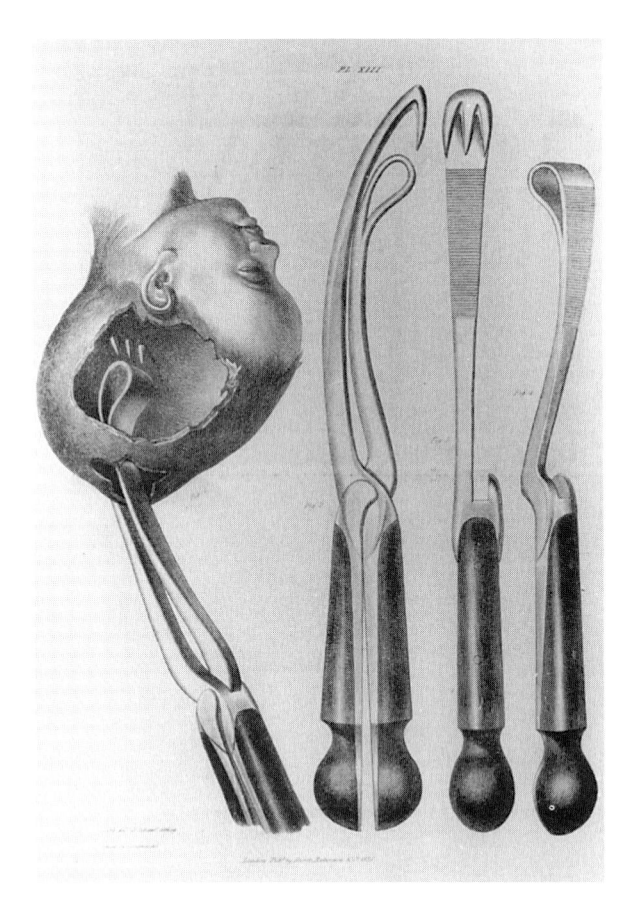

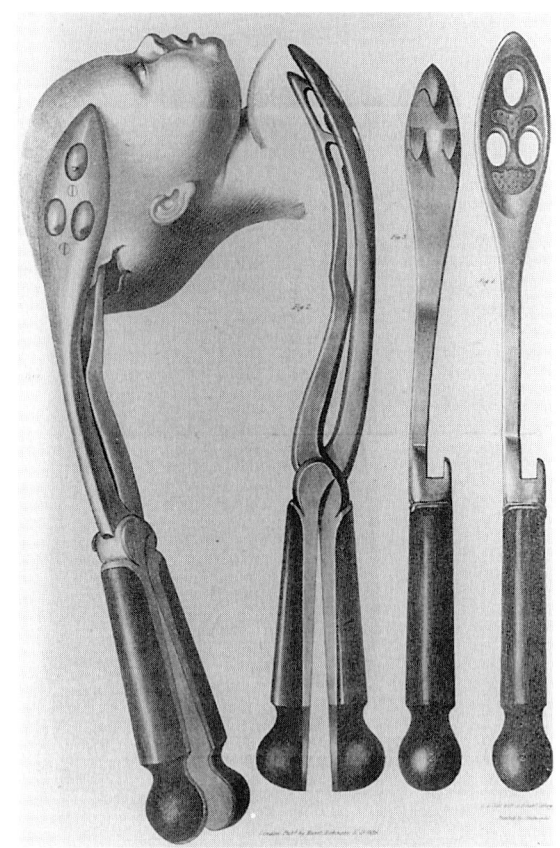

FIGURES 18.28–18.30.
Davis's guarded crotchets in use (Davis, 1825).
18.28: Plate XIII: external head crotchet. 18.29:
Plate XIV: internal head crotchet. 18.30: Plate
XVI: body crotchet.

the cranium Davis designed an alternative guarded crotchet (Figures 18.25, 18.28) to be used in this way, the guard being spoon-shaped with a rasp-like interior surface. Davis received a gold medal from the Society for the Encouragement of the Arts and Sciences in London for his invention, his guarded crotchets being significantly safer for the mother (and obstetrician) than any others invented thus far. This incensed R. Rawlins of Oxford, who claimed to have described the same instruments in 1793. Rawlins's design, however, was in fact dissimilar and cruder (1817).

For the rare cases where there was difficulty in delivery of the trunk David Davis also devised *body crotchets* (Figures 18.27, 18.30). These were used in exactly the same manner as the guarded head crotchets but were applied to the trunk of the fetus after decapitation.

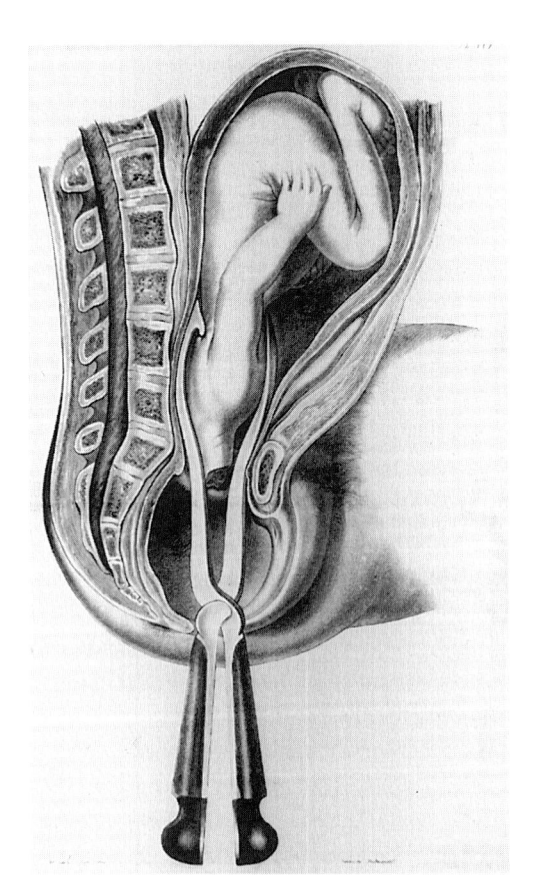

230 CHAPTER 18

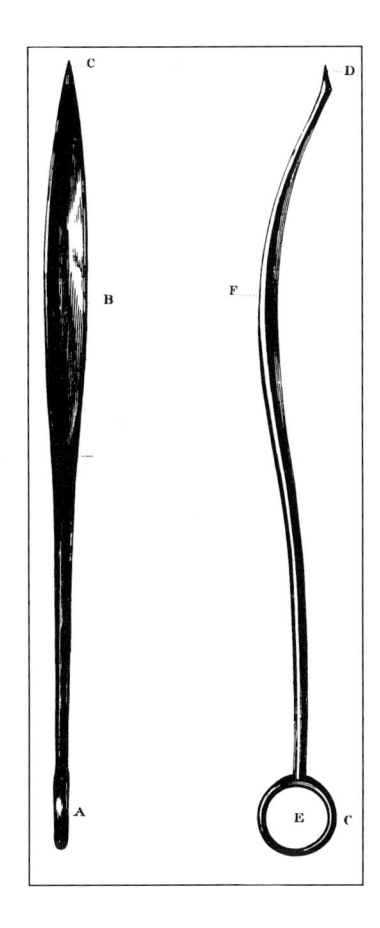

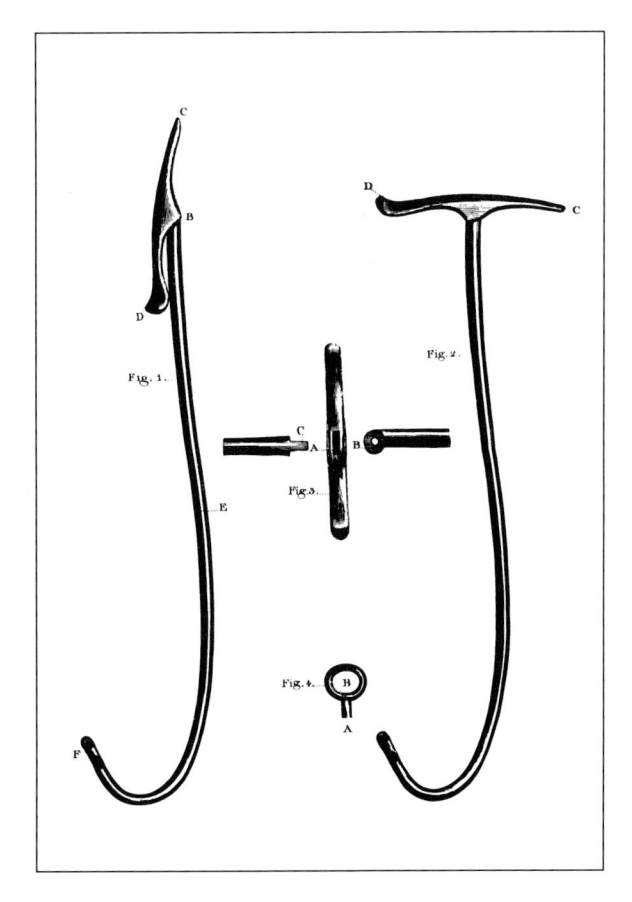

Other Extractors

Most of the extractors in common use (the obstetric forceps excluded) in the late eighteenth through early nineteenth centuries were potentially dangerous and/or inefficient. While craniotomy forceps (see Chapter 19) were sometimes used for traction also, they were unsatisfactory for this purpose. However, cranioclasts provided a better grip and were used more commonly. It is not surprising that a number of novel, and sometimes ingenious, extractors were devised, but none endured. Mauriceau's *tire-tête* and Ould's *terebra occulta*, modified by Burton, have been referred to above.

Johnson (1769) devised his own instruments, which he thought should deal with most problems. These comprised a perforator, or director, (Figure 18.31), 229 millimeters (9 inches) long with a curved and grooved blade; and a multipurpose device, which he called the "embryulcus," or "eductor," 203 millimeters (8 inches) long (Figure 18.32), utilizing the same principle as in the extractor recommended by Burton (Figure 18.20 [4]). The embryulcus was introduced by sliding it along the groove in the director after the head had been perforated. When the handle of the embryulcus was pulled back the hinged crossbar would come to lie transversely within the skull. The opposite end of the embryulcus served as both handle and crotchet. So if the initial procedure failed the instrument was reversed and the hook inserted into an orbit, the roof of the mouth, or under the chin. As a last alternative the crotchet terminated in a ring that could be used to introduce a fillet. The swivel end was also used to extract the head after decapitation and delivery of the trunk by passing the swivel end through the foramen magnum.

Henry Edward Eastlake, a physician accoucheur at the St. Marylebone General Dispensary in London, was one obstetrician who objected to the increasing use of craniotomy forceps and cephalotribes (see below) rather than crotchets and devised his own drill-crotchet (1868) (Figure 18.33). This

FIGURES 18.31, 18.32.
Johnson's perforator (or director) and embryulcus (RCOG). 18.31: The shaped-spear perforator with a groove to facilitate introduction of the embryulcus. 18.32: Johnson's embryulcus.

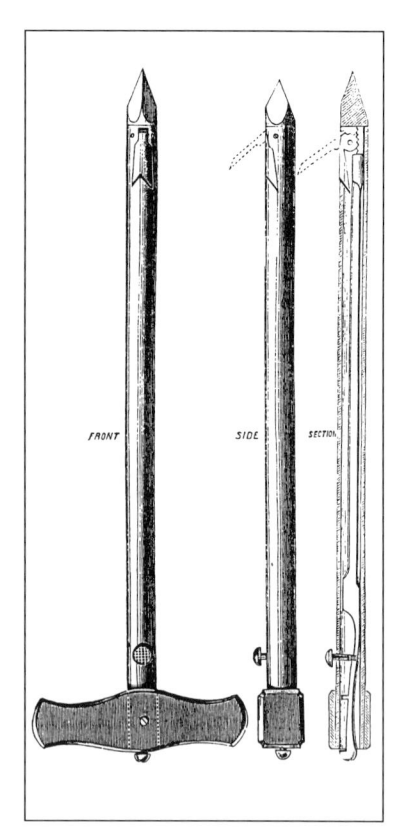

FIGURE 18.33.
Eastlake's drill crotchet. The protrusion of the hinged crotchet bar below the trocar point is controlled by a sliding rod with a terminal rack and pinion. (Eastlake, 1868)

FIGURE 18.34.
Newham's Guide Hook. A double-ended instrument with detachable handle. Newham claimed that it could also be used as a perforator. (Newham, 1865)

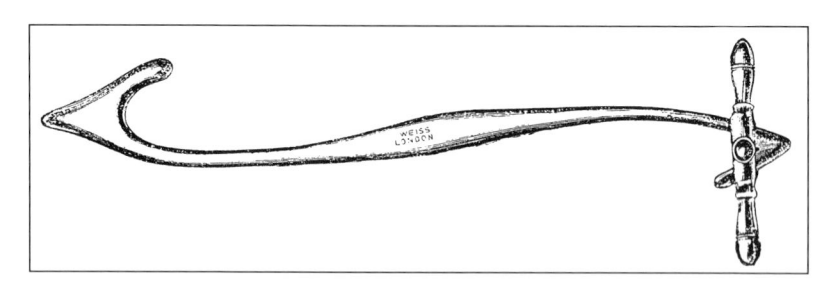

was based on the same principal as Burton's instrument, which could be used as a drill perforator and/or a crotchet. A hollow cylinder terminated in a trocar point. An internal rod with a terminal rack and pinion controlled the angle at which the crotchet bar protruded. His suggestions for its use, which were extensive and included application through a partially dilated cervix, were all in the conditional tense and he gave no account of practical experience.

Samuel Newham of Bury St. Edmunds devised a double-ended "Guide Hook" (Figure 18.34) for which he claimed many uses and advantages (1865). The many circumstances for the use of the instrument, apart from the conventional function as a tractor, included: perforation through the mouth or orbit; insertion into the perforated head to dilate the opening; as an extractor by inserting it into the foramen magnum; as an eviscerating tool; and as a means of rotating the head. A handle could be attached to the smaller end of the hook to facilitate traction.

In spite of Newham's self congratulation—"I feel great satisfaction myself in possessing so useful an addition to my *armamentarium obstetricum*, and confidently advise every accoucheur to add the guide-hook to his collection of instruments."—the instrument does not seem to have found any significant favor, probably because most of the procedures for which Newham advocated it were old fashioned and were being superseded.

Vertebra Hooks

The vertebra hook was a sharp instrument used for traction after decapitation but never found much favor, probably because, being so slender, it was liable to slip and cause maternal tears.

Oldham's hooks of 1855 (Figure 18.35) had a long, fine stem with a hook set at an acute angle. They were designed to

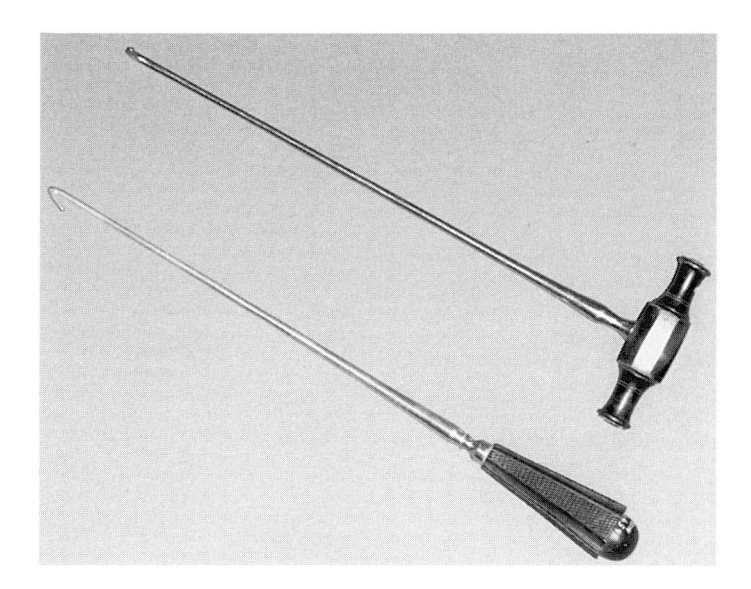

FIGURE 18.35.
Oldham's vertebra hooks. These could be used for traction or to steady the decapitated head. (Science Museum, London)

take hold of the foramen magnum when the cranium was to be broken up in order to give a hold for the crotchet or craniotomy forceps.

• • •

Dangerous and inefficient as many of these instruments were, they fulfilled a purpose when all else had failed, the baby was dead, and the mother's condition was critical. The time when any serious consideration would be given to Caesarian section in the presence of a dead baby was a long way off. Indeed Caesarian section was so dangerous that it was rarely considered when the baby was still alive. In the latter half of the nineteenth century considerable thought and effort was devoted to other instruments for extraction.

COMMINUTORS AND COMMINUTOR-EXTRACTORS

19 Although the concept of crushing the fetus to facilitate extraction was known since ancient times (see Rueff's *rostrum anatis* [Introduction]), it was not until the nineteenth century that instruments were designed specifically for these purposes. By the second half of the century a wide variety was available, many of which continued to be used in to the twentieth century. A. R. Simpson used the term *comminutor* ("crushing instrument") to include a range of instruments. He described five groups of head comminutors in approximately historical sequence. These were (1) craniotomes (craniotomy forceps); (2) cephalotribes (head crushers); (3) cranioclasts, often referred to also as craniotomy forceps (for crushing the base of the skull); (4) cephalotomes (for cutting or sawing); and (5) basilysts (to break up the base of the skull) (1884b).

Craniotomy Forceps

The concept of craniotomy forceps was reintroduced to common practice toward the end of the eighteenth century. Initially practitioners used various types of forceps, such as toothed lithotomy forceps, which they usually borrowed from the surgeons or lithotomists, to break up the skull bones.

Later variations of these crushing forceps included Mesnard's *tenette à conducteur* (1753) and the forceps of Lyon (Figure 19.1), both widely used in Europe and recommended strongly by Alexander Hamilton. While they were used primarily for breaking down the skull bones by *morcellement* they played some part as extractors.

Although craniotomy forceps were gaining popularity in Britain in the early nineteenth century they were not universally favored, perhaps because of growing recognition that crushing tools might be useful and possibly less dangerous. Rigby the Younger, for example, much preferred to use the common curved forceps (1841). A selection of English nineteenth-century craniotomy forceps is shown in Figure 19.2. Heavier and more complex designs often referred to as craniotomy forceps are described below under the section entitled "Cranioclasts."

The main design problem of the craniotomy forceps was to reconcile the functions of crusher and tractor. Ziegler tried to overcome this with an instrument with interchangeable blades for the two different functions (Figure 19.3). This could be used in one mode as a cranioclast and, with the alternative blade, as an extractor (1848–1849). The craniotomy blade had small teeth on its inner surface, a feature found in heavier cranioclasts of the time.

In America craniotomy was performed from at least the 1880s (Speert, 1980). In the first one thousand deliveries at the Sloane Maternity Hospital that occurred between 1888 and 1890, three craniotomies were performed, but no Caesarian sections. At the Sixteenth Annual Meeting of the American Gynecological Society in 1891 Robert P. Harris of Philadelphia made a plea for greater resort to Caesarian section. Henry Garrigues dissented with a remarkable outburst.

> As to the question, Are we justified in destroying the life of the living child? I would say that in my opinion we are. In spite of all the progress which Caesarean section has made, it still has a much greater mortality than has craniotomy.... We

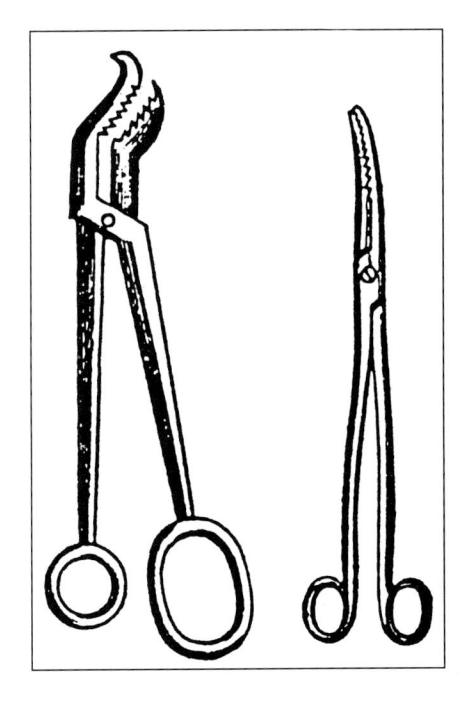

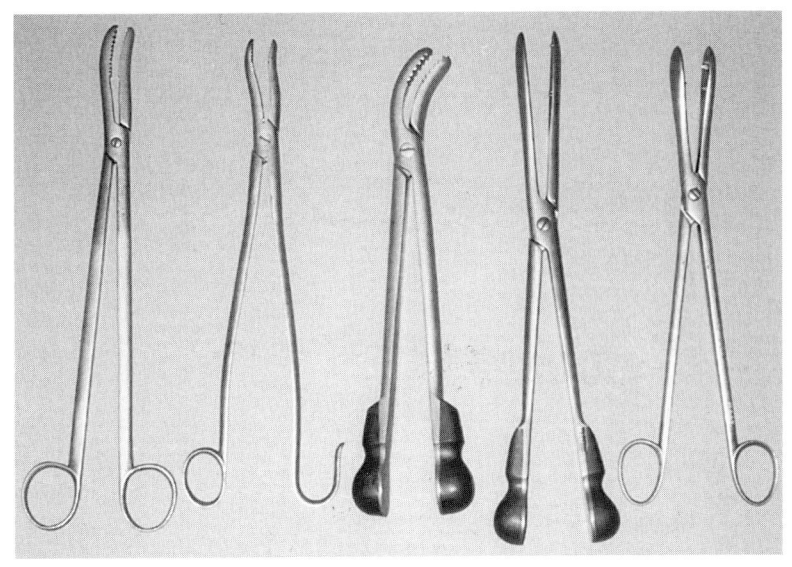

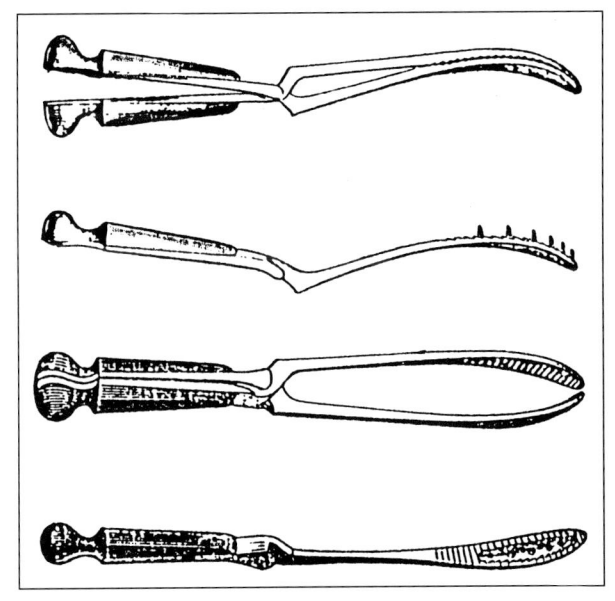

FIGURE 19.1 (ABOVE LEFT).
Mesnard's and Lyon's forceps. With the Mesnard *tenette à conducteur* (left), the longer blade was inserted in the cranium and the shorter blade outside. The Lyon forceps (right), intended for morcellement, was used with the outer blade between the scalp and the cranial bones. (A. R. Simpson, 1884b)

FIGURE 19.2 (ABOVE).
British nineteenth-century craniotomy forceps. There are many variations in design detail but they were usually of heavy construction with marked serrations on the blades (left). Some (right) have spoon-shaped blades with teeth. (RCOG)

FIGURE 19.3 (LEFT).
Ziegler's craniotomy and extracting forceps. The concave blade is used with either the toothed craniotomy blade or with the fenestrated extractor blade. (Ziegler, 1848–1849)

sacrifice the child; but then we know that almost all those cases occur among the poorest classes; that a large number of these children die within one year; that scarcely one-half live five years, and that life for many of the survivors is misery. Taking all these facts into consideration, I do not hesitate to perform craniotomy, even on the living child, when it is necessary in order to save the mother.

Simple but strong craniotomy forceps continued to be in general use in the late nineteenth century in America, as shown by the range of instruments illustrated in George Tiemann's 1889 catalogue (Figure 19.4).

COMMINUTORS AND COMMINUTOR-EXTRACTORS   235

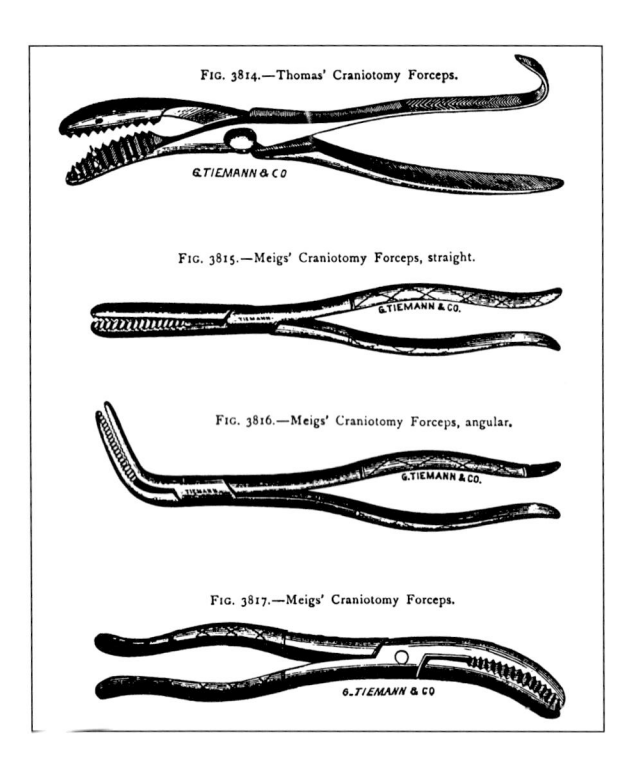

FIGURE 19.4.
American craniotomy forceps. A selection from the Tiemann catalogue. (Tiemann, 1889)

Punch Forceps for Craniotomy

When it was clear that there was no prospect of delivery of a live baby, David Davis was anxious to ensure that instrumental delivery should be achieved with minimal risk to the mother and his destructive instruments were designed to this end. Davis's osteotomists, or bone pliers (Figures 19.5–19.7), were advocated in extreme cases of pelvic distortion where other methods of delivery had failed. The original instrument (Figures 19.5, 19.6) combined the principles of both a punch and scissors and allowed the fetal skeleton to be broken down into fragments of about half an inch in diameter "with the most perfect impunity to the structure of the parts of the mother concerned in the operation." The use of osteotomists, he claimed, reduced the need for Caesarian section almost to zero (1825).

Davis's original oval punch was later supplemented by a longer blade designed to make long sections through, and in different directions across, the fetal skull (Figures 19.5, 19.7). Considerable cutting force was possible and, with the oval version, portions of bone 19 to 24 millimeters (.75 to 1 inch) were easily removed from the base of the skull as well as the parietes. Davis warned that the practitioner must guard against "his own fingers from being included within its uncompromisingly destructive action."

This principle of the punch was adopted later by Anderson of Liverpool, whose punch forceps had a spring-loaded handle for single-handed operation and an attached vulcanized tube to accept the debris (1870) (Figure 19.8).

The Role of Craniotomy

The differing practices in relation to the use of forceps and craniotomy are well illustrated by J. Hall Davis's data from eminent obstetricians of the time, which is contained in his *Illustrations of Difficult Parturition* (1858) (Table 19.1).
In spite of pleas by W. Tyler Smith (1815–1873), Physician Accoucheur, St. Mary's Hospital, London, to abolish the operation (1860), it remained popular in Britain but not on the Continent. Smith quoted figures previously gathered by

TABLE 19.1. The Frequency of Forceps Delivery and Craniotomy in Various British Practices (J. Hall Davis, 1858)

	Forceps	Craniotomy	Ratio Forceps:Craniotomy
J. Y. Simpson	1 in 472	1 in 1417	1:0.3
Lever	1 in 518	1 in 186	1:2.8
Churchill	1 in 546	1 in 149	1:3.7
Ramsbotham	1 in 611	1 in 805	1:0.8
Collins	1 in 617	1 in 141	1:4.4

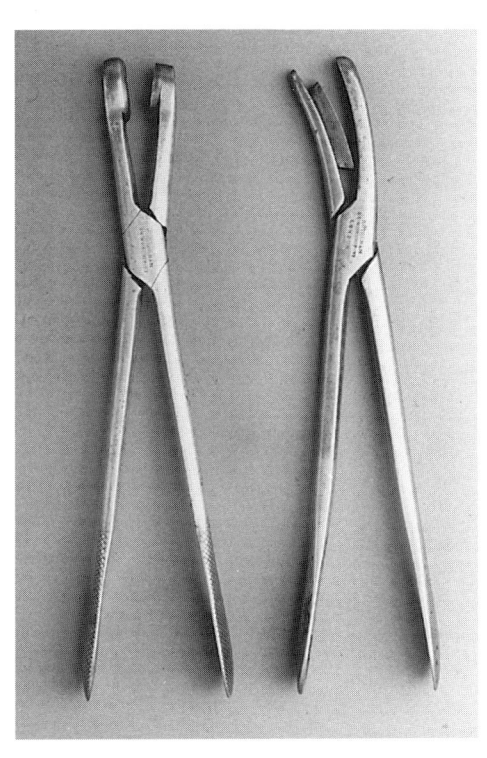

FIGURE 19.5 (LEFT).
Davis's osteotomists. The oval-bladed version (left) is the original design. The longitudinal version (right) was introduced later. (RCOG)

FIGURE 19.6 (BELOW LEFT).
Davis's oval osteotomist in use. Plate XVIII: The technique for piecemeal removal of the cranium is shown. (Davis, 1825)

FIGURE 19.7 (BELOW RIGHT).
Davis's longitudinal osteotomists. Plate XIX: These enable bigger pieces of cranium to be removed but, unlike the oval osteotomist, were not usable to destroy the basal bones. (Davis, 1825)

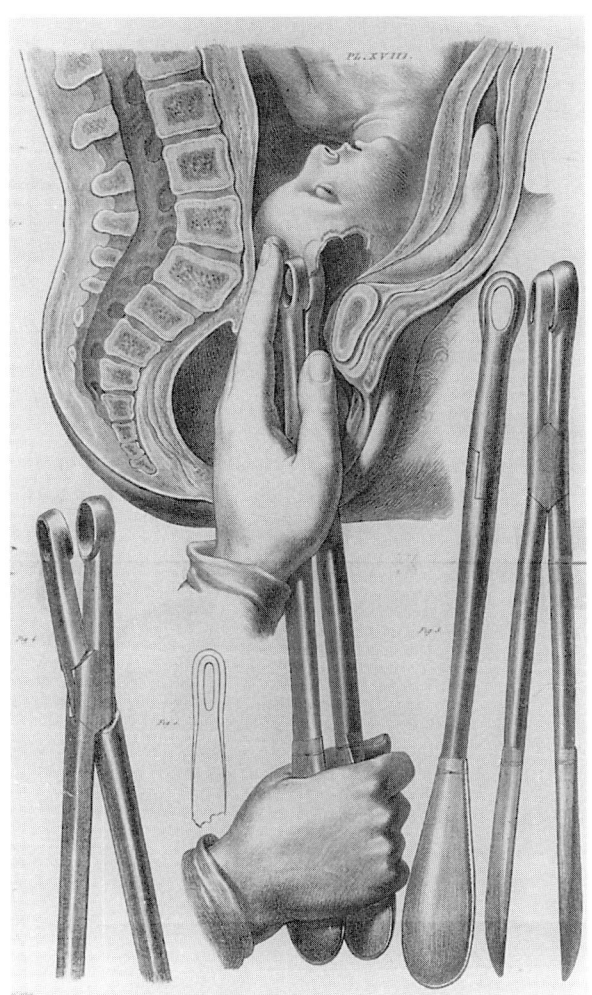

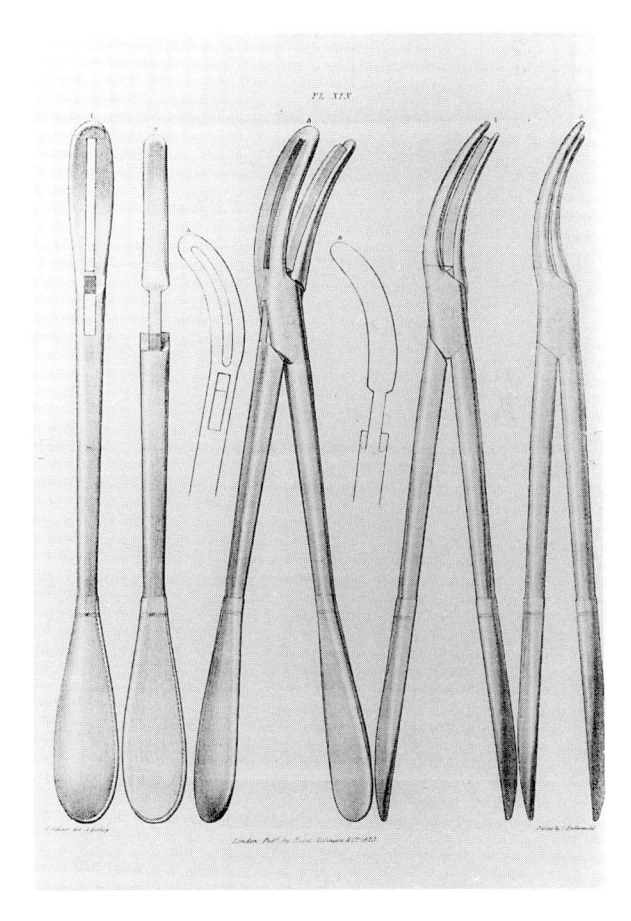

COMMINUTORS AND COMMINUTOR-EXTRACTORS

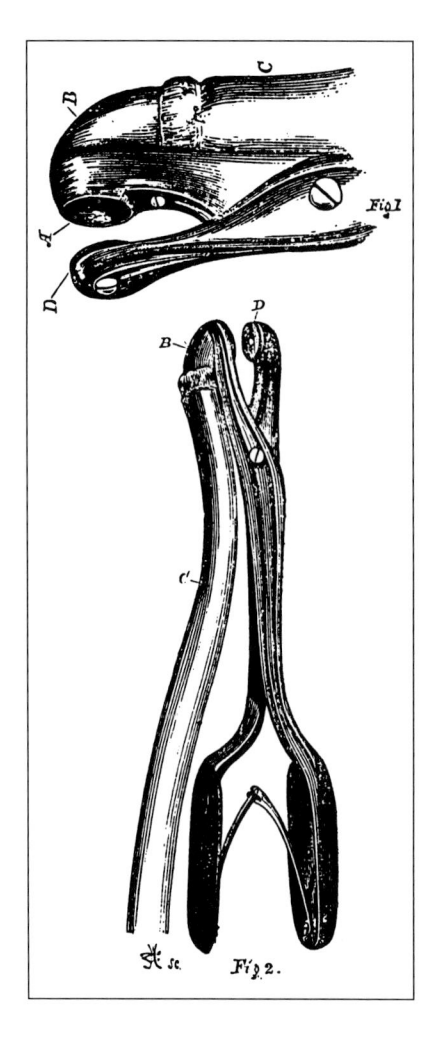

FIGURE 19.8.
Anderson's cranium punch forceps. A later development of Davis's osteotomists. (T. Anderson, 1870)

Lee (1844, 1875). He estimated the frequency of craniotomy in Britain as 1 in 340 births, twice that of France and four times that of Germany. Among the lowest figures were Baudelocque's 1 in 2898, in Paris, for he was apparently well known for his antagonism to the operation.

Later, Archibald Donald (1860–1937) of St. Mary's Hospital in Manchester attempted to put the role of craniotomy in perspective. He believed that the incidence of the operation had declined because delivery was more often achieved with axis-traction forceps in the lesser degrees of pelvic contraction and there was greater recourse to Caesarian section in the presence of a more severely contracted pelvis. He enumerated the circumstances in which the operation was justified:

(1) when persistent attempts with the forceps had failed. He advocated leaving the forceps on the head, perforating between the blades, and tightening the forceps to get a good traction grip;

(2) when podalic version had been performed and the head could not be extracted;

(3) when there was certainty or great probability that the child was dead, or there was fetal deformity that rendered the chance of surviving slender; and

(4) when there was maternal illness of a degree that would have made Caesarian section almost certainly fatal (1890).

Cephalotribes

Cephalotribes (head crushers) first appeared early in the nineteenth century and became widely used toward the middle of the century. They were powerful devices with a screw and wing nut on the handles and were designed with great mechanical advantage to crush and flatten the skull. They could also be used as extractors. Therefore, when they were intended for both purposes, compromises in design were required, especially in the shape and curve of the blades. Initially they were applied without preliminary perforation of the head but prior perforation soon became the preferred technique. Considering their brutal construction and unwieldiness they became remarkably popular. At the *Conversazione* of the Obstetrical Society of London in 1866 some seventeen different models were exhibited (Meadows, 1867).

The credit for the original instrument is generally ascribed to Assalini. His instrument, the *conquasator capitis* (Figure 19.9), comprised two heavy, solid, curved blades, joined at the ends of the handles (parallel blades as in his forceps) by a bar fixed to one side that fit into a slot on the other side, with a strong screw compressor one third of the way along the shaft. It was used for crushing the face and the base of the skull when the true conjugate was much less than 76 millimeters (3 inches) or for extraction after decapitation (1811). The only other parallel-bladed instrument traced was shown by Lazarewitch of Kharkov at the Obstetric Society in 1866 (Meadows, 1867). The model upon which most later developments were based was the instrument devised by L.-A. Baudelocque, J. L. Baudelocque's father (1836).

European Practice

European practice, particularly in the Viennese school, was well reviewed by Paul Fortunatus Mundé (b. 1846), Attending Physician, West Side German Dispensary, New York, and

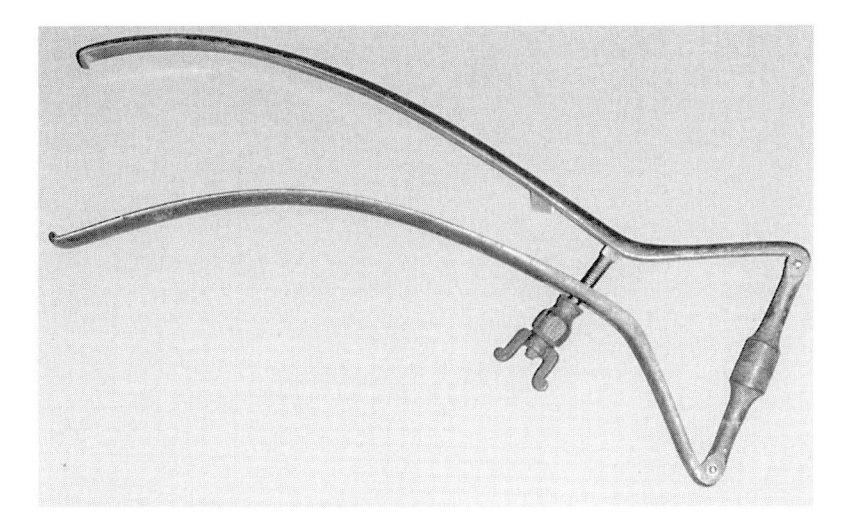

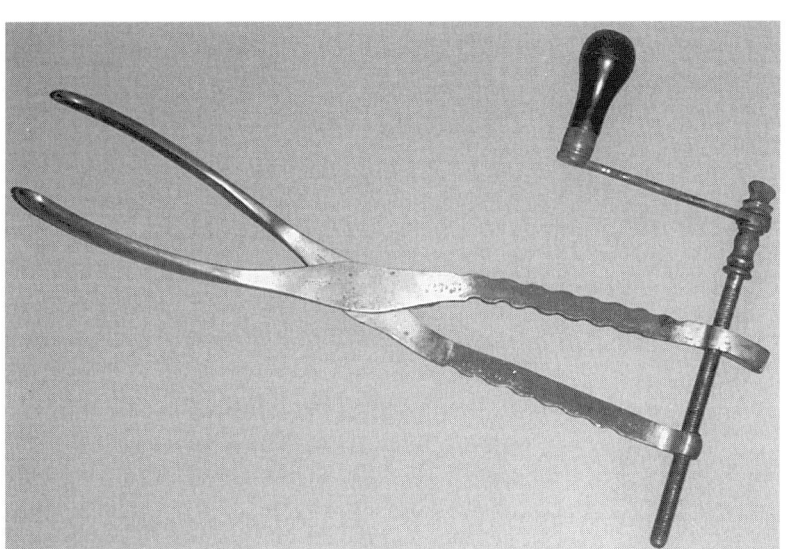

FIGURE 19.9.
Assalini's *conquasator capitis.* In spite of the heavy construction the crushing force is limited by the leverage system. (Royal College of Surgeons)

FIGURE 19.10.
Baudelocque's cephalotribe. The heavy (3.2kg) instrument was so powerful that it was used without preliminary perforation. (Trinity Centre for Health Sciences, Dublin)

a former assistant to Scanzoni. In his view the cephalotribe had "in all countries except England, maintained its superiority, and been universally acknowledged and used as the most convenient, efficient, and least dangerous instrument for the compression and extraction of the foetal head after perforation in cases of deformed pelvis" (1873). The cephalotribe soon became the favorite method of comminution on the Continent, with many modifications in design, a common feature being curved blades that reflected their extractive function. However there were dissenters even on the Continent. When the cephalotribe was used almost exclusively in cases that could not be delivered with forceps, Carl Hennig (b. 1825) of Leipzig (see Wiener, 1878) showed by experiment that while the instrument diminished the diameter of the head in one direction it increased it in all others and, in spite of designing his own instrument (see below), he regarded it as inherently dangerous.

L.-A. Baudelocque designed his cephalotribe as a consequence of being appalled after witnessing the extensive trauma and death of a patient with a true conjugate of 63 millimeters (2.5 inches) who was delivered by the use of perforators and crotchets. His instrument, which had a winch handle, was 610 millimeters (24 inches) long and its weight was over 3.2 kilograms (7 pounds) (Figure 19.10). It was designed to crush both the parietes and the base of the skull, forcing the brain through the nose, orbits, and mouth. The skin and integuments remained intact to form a protective sac and thereby reduce maternal injury from fetal bone fragments. It is of some interest that Baudelocque embarked on this crushing procedure without prior perforation, contrary to the perceived wisdom of the time, and he envisaged that his instrument would replace the perforator and crotchet. He first described the instrument in 1829. In 1833, he was honored by the Academy of Sciences of Paris with a prize of

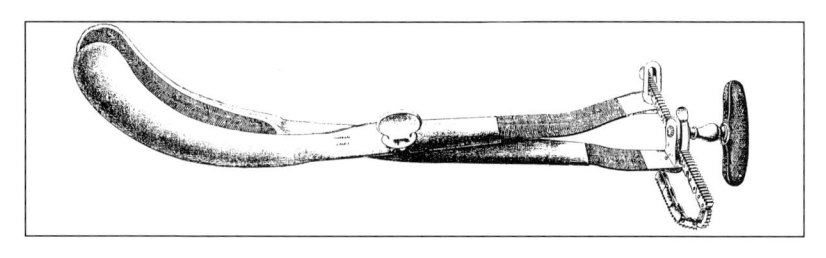

FIGURES 19.11–19.13.
Some late nineteenth-century European heavy cephalotribes. 19.11: Pajot: This has a simple chain-ratchet mechanism (Pajot, 1863). 19.12: Hennig's *Kephalotryptor à crochets*: The movable crotchets on the inner surfaces of the blades are controlled by hooks on the handles (Hennig, 1859). 19.13: Kilian: A robust device of even greater mechanical potential. (Kilian, 1835)

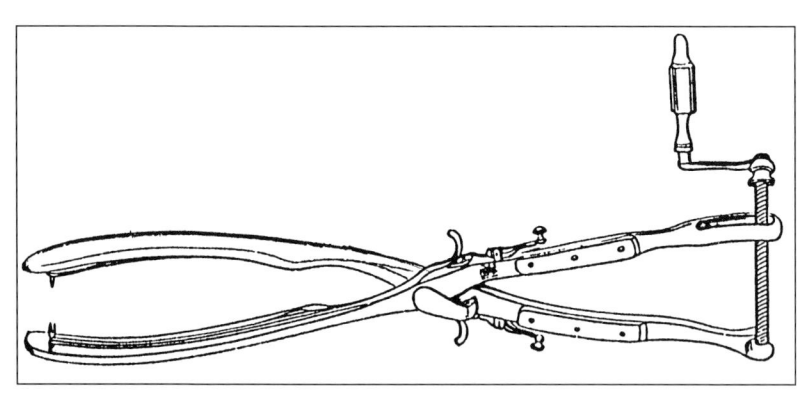

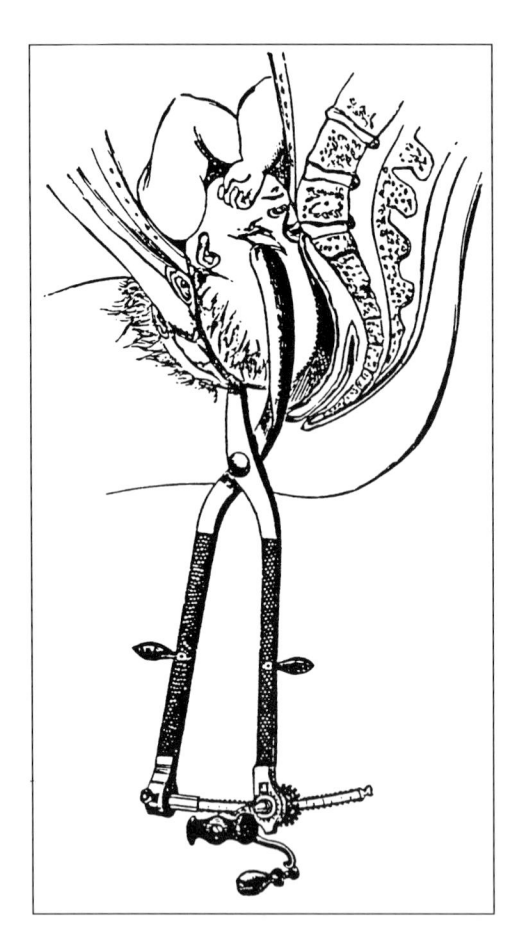

two thousand francs, although a published description of his instrument and its use in fifteen cases did not appear until 1836.

Many variations of heavy instruments that followed the Baudelocque tradition were eventually available. Pajot's cephalotribe (1863) (Figure 19.11; see also Ritchie, 1865), also originating in Paris, was of even heavier construction but had a simpler chain ratchet mechanism on the ends of the handles for compression. Pajot gave detailed instructions for its use and application. His method was to crush the head, three or four times if necessary, but not to apply traction. Following the passage of the head the thorax could be treated in a similar manner.

Hennig invented his *Kephalotryptor à crochets* in 1865 and exhibited it at the Obstetrical Society in 1866 (Figure 19.12). It was a massive instrument, 610 millimeters (24 inches) long, and operated by a winch similar to that of Baudelocque. In addition two crotchets were concealed on the inner surfaces of the blades and they could be advanced or retracted by two hooks on the handles.

Kilian of Bonn also favored a massive instrument that was 635 millimeters (25 inches) long (Figure 19.13). The compression force was obtained by a winch and pinion in one handle working on a rack attached to the other handle. Kilian claimed to have broken up the skull into fifty-four pieces with a single application of the instrument! (1835)

Nicolas Charles Chailly-Honoré (1805–1866), unlike Baudelocque, considered that perforation should always be carried out prior to use of the cephalotribe and this became

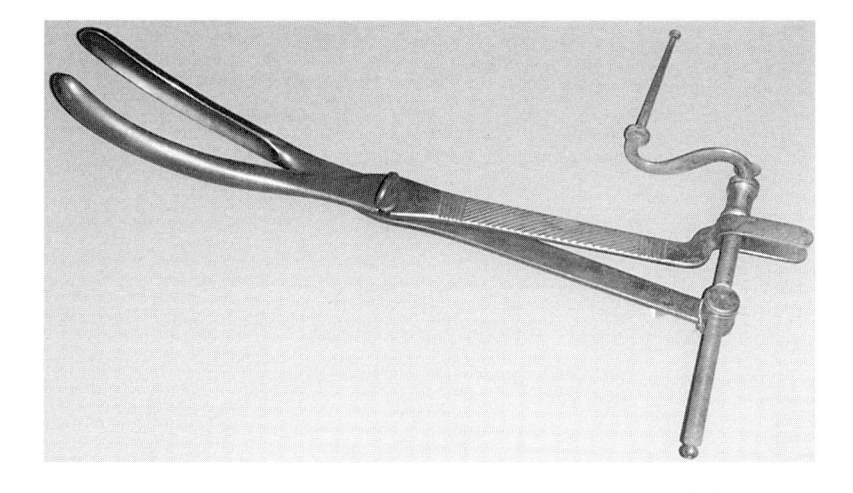

FIGURE 19.14.
Rizzoli's cephalotribe. An Italian lighter version of Baudelocque's cephalotribe. (Royal College of Surgeons)

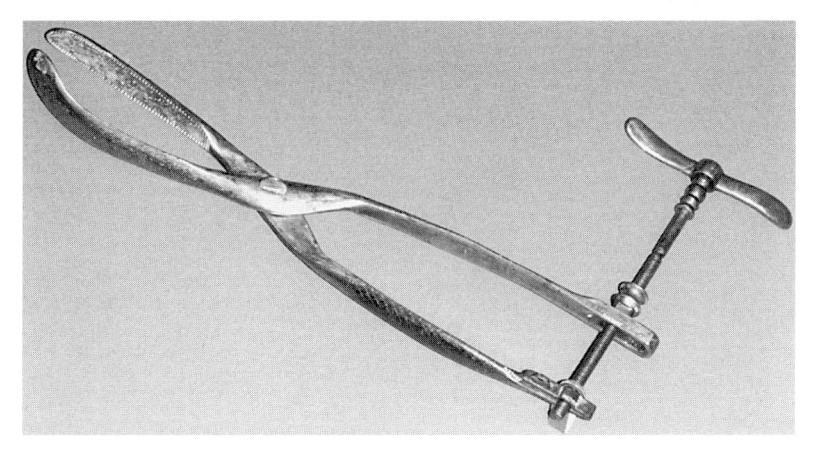

FIGURE 19.15.
Locarelli's cephalotribe. Another lighter Italian instrument. (Science Museum, London)

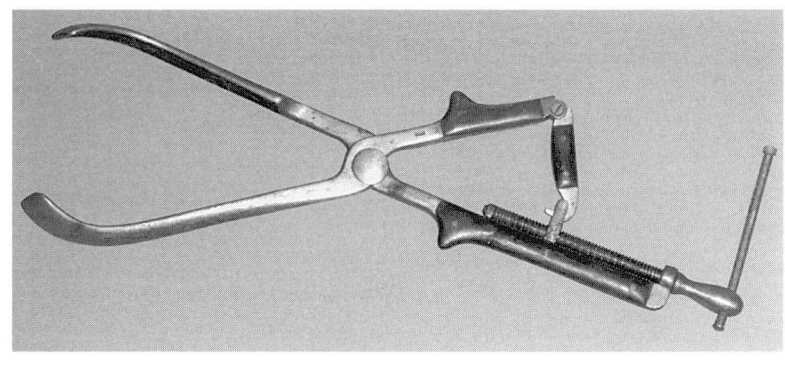

FIGURE 19.16.
Braun's cephalotribe. Note the Brunninghausen lock and the complex mechanics. (Trinity Centre for Health Sciences, Dublin)

the usual practice, making possible the use of lighter instruments (1844). One of the earlier lighter designs came from Rizzoli of Bologna (1856). Although based on the Baudelocque instrument it was only 495 millimeters (19.5 inches) long and weighed only 1.6 kilograms (3 pounds, 9 ounces) (Figure 19.14; see also Meadows, 1867). A similar instrument was marketed by Locarelli (Figure 19.15).

The Viennese school also preferred cephalotripsy to the use of the crotchet. The skull was perforated with the Mende's trephine (Figure 18.14). Braun's cephalotribe (see Ritchie, 1865) (Figure 19.16) was relatively light by European standards and was 406 millimeters (16 inches) long, with a Brunninghausen button-and-slot articulation. The maximum width of the blades was just over 50 millimeters (2 inches). The inner surface was serrated, with three longitudinal ridges to improve the grip. A rather complex winding mechanism to close the blades comprised a hinged joint and hook on one handle that fit into a nut on a long screw on

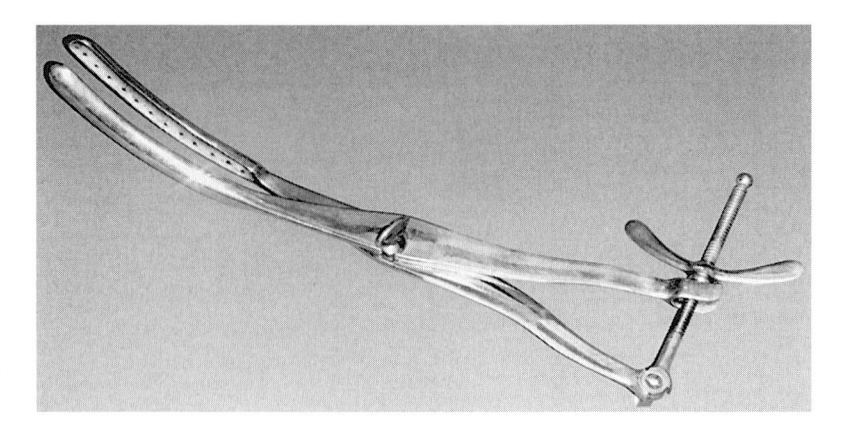

FIGURE 19.17.
Blot's cephalotribe. The blades are long and curved, with serrations on the concave inner surface. (Science Museum, London)

FIGURE 19.18.
Scanzoni's cephalotribe. The design limits the amount of compressive force, as in Assalini's instrument. (Royal College of Surgeons)

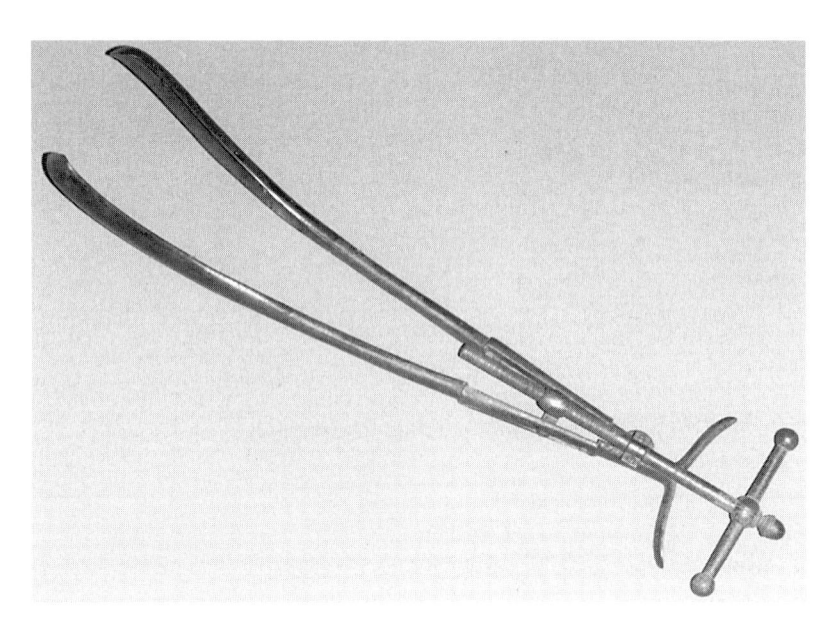

the other handle. When Charles George Ritchie (1842–1875) presented the Pajot and Braun instruments, together with Braun's perforator, at the Obstetrical Society of London in 1865, Robert Barnes and Graily Hewitt both preferred the Braun instrument.

Blot's (1855) and Scanzoni's (1853) cephalotribes (Figures 19.17, 19.18) both had curved blades. Scanzoni's instrument was about 535 millimeters (21 inches) long. The blades had a pelvic curve and were sharply curved inward to meet at their extremities, the maximum distance between the blades being 38 millimeters (1.5 inches). The inner surfaces of the blades were concave with a longitudinal ridge.

British Practice

As with the forceps, cephalotribes of different types were developed in Britain and on the Continent, the latter generally being heavier, unwieldy, and formidable in appearance. However, cephalotripsy was hardly ever practiced in Britain until the 1860s. Even as late as 1866 the influential Fleetwood Churchill in the fifth edition of his textbook, *On the Theory and Practice of Midwifery*, concluded that "[i]t would require unusual hardihood to venture upon the latter instrument [the cephalotribe] in private practice in this country."

A. R. Simpson brought Scanzoni's cephalotribe back to Britain in 1858 and gave it to his uncle, J. Y. Simpson, who used it, favored it, and modified it, making it much lighter and shorter (400 millimeters/14.5 inches), with only a slight pelvic curve (Figure 19.19, left). When he first exhibited his new design to the Edinburgh Obstetric Society in 1864 (Simpson, 1867), he had not actually used it. He then decried the cranioclast in favor of his cephalotribe. He emphasized the high mortality with the cranioclast, quoting Churchill's figures, and related several anecdotes, including a case of A. R. Hamilton's in which Hamilton took eight hours to remove the whole arch of the cranium with the cranioclast. The outcome for the patient was not stated but

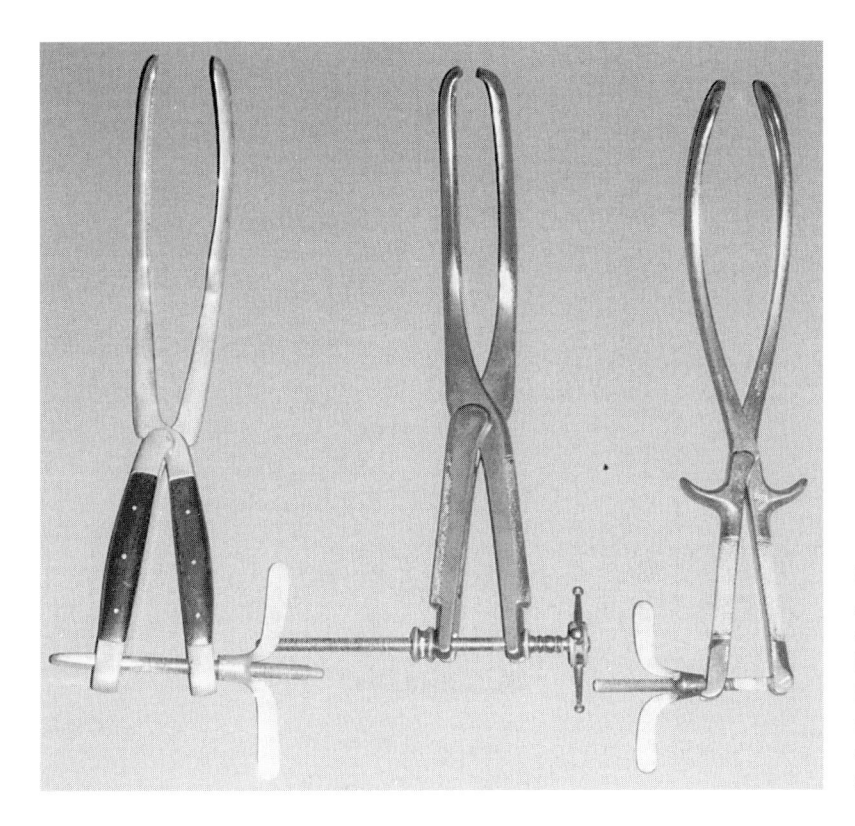

FIGURE 19.19.
J. Y. Simpson's, Hicks's, and Smith's cephalotribes. Simpson's instrument (left) was a lighter, shorter version of the original Baudelocque. Braxton Hicks (center) reverted to nearer the heavy Continental style. Smith (right) adopted the fenestrated blade (page 245). (Science Museum, London)

the exhausted Hamilton had to be rolled in blankets and carried home!

Braxton Hicks described his own cephalotribe (Figure 19.19, center), similar to that of J. Y. Simpson, which he subsequently modified and strengthened with a powerful detachable screw on the handles and blades that approximated almost as much as the French versions. His instrument, with incurved tips, was designed to provide efficient traction and to obtain a good grip without having to use great force to crush the base of the skull (1869). The previous practice had been to remove the cephalotribe, which allowed some reexpansion of the skull, and to complete the delivery with crotchet or craniotomy forceps. An alternative was to wait for some hours to see if the natural powers produced any advance, or even longer to allow decomposition to assist. According to Hicks the latter had been advocated by Pajot.

Mathews Duncan (1869, 1870) was critical of the British cephalotribes based on J. Y. Simpson's short-handled model, which he considered ill-adapted to their primary purpose of crushing because the blades were too long and flexible and, when closed, were too far apart, an opinion shared by the French. Mathews Duncan compared the measurements of a typical Parisian (modified Baudelocque) instrument with the design in common use in Edinburgh (J. Y. Simpson) and designated them as long-handled and short-handled respectively. The long-handled version measured 520 millimeters (20.5 inches) overall, compared with 368 millimeters (14.5 inches) for the short version. The difference was almost entirely in the length of the handles—268 millimeters (10.5 inches) compared with 127 millimeters (5 inches). The maximum gaps between the blades were, respectively, 18 millimeters (0.5 inches) and 32 millimeters (1.25 inches). Duncan devised his own instrument (Figure 19.20) based on the Parisian pattern but with a simplified pivot that had a broad top, a stronger screw, and a reduced pelvic curve. The handles were broader and thinner. Braxton Hicks was quick to respond to Duncan's criticisms and, in the British tradition, saw virtue in the lighter instruments for most occasions. In fact, Hicks demonstrated a stronger version of his original design so it seems that a compromise had been reached (1869).

George H. Kidd of Dublin (Chapter 6), who had been introduced to J. Y. Simpson's cephalotribe by A. R. Simpson and used it for some time, preferred straight blades, which were easier to apply and gave a better grip (Figure 19.21). Like many of the Continental practitioners, such as Pajot, he favored multiple applications of the blades. He reported a successful delivery of a woman with a reputed true conjugate of 45 millimeters (1.75 inches) (1867).

Although cephalotripsy did continue to be employed in Britain, the foremost writers in the latter part of the eighteenth century gave it little support. William Leishman (1834–

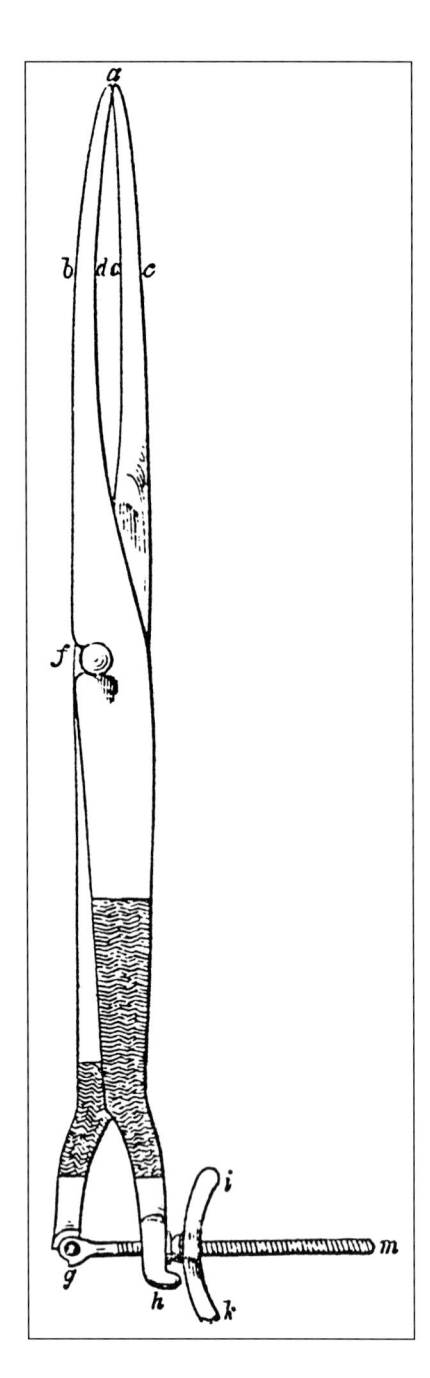

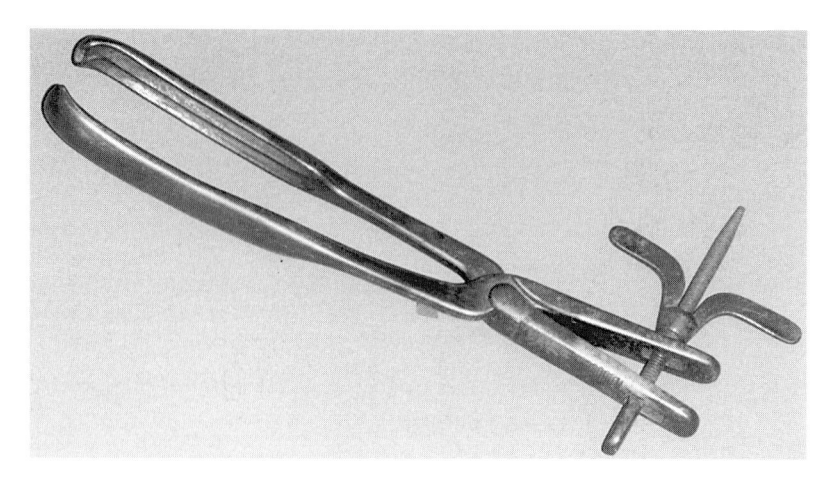

FIGURE 19.20 (LEFT).
Mathews Duncan's cephalotribe. Duncan was critical of his mentor's and related designs and reverted to the Parisian style. (Duncan, 1870)

FIGURE 19.21 (ABOVE).
Kidd's cephalotribe. This also is a reversion to the straight Continental blades which, he claimed, gave a better grip. (Royal College of Surgeons)

1894), Professor of Midwifery, University of Glasgow, gave a very detailed description and critique of destructive operations with a very conservative attitude to their use, especially cephalotripsy, even though he quoted the mortality from Caesarian section at that time as 85 percent (1880). F. H. Ramsbotham, in the 1867 edition of his textbook, made no mention of the procedure.

American Practice

Various models of the cephalotribe were in common use in America in the late nineteenth and into the twentieth century as is illustrated by the writings of the time (Wallace, 1878; Lusk, 1882; Crockett, 1907), but it seems that in general practitioners were content to use designs imported from Europe. George Tiemann's catalogue of 1889 lists only one original American design, that of Lusk, although Ellerslie Wallace of Jefferson Medical College of Philadelphia, described his modification of European designs, which he did by adding teeth to the inner surfaces of the blades (1878).

Lusk believed that the cephalotribe was not held in the esteem that it merited. He considered that it was unproductive to try to promote a single instrument, which could "lead to embarrassment and failure," and that all obstetricians should have a range of instruments (1869). His own instrument is described below under "Fenestrated Cephalotribes."

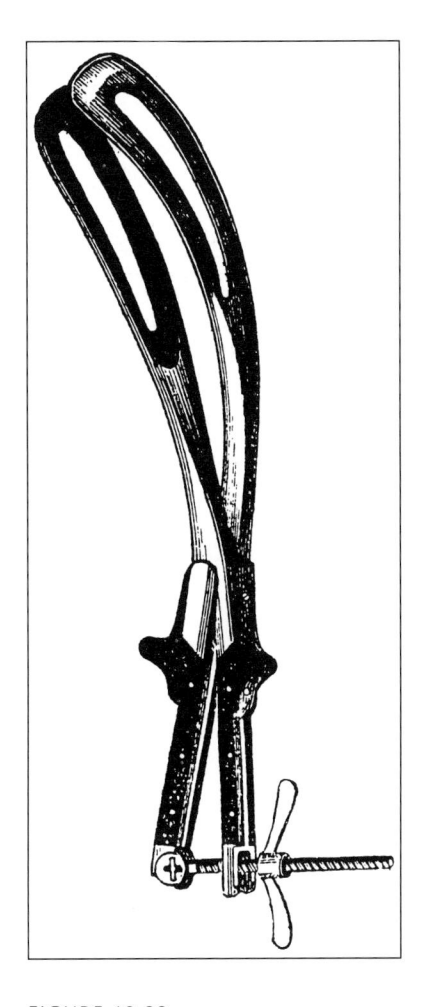

FIGURE 19.22.
Martin's fenestrated cephalotribe. This is probably the first fenestrated cephalotribe. Although it originated in Berlin it has many British features. (Martin, 1873)

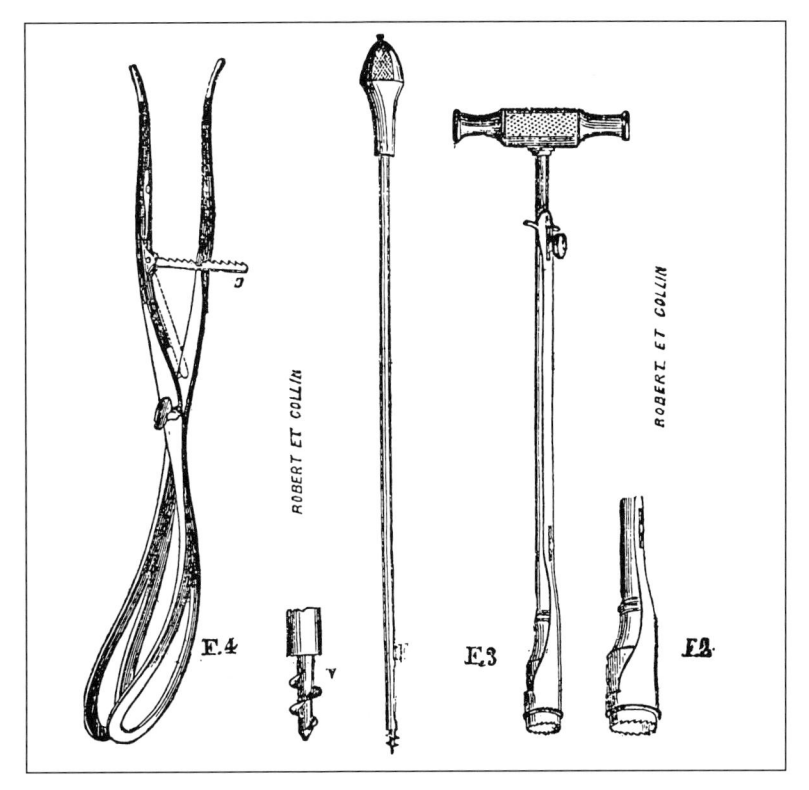

FIGURE 19.23.
Guyon's instruments. The cephalotribe (left) has relatively flexible fenestrated blades. The corkscrew pointed stylet (center) is screwed into the sphenoid and acts as a guide for the trephine (right). (Guyon, 1867)

Fenestrated Cephalotribes

Another development seen in Britain and America and on the Continent was the fenestrated blade. Eduard Martin of Berlin (Chapter 5) may have been the originator of this for his design was shown at the *Conversazione* of 1866 (Meadows, 1867) and was described by his son, A. E. Martin, when he presented the original instrument to the Obstetrical Society of London in 1872. It was 430 millimeters (17 inches) in length, with an English lock and a wing nut and screw on the handle (Figure 19.22). The blades were double-curved and fenestrated. The president of the Obstetrical Society at the time was Braxton Hicks and not surprisingly he endorsed the use of the cephalotribe, which he believed would ultimately almost entirely supersede other instruments for use after perforation.

About the same time Jean Casmir Felix Guyon (b. 1831) of Paris presented a much lighter design with more flexible blades (Figure 19.23), which was used after perforation and trephining (1867; see also Kalindero, 1870). It was more of a modified long forceps with blades which approximated to 30 millimeters (1.25 inches) at their widest part. Although it was called a cephalotribe the compression force must have been limited. It might also be considered as a basilyst since an essential part of the procedure was to screw the corkscrew-pointed stylet into the sphenoid and use it as a guide for the smaller trephine to drill out a disk of the skull base, a procedure that could be repeated two or three times if necessary.

James Smith of Belfast used straight fenestrated blades with the inner surfaces serrated. These features allowed the

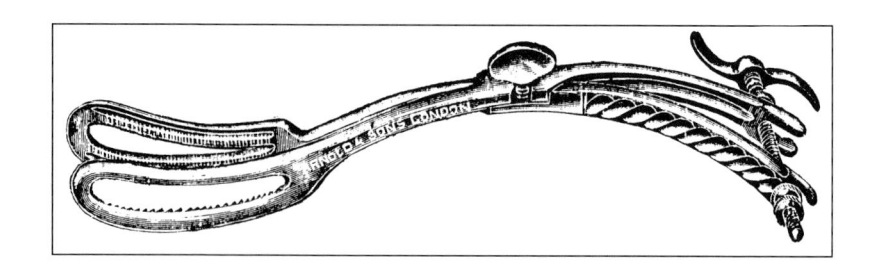

FIGURE 19.24.
Fancourt Barnes's fenestrated cephalotribe. The curved handle is intended to improve the direction of traction and serves as a perineal step. (Barnes and Barnes, 1885)

FIGURE 19.25.
Lusk's cephalotribe. An amalgam of desirable features from older designs. (Lusk, 1869)

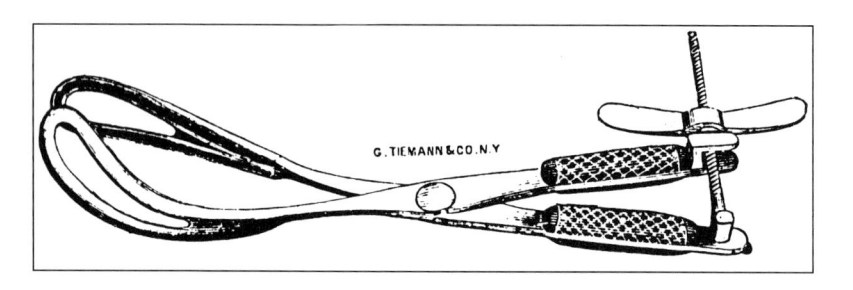

FIGURE 19.26.
Valette's cephalotribe. A three-bladed instrument of complex design and great strength. (Tarnier, 1870)

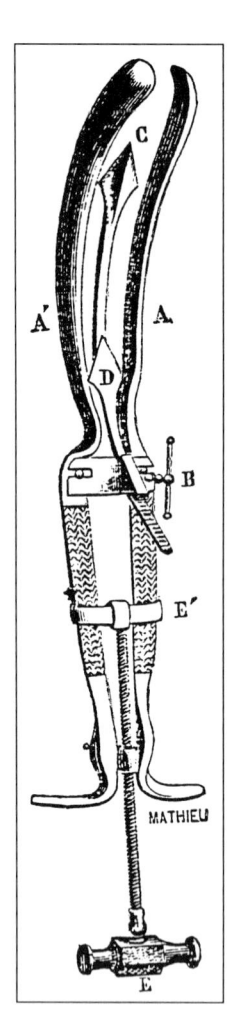

head to bulge through the fenestra and gave a better grip for extraction. The instrument was only 380 millimeters (15 inches) long, with short handles (Figure 19.19, right). Smith expounded upon the Continental virtue of weight, not only in the instrument but also in the maternity physician. He claimed that to be efficient the physician "should overbalance 12 stone whilst the occupant of the masters chair should counterpoise at least 16 stone" (1884).

Fancourt Barnes's instrument (Figure 19.24; see also Arnold and Sons, 1885) had a third curve on the principle of an axis-traction forceps that reduced the amount of traction force required. Robert Barnes claimed that this was the best cephalotribe available, combining lightness with power (1869a).

In America Lusk made a thoughtful analysis of the mechanism of cephalotripsy and recombined what he considered to be the best features of older models that had stood the test of time, minimizing the more repulsive features that he believed had constituted an impediment to their adoption. His cephalotribe (Figure 19.25) was of similar principle to but was lighter than most designs of the time. Fenestrated blades had an outer measurement of 57 millimeters (2.25 inches). The cephalic and pelvic curves made them stronger and more efficient for extraction, as in the Prague design. The articulation was of the Brunninghausen type and the handles were fitted with a wing nut and screw (1869). Lusk described its use in more detail in the 1882 edition of his book, *The Science and Art of Midwifery*. After perforation he did not wait for putrefaction to occur but proceeded to extraction as soon as the cervix was sufficiently dilated for "safety."

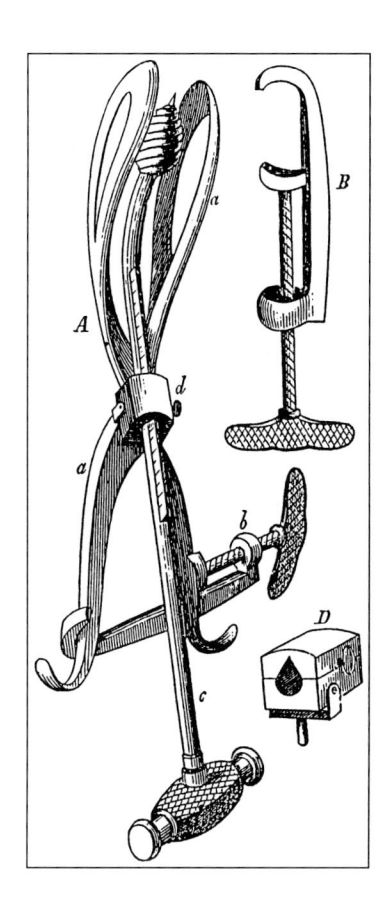

FIGURE 19.27.
Lollini's cephalotribe. The design has features in common with the basilyst. (Tarnier, 1870)

Combined Instruments

Cephalotribes that functioned also as perforators, comminutors, and extractors, became widely known. Examples of these were shown and explained by Tarnier (1883). The earliest was devised by Valette of Lyons in 1857, based on the *forceps lyonnais* (Figure 19.26). It was a complex three-bladed instrument that incorporated a perforator worked by a screw mechanism and a novel worm-screw device for apposing the blades.

In 1867 another combined instrument was invented by the brothers Lollini, instrument makers in Bologna, Italy, but it is more properly considered as a basilyst (Figure 19.27) as its function was primarily to crush the base of the skull. The instrument comprised very heavy curved fenestrated blades and a rather crude clamp with a screw mechanism to draw the handles together. A pear-shaped, graduated screw perforator to insert into the base of the skull with a cross handle was attached by a block to the joint of the blades. Both the Valette and Lollini instruments were remarkable for their solid construction and their capability of a powerful compression force because of their mechanical design. Lollini's instrument also served as an ordinary forceps.

Cranioclasts

Cranioclasts had their origin in Britain and were not introduced until some time after cephalotribes were in general use in Europe. They are essentially large-bladed craniotomy forceps of a more sophisticated and functional design. In the published descriptions and instrument catalogues they are frequently called craniotomy forceps. They were designed to crush the base of the skull, which in the very narrow pelvis often caused difficulty even after craniotomy of the vault bones.

The usual procedure of the time for severe cases of disproportion was to perforate the forecoming head but it was often difficult to diminish the base of the skull adequately. To overcome this difficulty Braxton Hicks's (1867) method of converting the presentation to a face by means of a hook fixed in the orbit was usually adopted. This method was subsequently superseded by the use of the cephalotribe. Donald, however, was a strong advocate of podalic version, followed by perforation through the roof of the mouth and traction on the trunk with, if necessary, cephalotripsy. He claimed that the base of the skull was more effectively broken up and the head was well fixed during the procedure (1890).

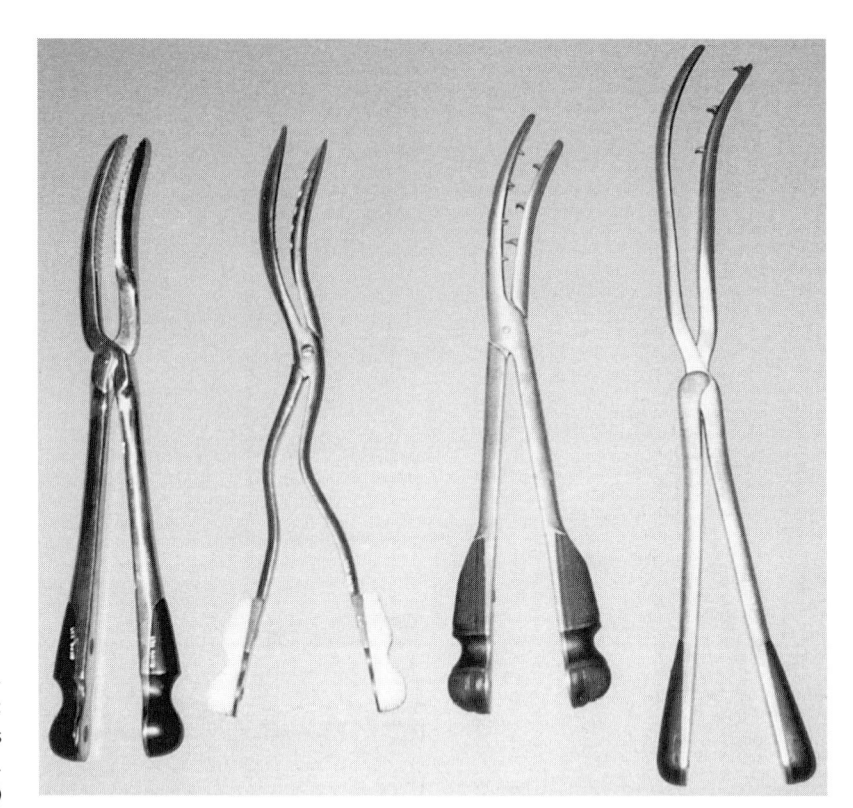

FIGURE 19.28.
Early British cranioclasts. From left to right: Lever, Conquest, Holmes, Ramsbotham. Holmes and Ramsbotham both added sharp teeth. (RCOG)

FIGURE 19.29.
Close up of the blades of Holmes's and Ramsbotham's cranioclasts. (RCOG)

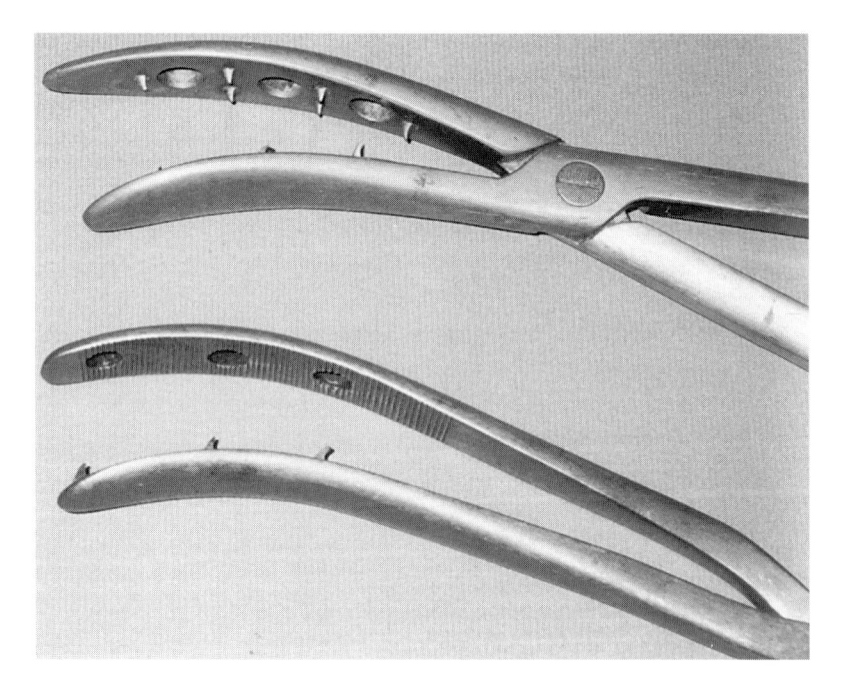

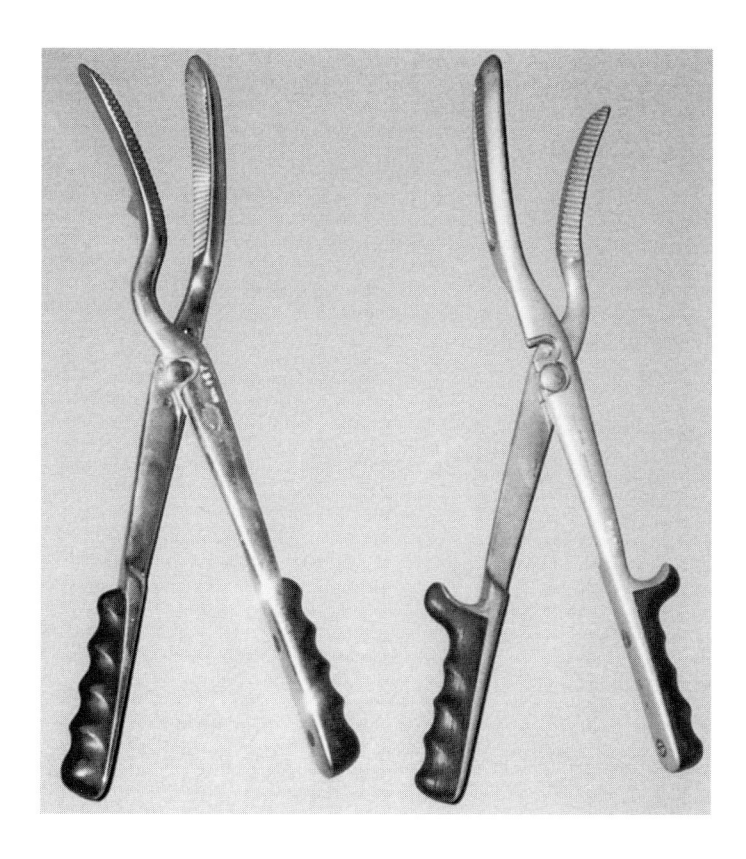

FIGURE 19.30.
Simpson's original and improved cranioclasts. The original model (left) has a single joint and no finger lugs. The improved model (right) has a second joint for cases of gross distortion and finger lugs for greater traction power. (RCOG)

Correspondence in the medical press of the time suggests much rivalry as to who could deliver through the smallest pelvis, but earlier claims such as Osborn's to have delivered successfully through a true conjugate of 38 millimeters (1.5 inches) were usually met with disbelief, the more polite critics pointing to the inaccuracy of pelvimetric assessment (Chapter 22).

Early in the nineteenth century stronger craniotomy forceps designs with greater mechanical advantage were appearing, some of which are shown in Figure 19.28, although they were not strictly cranioclasts.

Conquest illustrated his own cranioclast in a paper in 1820 (Conquest, 1820b) and recorded in the sixth edition of his *Outlines of Midwifery* (1837) procedures to reduce the bulk of the head by what he called *cephalatomia*. He recalled that Haighton in his lectures exhibited a pair of lithotomy forceps that he regarded as being a valuable substitute for the crotchet in some cases. Conquest designed his own instrument (Figure 19.28) but spoke favorably of David Davis's model, which had large teeth on the inner surface of one blade and three corresponding cavities on the other blade, a feature also seen in Holmes's and Ramsbotham's forceps (Figures 19.28, 19.29). Conquest concluded that, because of safety, simplicity, ease of application, and adaptability, the cranioclast would eventually supersede the crotchet. Even the conservative Blundell opted for Holmes's forceps (1834).

The purpose of the sharp teeth was to get a better grip on the tissues but, especially if the fetus was macerated, pieces of head were often torn away, leaving dangerous spicules of bone likely to lacerate the birth canal and make extraction with any other instrument difficult. Many obstetricians therefore reverted to toothless forceps with a serrated surface. Generally the instruments were also used for traction when necessary but to optimize this function it was necessary that the blades be parallel and have internal serrations to ensure a firm grasp and avoid tearing the scalp.

According to A. R. Simpson (1884b), J. Y. Simpson, in his *Clinical Lectures* (1872), detailed a case in 1858 in which he had perforated and comminuted the fetal head with craniotomy forceps and then awaited further progress. The head descended into the pelvis and after delivery he observed that the base of the skull was fractured (accidentally). This made him realize the importance of reducing the base of the skull and he designed an instrument that would achieve this, which he called a *cranioclast* (Figure 19.30). This terminology conforms with A. R. Simpson's classification, indicating that the function of the instrument was wider than that of the early craniotomy forceps. However many subsequent designs of cranioclasts were referred to as craniotomy forceps and vice versa.

J. Y. Simpson's original cranioclast comprised two blades with a crossover button and groove joint and handles simi-

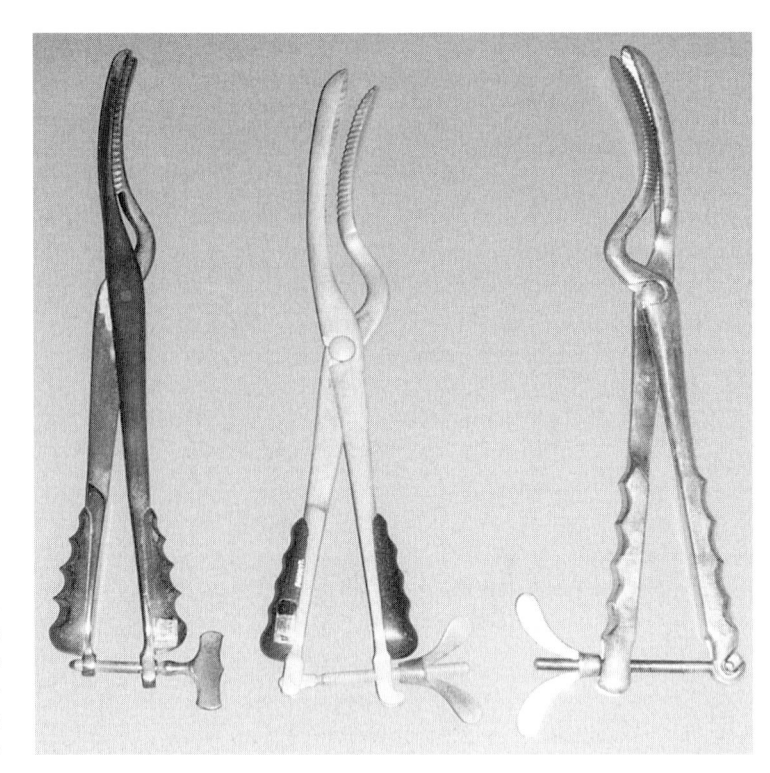

FIGURE 19.31.
Barnes's cranioclasts. There are many variations but the essential distinguishing features are the shape of the first blade, designed to accommodate scalp folds, and the screw at the end of the handles. (Science Museum, London)

FIGURE 19.32.
Hall Davis's cranioclast. The blades have deep serrations and grooves. The handles have a ratchet catch. (Science Museum, London)

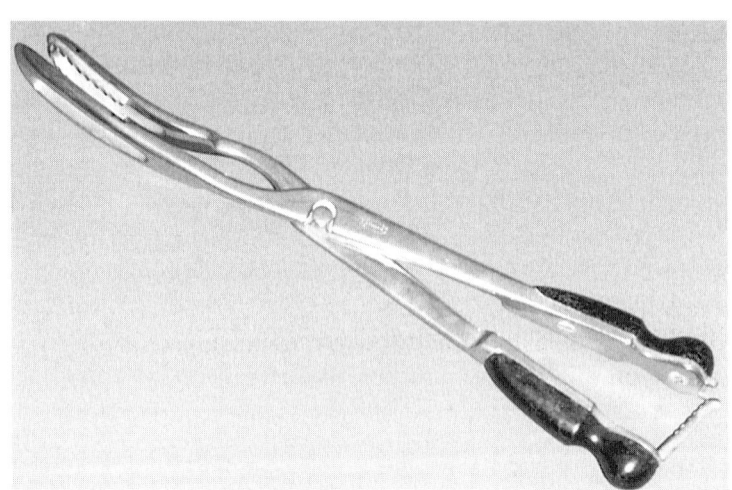

lar to those of his long forceps. The larger blade was fenestrated and grooved and was applied to the outer surface of the head, while the smaller was solid and ridged and was applied inside the cranium. The mode of use, after perforation and application, was to twist the instrument and wrench off portions of the cranial bones. His early model did not have finger lugs for traction but these were added later. He also added a second groove joint to facilitate locking in cases of gross distortion.

In the second half of the nineteenth century a wide range of minor variants based on J. Y. Simpson's patterns appeared. Generally there was a preference for the Brunninghausen button-and-slot articulation because this allowed the blades to be inserted independently and easily locked afterward.

Robert Barnes built on the designs of his predecessors and included what was called an "elbow" on the inner surfaces of the base of the blades to accommodate the scalp fold and therefore allowed deeper penetration of the blades and a

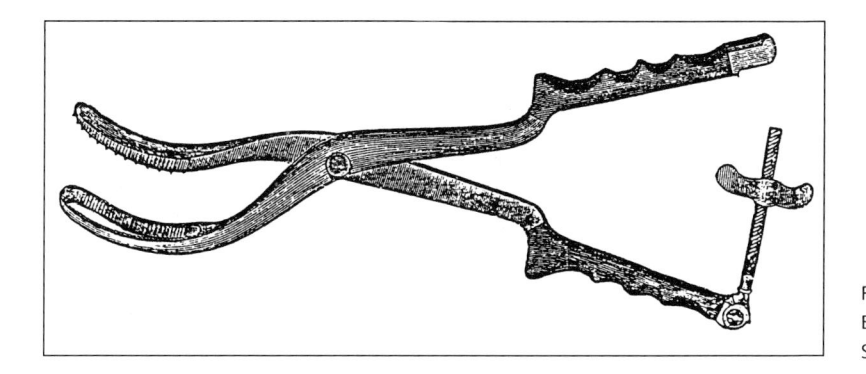

FIGURE 19.33.
Braun's cranioclast. A heavier version of Simpson's instrument. (Braun, 1859)

better grip. He also added a screw mechanism at the extremities of the handles to give a strong grip and fixation (1864) (Figure 19.31).

Hall Davis's forceps had deep serrations on the male blade that fit into corresponding grooves on the female blade (1865). He later added a ratchet catch at the tips of the handles (Figure 19.32).

European Practice

Simpson's instrument was much tried on the Continent, especially in Vienna, but generally met with disfavor, being considered as just an improved bone forceps and inferior to the cephalotribe.

However, Carl Braun of Vienna (see Mundé, 1873) took up Simpson's idea, envisaging the original instrument principally as a tractor, for which purpose it was preferable to the cephalotribe. His version of Simpson's instrument (Figure 19.33) was longer (445 millimeters/17.5 inches) and stronger and, like Barnes, for compression he added a screw and a wing nut to the handle to increase the mechanical advantage. Following this the cranioclast became adopted in Germany and most of the rest of Europe, in many places superseding cephalotripsy. Mundé proposed the term *craniotractor,* thus emphasizing its main function in Continental practice (1873).

Basilysts and Related Instruments

In general, there was dissatisfaction with the cranioclast's ability to crush the base of the skull adequately, especially among obstetricians who attempted delivery through grossly contracted pelves. One of the first obstetricians to emphasize the importance of reducing the base of the skull as well as the vault was Guyon of Paris (1867), whose apparatus is described above under the section "Cephalotribes." A variety of devices that turned out to be unsatisfactory in practice were reviewed by A. R. Simpson (1880, 1884b).

The first reasonably practical device designed specifically for crushing the base of the skull was that of L. J. Hubert from Louvain, who in 1860 suggested to the Academy of Medicine in Brussels an instrument for what he called *sphenotresia,* later called *transforation* (1860a). This instrument was an olive-shaped screw on a long shaft that was screwed into the base of the skull, the same principle as the *terebellum* described earlier by Antoine Louis Dugès (1797–1838), a professor at the Faculty of Medicine in Montpellier, with the addition of a thin, unfenestrated blade (1826). This blade was hinged to the main shaft and then passed over the head. It had a terminal groove that fit over the tip of the screw (Figure 19.34). L. J. Hubert's son, E. Hubert, subsequently reported favorably on its use in practice (1878).

The problem of, and need for, crushing the base of the skull were extensively reviewed and the earlier instruments were further developed by A. R. Simpson (1880, 1884a,b) in his *basilyst* (Figure 19.35), which had the advantage of simplicity. The basilyst was used for perforating the vault and then, if required, it was advanced to perforate the base of the skull. The improved version of 1884 had a double thread and was split to the point. The virtue of Simpson's procedure was that it was entirely intracranial and therefore there was less risk of damage to the maternal soft tissues. He also claimed that it could be used successfully even when there was insufficient space to insert a cephalotribe. Simpson favored the basilyst as a tractor and later added a blade to facilitate this (Figure 19.36).

Tarnier's three-bladed *basiotribe* was intended to break up the base and crush it (1883) (Figure 19.37). This device had a gimlet end but, like his axis-traction forceps, was soon found to be too complicated for general use. Another complex and unrelenting device was that of the Lollini brothers, described previously (Figure 19.27).

Pierre-Victor Alfred Auvard (b. 1855) (1884), Georg Winter, and others devised three-bladed instruments (Figures 19.38, 19.39) combining the principles of the cranioclast and cephalotribe, the design being further modified by Robert

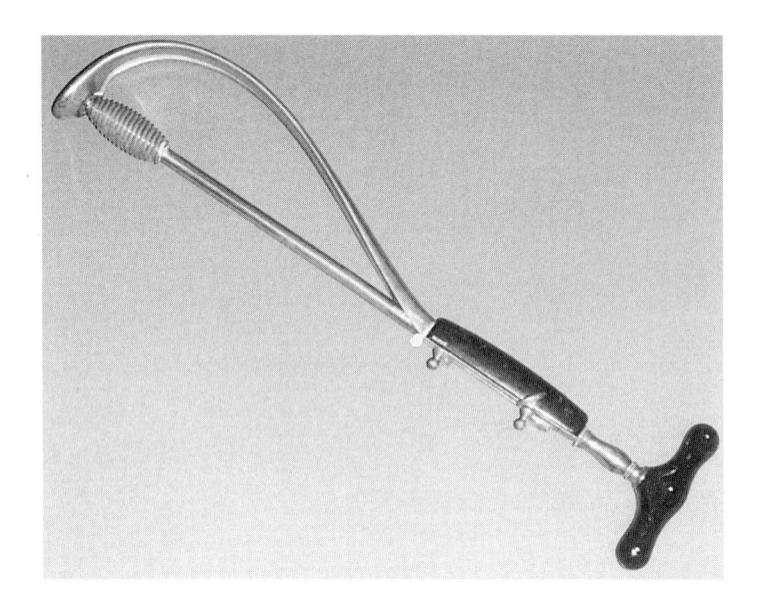

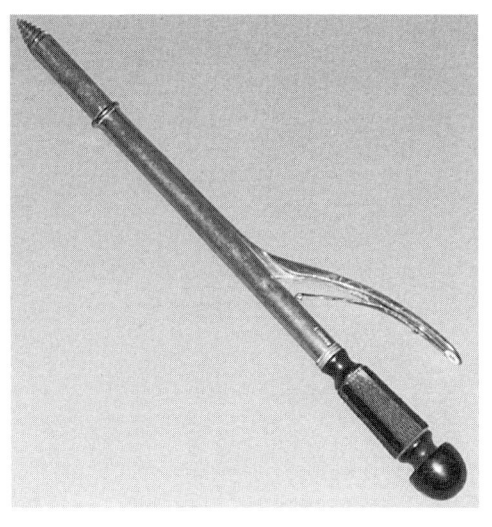

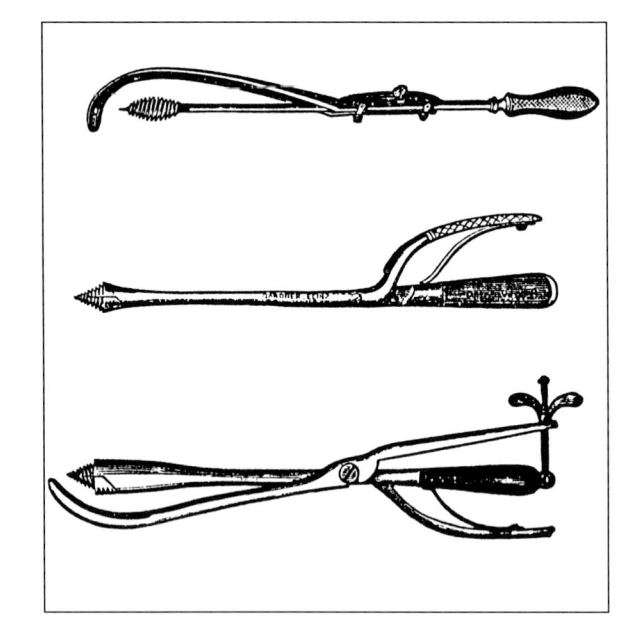

FIGURE 19.34 (ABOVE LEFT).
J. Hubert's transforator. The olive-shaped end is screwed into the base of the skull and the hinged blade is passed over the head. (Science Museum, London)

FIGURE 19.35 (ABOVE).
A. R. Simpson's basilyst. (Science Museum, London)

FIGURE 19.36 (LEFT).
Basilysts and basilyst-tractor. Top: Hubert's transforator. Center: Simpson's improved basilyst. It has a double thread and is split to the point. Bottom: Simpson's basilyst-tractor. (Simpson, 1884a)

Jardine (1862–1932), Professor of Midwifery, St. Mungo's College, Glasgow (1903). The center pointed and serrated blade was used for perforation and then screwed into the foramen magnum. The two outer blades were then applied successively over the face and occiput, crushing the skull against the retained middle blade.

• • •

There is little doubt that these comminutors and extractors, in spite of the massive and formidable appearance of many of them, fulfilled a function and need in the late nineteenth century and into the twentieth century. Providing they were properly applied in appropriate cases they must have been much safer than the crotchets and other crude instruments that preceded them. The use of these instruments only began to wane as Caesarian section became a safer procedure and a more acceptable option.

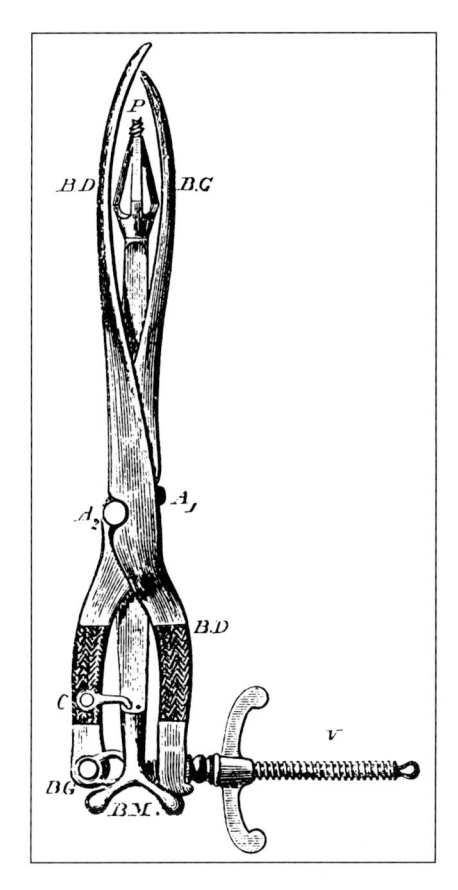

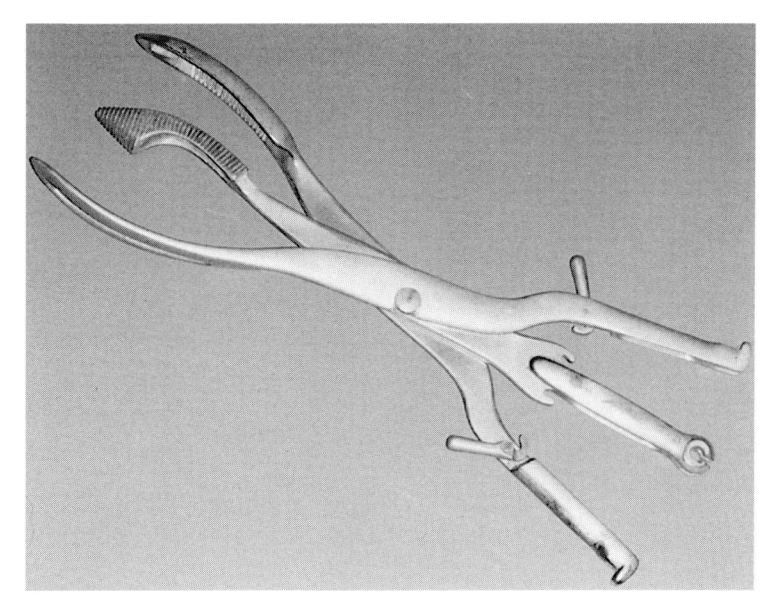

FIGURE 19.37 (LEFT).
Tarnier's basiotribe. One of Tarnier's ingenious devices that was too complicated to use in practice. (Parvin, 1890)

FIGURE 19.38 (ABOVE).
Auvard's basiotribe. A combination of cranioclast and cephalotribe. The center blade is for perforation and screwing into the foramen magnum. The crushing outer blades are then applied. (The screw compressor is missing from the handle). (Science Museum, London)

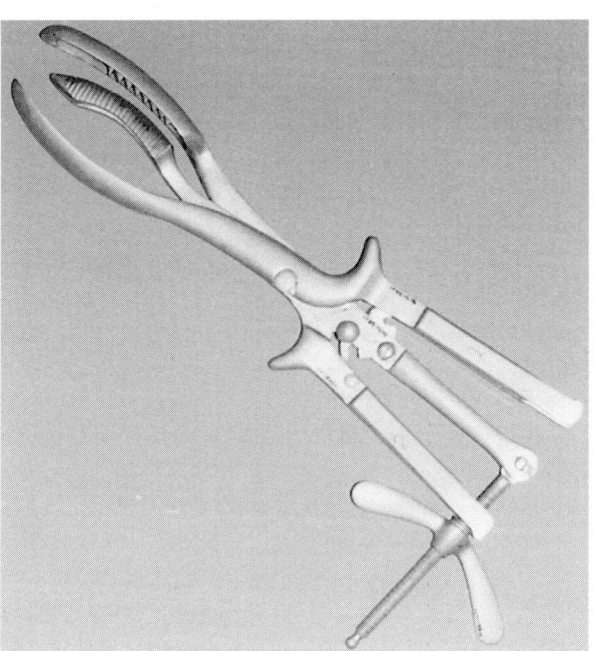

FIGURE 19.39.
Winter's combined cranioclast and cephalotribe. (Science Museum, London)

COMMINUTORS AND COMMINUTOR-EXTRACTORS 253

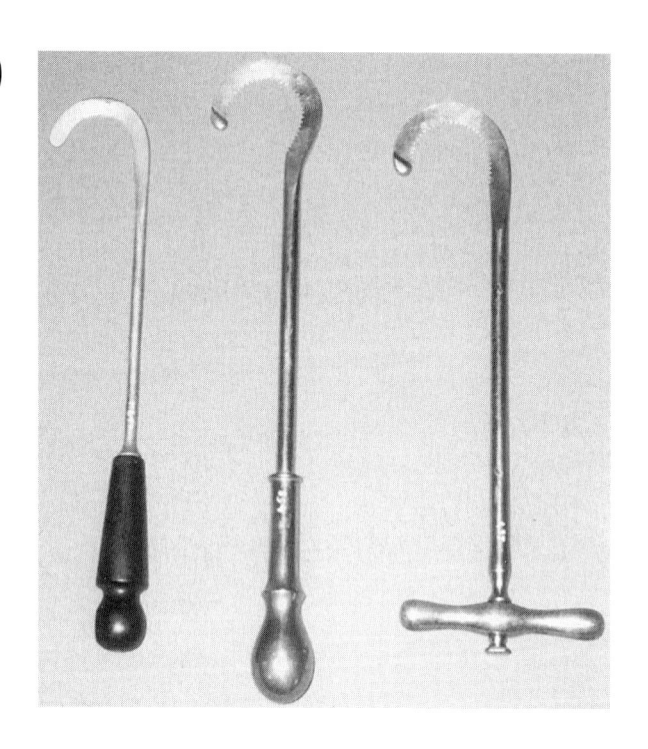

EMBRYOTOMY

20

FIGURE 20.1.
British decapitators. Ramsbotham's (left) has a sharp knife edge. Lever's (center) and Targett's (right) have sawtooth cutting edges. The handle on Targett's instrument is detachable and fits other accessories. (RCOG)

Alternative methods of dealing with gross obstruction, short of Caesarian section, included preliminary decapitation. The possibility of decapitation with a simple chain saw was suggested as early as 1786 by Aitken, but purpose-designed instruments taking up this idea did not appear until much later.

In Britain the common decapitators were of a "scythe" design, hooked instruments with an inner cutting blade, with either a knife or saw-toothed edge (Figure 20.1). Ramsbotham's (1867) decapitator was typical of the knife-edged variety (Figure 20.1, left). Many examples had the added refinement of a handle flattened on one side to indicate the direction of the blade. Lever's and Targett's (1863–1890) instruments were of the same shape as Ramsbotham's but had saw-toothed cutting edges. Widely illustrated in the catalogues of the time, Targett's instrument had a transverse bar handle and this was frequently made to be detachable as part of a set comprising decapitator, blunt hook, and crotchet.

In Vienna the practice was to use heavy embryotomy scissors with the blade set at an obtuse angle, then severing the spine as close as possible to the foramen magnum. Carl Braun used a simple angled hook, or *decollator,* which was passed around the neck and the head was severed by a twisting action (Figure 20.2). However, this instrument received little attention until it was popularized by his younger brother, G. A. Braun (1861).

Cephalotomes and Embryotomes

Cephalotomes are instruments for cutting or sawing the head to reduce its size. However, they were more commonly used for decapitation. Robert Barnes suggested the use of a popular gynecological instrument of the time, the wire écraseur,

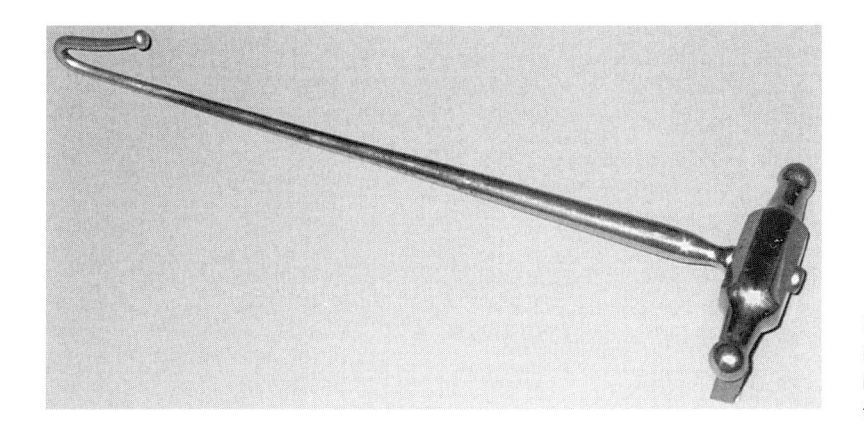

FIGURE 20.2.
Braun's *decollator*. Decapitation was achieved by passing the hook round the neck and twisting. (RCOG)

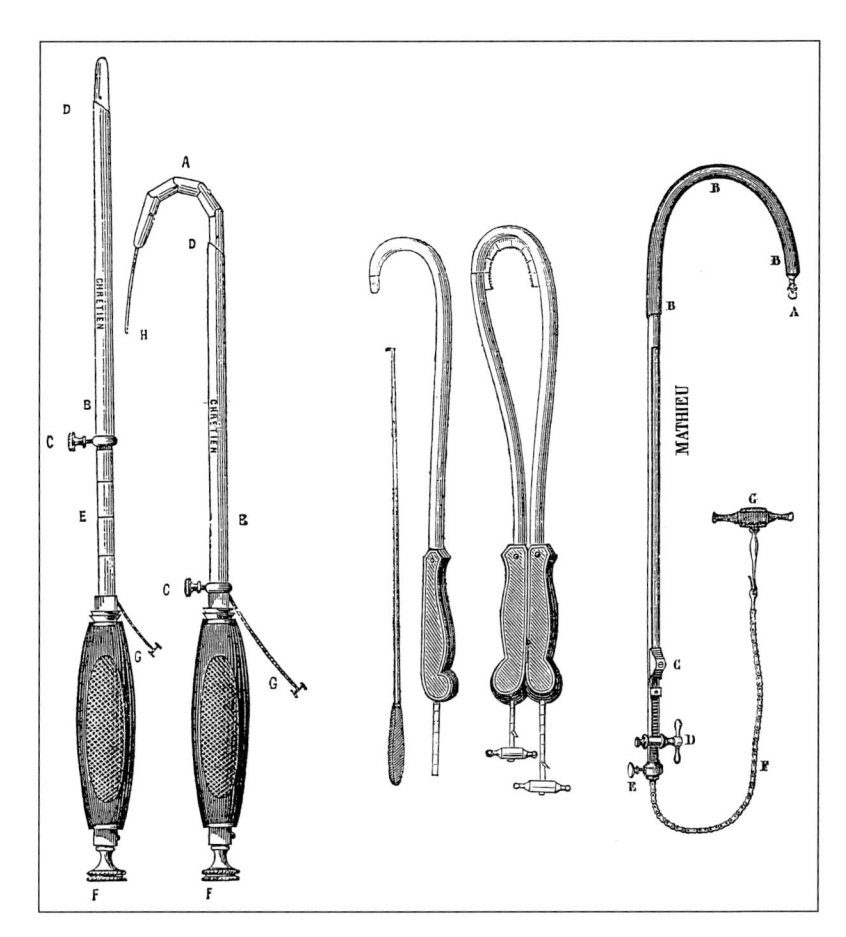

FIGURE 20.3.
Crotchet decapitators. Left: Wasseige's articulated embryotome with wire saw. Center: Van der Ecken's embryotome. The handles are separate. An articulated saw is passed up through one handle and brought down through the other. Right: Stanesco's embryotome. A chainsaw is driven through the cannula by a rack and pinion (D). (Charpentier, 1883)

for cutting through the head (1886). Barnes also advocated the use of a wire écraseur for a procedure he called *lamination*—slicing the head in different directions (1870)—which Tarnier also advocated (see below). The écraseur was apparently unsuccessful but wire saws, such as the Gigli saw (originally designed for symphysiotomy but recommended by Gigli for embryotomy in 1897 [see Chapter 21]), proved to be effective and their use continued well into the twentieth century. The most popular and enduring instrument of the twentieth century was the Blond-Heidler saw, invented by the Viennese physicians Kasper Blond (1889–1964) (1923) and Hans Heidler (1889–1955).

Various devices were used for passing wires or flexible saws round the neck, limbs, and trunk, many of which were described by Charpentier (1883). Some of these are shown in Figure 20.3.

In many cases of gross pelvic contraction, with a true conjugate of around 38 millimeters (1.5 inches), it could be difficult to deliver the shoulders or the trunk after reducing the size of the head. Simple division of the clavicles

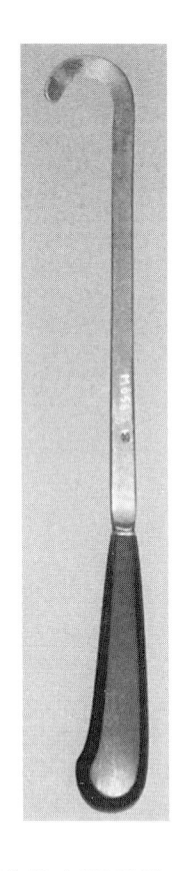

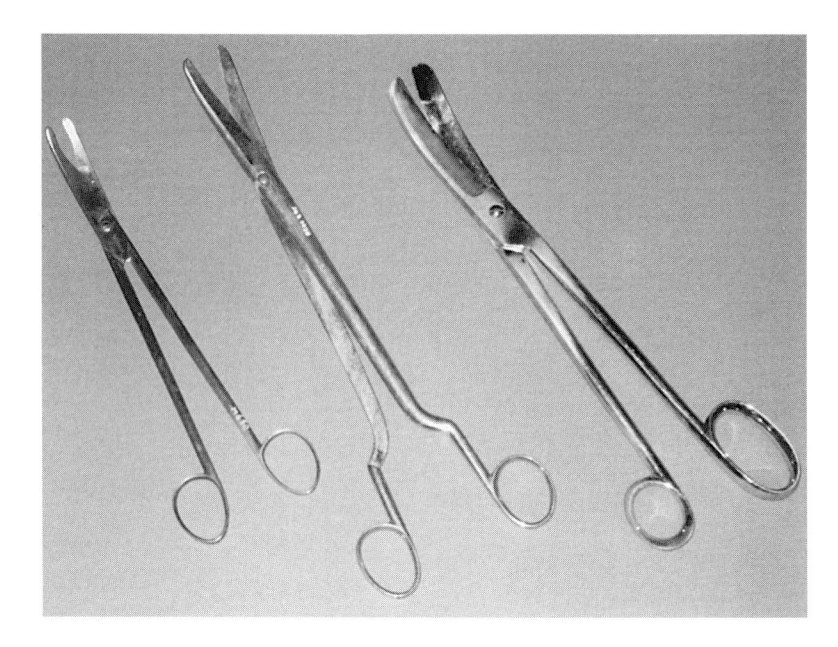

FIGURE 20.4 (ABOVE).
Curved embryotomy knife. (RCOG)

FIGURE 20.5 (ABOVE RIGHT).
Embryotomy/cleidotomy scissors. The pair on the left have concave cutting edges. (RCOG)

FIGURE 20.6 (RIGHT).
Scanzoni's *Auchenister*. A single, hinged blade is protected by the crotchet. (Scanzoni, 1853)

FIGURE 20.7 (CENTER RIGHT).
Lazarewitch's embryotome. Pincer blades are opened and closed by a screw and wing nut in the handle. (Thomas, 1879)

FIGURE 20.8 (FAR RIGHT).
Jacquemier's crotchet. There are two flexible cutting tools that fit into the grooved crotchet, a steel blade for soft tissue, and a chainsaw (illustrated) for bone. (Charpentier, 1883)

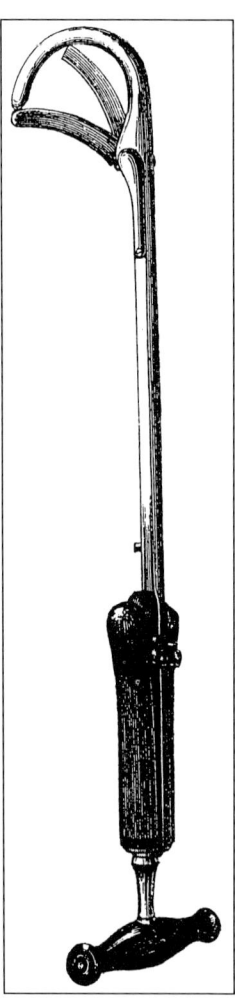

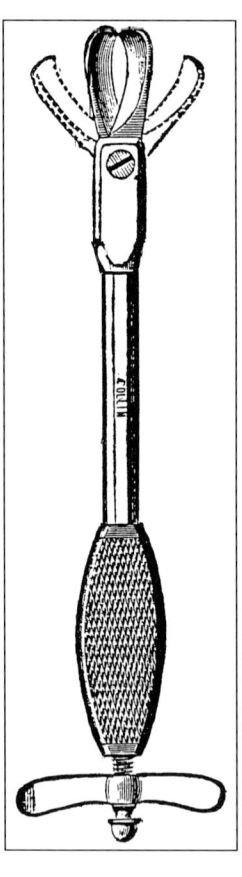

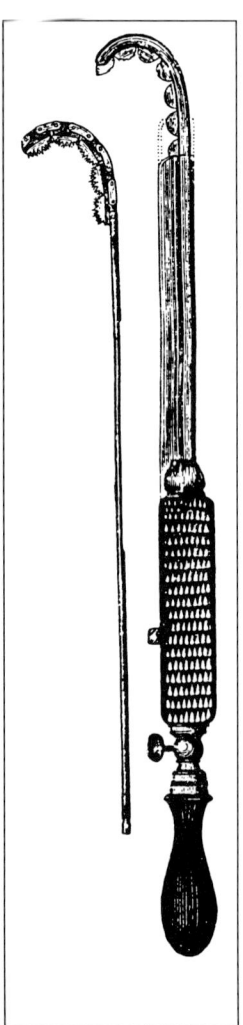

256 CHAPTER 20

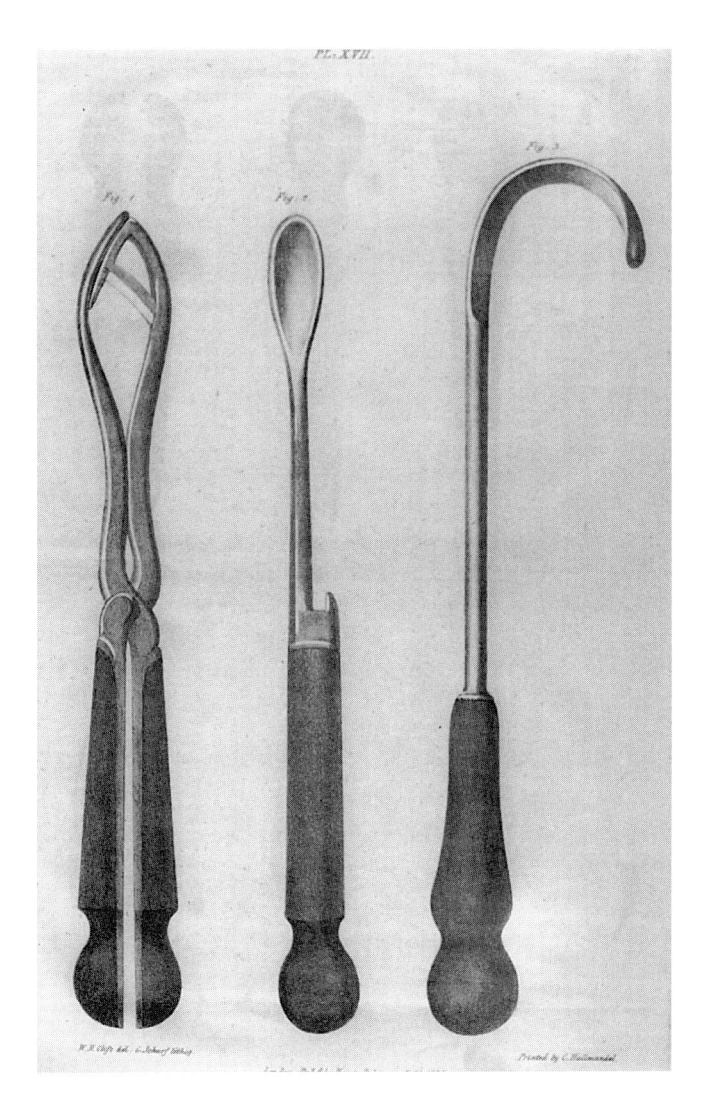

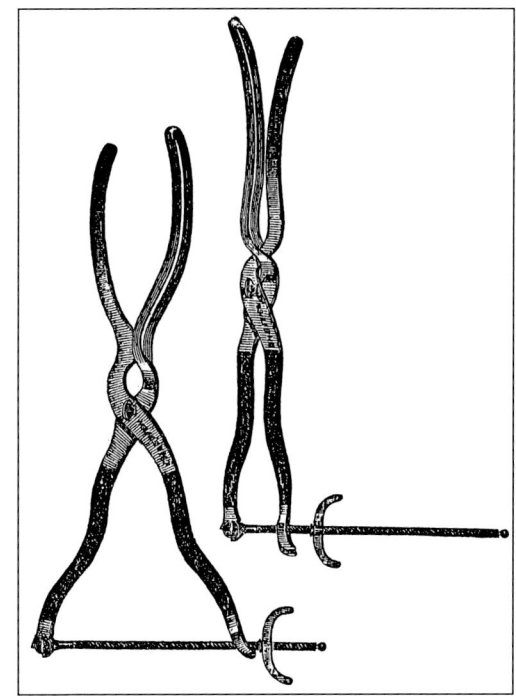

FIGURE 20.9 (LEFT).
Davis's guarded embryotomy knife. The cutting blade is protected by a crotchet (left) and a second spoon-shaped blade (center). On the right is a conventional "scythe" decapitator. (Plate XVII, Davis, 1825)

FIGURE 20.10 (ABOVE).
Wasseige's *lamineur céphalique*. The blades divide more by crushing than cutting but can also be used for traction. (Wasseige, 1876)

(cleidotomy) could relieve the obstruction but disruption of the thorax and/or abdominal contents might have been required as a result. In earlier times this disruption was achieved by ripping with a sharp crotchet. Later long-handled knives (Figure 20.4) and strong scissors (Figure 20.5) were in common use.

Subsequently more sophisticated instruments for embryotomy were introduced, such as Scanzoni's *Auchenister* (Figure 20.6), a crotchet design incorporating a single hinged blade (1853). Lazarewitch's embryotome (Figure 20.7) had two claw-like pincer blades (1869a).

Jean Marie Jacquemier of Paris invented a hook-shaped crotchet with a groove along its length into which fit a smooth strip of steel for cutting soft tissues (Figure 20.8). It also had an interchangeable chain saw for cutting through the spinal column. The cutters were operated by a sliding knob in the handle (1861–1862).

David Davis referred to piecemeal destruction of the fetus as *embryulcia*, rather than using the French term, *morcellement*, and he advocated caution in its use: "The child's life, however, must not be hastily yielded up, nor until nature and art shall have exerted their utmost and united resources; until the most powerful efforts of the one, and the best devised expedients of the other, shall have been fairly and deliberately exerted without effect" (1825).

Davis's guarded embryotomy knife comprised two jointed blades, one of which had a knife edge; the other blade acted as a guard (Figure 20.9). Davis's osteotomists were widely used and modifications appeared, such as that of Tempest Anderson (1870). These were intended primarily for craniotomy (see Chapter 19, Figure 19.8).

In Liège Wasseige (1877) devised a *lamineur céphalique* (Figure 20.10) which was a cross between a cranioclast and an osteotomist. Joulin's *diviseur céphalique* (Figure 20.11) was

EMBRYOTOMY 257

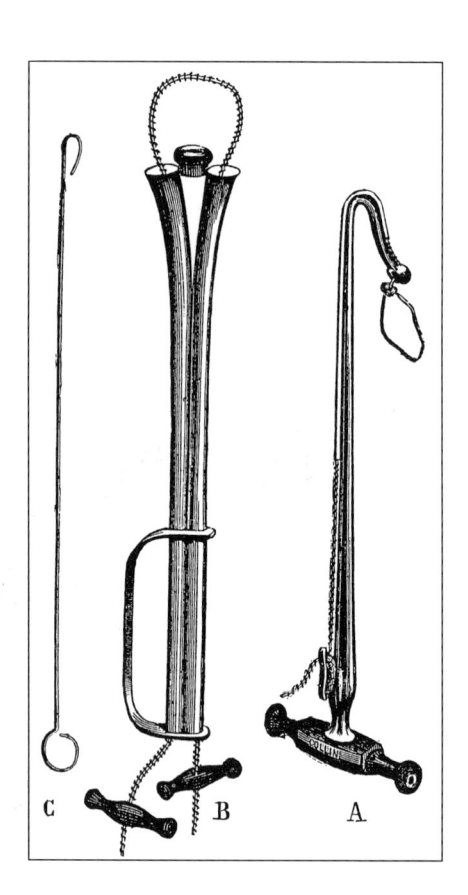

FIGURE 20.11.
Joulin's *diviseur céphalique*. The flexible saw has two introducers, one for soft tissue and one for bone. (Joulin, 1867)

FIGURE 20.12.
P. Thomas's embryotome. A modified Braun's hook (*A*) is used as an introducer for the cutting wire, which is threaded through a double cannula (*B*) using a wire hook (*C*). (Charpentier, 1883)

FIGURE 20.13.
Tarnier's embryotome. A complex device and forerunner of his *forceps-scie*. (Charpentier, 1883)

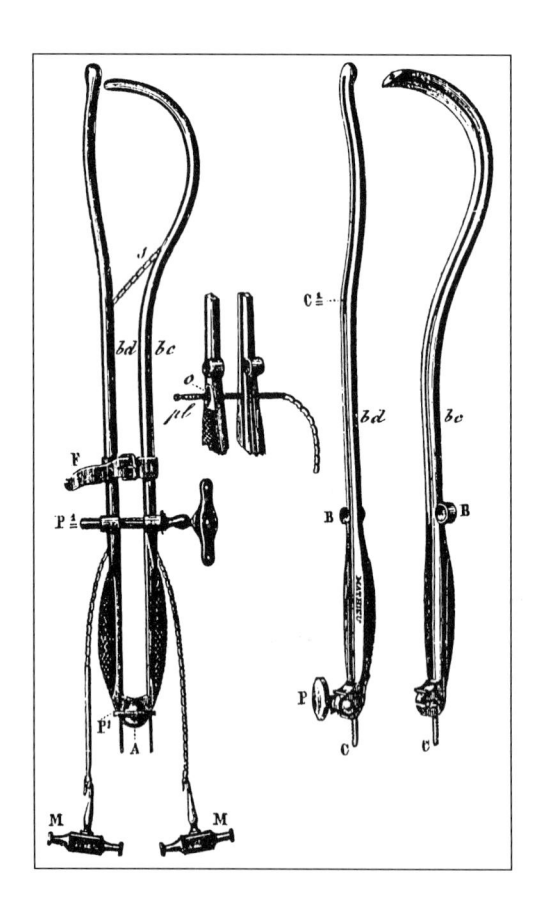

a purpose-designed écraseur with a separate introducer for the flexible saws, one of which was designed for bone and the other for soft tissue (1867).

Pierre Thomas (b. 1851) of Paris designed some simple snare instruments for various embryotomy procedures, one of which is illustrated in Figure 20.12. A modified Braun hook was used to guide a strong thread around the neck, with which a wire or chain écraseur could be drawn through a double tubular vaginal protector, aided by a fine hook (1879).

Tarnier's embryotome was, like so many of his instruments, ingenious but complicated (Figure 20.13). His instrument was a forerunner of the *forceps-scie*, discussed below.

Forceps-Scie

Jean Baptiste van Huevel (1802–1883) of Brussels and Tarnier both designed forceps that incorporated chain saws, the former being most commonly described and illustrated in the textbooks of the time. The Van Huevel forceps, invented in 1842 (Meadows, 1867), was a massive instrument over 585 millimeters (23 inches) long and incorporated a saw in grooves on the inner surfaces of the blades for slicing the head or trunk (Figure 20.14). It was ingeniously designed so that the saw could be introduced after the blades had been applied by means of a metal strip chain carrier that slid back

258 CHAPTER 20

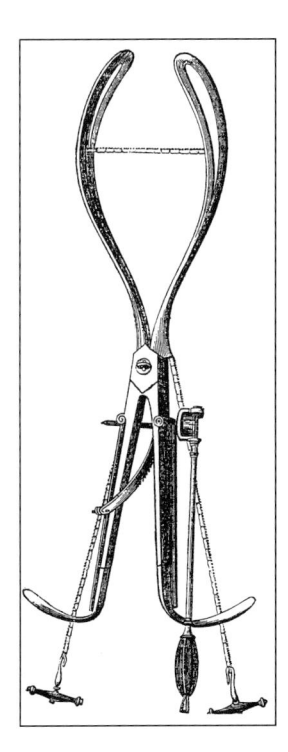

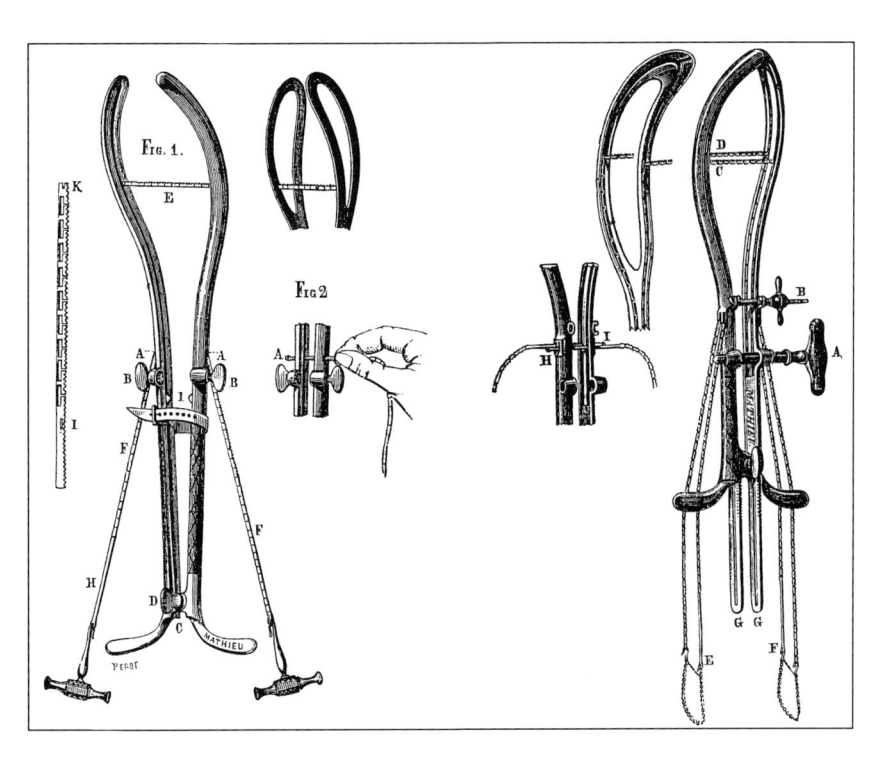

FIGURE 20.14.
Van Huevel's *forceps-scie*. The chainsaw is attached to metal strips running into each blade. The saw assembly is connected to a wheel and ratchet mechanism. (Charpentier, 1883)

FIGURE 20.15.
Tarnier's *simple* and *double forceps-scie*. The *simple* version (left) is based on Lyon's parallel forceps, with a chainsaw running in grooves in one arm of each blade. The *double* version (right) has a chain in each arm of the blades. (Charpentier, 1883)

In the innovative mechanical climate of the nineteenth century embryotomy instruments in general became more complex in design and were more difficult to use, clean, and later, to sterilize. It is not surprising, therefore, that many of them were destined to have a short life in practice. The instruments that survived and continued to be used throughout the era of relatively safe Caesarian section as an alternative method of delivery and well into the twentieth century were the simpler decapitators used in Britain, such as those of Lever and Targett.

and forth in the grooves. A full description of its use is given by Meadows (1867). Lighter and simpler versions of the Van Huevel forceps were shown at the 1866 Obstetric Society *Conversazione* by de Billi of Milan and by Professor Faye and Mette of Christiania.

Tarnier's "simple" *forceps-scie* was based on the Thenance parallel forceps (see Chapter 10) but he went a stage further with a second model that incorporated two chains (Figure 20.15). These instruments were destined to finish up as obstetric curiosities.

. . .

SYMPHYSIOTOMY AND PUBIOTOMY

Symphysiotomy in Europe

Division of the symphysis pubis, or symphysiotomy, is a procedure that was adopted in an attempt to increase the pelvic diameters in order to facilitate delivery in cases of disproportion. An alternative procedure, with the same objective, was pubiotomy (or hebotomy), in which the pubic bone itself was divided. According to Baudelocque, symphysiotomy was first suggested by Severin Pineau in the sixteenth century but was not performed on a living patient until 1777 by Sigault, with a "successful" outcome for both mother and child, although the mother's bladder and urethra were severely damaged. It was hoped that symphysiotomy would replace craniotomy in the management of obstructed labor but the latter was often required in addition to symphysiotomy. Sigault, while still a student, first presented his idea to the Royal Academy of Paris in 1768, but no one considered the operation justifiable. However, undaunted by this rebuff, Sigault planned and performed the operation on Madame Souchot, a rachitic dwarf, 3 feet, 8 inches in height, who had lost four children previously as the result of traumatic deliveries. Sigault carried out the operation in collaboration with A. le Roy, who had earlier shown that post mortem division of the symphysis allowed the pubes to be separated by 63 millimeters (2.5 inches). Le Roy subsequently published an account of the procedure (1778). When Sigault presented his case to the Faculty of Medicine in Paris, the applause given to him was said to be "extravagant," a medal was struck to mark the occasion, and a royal pension was granted. However the Academy of Surgery were opposed to the publicity and fame accorded on the basis of one dubious case and as a consequence professionals were divided into "Caesarianists" and "Symphysiotomists."

The technique of symphysiotomy appeared to be seductively simple and was widely adopted on the Continent but the reality of its difficulty soon became evident. Inevitably the procedure was abused. It was often performed unskillfully so that lives were lost and in many cases permanent disability, commonly from bladder injuries, resulted. The main problems arose because mere division of the symphysis gave little extra space. Therefore forceful distraction, separating the pubes by as much as 75 to 100 millimeters (3 to 4 inches), was often undertaken, resulting in damage to the sacroiliac joints, sometimes even to the sciatic nerve, as well as a stretching of the pelvic viscera. The entire procedure was also accompanied by a great deal of pain. In any case the initial obstetric problem was commonly obstruction due to rhachitic flattening of the pelvic brim and the operation had little effect on the antero-posterior diameter. Consequently, by the end of the eighteenth century the procedure was hardly ever performed, except in Italy. J. L. Baudelocque in particular, having initially seen some merit in the procedure, carried out a detailed analysis of all reported cases and of a number of cadaver experiments. This led him to conclude that in many cases the indication for the operation was doubtful, that Caesarian section was preferable in major degrees of pelvic contraction if the baby was alive, and that when the contraction was less forceps could achieve delivery equally well with less trauma to the mother (1790).

R. P. Harris provided an extensive historical review of the European literature in 1883. Between 1777 and 1858, the operation was promoted as an alternative to Caesarian section and was used in extreme degrees of pelvic contraction. Maternal mortality following the procedure was 37 percent and fetal mortality 67 percent. In the period between 1866 and 1880 the operation was mainly confined to more experienced operators in Naples, where opposition of the Papal Church to destructive operations was strong. The maternal mortality fell to 20 percent and fetal mortality to 18 percent. In 1891 only twelve operations were recorded, all in Naples. The relatively good results could be attributed to attention to detail, careful pelvic mensuration, and the advent of antisepsis. There was some revival of the procedure in Europe toward the end of the nineteenth century, with ever-improving results as cases were better selected, that is, when the pelvis was just too small for forceps delivery.

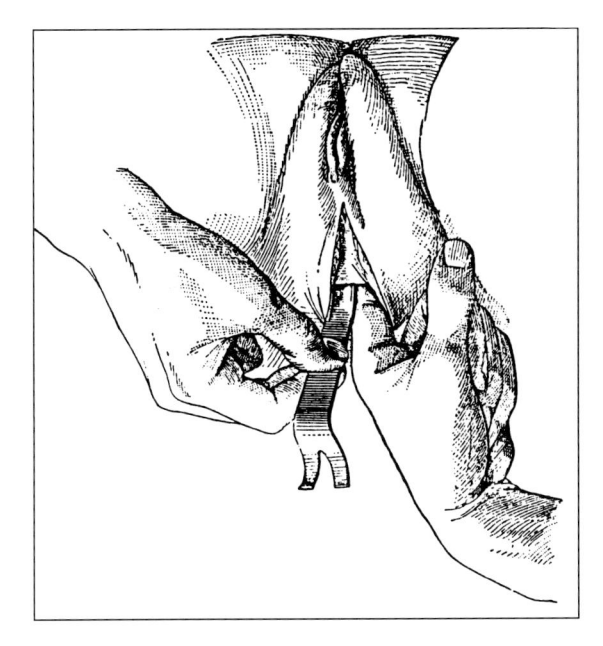

T. G. Thomas (1907) outlined the techniques that had been employed in different countries in Europe in the late nineteenth century. The French, like the Germans, favored an open technique, with an incision starting 38 millimeters (1.5 inches) above the symphysis and extending almost to the clitoris. The recti were separated to allow a finger to be passed down behind the symphysis to push the catheterized bladder and urethra to one side (Figure 21.1), after which a grooved director was introduced. The incision was made either from the outside in with a short, thin-bladed knife or from the inside out using a sickle-shaped knife (Figure 21.2).

The Italian method involved a smaller incision and minimal separation of the recti. A curved knife was introduced behind the symphysis, using the finger as a guide, and the joint was cut from below upward and behind forward, using a sawing motion.

The later Neapolitan technique, described by Henry Jacques Garrigues (b. 1831), Professor of Obstetrics at the New York Postgraduate Medical School, was to make a sub-

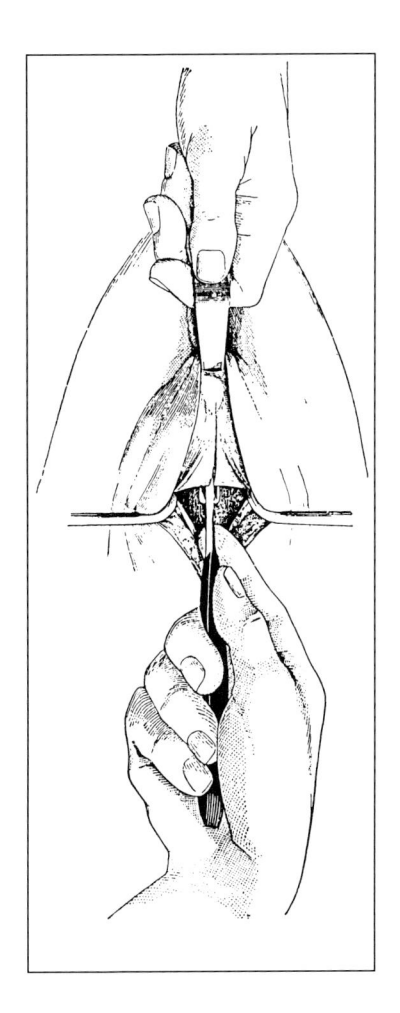

FIGURES 21.1, 21.2.
Symphysiotomy: the French technique. 21.1: The recti are separated and a grooved director introduced. 21.2: A sickle-shaped knife is used to cut from within outward. (Thomas, 1907)

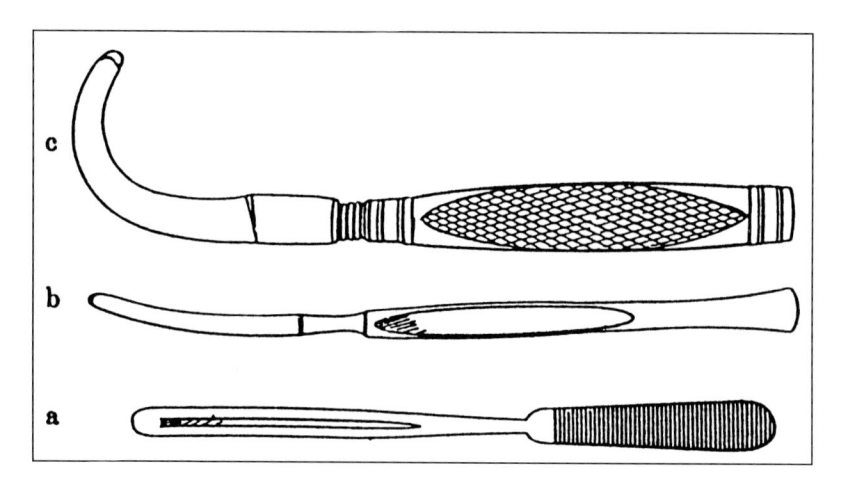

FIGURE 21.3.
Instruments used by Garrigues. a: Hay's director.
b: bistoury. c: Galbiatta's *falcetta*.

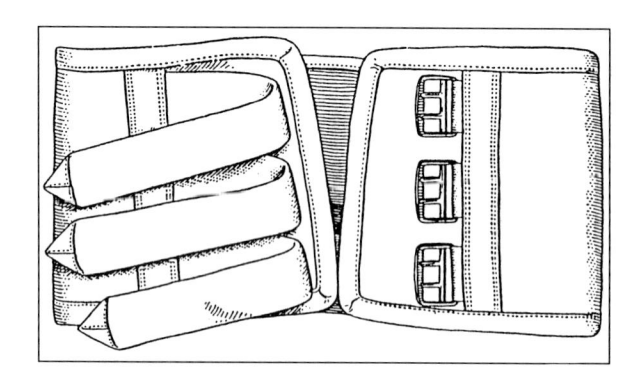

FIGURE 21.4.
Garrigues's binder. (Garrigues, 1893)

cutaneous cut with a *falcetta* (a sickle-shaped bistoury, Figure 21.3, c), dividing the ligaments from below upward. The joint was not forced apart and labor was allowed to progress. Forceps were applied in about 25 percent of the cases. (See also "Symphysiotomy in America" below.)

Pubiotomy (Hebotomy)

According to Thomas cutting through the bone to one side of the joint was first described in the early nineteenth century by Champion Bar de Luc, using a flexible saw, such as that described by Aitken (1786), or the later flexible saw of Gigli (see below). Van de Velde claimed that hebotomy was a safer operation because the supports of the bladder and urethra were not disturbed, there was less danger of soft tissue trauma and hemorrhage, and healing was better (see Thomas, T. G., 1907).

In the late nineteenth century Leonardo Gigli of Florence (1863–1908) published an account of his "string saw," which had been developed after experiments with various roughened wires on cadavers. His technique was based on the classic open approach and introduction of the saw from above downward. He incised the upper third of the symphysis and then used his flexible saw to cut obliquely through the pubis "with a few strokes, easily and with great safety, as though the bone were not being sawed but cut with a knife." Gigli believed that hebotomy was safer and that symphysiotomy was surgically incorrect because the joint was opened and was contiguous to a wounded surface, with consequent greater risk of sepsis (1893, 1894).

Symphysiotomy in America

In America symphysiotomy was condemned from the outset. Dewees, who wrote and annotated an abridged translation of Baudelocque's textbook (Baudelocque, 1823), felt that

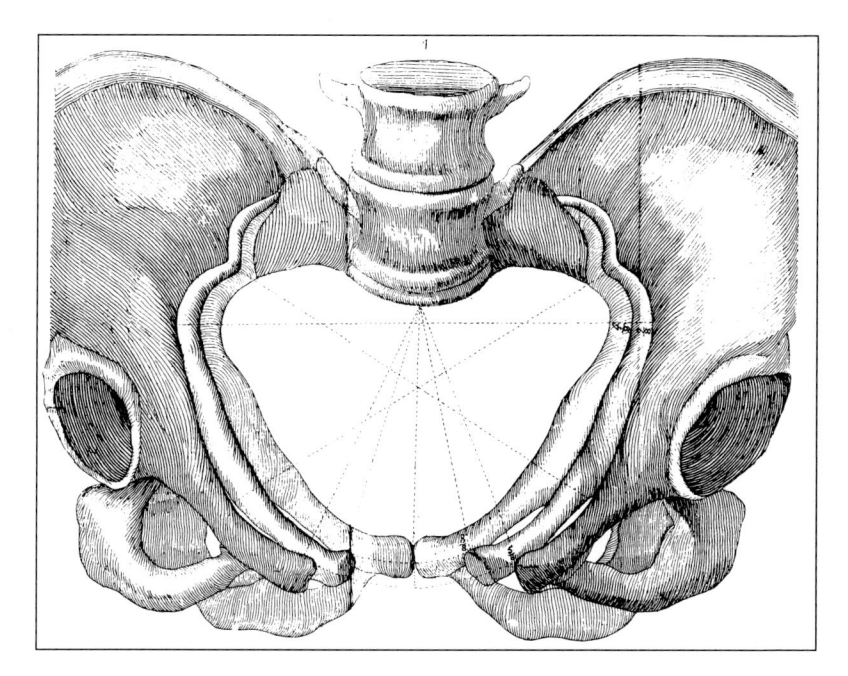

FIGURE 21.5.
Change in pelvic capacity after "pelvimity." Aitken's diagram, derived from Baudelocque. He points out that there is proportional laceration of the posterior symphyses. (Aitken, 1786)

Baudelocque did not go far enough with his condemnation of the procedure and deleted the operation from Baudelocque's list of techniques for managing cephalopelvic disproportion. In a footnote Dewees commented that Baudelocque had "contributed much to the cause of humanity, by bringing this horrible operation into complete disgrace." No doubt as a result of this it was not until 1892, according to Thomas (1907), that the first symphysiotomy in America was performed by Charles Jewett. Garrigues had been impressed by Harris's account of Italian practice and purchased a *falcetta* from Italy, with which he experimented on cadavers. However, it was nearly ten years before he eventually carried out an operation on a patient and, in fact, did not use the *falcetta*. After making a 100-millimeter (4-inch) incision extending down between the labia majora and minora he used a Hay's director to separate the tissues behind the symphysis and a simple curved bistoury to divide the symphysis from behind forward and above downward (Figure 21.3 a,b). He also devised a binder (Figure 21.4) to stabilize the pelvis postoperatively (1893). Garrigues subsequently reported enthusiasm from members of the American Gynecological Society and a great demand for copies of his *falcetta*. However, the introduction of symphysiotomy in America was destined to be relatively short-lived for it did not find favor with the influential Whitridge Williams. In his 1903 textbook he wrote, "I do not expect to perform symphyseotomy [*sic*] under any circumstances, and consider that the present enthusiasm for it will eventually disappear."

Symphysiotomy in Britain

Symphysiotomy was first performed in Britain by Welchman in 1782 but both mother and baby perished (1790). He used a common dissecting knife, cutting from the inside out, and afterward bound the pelvis with a broad bandage. His son removed the pelvis after the woman died and measured the true conjugate as 57 millimeters (2.25 inches) and the distance between the tuberosities as 38 millimeters (1.5 inches). It was noted that the bones were very soft, and the description was typical of severe osteomalacia, so this may have contributed to the relative facility of the delivery. The procedure never found great favor in Britain and was disapproved of by William Hunter, whose experiments showed that simple division of the symphysis pubis gained very little space and that forceful displacement of as little as 38 millimeters (1.5 inches) endangered sacroiliac ligaments and joints and the bladder. He also showed that the pubis had to be separated by 76 millimeters (3 inches) to increase the true conjugate by 25.5 millimeters (1 inch) (1778). Leake experimented, with colleagues, on a cadaver and found the procedure to be technically simple; he achieved a separation of 54 millimeters (2.125 inches) (1781). Similar experiments had been carried out by a number of Continental surgeons and were reported by Baudelocque. A similar experiment was also illustrated by Aitken (1786) (Figure 21.5).

Although Leake spoke favorably of symphysiotomy he never recorded a personal case. Aitken had many objections to the procedure but nevertheless invented a flexible knife to cut from the outside in and also a flexible saw for use in

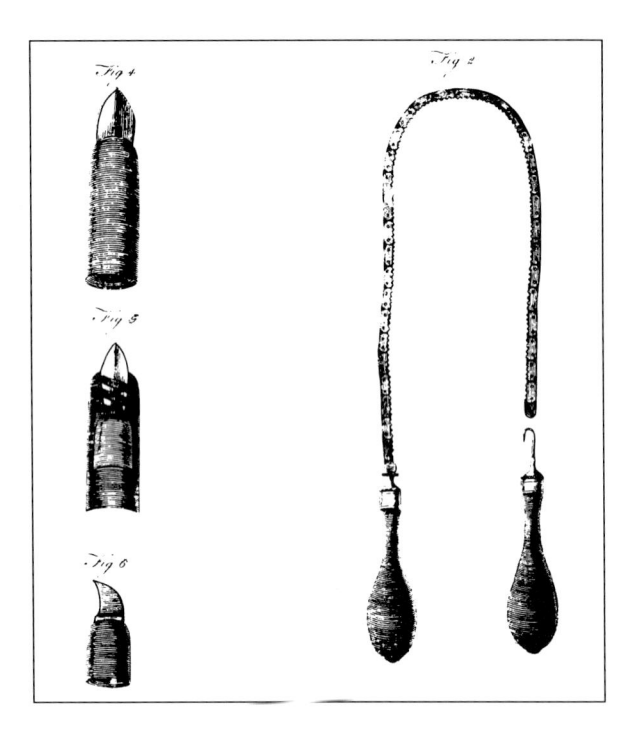

FIGURE 21.6.
Aitken's flexible saw. One of the handles is removable to allow insertion retropubically (Figure 2). Also shown are a thimble-type spring-loaded embryotomy knife (Figures 4 and 5) and a finger scalpel (Figure 6). (Aitken, 1786)

cases where the joint was ossified (Figure 21.6). He also later proposed the modified procedure of pelviotomy (pubiotomy). By pelviotomy he meant bilateral division of the pubes, thereby releasing a section, including the symphysis, about four inches wide. Osborn, Denman, Burns (1809), Merriman (1826), and many others were all opposed to the procedure. Osborn's *Essay on Laborious Parturition* (1783) is a long dissertation against symphysiotomy and Denman's *Essay on Difficult Labours* (1787–1790) is another lengthy work whose main thrust was to counsel against symphysiotomy. At this time the British preference generally was to try and avoid disproportion by limiting the size of the baby at birth through premature induction of labor or through restriction of the maternal diet (Lucas, 1794; see also Chapter 17).

Conquest, in his *Outlines of Midwifery*, summarily dismissed the operation: "It is scarcely necessary to say any thing on this third method of relief, which was proposed by Monsieur Sigault in the year 1767 [sic], because the result of nearly *fifty* recorded cases was so disastrous, that the operation has been long since abandoned" (1820a).

An appropriate epitaph also came from Merriman, who stated that "the remembrance of it can now be beneficial, only as it may serve to caution us against the inconsiderate and hasty adoption of modes of practice, unsupported by just reasoning, and unsanctioned by experience" (1826).

. . .

In spite of the limited Continental revival of symphysiotomy late in the nineteenth century there was little interest in Britain. Harris made a plea for the practice of symphysiotomy, based on the Italian and other data of recent years that he had published previously, at a meeting of the Obstetrical Society of London in 1894. He emphasized the need for a rational basis for the operation and said that the operation should be performed in good time; that the true conjugate must be accurately measured and not be less than 70 millimeters (2.75 inches); and that the child should be delivered unhurriedly by forceps in correct cephalic application. Following Harris' presentation there was much pontification, based more on theory than practical experience, with claims for the relative safety of Caesarian section, where the improbable claim was made that this procedure had a maternal mortality rate as low as 10 percent and therefore compared favorably with symphysiotomy. Yet 125 years later the operation was still being practiced, with a further revival in the twentieth century, particularly in Dublin (Browne, 1947), and it was seen as an alternative to Caesarian section in undeveloped countries.

PELVIMETRY

One of the outcomes that was a result of the more objective scientific approach to obstetrics that was gathering momentum in the mid-eighteenth century, as well as the abandonment of the notion that the fetus had an active role in escaping from the uterus, was the development of pelvic mensuration in relation to difficult labor. Initially this was done by digital pelvic examination, assessing specific diameters, but more objectivity was obtained by the use of measuring rods, calipers, and other devices. This was known as internal pelvimetry but it was soon recognized that an approximation of the capacity of the birth canal could be obtained less intrusively from external measurements of the bony pelvis. As in other fields two of the outstanding pioneers were Smellie and Levret, who both described in detail the pelvic deformities due to rickets. Levret gave a complex description of pelvic planes and axes in 1753 in his *L'Art des accouchemens* and in the following year Smellie, in *A Sett of Anatomical Tables*, concentrated on the clinical applications of his studies of the pelvis. He was the first to describe the diagonal conjugate and its significance. In particular he noted that the largest diameter was the transverse diameter of the brim and that difficulties arising from contracted pelvis were usually encountered at the brim, in contradistinction to Levret's observations. R. W. Johnson was one of the first writers to give detailed instructions for digital assessment of pelvic measurements and capacity during labor, with guidelines on appropriate interventions (1769).

An instrument for internal pelvimetry was devised toward the end of the eighteenth century by P. V. Coutouly (Figure 22.1). It comprised two straight, graduated rods, one sliding in a groove in the other and both having terminal spoon-shaped ends set at right angles. The instrument was introduced beneath the pubic arch and one limb was advanced until it reached the sacral promontory.

J. L. Baudelocque was responsible for one of the first purpose-designed calipers, his *compas d'épaisseur*, designed to measure the external pelvic diameters. He emphasized the importance of the antero-posterior diameter of the pelvic inlet and introduced the concept of measuring the external conjugate (which came to be known as *Baudelocque's diameter*), measured from the tip of the spine of the fifth lumbar vertebra to the middle of the symphysis pubis, as an index of the true conjugate, which was arrived at by deducting 75 millimeters (3 inches) from the external conjugate. In spite of this inaccuracy and the criticism of the principle by a number of obstetricians, external pelvimetry took a firm hold because it was simpler, more convenient, and more comfortable for the patient than internal manual pelvic assessment. Baudelocque, in his *L'Art des accouchemens* (1789), illustrated the combined use of his external pelvimeter with Coutouly's rod (Figure 22.2).

Pelvimeters were slow to be adopted in Britain. Aitken (1786) advocated Coutouly's pelvimeter and also devised his own, which was suitable for both internal and external mensuration (Figure 22.3). In addition he used a graduated silver catheter for measuring the diagonal conjugate. Even so digital assessment remained the standard practice in Britain in the late eighteenth and early nineteenth centuries.

Nineteenth-Century Pelvimeters

During the nineteenth century there were many designs of both internal and external caliper-type pelvimeters of vary-

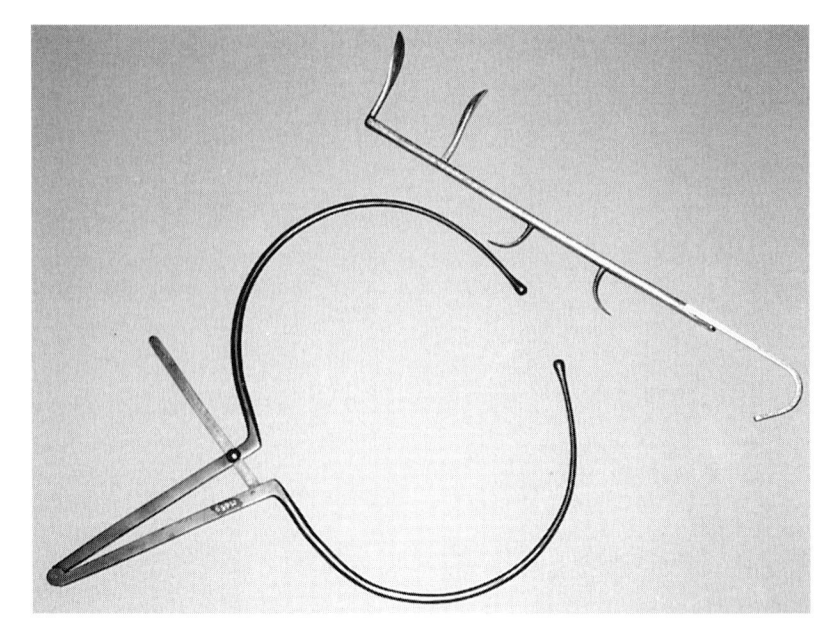

FIGURE 22.1.
Coutouly's internal pelvimeter, Mathews Duncan's external pelvimeter. Mathews Duncan's pelvimeter was virtually indistinguishable from that described by Baudelocque nearly one hundred years earlier. (RCOG)

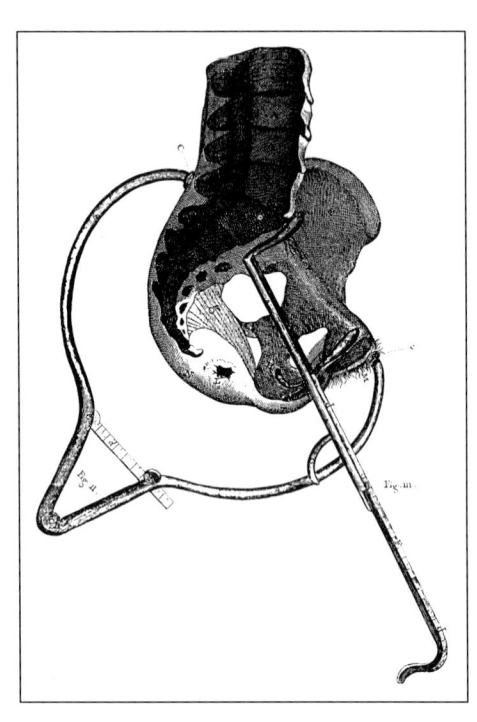

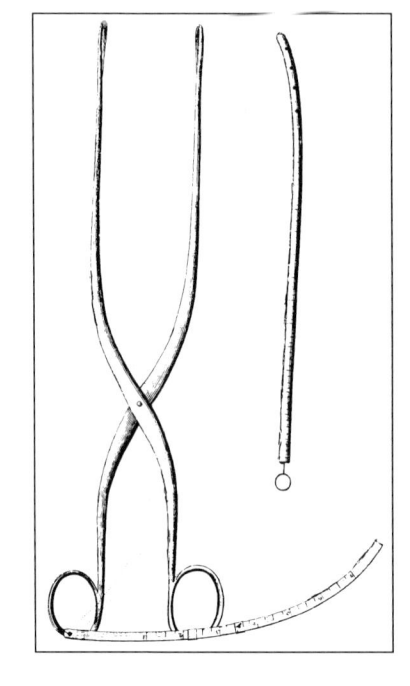

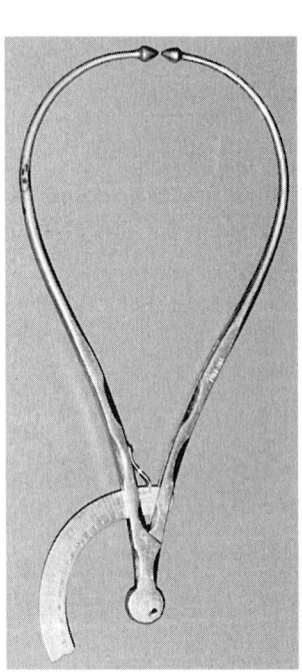

FIGURE 22.2.
Coutouly's and Baudelocque's pelvimeters used in combination. Coutouly's pelvimeter (Figure III) comprises a rod P with a graduated scale F, which slides into an outer grooved rod A. Each rod has a shaped end at right angles which impinge on the sacral promontory and the symphysis pubes. Baudelocque's pelvimeter (Figure II) is used principally to measure the external conjugate. (Baudelocque, 1789)

FIGURE 22.3.
Aitken's pelvimeter. A rather crude scissors device. The graduated catheter (right) was used to measure the diagonal conjugate. (Aitken, 1790)

FIGURE 22.4.
Martin's pelvimeter. (Science Museum, London)

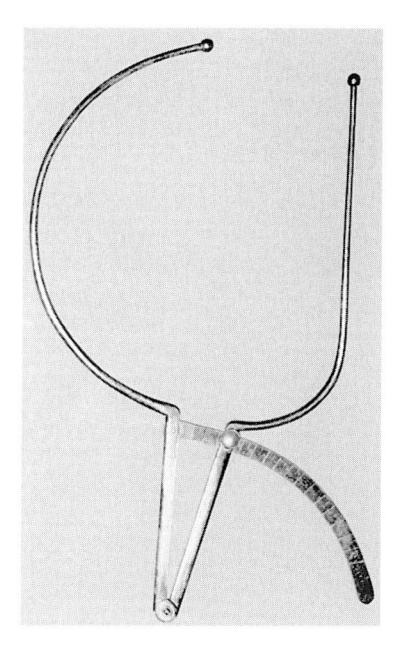

FIGURE 22.5.
Pelvimeter by Milliken. (Science Museum, London)

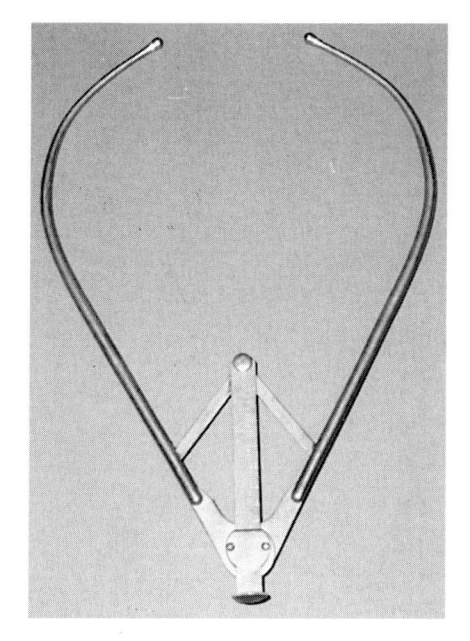

FIGURE 22.6.
Collyer's pelvimeter. Marketed by Mayer and Meltzer as "Readeasy." (RCOG)

ing degrees of complexity, the latter nearly all being of European origin and usually accompanied by lengthy instructions as to their use. D. W. H. Busch illustrated thirty-one different pelvimeters (1841) and Witkowski illustrated fifty-six (1887). At the *Conversazione* of the Obstetrical Society of London in 1866 some nineteen pelvimeters were exhibited (Meadows, 1867). More detail concerning these instruments can be obtained from these works and the representative selection illustrated here is chosen to show the range and ingenuity of instruments.

External Pelvimeters

External caliper-type pelvimeters were nearly all designed on the Baudelocque principle and differed only in detail. A version that was widely illustrated in the textbooks of the time was that designed by Dugès of Montpelier in 1826, which did not differ significantly from Baudelocque's instrument. Also a number of instrument makers offered pelvimeters apparently of their own design, most being variations on the Baudelocque theme, varying in the shape of the arms and/or the measuring scale. Martin of Berlin designed a pear-shaped version that was widely used (1862) (Figure 22.4).

In Britain pelvimeters did not come into common use until the second half of the nineteenth century but they were of the same general design, common examples being those of Mathews Duncan (1875) (Figure 22.1), and Collyer (Figure 22.6), while the instrument makers Arnold produced a more refined version with better detail (Figure 22.7).

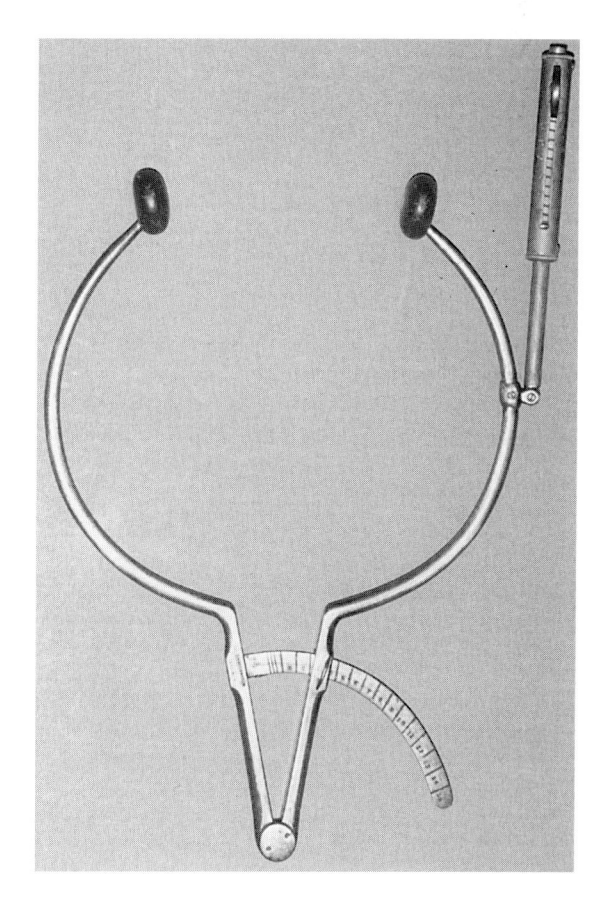

FIGURE 22.7.
Pelvimeter by Arnold. (Science Museum, London)

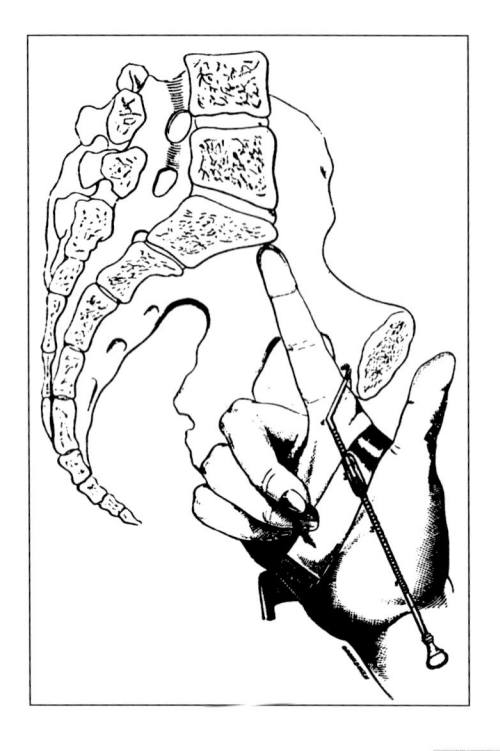

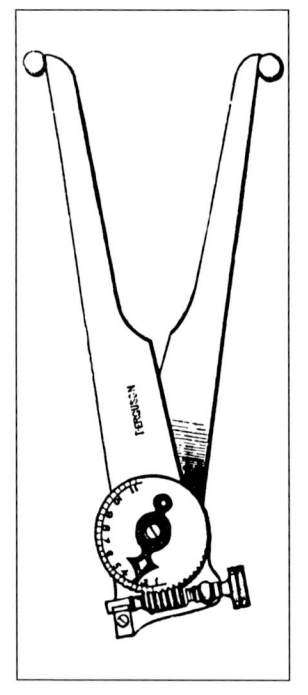

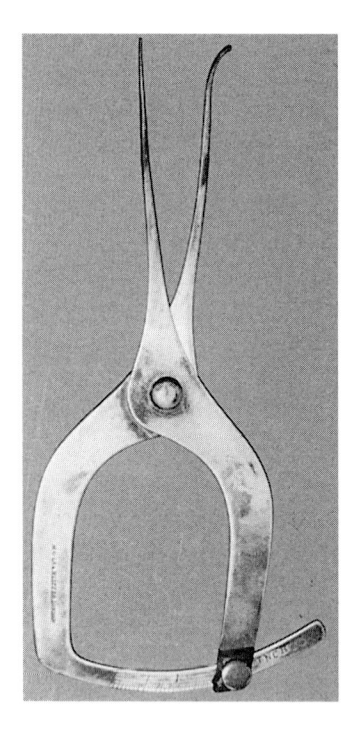

FIGURE 22.8 (ABOVE).
Greenhalgh's internal pelvimeter. A simple variant of an older idea. (Meadows, 1867)

FIGURE 22.9 (ABOVE CENTER).
Internal pelvimeter by Ferguson. (Meadows, 1867)

FIGURE 22.10 (ABOVE RIGHT).
Internal pelvimeter by Mayer and Meltzer. (Science Museum, London)

FIGURE 22.11 (RIGHT).
Cadran's pelvimeter for measuring the subpubic arch. (Science Museum, London)

FIGURE 22.12 (FAR RIGHT).
Earle's pelvimeter. (Science Museum, London)

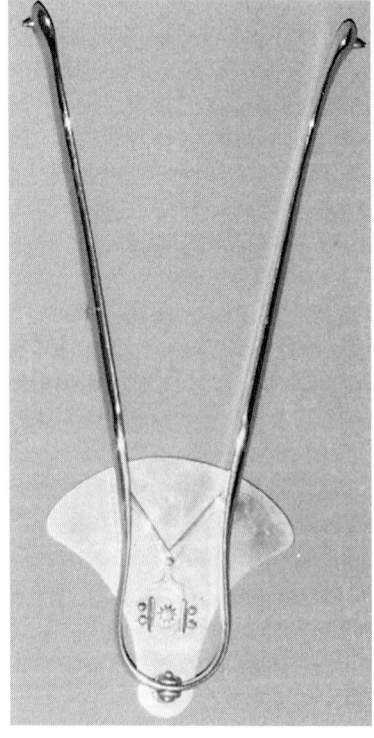

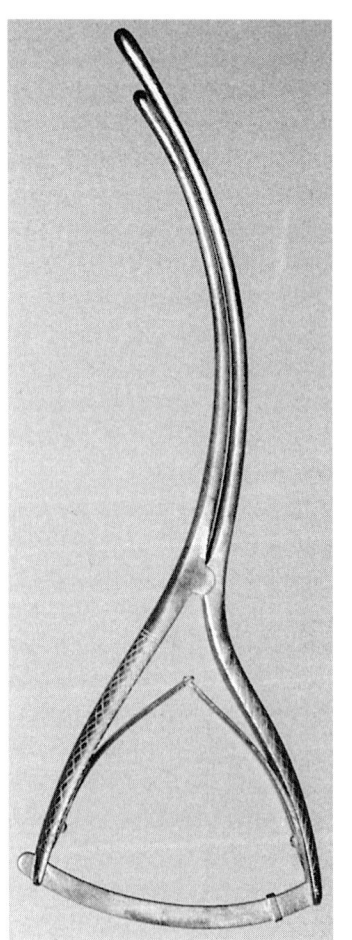

FIGURE 22.13.
Harris's pelvimeter. (Greenhalgh, 1865)

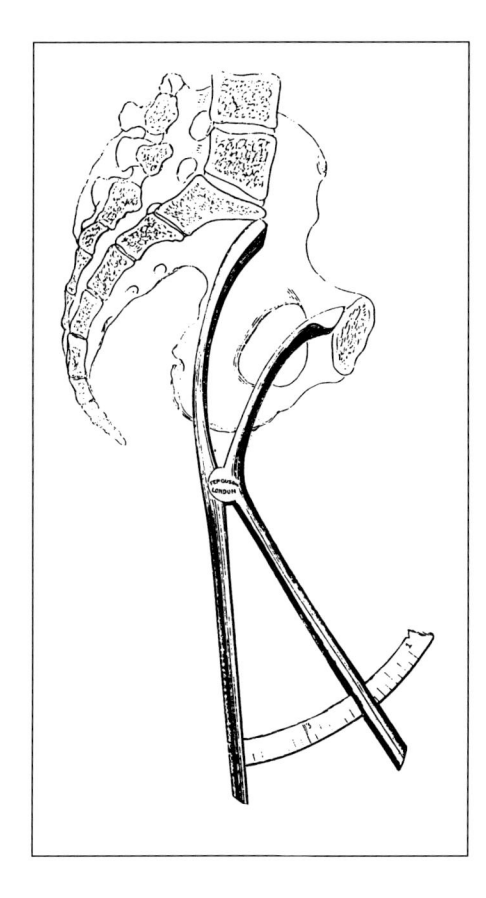

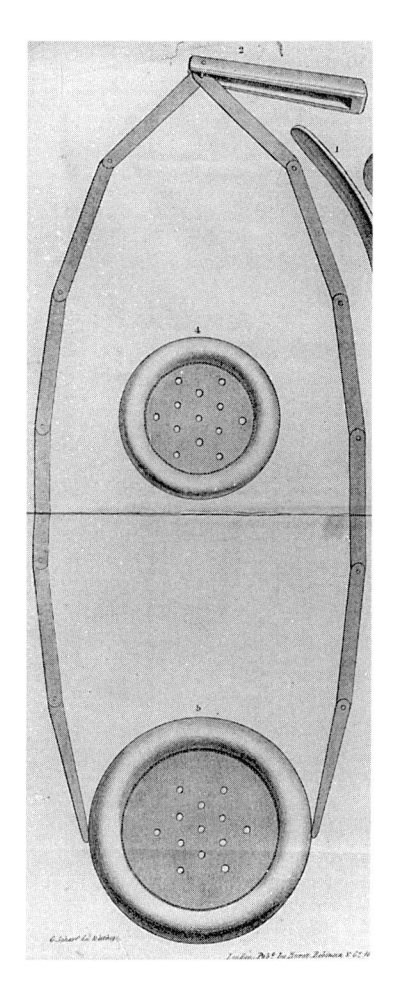

FIGURE 22.14.
Davis's pelvimeter. Each limb of the caliper has six hinged segments. (Davis, 1825)

Internal Pelvimeters

British Greenhalgh had a simple device which was in effect an extension to the index finger and is shown in use in Figure 22.8 (1865). It was the development of an idea of a graduated conical thimble, first proposed by Francesco Asdrubaldi (1756–1832) of Rome in 1795 and described in his *Treatise* of 1812.

However, most British internal pelvimeters were simple calipers and some were only used for assessing the subpubic arch by measuring the intertuberous diameter. In 1850, the London instrument maker Ferguson designed an internal pelvimeter that resembled a compass with a circular scale and a tangent screw (Figure 22.9). He exhibited it at the Obstetric Society *Conversazione* in 1866 (Meadows, 1867). Other similar designs are shown in Figure 22.10 by the London instrument makers Mayer and Meltzer and in Figure 22.11.

In an article published in 1862, James I. Lumley Earle (1840–1870), Resident Surgeon-Accoucheur to the General Dispensary, Birmingham, referred to the general prejudice against pelvimetry because of the inconvenience it caused. His pelvimeter was a simple device comprising two curved blades (to follow the curve of the sacrum). They had terminal bulbs and a spring-loaded handle with a measuring plate at the end, which was hinged on one handle and passed through a slot in the other handle (Figure 22.12). He later modified the instrument by reducing the curve and making the anterior arm shorter. Earle claimed great accuracy of measurement, with facility of application and little inconvenience. E. Murphy, in 1862, and R. P. Harris, in 1858, designed similar internal pelvimeters but it was not until 1865 that Greenhalgh claimed pride of place for Harris's instrument (Figure 22.13) on behalf of his colleague, by which time Earle's design was widely used.

Davis's portable calipers were more complex, each limb having six hinged, riveted segments (Figure 22.14), but this seems to have been little more than a design exercise that illustrated Davis's inventiveness rather than a practical instrument, for the author himself dismissed pelvimetry, saying that he did not "attach much value to any kind of artificial pelvimeter" (1825).

FIGURE 22.15 (RIGHT).
Stein's pelvimeters. The *grand pelvimètre* (Figures 1 and 2) has interchangeable ends on the short limb. The *petit pelvimètre* (Figure 3) is a measuring rod of the Coutouly type.(Stein, 1793)

FIGURES 22.16 (BELOW LEFT), 22.17 (BELOW CENTER).
Howitz's internal pelvimeter. Figure 22.16 shows a detail of the construction (Meadows, 1867). Figure 22.17 shows the detail of the scales. The two scales have to be read with the instrument *in situ*. After removal the readings are reset and the length of the crossbar measured directly. (RCOG)

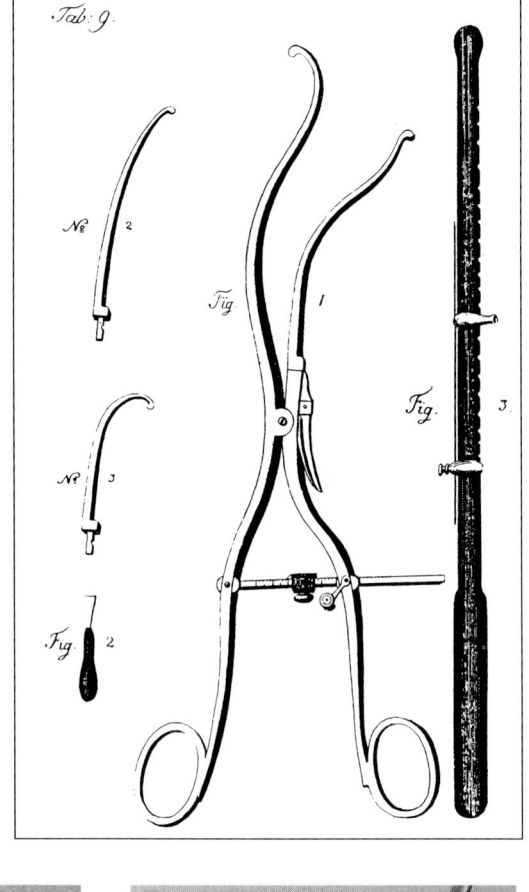

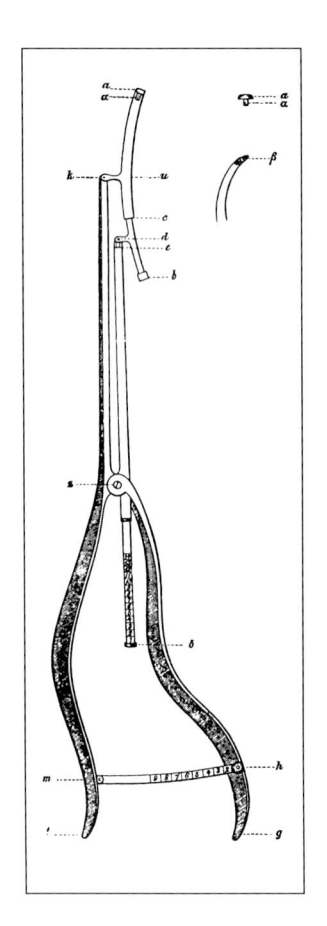

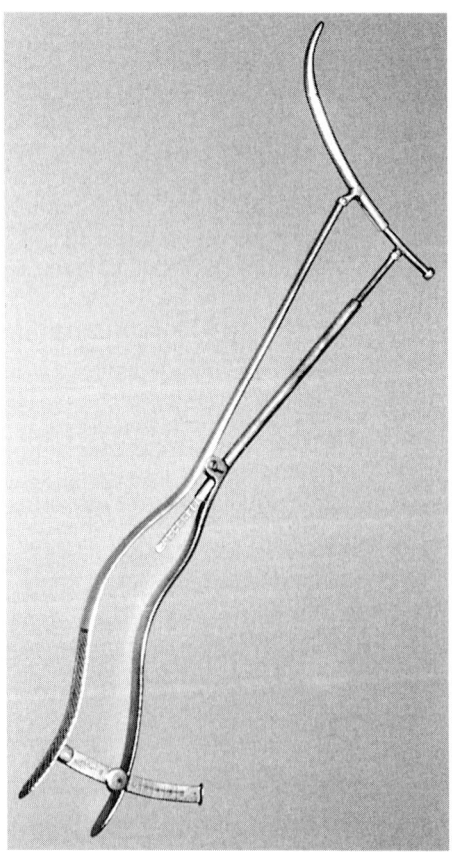

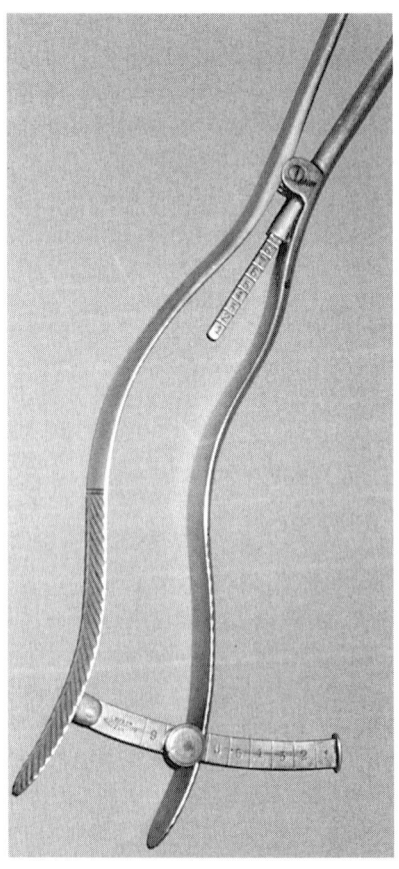

FIGURE 22.18 (BELOW RIGHT).
Howitz's internal pelvimeter. Detail of construction. (RCOG)

270 CHAPTER 22

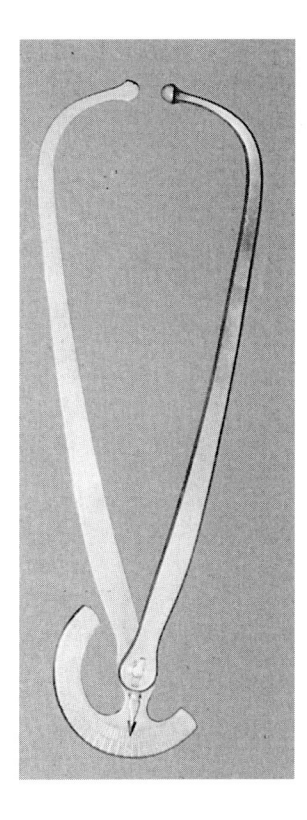

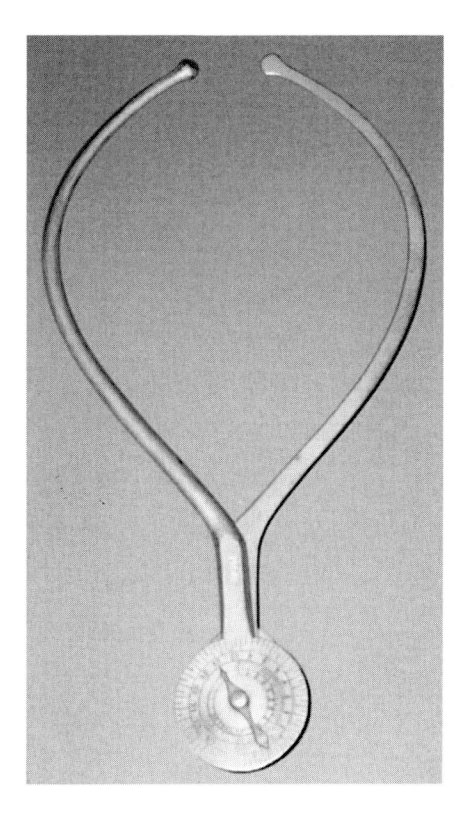

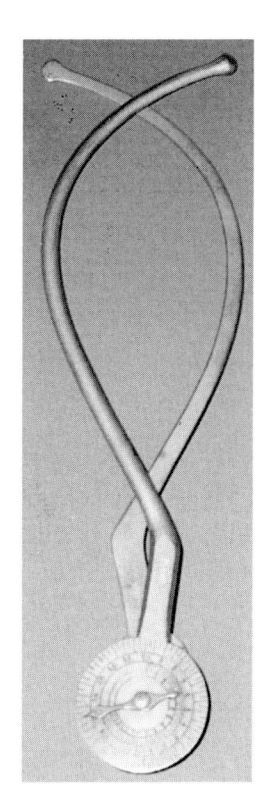

European A simple caliper instrument similar to the later British instruments, which he termed a *grand pelvimètre*, was designed by G. W. Stein and was supplemented by a measuring rod of the Coutouly type, the *petit pelvimètre* (Figure 22.15). It was used primarily for assessing the need for Caesarian section (1793).

Frantz J. A. C. Howitz's (b. 1828) pelvimeter was first described in Copenhagen in 1861 and was shown at the Obstetric Society in 1866. It was a complex device (Figures 22.16–22.18), with two measuring scales that had to be read with the instrument in position. It was then withdrawn and reset in the same position so that the length of the telescopic crossbar could be measured directly. Details of its use are given by Meadows (1867).

Combined Internal and External Pelvimeters

Early combined internal and external pelvimeters were simple adaptations of the basic caliper design. As shown in figures 22.19, 22.20, and 22.21, these instruments allowed the limbs to cross over and had a scale that could be read in both directions. They were simple, functional instruments but were cumbersome for internal pelvimetry.

Van Huevel constructed a caliper-type instrument with a telescopic projection on one limb. It was intended for mea-

FIGURE 22.19 (ABOVE LEFT).
Collins's internal and external pelvimeter.
(Science Museum, London)

FIGURES 22.20 (ABOVE),
22.21 (ABOVE RIGHT).
Boyer's internal and external pelvimeter. The flat adjoining surfaces of the calipers allows them to cross for internal pelvimetry. (RCOG)

FIGURE 22.22 (RIGHT). Rizzoli's multifunction pelvimeter. (Royal College of Surgeons)

FIGURE 22.23 (BELOW LEFT). Charrière's (Collins's) internal and external folding pelvimeter. (Meadows, 1867)

FIGURE 22.24 (BELOW RIGHT). Lazarewitch's pelvimeter. For external pelvimetry the convex arms A,B are used. For internal measurements these are replaced by the arms C,D. An additional scale G is used to measure the angle of inclination of the pelvic brim. (Meadows, 1867)

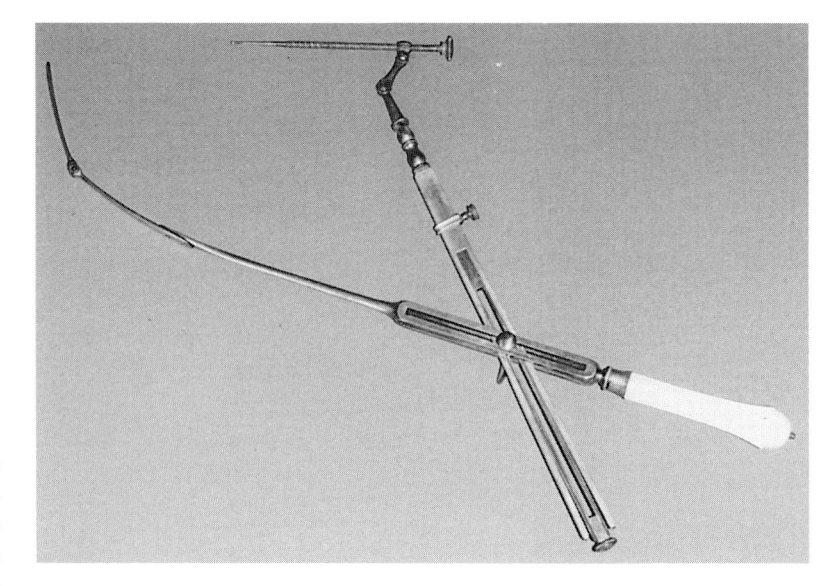

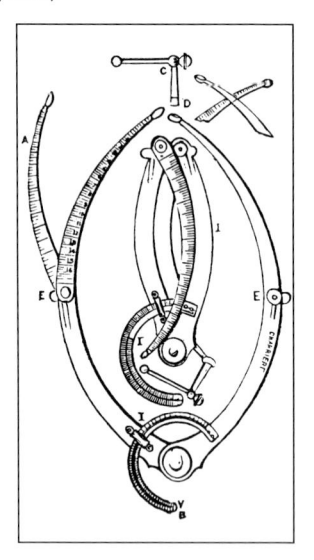

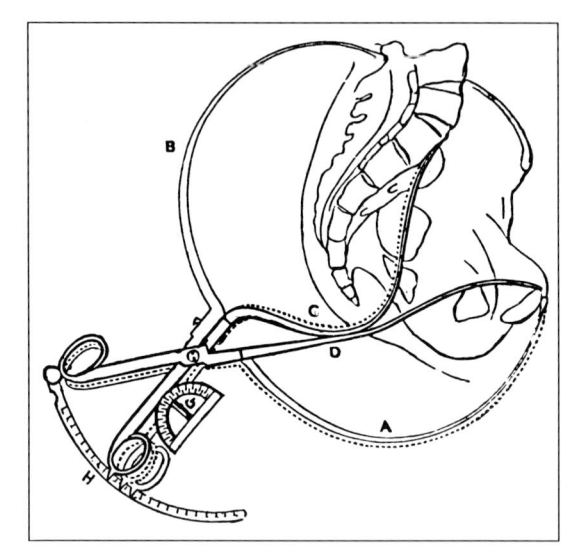

suring the external conjugate and also the thickness of the symphysis pubis. The somewhat complicated operation is described by Meadows (1867). An ingenious but not very practical modification of this instrument was made by Rizzoli of Bologna in 1856 to make it function as both a full internal and an external pelvimeter (Figure 22.22). The length of each of the two arms could be varied at will and fixed with screws. It could be used as an internal pelvimeter or to measure from the sacral promontory internally to the anterior surface of the symphysis pubis. The shape, joints, and sharp screw end on one limb made it difficult to use.

The instrument maker Charrière in Paris devised a complex, multipurpose instrument in 1862 that was meant to combine the properties of several pelvimeters then in use. He showed it at the Obstetrical Society in 1866 (Figure 22.23).

It could be used as an external pelvimeter, in the Baudelocque manner; for the measurements made with the Van Huevel instrument; or as an internal pelvimeter (Meadows, 1867). It was subsequently marketed in Britain as Collins's folding pelvimeter.

Another universal pelvimeter was shown for the first time at the Obstetric Society *Conversazione* by Lazarewitch of Kharkoff, for which he claimed that virtually any external or internal diameter could be measured (Figure 22.24).

In the quest for precision an even more complicated apparatus was described by Germann of Leipzig (1862). It comprised seven jointed pieces and a board fixed to the pelvis with a bandage. A construction of similar complexity, ascribed to Küstner, was illustrated by Witkowski (1887) (Figure 22.25).

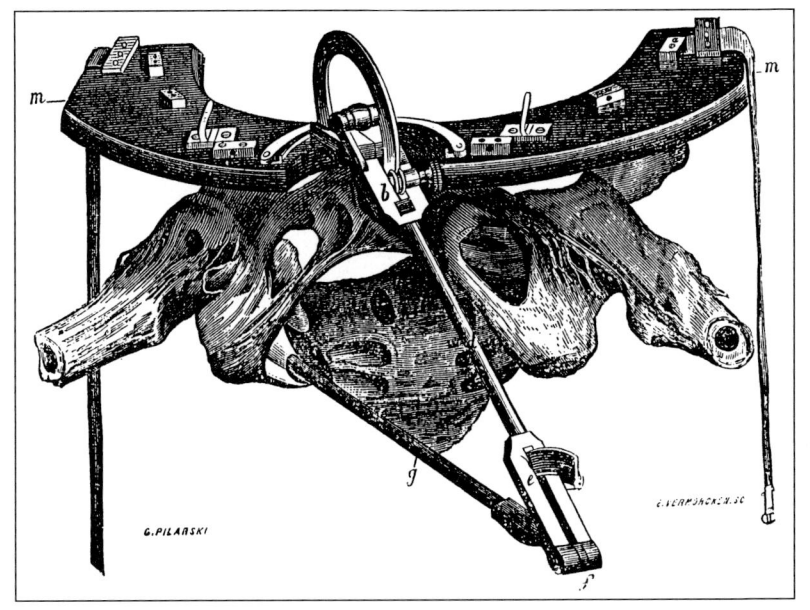

FIGURE 22.25.
Kustner's pelvimeter. A complex device that was strapped to the pelvis. (Witkowski, 1887)

FIGURES 22.26, 22.27.
Digital pelvimetry illustrated by Ramsbotham. The first method is only of value if the conjugate is less than 76mm (3ins), while the second requires the introduction of the whole hand into the vagina. (Ramsbotham, 1856)

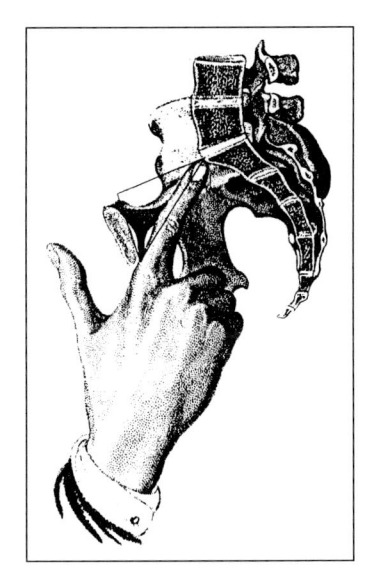

In spite of this widespread ingenuity and quest for precision, pelvimetry was not universally accepted with acclaim in Britain, even by advanced thinkers of the time. Churchill enumerated the various pelvimeters then available but said that they were rarely, if ever, used in Britain and he continued to repeat the old adage that the finger was the best pelvimeter (1866). Further, with the benefit of chloroform the whole hand could be put in the pelvis. Indeed, such was the common practice in the assessment of women who had previously experienced an obstructed labor.

F. H Ramsbotham also concluded that "such contrivances . . . have by no means met with the sanction of British practitioners in general; but they are in the habit of depending for this information on examinations conducted by the fingers or the hand" (1856) (Figures 22.26, 22.27).

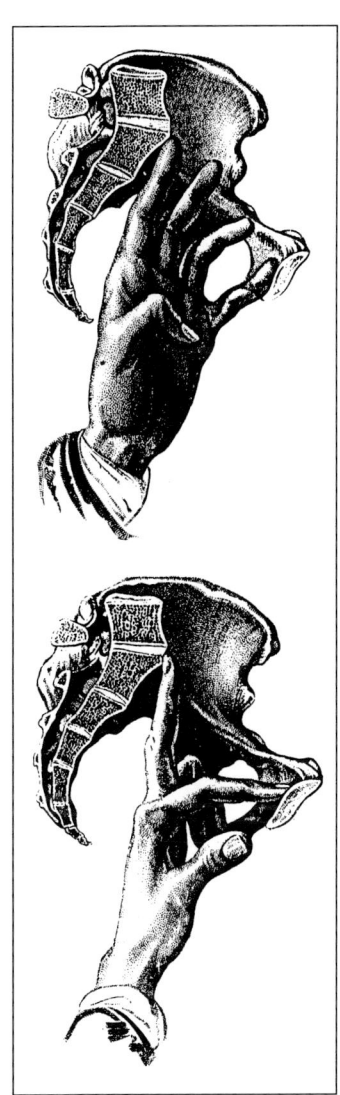

PELVIMETRY 273

Nevertheless, external pelvimeters continued to be used into the middle of the twentieth century and three measurements were considered to be of importance: (1) the external conjugate, (2) the distance between the anterior superior iliac spines, and (3) the maximum distance between the iliac crests. Radiological pelvimetry was introduced in Europe at the end of the nineteenth century but did not become generally adopted until the middle of the twentieth century, as the result of improvements in technology and the detailed studies of William Edgar Caldwell (1880–1943), Professor of Clinical Obstetrics, Columbia University, New York, and Howard Carman Moloy (1903-1953) of the Sloane Hospital l(1933, 1935, 1940), and those of Herbert Thoms (1885–1972), Professor of Obstetrics and Gynecology at Yale (1922). It was not until this time that the eighteenth-century calipers found their way to the museums.

Intrauterine Craniotomy

In a paper published in 1875, Mathews Duncan repeatedly drew attention to the remarkable neglect of the use of intrauterine craniometry, which he regarded as the natural complement to pelvimetry, claiming that it "[afforded] the accoucheur with information of the highest value." He underlined the importance of the clinical history in the assessment of disproportion, including the racial and genetic characteristics of the parents, parity, duration of pregnancy, as well as the importance of palpation of the anterior fontanel and sagittal suture. While he did not suggest any specially designed instrument for intrauterine craniometry, he did advocate application of the forceps and assessment of cephalic size by the degree of divergence of the handles. In the discussion following Mathews Duncan's paper, A. R. Simpson observed that Osiander had advocated a similar practice and had a measuring index attached to the handles of his forceps. This was effectively an attempt at revival of the labimeters that had been common in Europe in the early part of the eighteenth century (Chapter 5). Although the argument for craniometry was sound and logical the procedure never gained any great degree of popularity and most obstetricians were content to base their judgments on incomplete information.

. . .

The long saga of endeavoring to assess the capacity of the birth canal accurately and to prognosticate on the outcome of labor was too often dominated by striving for a degree of precision that was not achievable and was practically unnecessary. Mechanical innovation began to dominate design, resulting in the production of many complex curiosities. Significant further developments had to await the coming of radiology and even than it was many decades before reliable assessment became possible. By this time the perceived need for accurate pelvic mensuration was already on the wane.

MEASUREMENTS OF 17TH–EARLY 20TH CENTURY OBSTETRIC FORCEPS IN THE COLLECTION OF THE ROYAL COLLEGE OF OBSTETRICIANS AND GYNAECOLOGISTS

Measurements in millimeters
Mean radius of curvature by method of Hibbard and McKenna (1990)
Measurements do not necessarily coincide with original measurements quoted in the text because of manufacturing variations
* Brackets indicate illustration from another collection
NOT MEAS. stands for NOT MEASURABLE

CAT. NO.	FIGURE (*)	DESIGN	DATE FIRST DESCRIBED	OVERALL LENGTH	BLADE LENGTH	BLADE + SHANK LENGTH	HANDLE LENGTH	DISTANCE BETWEEN TIPS	MAX. DISTANCE BETWEEN BLADES	MEAN RADIUS OF CEPHALIC CURVE LEFT	RIGHT
18C BRITISH STRAIGHT FORCEPS											
279	2.5, 2.6	Chapman	1735	390	245	-	145	2	60	161	166
511	(2.8)	Walker	1736	348	203	-	145	3	62	133	125
ASCRIBED TO SMELLIE											
278	3.2	Smellie (wooden)	?	285	140	-	165	14	56	120	118
510		Smellie (short)	1751	284	174	-	110	20	73	106	110
282	3.7	Smellie (long)	1751	310	175	-	135	12	61	128	130
306a		Smellie (long)	1751	325	210	-	115	37	69	209	221
501	3.7	Smellie (long)	1751	315	205	-	110	15	65	146	152
502		Smellie (long)	1751	318	203	-	115	20	70	112	110
306b		Smellie type (short)	?	290	170	-	115	2	61	134	138
306c		Smellie type (short)	?	295	180	-	115	0	66	95	92
ORME/LOWDER/HAIGHTON											
503	4.2	Orme	1770–80	256	146	-	110	45	77	NOT MEAS.	
504		Orme	1770–80	256	136	-	120	50	78	NOT MEAS.	
146		Orme/Lowder	late 18c	272	162	-	110	35	73	183	115
305		Orme/Lowder	1780–90	280	160	-	120	33	78	115	109
419		Orme/Lowder	1780–90	290	160	-	130	38	77	NOT MEAS.	
505	4.2	Lowder	1780–90	287	172	-	115	24	71	128	123
281	4.2	Haighton	ca. 1790	280	160	-	120	7	67	107	101
506		Haighton	ca. 1790	292	177	-	115	15	63	143	148
507		Haighton type	late 18c.	292	172	-	120	5	61	116	116
508		Haighton type	late 18c.	314	189	-	125	15	68	130	141
OTHER 18C STRAIGHT											
509	4.3	Denman type	late 18c.	280	160	-	120	22	75	101	100
312		Denman type	late 18c.	275	160	-	110	23	73	98	97
357		Denman type	late 18c.	288	178	-	110	17	75	115	117
144	4.11	Aitken	1784	265	170	-	95	MIN. 42 MAX. 62	MIN. 77 MAX. 88	109	120

APPENDIX 275

CAT. NO.	FIGURE (*)	DESIGN	DATE FIRST DESCRIBED	OVERALL LENGTH	BLADE LENGTH	BLADE + SHANK LENGTH	HANDLE LENGTH	DISTANCE BETWEEN TIPS	MAX. DISTANCE BETWEEN BLADES	MEAN RADIUS OF CEPHALIC CURVE LEFT	RIGHT
18C BRITISH CURVED FORCEPS											
418		Smellie	1751	280	165	-	115	9	71	110	115
512	3.7 12.1	Smellie	1751	316	186	-	120	10	70	137	151
513	(2.9)	Pugh	1754	345	202	-	140	37	60	220	220
514		Pugh	1754	344	209	-	135	18	73	140	148
156		Clark	late 18c.	273	158	-	105	24	79	118	117
517		Clark	late 18c.	283	168	-	115	20	75	108	101
518		? Clark	late 18c.	288	173	-	115	20	74	119	119
276	4.6	Osborn	1792	284	164	-	120	21	73	140	140
516		Osborn type		289	174	-	115	21	75	118	120
515	4.7	Thynne	late 18c.	297	182	-	115	45	77	145	150
EDINBURGH SCHOOL											
309		Johnson	1769	282	162	-	120	32	74	102	104
551	4.9 12.1	Johnson	1769	270	165	-	105	22	76	98	94
310b		Johnson type		281	166	-	115	54	82	197	181
356		Johnson type		301	176	-	125	33	76	107	107
310a		Young	ca. 1780	276	176	-	110	22	77	107	97
552	4.9	Young	ca. 1780	302	198	-	110	22	75	144	151
311		Hamilton	1793	290	175	-	115	15	70	121	123
553	8.9	Hamilton	1793	283	163	-	120	26	70	101	102
554	4.9 8.9 8.11	Hamilton	1793	300	185	-	115	30	75	113	103
548		Edinburgh type	Late 18c.	310	175	-	135	29	78	124	119
549		Edinburgh type	Late 18c.	297	177	-	120	3	83	105	107
550		Edinburgh type	Late 18c.	289	174	-	115	18	65	110	101
INTERLOCKING BLADES											
277	8.27 8.29	J.Beatty	ca. 1829	300	175	-	125	20	87	104	101
559	8.30	Barclay	1872	345	150	215	130	25	75	122	124
560		Barclay	1872	348	155	218	130	25	76	129	135
153		Ziegler (straight)	ca. 1850	316	145	210	110	30	68	124	121
261		Ziegler (straight)	ca. 1850	340	175	225	115	22	74	168	132
353		Ziegler (straight)	ca. 1850	322	150	207	115	27	71	128	137
556	8.28	Ziegler (straight)	ca. 1850	340	155	220	120	20	77	117	122
RH 10		Ziegler (straight)	ca. 1850	310	153	182	128	19	64	134	119
555	8.28 8.29	Ziegler (curved)	ca. 1850	355	155	214	140	24	76	142	138
251		Ziegler (curved)	ca. 1850	313	133	183	130	33	68	126	114
260	8.28	Ziegler (asymmetric)	ca. 1850	347	160	217	130	43	72	161	151
557		Ziegler type	2nd half 18c.	310	155	195	115	18	74	118	118
558		Ziegler type	2nd half 18c.	302	135	182	120	24	65	103	109

CAT. NO.	FIGURE (*)	DESIGN	DATE FIRST DESCRIBED	OVERALL LENGTH	BLADE LENGTH	BLADE + SHANK LENGTH	HANDLE LENGTH	DISTANCE BETWEEN TIPS	MAX. DISTANCE BETWEEN BLADES	MEAN RADIUS OF CEPHALIC CURVE LEFT	RIGHT

19C BRITISH SHORT STRAIGHT FORCEPS

CAT. NO.	FIGURE	DESIGN	DATE	OVERALL	BLADE	BLADE+SHANK	HANDLE	TIPS	BLADES	LEFT	RIGHT
RH1	(4.10)	Collins	ca. 1830	278	148	-	130	40	83	95	94
147	6.11	J.Y. Simpson (short)	ca. 1840	240	175	-	65	25	67	128	127
148	6.11, 6.26	J.Y. Simpson (short)	ca. 1840	245	180	-	65	18	72	127	121
197		J.Y. Simpson (short)	ca. 1840	247	187	-	60	18	68	117	118
RH8		J.Y. Simpson (short)	ca. 1840	249	132	-	71	31	75	111	108
365	(6.20)	Braithwaite	1869	285	145	190	95	21	72	121	126
274		Unidentified	early 19c.	296	181	-	115	19	75	127	127
250		Unidentified	late 19c.	280	175	-	105	35	80	127	121
522		Unidentified	mid 19c.	303	183	-	120	20	68	137	134
101		Unidentified		287	177	-	110	40	88	96	116

19C BRITISH INTERMEDIATE AND LONG STRAIGHT FORCEPS

CAT. NO.	FIGURE	DESIGN	DATE	OVERALL	BLADE	BLADE+SHANK	HANDLE	TIPS	BLADES	LEFT	RIGHT
151		Conquest	1820	328	204	-	124	24	75	183	198
520		Conquest	1820	327	202	-	125	10	65	180	175
521	8.12	Conquest	1820	342	215	-	127	14	65	222	217
RH7		Conquest	1820	337	137	-	135	10	72	172	158
524	9.11	Radford asymmetric	1825	L 325 / R 344	150 / 170	245 / 264	80 / 80	- / -	75	125	123
248		Radford asymmetric	1825	L 330 / R 350	170 / 190	255 / 275	75 / 75	- / -	80	125	162
355		Blundell	ca. 1830	366	150	230	136	21	72	143	142
525		? Blundell ? Waller	mid 19c	360	155	220	140	22	70	120	122
202		Ramsbotham "short"	1832	283	163	-	120	22	75	110	108
265	6.17	Churchill	1840	348	210	-	138	25	72	207	207
RH2		Churchill	1840	315	185	-	130	25	75	125	116
152	6.17	T.E. Beatty	ca. 1842	305	195	-	115	75	25	123	110
RH3		T.E. Beatty	ca. 1842	312	192	-	120	30	75	157	156
526	6.17	Hewitt type	1861	320	215	-	115	25	78	143	148
RH4		Murphy	1862	317	167	197	120	22	80	115	112
201	(6.19)	Murphy	1862	327	170	212	115	23	77	123	120
264		Unidentified	late 19c.	393	108	243	150	26	81	188	157
262		Unidentified–hinged blades		380	160	255	125	18	80	124	126

APPENDIX 277

CAT. NO.	FIGURE (*)	DESIGN	DATE FIRST DESCRIBED	OVERALL LENGTH	BLADE LENGTH	BLADE + SHANK LENGTH	HANDLE LENGTH	DISTANCE BETWEEN TIPS	MAX. DISTANCE BETWEEN BLADES	MEAN RADIUS OF CEPHALIC CURVE LEFT	RIGHT

J. Y. SIMPSON AND RELATED LONG CURVED FORCEPS

CAT. NO.	FIGURE	DESIGN	DATE	OVERALL	BLADE	BLADE+SHANK	HANDLE	TIPS	BLADES	LEFT	RIGHT
149	6.26	J.Y. Simpson	1848	350	160	220	130	39	80	150	137
198		J.Y. Simpson	1848	347	157	212	135	25	78	148	145
256		J.Y. Simpson	1848	345	155	210	135	24	77	133	137
266		J.Y. Simpson	1848	353	153	213	140	21	76	136	139
354		J.Y. Simpson	1848	346	156	211	135	24	78	142	146
422		J.Y. Simpson	1848	352	132	225	127	14	75	101	112
RH9		J.Y. Simpson	1848	350	154	215	135	27	76	122	127
204	6.30	Barnes	1866	370	165	240	130	21	75	162	162
205		Barnes	1866	370	160	235	135	25	78	133	199
258		Barnes	1866	375	165	245	130	17	75	155	155
263		Barnes	1866	370	160	240	130	19	80	132	128
324		Barnes	1866	370	160	235	135	25	78	133	119
543		Barnes	1866	373	170	243	130	8	77	132	122
544		Barnes	1866	370	170	245	125	25	75	150	153
545		Barnes	1866	370	170	240	130	31	75	152	154
546		Barnes	1866	370	170	240	130	16	76	137	125
RH 11		Barnes	1866	376	173	246	130	22	74	166	162
200	6.31	Anderson	1879	376	161	241	135	21	76	141	136
254		Anderson	1879	365	155	235	130	25	90	139	132
367		Anderson	1879	373	170	240	133	20	72	151	153
547		J.Y. Simpson type–hinged shanks	late 19c.	357	155	227	130	20	73	118	117

OTHER 19C BRITISH CURVED FORCEPS

CAT. NO.	FIGURE	DESIGN	DATE	OVERALL	BLADE	BLADE+SHANK	HANDLE	TIPS	BLADES	LEFT	RIGHT
538	(6.23)	Ramsbotham	1832	330	160	215	115	26	76	140	143
539		? Simpson modification of Ramsbotham	mid 19c.	347	170	227	120	27	76	132	141
206		Radford	1839	372	177	237	135	24	77	159	161
536		Radford	1839	355	170	225	130	25	75	126	118
537	6.22	Radford	1839	365	180	235	130	14	75	141	153
145	(6.28)	Mathews Duncan	1861	320	170	210	110	25	81	124	124
541		Mathews Duncan	1861	323	160	213	110	27	72	148	142
272		Unidentified	mid 19c.	290	175	-	115	59	84	157	154
275		Unidentified	mid 19c.	343	203	-	140	18	62	220	220
540		Unidentified	mid 19c.	382	170	252	130	23	77	127	137
542		Unidentified	early–mid 19c.	354	165	214	140	30	75	134	130

CAT. NO.	FIGURE (*)	DESIGN	DATE FIRST DESCRIBED	OVERALL LENGTH	BLADE LENGTH	BLADE + SHANK LENGTH	HANDLE LENGTH	DISTANCE BETWEEN TIPS	MAX. DISTANCE BETWEEN BLADES	MEAN RADIUS OF CEPHALIC CURVE LEFT RIGHT
DAVID DAVIS										
528		Davis I ("COMMON" FORCEPS) unhinged	1823	303	160	203	100	11	64	168 166 APPROX.
529	6.1	Davis I ("COMMON" FORCEPS) hinged	1823	300	170	200	100	25	70	183 166 APPROX.
530	6.1	Davis II – blades of unequal breadth	1823	307	165	207	100	14	64	152 119
531	6.1	Davis II – blades of unequal breadth	1823	308	170	203	105	14	62	124 150 APPROX.
532	6.1	Davis III – blades of unequal length L R	1823	238 297	88 147	128 187	110 –	– –	65 –	NOT MEAS. 90
533	6.1	Davis III – blades of unequal length L R	1823	304 255	144 95	194 145	110 –	– –	65 –	80 NOT MEAS.
534	6.1	Davis IV – straight blade for use with Davis III	1823	274	130	169	105	–	–	NOT MEAS.
535	6.1	Davis V – jointed blade	1823	375	190	260	115	–	–	NOT MEAS.
157		Davis type	mid 19c.	305	210	–	95	35	65	179 159 APPROX.
527		Davis type	mid 19c.	296	181	–	115	15	62	137 134 APPROX.

EUROPEAN FORCEPS

CAT. NO.	FIGURE (*)	DESIGN	DATE FIRST DESCRIBED	OVERALL LENGTH	BLADE LENGTH	BLADE + SHANK LENGTH	HANDLE LENGTH	DISTANCE BETWEEN TIPS	MAX. DISTANCE BETWEEN BLADES	MEAN RADIUS OF CEPHALIC CURVE LEFT RIGHT
246	2.15	Dusée	early 18c.	387	127	167	210	64	82	NOT MEAS.
308		Dusée	early 18c.	420	150 APPROX.	a. 210 b. 210	a. 200 b. 140	a. 18 b. 42	a. 83 b. 113	86 86 APPROX. APPROX.
307	3.14 3.15	Levret Type III	ca. 1762	395	325	–	70	0	70	161 164
196	(5.8)	A. Dubois	1791	470	275	–	200	5	65	192 189
247		A. Dubois	1791	382	225	–	155	32	60	NOT MEAS.
562		? Starke	? 1785	350	200	–	150	31	80	125 128
154	10.14	Assalini (straight)	1811	295	145	–	–	VARIABLE	VARIABLE	115 115
564		Assalini (curved)	1811	322	187	–	–	VARIABLE	VARIABLE	154 154
136	10.14	Assalini (curved)	1811	337	222	–	–	VARIABLE	VARIABLE	147 143
155	10.14	Assalini (curved)	1811	295	145	–	–	VARIABLE	VARIABLE	123 127
257		Assalini (curved)	1811	311	156	–	–	VARIABLE	VARIABLE	122 127
150	5.24	Stolz	ca. 1839	435	240	–	190	12	73	123 124
103	5.25	Spiegelberg	mid 19c.	370	250	–	120	26	79	146 142
565	(5.8)	P. Dubois	ca. 1850	470	220	–	250	6	71	118 122
142	5.22	Naegele	ca. 1850	380	230	–	150	45	85	153 209
420		Naegele	ca. 1850	395	215	–	180	12	70	126 134
455		Naegele	ca. 1850	370	215	–	155	12	68	121 118
RH 15		Naegele	ca. 1850	358	200	–	158	0.5	61	128 136
566	10.21	Lazarewitch (parallel)	ca. 1860	283	148	188	95	16	71	99 96
563	5.23	J. D. Busch	late 18c.	398	248	–	150	4	77	104 106
567		Prague School	19c.	366	211	–	155	23	61	134 119
568	5.1	Prague School	19c.	401	321	–	180	15	67	151 153

CAT. NO.	FIGURE (*)	DESIGN	DATE FIRST DESCRIBED	OVERALL LENGTH	BLADE LENGTH	BLADE + SHANK LENGTH	HANDLE LENGTH	DISTANCE BETWEEN TIPS	MAX. DISTANCE BETWEEN BLADES	MEAN RADIUS OF CEPHALIC CURVE LEFT	RIGHT
AMERICAN FORCEPS											
407	7.14	Elliot	1858	390	-	230	160	18	71	130	128
415	7.20	Tucker-McLane (Luikart modification)	1885	397	147	247	150	26	74	103	96
416		Barton	1925	364	150	230	150	35	85	101	109
404		Barton, with traction rod	1925	368	155	208	160	35	88	120	120
459		Barton, with traction rod	1925	375	175	260	115	35	90	130	100
AXIS-TRACTION FORCEPS											
STEPPED SHANKS											
141	12.10	Galabin	1877	410	150	230	190	19	73	124	118
199	12.12	Wagstaff	ca. 1890	330	180	230	100	16	67	135	122
362		Wagstaff	ca. 1890	332	172	205	118	16	68	116 APPROX.	118
461		Wagstaff	ca. 1890	335	185	215	120	21	75	128	128
TARNIER-TYPE FORCEPS AND MODIFICATIONS											
RH 12		Tarnier (early model)	1877	352	152 APPROX.	258	94	9	65	132	136
363	13.4	Tarnier	ca. 1880	380	175 APPROX.	245	140	20	62	139	134
249	13.7 13.8 13.9	A. R. Simpson	1879	348	155	215	133	28	78	136	128
RH 13		A. R. Simpson	1879	370	162	230	140	19	80	142	144
268		Milne Murray	1897–99	370	160	230	140	28	78	175	179
401		Milne Murray	1897–99	362	160	220	142	23	69	157	158
408	13.11 13.12 13.13	Milne Murray	1897–99	370	165	235	135	28	77	134	134
421		Milne Murray	1897–99	382	170	242	140	28	89	136	134
RH 14		Milne Murray	1897–99	364	156	224	140	32	80	135	145
267		Milne Murray/ A. R. Simpson hybrid	late 19c.	370	165	230	140	28	78	175	179
271		Milne Murray/ A. R. Simpson hybrid	late 19c.	360	155	215	145	23	80	127	134
402		Milne Murray/ A. R. Simpson hybrid	late 19c.	370	165	225	145	28	77	150	149
462		Milne Murray/ A. R. Simpson hybrid	late 19c.	360	160	220	140	22	75	134	136
270		? Milne Murray	late 19c.	370	160	235	135	24	78	152	136

CAT. NO.	FIGURE (*)	DESIGN	DATE FIRST DESCRIBED	OVERALL LENGTH	BLADE LENGTH	BLADE + SHANK LENGTH	HANDLE LENGTH	DISTANCE BETWEEN TIPS	MAX. DISTANCE BETWEEN BLADES	MEAN RADIUS OF CEPHALIC CURVE LEFT	RIGHT
OTHER AXIS-TRACTION FORCEPS											
403	14.4, 14.5	Barnes-Neville	ca. 1896	385	165	255	130	42	80	173	166
423	14.5	Anderson-Neville	ca. 1896	423	166	246	130	23	82	126	132
424		Anderson-Neville	ca. 1896	376	166	246	130	26	87	130	124
425		Anderson-Neville	ca. 1896	368	158	238	130	26	83	123	118
426		Anderson-Neville	ca. 1896	380	165	250	130	29	79	152	150
427		Anderson-Neville	ca. 1896	366	156	236	130	27	80	119	126
366	14.5	Greville	ca. 1904	382	157	242	140	20	81	134	132
143		Breus	1882	390	165	245	145	50	93	136	128
428		Cameron	1893	312	155	197	115	0	39	170	152
434		Porter Mathew	1898	298	150	230	68	20	70	121	111
464		Porter Mathew	1898	295	175	235	60	25	70	171	170
259		Bonney	1902	365	150	225	135	27	73	132	125
405		Haig Ferguson	1911	330	160	230	100	33	82	130	128
417		Haig Ferguson	1911	326	150	215	111	24	81	119	125
463		Haig Ferguson	1911	330	160	230	100	33	82	138	129
435		Kielland *Original*	1910–16	405	180	270	120	19	83	120	120
255		Kielland *Original*	1910–16	405	180	245	160	40	77	126	126
296		Unidentified		388	210 APPROX.	258 APPROX.	130 APPROX.	42	83	142	147

BIBLIOGRAPHY

Aitken, D. W. 1893. New Midwifery Forceps. *British Medical Journal*. 1: 76.

Aitken, J. 1784. *Principles of Midwifery, or Puerperal Medicine*. First edition. London: Murray. Third edition, 1786.

Albucasis. *Chirurgia*. *See* Spink and Lewis, 1973.

Amand, P. 1715. *Nouvelle Observations sur la pratique des accouchemens*. Second edition. Paris: D'Houry.

Anderson, C. L. 1879. Modification of Midwifery Forceps. *Obstetrical Journal*. 6: 720.

Anderson, T. 1870. An Instrument for Piecemeal Extraction of the Foetus. *Medical Times and Gazette*. 2: 435–436.

Arnold and Sons. 1885, 1889. *Catalogue of Surgical Instruments and Appliances*. London.

Arnott, N. 1829. *Elements of Physics or Natural Philosophy*. Volume I. Fourth edition. London: Longman, Rees, Orme, Brown and Green. Pages 332–334 (Part III, Section II), 650–653 (Part II, Section V).

Asdrubaldi, F. 1812. *Trattato generale di ostetricia, teoretica e prattica*. Second edition. Rome: de Romanis.

Assalini, P. 1811. *Nuovi stromenti di ostetricia e loro uso*. Milan: Stamperia reale.

Auvard, A. 1884. *De la pince à os et du crânioclaste*. Paris: O. Doin.

Aveling, J. H. 1870. On the Advantages to Be Gained from Curving the Handles of the Midwifery Forceps. *British Medical Journal*. 2: 528.

———. 1872. *English Midwives, Their History and Prospects*. Reprinted with a biographical sketch of the author by John L. Thornton. London: Elliott, 1967.

———. 1874. An Account of the Earliest English Work on Midwifery and the Diseases of Women. *Obstetric Journal of Great Britain and Ireland*. 2: 73–83.

———. 1882. *The Chamberlens and the Midwifery Forceps*. London: Churchill.

———. 1879. The Curves of the Midwifery Forceps; Their Origins and Uses. *Transactions of the Obstetrical Society of London*. 20: 130–151.

Avicenna. *Liber Canonis*. *See also* Grunner, 1970.

Baglioni, S. 1937. Conoscevano gli antichi l'uso del forcipe ostetrico. *Fisiologia e medicina*. 8: 169–175.

Ballantyne, J. W. 1906. The "Byrthe of Mankynde" (It's [sic] Author and Editions). *Journal of Obstetrics and Gynaecology of the British Empire*. 10: 297–325.

———. 1907. The "Byrthe of Mankynde" (It's [sic] Contents). *Journal of Obstetrics and Gynaecology of the British Empire*. 12: 175–194, 255–274.

Barclay, J. 1872. A New Midwifery Forceps. *Lancet*. 1: 9–10.

Bard, S. 1808. *A Compendium of the Theory and Practice of Midwifery for Midwives, Students and Young Practitioners*. New York: Collins and Perkins.

Barker, F. 1877. Demonstration of Tarnier's forceps. *Medical Times and Gazette*. 2: 680.

———. 1878. Remarks on the Obstetric Forceps, with a Description and Demonstration of Tarnier's New Instrument. *American Journal of Obstetrics*. 11: 1–11.

Barnes, R. 1862. On the Indications and Operations for the Induction of Premature Labour and for the Acceleration of Labour. *Transactions of the Obstetrical Society of London*. 3: 107–141.

———. 1864. Craniotomy Forceps. *Transactions of the Obstetrical Society of London*. 5: 277–279.

———. 1869a. A New Method of Embryotomy. *Transactions of the Obstetrical Society of London*. 11: 126–128.

———. 1869b. Dr Barnes's Water-bags—Response to Dr Playfair's Letter. *Medical Times and Gazette*. 2: 446–447.

———. 1870. *Lectures on Obstetric Operations*. First edition. London: Churchill. Fourth edition, 1886.

———. 1878. Modification of Tarnier's Forceps. *Transactions of the Obstetrical Society of London*. 20: 163.

Barnes, R., and F. Barnes. 1885. *A System of Obstetric Medicine and Surgery*. Volume 2. London: Smith, Elder.

Bartlett, J. 1880. The Mechanics of the Obstetrical Forceps. *Chicago Medical Journal and Examiner*. 40: 225–249. See also Jaggard, 1886.

Baskett, T. F. 1996. *On the Shoulders of Giants: Eponyms and Names in Obstetrics and Gynaecology*. London: RCOG Press.

Baudelocque, A. C. 1833. *See* Bethel, 1853.

Baudelocque, J. L. 1776. *An in partu, propter augustiam pelvis, impossibili, symphysis ossium pubis secanda*. Paris.

———. 1781. *L'Art des accouchemens*. Paris: Méquignon. Second edition, 1789. Paris: Méquignon l'aîné.

———. 1790. *A System of Midwifery*. English translation of *L'Art des accouchemens* by J. Heath. London: Parkinson and Murray.

———. 1823. *An Abridgement of Mr Heath's Translation of Baudelocque's Midwifery, with Notes, by William P. Dewees, M.D.* Third edition. Philadelphia: Thomas Desilver.

Baudelocque, L.-A. 1836. *De la céphalotripsie, suivie de l'histoire de 15 opérations de ce genre*. Paris: Dupuy.

Baumers, M. R. 1849. Mémoires sur les indications et les avantages d'un forceps courbé sur le plat. *Gazette médicale de Paris*. 4: 538–542, 558–564.

Beatty, J. 1829. Observations on the Use of Instruments in Cases of Difficult and Protracted Labour. Paper to the Association of Physicians (Dublin). Reprinted as Chapter 1 in Beatty, T. E. 1866. *Contributions to Medicine and Midwifery*. Dublin: Fannin.

Beatty, T. E. 1842. Contributions to Midwifery. No. IV: Cases Illustrative of the Use of the Forceps. *Dublin Journal of Medical Science*. 21: 337–363.

———. 1867. On Dr Barnes' Description of Dr Beatty's Forceps. *Medical Times and Gazette*. 2: 314–316.

Bedford, G. S. 1861. *The Principles and Practice of Obstetrics*. New York: Wood.

Benjamin, D. 1898. Some Practical Remarks on the Obstetric Forceps; a Description of a Modified Simpson's Forceps and Also a Traction Instrument. *American Obstetrical and Gynecological Journal*. 13: 248–255.

Bernard, C. 1836. Sur un nouveau forceps. *Bulletin de L'Académie Royale de Médicine* (Paris). 1: 177–178.

———. 1853. *Mémoire sur le forceps-assembli, ou nouveaux principes de construction et d'application du forceps*. Brussels: J. B. Tircher.

Bethell, J. P. 1853. Description of a New Obstetric Forceps Constructed upon Philosophical Principles. *American Journal of the Medical Sciences*. 27: 116–120.

Black, J. W., Editor. 1871. *Selected Obstetrical and Gynaecological Works of Sir James Y. Simpson*. Edinburgh: Adam and Black.

Bland, R. 1790. Some Account of the Invention and Use of the Lever of Roonhuysen. *Medical Communications of the Society for Promoting Medical Knowledge*. 2: 397–462.

———. 1794. *Observations on Human and on Comparative Parturition*. London: Johnson, Becket and Cuthel.

Blenkarne, W. L'H. 1889. An Improved Midwifery Forceps. *British Medical Journal*. 1: 423.

Blond, K. 1923. *Der Dekapitationsfingerhut. Zentralblat für Gynäkologie.* 47: 1097–1100.

Blot, H. 1855a. Nouveau craniotome. *Gazette des hôpitaux civils et militaires. Paris.* 28: 439.

———. 1855b. Correspondance. *Gazette médicale de Paris.* 10: 601.

Blundell, J. 1832. *Lectures on Midwifery, and the Diseases of Women and Children; As Delivered at Guy's Hospital.* London: Field and Bull.

———. 1834. *The Principles and Practice of Obstetricy, As at Present Taught by James Blundell. To Which Are Added Notes and Illustrations by Thomas Castle.* London: Cox.

———. 1839. *Lectures on the Principles and Practice of Midwifery.* Edited by Charles Severn. London: Masters.

———. 1840. *The Principles and Practice of Obstetric Medicine.* Revised by A. L. Lee and N. Rogers. London: Butler.

Blunt, J (pseudonym of S. W. Fores). 1793. *Man-Midwifery Dissected.* London: Fores.

Böehmer, A. 1746. *Artis obstetricariae compendium tam theoriam quam praxin.* Halle. (Cited in Doran, 1913a)

Boër, L. J. 1812. *Naturalis medicinae obstetricae libri septem.* Vienna: De Moesle. *See also* Carus, 1828.

Bossi, L. M. 1892. Sulla provocazione artificiale del parto. *Annali di ostetricia e ginecologia.* 14: 881–928.

———. 1900. Il mio instrumentoridotto a quatro branche. *Annali di ostetricia e ginecologia.* 21: 516–521.

Bourgeois, L. 1609. *Observations diverses sur la stérilité, perte de fruict, foecondité, accouchements et maladies des femmes et enfants nouveaux naiz.* Paris: Saugrain.

Braithwaite, J. 1869. Remarks on a Mode of Applying the Short Midwifery-Forceps, Productive of Less Pain to, and Disturbance of, the Patient Than That Usually Adopted. *British Medical Journal.* 2: 673–674.

Braun (von Ferwald), C. 1859. Ueber die neueren Methoden der Craniotomie des Fötus. *Zeitschrift der kaiserlich-königlichen Gesellschaft der Aerzte zu Wien.* 15: 33–37. *See also* Mundé, 1873; Ritchie, 1865.

———. 1886. Ueber die Vielseitige Verwendbarkeit einer deigestaltigen Geburtszange. *Wiener medizinische Wochenschrift. Sechsunddreissigster Jahrgang.* No. 9: 285–289.(Abstract: *See American Journal of Obstetrics.* 1886. 19: 1230–1231.)

Braun, G. A. 1861. Über das technische Verfahren bei vernachlässigten Querlagen und über Decapitationsinstrumente. *Wiener medizinische Wochenschrift.* 11: 713–716.

———. 1880. Ueber Tarniers Forceps. *Wiener medizinische Wochenschrift. Dreissigster Jahrgang.* No. 25: 681–685, 709–711. (Abstract: *See American Journal of Obstetrics.* 1881. 14: 186.)

Bredin, J. N. 1889. Midwifery Forceps. *Lancet* 1:83.

Breisky, A. *See* Das, 1929.

Breus, C. 1882. Ueber eine neue vereinfachte Construction der sogenannten Achsenzugzangen. *Archiv für Gynaekologie.* 20: 211–235. (Abstract: *See American Journal of Obstetrics* .1886. 19: 421–425.)

———. 1885. *Die Beckeneingangzangen.* Vienna: Toeplitz and Deuticke.

Browne, O. D. T. 1947. *The Rotunda Hospital 1745–1945.* Edinburgh: Livingstone.

Brulatour. 1817. Mémoire sur un nouveau genre de forceps. *Séance publique de l'École Royale de Médecine de Bordeaux.* 14–19. Bordeaux: Pierre Beaume.

Brunninghausen, H. J. 1802. *Uber eine neue von ihm erfindene Geburtszange.* Wurzberg.

Burge, J. H. H. 1880–1881. A New Obstetric Forceps; Multiple, Adjustable and Readjustable. *Proceedings of the Medical Society of Kings County, Brooklyn.* 5: 23–27. *See also* Tiemann, 1889.

Burns, J. 1809. *The Principles of Midwifery.* First edition. London: Longman, Hurst, Rees and Orme. Tenth edition, 1843.

Burton, J. 1751. *An Essay towards a Complete New System of Midwifry.* London: Hodges.

———. 1753. *A Letter to William Smellie MD.* London: Owen.

Busch, D. W. H. 1841. *Atlas geburtshülflicher Abbildungen mit Bezugnahme auf das Lehrbuch der Geburtskunde.* Berlin: Hirschwald.

Busch, J. D. 1796. Beschreibung einer neuen Geburtszange, nebst einigen Beobachtungen über ihre Anwendung. *Archiv für der Geburtshülfe, Jena.* 6: 438–454.

———. 1801–1802. Beschreibung eines Labimeters zu meiner Geburtszange. *Archiv für der Geburtshülfe, Jena.* 2: 109–116.

Butter, A. 1735. The Description of a Forceps for Extracting Children by the Head When Lodged Low in the Pelvis of the Mother. *Medical Essays and Observations (Edinburgh).* 3: 325.

Caldwell, W. E. 1933. Anatomical Variations in the Female Pelvis and Their Effects in Labor with a Suggested Classification. *American Journal of Obstetrics and Gynecology.* 26: 479–505.

Caldwell, W. E., H. C. Moloy, and D. A. D'Esopo. 1935. Further Studies on the Mechanism of Labour. *American Journal of Obstetrics and Gynecology.* 30: 763–814.

———. 1940. The More Recent Conceptions of the Pelvic Architecture. *American Journal of Obstetrics and Gynecology.* 40: 558–565.

Cameron, M. *See* Kerr, 1908.

Campbell, C. J. *See* Poullet, 1883.

Campbell, W. M. 1899. The Midwifery Forceps as Used and Abused. *The Liverpool Medico-Chirurgical Journal.* 22: 1–24.

Cappie, J. 1863. Modification of Midwifery Forceps. *Edinburgh Medical Journal.* 8: 557–561.

———. 1872. On the Mode of Introducing the Midwifery Forceps, with Note of Their Modification. *Transactions of the Edinburgh Obstetrical Society 1869–71.* 2: 369–379.

Capuron. 1842–1843. Nouveau forceps à double articulation. *Bulletin d'AcadémieRoyale de Médecine de Paris.* 8:1136–1138.

———. 1843–1844. Note sur un nouveau forceps. *Bulletin d'Académie de Médecine de Paris.* 9: 757–759.

Carof, J. 1869. Notice sur un forceps à articulation libre. *Bulletin d'Academie Royale de Médecine de Belge (Bruxelles).* Third series. 3: 1216–1220.

Carus, C. G. 1828. *Lehrbuch der Gynäkologie.* Leipzig: Fleischer.

Carwardine, H. H. 1818. The Original Obstetric Instruments of the Chamberlins[sic]. *Transactions of the Medico-Chirurgical Society.* 9: 181–184.

Cazeaux, P. 1850. *Traité théorique et pratique de l'art des accouchements.* Third edition. Paris: Chamerot.

———. 1868. *A Theoretical and Practical Treatise on Midwifery.* English translation of seventh French edition of *Traité théorique et pratique de l'art des accouchements* by W. R. Bullock. Philadelphia: Lindsay and Blakiston.

Cazeaux, P., and E. Tarnier. 1885. *The Theory and Practice of Obstetrics.* English translation of *Traité théorique et pratique de l'art des accouchements.* Edited by R. J. Hess. Seventh English edition. London: Lewis.

Chailly-Honoré, N. C. 1844. *A Practical Treatise on Midwifery.* Translated from the French and edited by Gunning S. Bedford. New York: Harper.

Chalmers, J. A. 1971. *The Ventouse.* London: Lloyd Luke.

Chamberlen, H. 1673. T*he Accomplisht Midwife Treating of the Disease of Woman with Child, and in Childbed.* English translation of Mauriceau, *Des maladies des femmes grosses.* London: Billingsley.

Chamberlen, P. 1647. *A Voice in Rhama; or the Crie of Women and Children.* London.

Chapman, E. 1733. *An Essay on the Improvement of Midwifery.* London: William Bentley for John Marshall.

———. 1735. *A Treatise on the Improvement of Midwifery.* Second edition. London: Brindley, Clarke and Corbett. Third edition, 1753. London: Brindley and Hodges.

Charpentier, A. 1883. *Traité pratique des accouchements.* First edition. Paris: Baillière.

Charrière. *See* Meadows, 1867.

Chassagny, M. 1860–1861. Du forceps à traction soutenue et à pression progressive. *Bulletin de L'Académie Impériale de Médicine* (Paris). 26: 414–417.

———. 1863. Du forceps à traction soutenue et à pression progressive; réponse à quelques objections. *Gazette médicale de Paris.* 28: 208—210, 309—311, 354—355.

———. 1871. *Méthode des tractions soutenues; le forceps considéré comme agent de préhension et de traction; preuves experimentales de la non-identité d'action des diverses variétés de forceps.* Paris: Masson et fils.

———. 1875. Un mot sur la modification apportée aux tractions sur le forceps. *Lyon médical.* 19: 655–661.

———. 1884. Au sujet du dernier forceps de M. Poullet. *Archives de tocologie des maladies des femmes* (Paris). 11: 783–805.

———. 1885. Nouveau forceps. *L'Union médicale de Paris*. 40: 844–847.

———. 1891. *Fonctions du forceps*. Paris: Baillière.

Christie, D. 1878. On a New Form of the Long Forceps, and An Apparatus to Control Uterine Haemorrhage. *Glasgow Medical Journal*. 10: 262–266.

Churchill, F. 1841. *Researches on Operative Midwifery*. Dublin: Keene.

———. 1866. *On the Theory and Practice of Midwifery*. Fifth edition. London: Renshaw.

Clark(e), John. *See* Doran, 1921.

Cleeman, R. A. 1878. A Pelvic Curve in the Shank of the Obstetric Forceps. *American Journal of Obstetrics*. 11: 341–347.

Cleveland, W. F. 1868. A Modified Perforator. *Transactions of the Obstetrical Society of London*. 9: 56.

Collins, R. 1836. *A Practical Treatise on Midwifery*. London: Longman, Rees, Orme, Browne, Green and Longman.

Conquest, J. T. 1820a. *Outlines of Midwifery*. First edition. London: Anderson. Sixth edition, 1837. London: Longman, Orme, Brown, and Green.

———. 1820b. Practical Remarks on Obstetric Instruments. *London Medical Repository*. 13: 185–192.

Coutouly, P. V. 1807. *Mémoires et observations sur divers sujets relatifs à l'art des accouchemens*. Paris: Laurens Snr.

———. 1808. Mémoire sur le forceps brisé. *Journal général de médecine, de chirurgerie et de pharmacie* (Paris). 32: 45–73.

Crainz, F. 1941. Einige wenig bekannte italienische Prioritäten in der Geburtshilfe und Gynäkologie. *Zentralblatt für Gynäkologie*. 65: 1452–1466.

———. 1977. *An Obstetric Tragedy*. London: Heinemann.

Crockett, Montgomery A. 1907. Destructive Operations. In *The Practice of Obstetrics in Original Contributions by American Authors*. Edited by Reuben Peterson. London: Henry Kimpton.

Crummer, Le R. 1926. The Copper Plates in Raynalde and Geminus. *Proceedings of the Royal Society of Medicine*. 20: 1–4.

Cullingworth, C. J. 1892. The Axis-Traction Forceps. *Lancet*. 2: 1325–1327.

Das, K. 1929. *Obstetric Forceps: Its History and Evolution*. Calcutta: The Art Press. Reprint Leeds: Medical Museum Publishing, 1993.

Davis, D. D. 1825. *Elements of Operative Midwifery*. London: Hurst Robinson.

Davis, J. H. 1858. *Illustrations of Difficult Parturition*. London: Churchill.

———. 1865. Craniotomy Forceps. *Transactions of the Obstetrical Society of London*. 6: 123–125.

Debenham, R. K. 1867–1868. Description of a Whalebone Fillet for Facilitating Lingering Labour. *Clinical Lectures and Reports of the London Hospital*. 4: 506.

Delore, X. 1867. Du forceps au point de vue historique et critique. *Journal de médecine de Lyon*. 7: 441–452.

Demelin, L. 1899. Du forceps. *L'Obstétrique* (Paris). 4: 257–268, 384–399.

Denman, T. 1787–1790. *An Essay on Difficult Labours*. London: Johnson.

———. 1788. *Introduction to the Practice of Midwifery*. First edition. London: Johnson. Seventh edition, with biography, 1832. London: Cox, Burgess and Hill.

———. 1815. *Aphorisms on the Application and Use of the Forceps and Vectis*. Fifth edition. London: Cox.

De Vischer, J., and H. Van de Poll. 1753. *Het ontdekt Roonhuysiaansch geheim in de vroedkunde nade opgehelderd en bevestigt*. Leiden: Heiligert.

Dewees, W. B. 1892. New Axis-Traction Obstetric Forceps. *Journal of the American Medical Association*. 19: 32–33.

———. 1895. A New Axis-Traction and Anti-Craniotomy Forceps. *Transactions of the American Association of Obstetrics and Gynecology (1894)*. 7: 477–480. See also *American Journal of Obstetrics*. 1894. 31: 134–136.

Dewees, W. P. 1811. *An Abridgement of Mr Heath's Translation of Baudeloque's [sic] Midwifery, with Notes*. Philadelphia: Dobson.

———. 1824. *Compendious System of Midwifery*. Philadelphia: Carey, Lea and Carey. Tenth edition, 1843. Philadelphia: Lea and Blanchard.

———. 1825. *A Compendious System of Midwifery*. London: Miller.

Dewhurst, J. 1980. *Royal Confinements*. London: Weidenfeld and Nicolson.

De Wind, P. 1751. *'t Gek, emd Hoofd geredt*. Middelburg: Gillisen.

Donald, A. 1890. Methods of Craniotomy. *Transactions of the Obstetrical Society of London*. 31: 28–42.

Doran, A. 1912a. Dusée: His Forceps and His Contemporaries. *Journal of Obstetrics and Gynaeology of the British Empire*. 22: 119–142.

———. 1912b. Dusée, De Wind and Smellie: An Addendum. *Journal of Obstetrics and Gynaecology of the British Empire*. 22: 203–207.

———. 1913a. A Demonstration of Some Eighteenth Century Obstetric Forceps. *Proceedings of the Royal Society of Medicine (Section of the History of Medicine)*. 6: 54–77.

———. 1913b. Burton ("Dr. Slop"): His Forceps and His Foes. *Journal of Obstetrics and Gynaecology of the British Empire*. 23: 3–24, 65–86.

———. 1913c. Mursinna: Osiander: Weissbrod. A Study of Forceps. *Journal of Obstetrics and Gynaecology of the British Empire*. 24: 1–11.

———. 1913d. Jointed Obstetric Forceps. *Journal of Obstetrics and Gynaecology of the British Empire*. 24: 197–210.

———. 1914. Some Eighteenth Century Foreign Obstetric Forceps in the Museum of the Royal College of Surgeons of England. *Transactions of the XVIIth International Congress of Medicine, Section XXIII, History of Medicine, 1913*. Pages 445–456. London: Henry Frowde (Oxford University Press) and Hodder and Stoughton.

———. 1921. *Descriptive Catalogue of the Obstetrical and Gynaecological Instruments in the Museum of the Royal College of Surgeons of England*. London: Royal College of Surgeons.

Dorland, W. A. N. 1896. *A Manual of Obstetrics*. London: Kimpton.

Douglas, John. 1736. *A Short Account of the State of Midwifery in London, Westminster, &c*. London.

Douglas, William. 1748. *A Letter to Dr Smellie. Shewing the Impropriety of his New-invented Forceps: As Also, the Absurdity of His Method of Teaching and Practising Midwifery*. London: Roberts.

Draper, W. 1875–1876. Folding Short Forceps. *Obstetrical Journal of Great Britain and Ireland*. 3: 715–718.

Dubois, A. *See* Kilian, 1856.

Dubois, P. 1849. *Traité complet de l'art des accouchemens*. Paris: Béchet Jeune.

Dugès, A. 1826. *Manuel d'obstétrique*. First edition. Paris: Gabon. Third edition, 1840. Paris: Baillière.

Duke, A. 1879. A New Tractor for Obstetric Forceps. *British Medical Journal*. 1: 189.

———. 1880. Aid in Forceps Delivery. *British Medical Journal*. 11: 693.

Duncan, J. Mathews. 1849. The Controversy Respecting the Invention of the Air-Tractor. *London Medical Gazette*. 8: 609.

———. 1869. On the Cephalotribe. *Transactions of the Obstetrical Society of London*. 11: 42–43.

———. 1870. On the Construction of the Cephalotribe. *Transactions of the Edinburgh Obstetrical Society(1868)*. 1: 1–20.

———. 1875. Note on Intrauterine Craniometry. *Transactions of the Edinburgh Obstetrical Society*. 4: 116–121.

———. 1876. Against the Pendulum Movement in Working the Midwifery Forceps. *Edinburgh Medical Journal*. 21: 683–686.

———. 1887. Discussion on Tarnier's Forceps. *Transactions of the Obstetrical Society of London*. 19: 223–227.

Duns, J. 1873. *Memoir of Sir James Y. Simpson, Bart*. Edinburgh: Edmonston and Douglas.

Eardley-Wilmot, R. 1874. On the Fillet or Loop As an Obstetric Aid. *Transactions of the Obstetrical Society of London*. 15: 172–177.

Earle, J. I. L. 1862. New Pelvimeter. *Transactions of the Obstetrical Society of London*. 3: 145–146.

Eastlake, H. 1868. On the Indications for the Employment of a Drill Crotchet; Its Special Advantages in Certain Forms of Labour, with a Description of the Instrument. *Transactions of the Obstetrical Society of London*. 9: 146–152.

Ecken, A. van der. 1845. Invention d'un nouveau crochet-scie. *Archives de la Médecine Belge*. 17: 203–209. *See also* Charpentier, 1883.

Edis, A. W. 1878. The Forceps in Modern Midwifery. *Transactions of the Obstetrical Society of London.* 19: 69–92.

Elliot, G. T. 1858. Description of a New Midwifery Forceps, Having a Sliding Pivot to Prevent Compression of the Foetal Head. *New York Journal of Medicine.* 5: 151–182.

Ermengem. *See* Hubert, E., 1884.

Evans. *See* Aitken, 1786.

Fabricius Hildanus, G. 1643 *Observationium et curationum medico-chirurgicarum centuriae.* Frankfurt-am-Main: Beyer. *See also* Jones, 1960.

Faye. *See* Meadows, 1867.

Felsenreich, T. 1886. Experiences with the Axis-Traction Forceps. *Journal of the American Medical Association.* 6: 144–146.

Ferguson. *See* Meadows, 1867.

Fisher, R. W. 1895. A New Axis-Traction Forceps. *Medical Record (N.Y.)* 47: 348.

Flamant, P. R. 1816. *Mémoire pratique sur les forceps.* Strasbourg: Levrault.

Forster, F. M. C. 1971. Robert Barnes and His Obstetric Forceps. *Australia and New Zealand Journal of Obstetrics and Gynaecology.* 11: 139–147.

Foulis, J. 1887. On Axis-Traction Forceps. *Transactions of the Edinburgh Obstetrical Society* (Session 1886–1887). 22: 189–198.

———. 1900. A New Handle for Axis Traction Forceps. *Transactions of the Edinburgh Obstetric Society.* 25:126

Franco, Pierre. 1556. *Petit traité contenant une des parties principalles de chirurgie, laquelle les chirurgiens hernières exercent.* Lyon: Antoine Vincent.

Fries. 1806. Beschreibung und Abbildung einer neuen Entbindungszange. *Lucina.* 3: 321–333.

Froriep, L. F. von. 1804. Über einen an meiner Geburtzange angebrachten Mechanismus. *Lucina.* 2: 1–7.

———. 1832. *Theoretisch-practisches Handbuch der Geburtshilfe.* Ninth edition. Weimar: Landes-Industrie-Comptoir.

Fry, H. D. 1889a. The Application of Forceps to Transverse and Oblique Positions of the Head—Description of New Forceps. *American Journal of Obstetrics.* 22: 722–724.

———. 1889b. A New Obstetric Forceps. *American Journal of Obstetrics.* 22: 1165–1169.

Gaitskell, W. 1823. A Case of Laceration of the Perinaeum, Urinary Bladder, and Rectum: with Observations on the Use and Abuse of the Vectis. *London Medical Repository.* 20: 376–381.

Galabin, A. L. 1877a. The Effects of Frequent and Early Use of Midwifery Forceps upon the Foetal and Maternal Morality. *The Obstetrical Journal of Great Britain and Ireland.* 5: 561–588.

———. 1877b. Axis Traction Forceps. *Transactions of the Obstetrical Society of London.* 19: 227–231.

Gardner, W. S. 1892. Mechanism of Axis-Traction Forceps. *American Journal of Obstetrics.* 26: 60–68.

Gariel, M.-M. 1852. *Note sur les pessaires à réservoir d'air en caoutchouc vulcanisé précédé de quelques réflexions sur les pessaires en général.* Paris: Varnout et Galante.

Garland, G. W. 1871. A New Instrument for Craniotomy. *Boston Medical and Surgical Journal.* 85: 69.

Garrigues, H. J. 1891. Discussion. *Transactions of the American Gynecological Society.* 16: 132–144.

———. 1893. Symphysiotomy; with the Report of a Successful Case. *American Journal of Medical Sciences.* 105: 286–298.

Gayton, W. 1863. On a New Mode of Securing the Handles of the Forceps during Delivery. *Medical Times and Gazette.* 2: 217–218.

Gebbie, D. A. M. 1981. *Reproductive Anthropology—Descent through Women.* Chichester: Wiley.

Geijl, A. 1905. *De geschiedenis van het Roonhuyiaansch geheim.* Rotterdam: Meindert Boogaerdt, Jr.

Germann. 1862. *See* Meadows, 1867.

Giffard, W. 1734. *Cases in Midwifery.* Revised and published by E. Hody, with illustrations. London.

Gigli, L. 1893. Della sezione della sinfisi con la sega in filo metallico (Drahtsäger). *Annales ostetricia e ginecologia.* 15: 557–560.

———. 1894. Taglio lateralizzato del pube. Suoi vantaggi—sua tecnica. *Annales ostetricia e ginecologia.* 16: 649–667.

———. 1897. Embriotomie col filo; decapitatzione; craniotomia a testa posteriore; riduzione della base fetale. *Annali di ostetricia, Milano.* 19: 913–920.

Giordano, S. 1865. Modificazioni al forcipe. *Giornale della R. Accademia di Medicina di Torino.* 18: 1–4.

Glaister, J. 1894. *Dr. William Smellie and His Contemporaries.* Glasgow: Maclehose.

Gordon, D. 1875. A New Kind of Midwifery Forceps. *Transactions of the Edinburgh Obstetrical Society (1871–74).* 3: 19–20.

Grattan, N. 1888. Axis-Traction Midwifery Forceps. *Lancet.* 1: 25.

Greenhalgh, R. 1865. Harris' Pelvimeter. *Transactions of the Obstetrical Society of London.* 6: 186–188.

———. 1866. On the Comparative Merits of the Caesarean Operation and Craniotomy in Cases of Extreme Distortion of the Pelvis. *Transactions of the Obstetrical Society of London.* 7: 270–289.

Grunner, O. C. 1970. *A Treatise on the Canon of Medicine.* New York: Kelley.

Guillemeau, J. 1609. *De la grossesse et accouchement des femmes.* Paris: Pacard.

———. 1612. *Childbirth, or the Happie Deliverie of Women.* English translation of *De la grossesse et accouchement des femmes.* London: Hatfield.

Guillon, J. B. *See* Maygrier, 1822

Guyon, J. C. F. 1867. Céphalotripsie intra-cranienne. *Gazette des hôpitaux civils et militaires. Paris.* No. 145: 577.

Hamilton, A. 1775. *Elements of the Practice of Midwifery.* London: Murray.

———. 1787. *Outlines of the Theory and Practice of Midwifery.* Second edition. Edinburgh: Elliott.

———. 1792. *Letters to Dr William Osborn from Alexander Hamilton.* Edinburgh: Hill and Murray.

———. 1806. *Outlines of the Theory and Practice of Midwifery.* Fifth edition. Edinburgh: Murray.

Hamilton, J. 1793. Observations on the Instrument Employed in the Practice of Midwifery, Commonly Called Lowder's Lever. *Medical Commentaries for the Year MDCCXCIII.* 8: 400–424.

———. 1794. *Select Cases in Midwifery; Extracted from the Records of the Edinburgh General Lying-in Hospital.* Edinburgh and London: Printed for the Benefit of the Hospital.

———. 1836. *Practical Observations on Various Subjects Relating to Midwifery.* Part 2. Edinburgh: Bell and Bradfute; London: Longman.

Hamon, L. 1864a. Forceps droit (ou à branches parallèles) simplifié. *Gazette des hôpitaux civils et militaires. Paris.* Septième année. No. 96, 381–382.

———. 1864b. Forceps droit (ou à branches parallèles) simplifié. *L'Union médicale de Paris.* 23: 343–345.

———. 1877. Simple note sur un appareil obstétrical à tractions mécaniques. *Bulletin général de thérapeutique.* 93: 130–132.

Harper, P. H. 1859. The More Frequent Use of the Forceps as a Means of Lessening Both Maternal and Foetal Mortality. *Transactions of the Obstetrical Society of London.* 1: 142–185.

Harris. *See* Greenhalgh, 1865.

Harris, R. P. 1872a. History of a Pair of Obstetric Forceps Sixty Years Old. *American Journal of Obstetrics.* 4: 55–59.

———. 1872b. The Forceps. *American Journal of Obstetrics.* 5: 340–353.

———. 1883. The Revival of Symphysiotomy in Italy, with Comparative Tables of the Early and Later Cases, Showing That the Operation Has Been More Frequently Performed in That Country in the Last Seventeen Years Than in All Europe in the Previous Eighty, and with Far Better Results. The Whole Subject Examined Historically and Clinically. *American Journal of the Medical Sciences.* 85: 17–32.

———. 1894. A Plea for the Practice of Symphysiotomy (Editorial). *Lancet.* 1: 675–676, 809–811.

Hartmann, R. 1870. Erklärung über seine Geburtszange. *St. Petersburger medizinische Zeitschrift.* 1: 353–355.

Haslam, W. D. 1887. New Midwifery Forceps. *British Medical Journal.* 1: 1104–1105.

Heidler, H. 1923. Zum Dekapitationsfingerhut von Kasper Blond. *Zentralblatt für Gynäkologie.* 48: 1815–1817.

Heister, L. 1724. *Chirugie.* Nuremberg: Raspe.

———. 1739. *Institutiones chirurgicae.* Amsterdam: Jansson-Waesberge.

———. 1743. *A General System of Surgery*. English translation of *Institutiones chirurgicae*. Part 2, Book 5, Chapter 153. London: Innys, Davis, Clarke, Manby and Whiston.

Hellier, J. B. 1912. A Pair of Midwifery Forceps of Early Eighteenth Century Pattern. *British Medical Journal*. 1: 1027–1028.

Hennig, C. 1859. Ueber perforation und Kephalotrypsis. *Monatschrift für Geburtskunde und Frauenkrankheiten*. 13: 40–59. *See also* Meadows, 1867.

Herbiniaux, G. M. 1794. *Traité sur divers accouchemens laborieux*. Brussels: Lemaire.

Herff. 1892. *See* Das, 1929.

Hermann, T. 1844. *Ueber eine neue Geburtszange zur Extraction des im Beckeneingange stehenden Kindskopfes*. Bern: Haller.

Hewitt, W. M. G. 1861. On Unusual Elongation of the Foetal Head as a Cause of Difficulty in the Application of the Ordinary Obstetric Forceps. *Transactions of the Obstetrical Society of London*. 3: 180–197.

Hibbard, B. M. 1993. William Smellie and William Hunter—A Century of Influence. *Hunterian Society Transactions, 1992–1993*. Pages 17–29.

Hibbard, B. M., and D. M. McKenna. 1990. The Obstetric Forceps — Are We Using the Appropriate Tools? *British Journal of Obstetrics and Gynaecology*. 97: 374—380.

Hicks, J. Braxton. 1867. The Cephalotribe. *British Medical Journal*. 2: 337–338.

———.1869. Some Remarks on the Cephalotribe. *Transactions of the Obstetrical Society of London*. 11: 43–52.

———. 1877. Discussion on Tarnier's forceps. *Transactions of the Obstetrical Society of London*. 19: 223–227.

Hilliard, R. H. 1880. Obstetric Forceps. *British Medical Journal*. 1: 287.

Hodge, H. L. 1864. *The Principles and Practice of Obstetrics*. Philadelphia: Blanchard and Lea.

Hody, E. *See* Giffard, W. 1734.

Hohl, A. F. 1855. *Lehrbuch der Geburtshülfe*. Leipzig: Engelmann.

Holland, Eardley. 1951.The Princess Charlotte of Wales: A Triple Obstetric Tragedy. *Journal of Obstetrics and Gynaecology of the British Empire*. 58: 905–919.

Holland, Edmund. 1886. New Axis-Traction Forceps for High Delivery. *British Medical Journal*. 1: 305.

Holmes, J. P. 1831. *Popular Observations on Diseases Incident to Females*. London: Jones.

Hopkins, J. 1826. *The Accoucheur's Vade Mecum*. Fourth edition London: Rayer.

Howard, W. T. *See* Simpson, A. R., 1883.

Hubert, E. 1877. Du forceps; théorie de la traction et nouveau forceps. *Journal des sciences médicales de Louvain*. 2: 145–157, 291–297.

———. 1878. *Cours d'accouchements*. Louvain: C. Peeters.

———. 1884. De quelques nouveaux forceps. *Revue de médecine*. 3: 389–392, 481–501.

———. 1889. Le nouveau forceps de M. Chassagny. *Revue médicale* (Louvain). 8: 533–546.

Hubert, L. J. 1860a. *Cours d'accouchements*. Louvain: E. Fonteyn.

———. 1860b. Notes sur l'équilibre du forceps et du levier et sur le choix à faire entre ces deux instruments. *Bulletin de l'Académie Royale de Médecine de Belgique*. Second series. 3: 346–352.

Huevel, J van. 1843. Description du forceps-scie ou nouveau céphalotôme. *Annales d'obstétrique de Paris*. 3: 393–405.

———. 1846. *Mémoire sur les divers moyens propres à délivrer la femme, en casse de rétrécissement du bassin, et sur le forceps-scie ou nouveau céphalotome, suivi d'un appendice comprenant la description abrégée de pelvimetre géométrique*. Brussels.

Hunter, W. 1778. *Reflections, Occasioned by a Decree of the Faculty of Medicine at Paris; Relative to the Operation of Cutting the Symphysis of the ossa pubis*. London: Cadell.

Huston, R. M. *See* Meigs, 1849.

Jacquemier, Jean Marie. 1861–1862. Embryotome cáché à lames mobiles et à chainons de scie. *Bulletin de L'Académie Impériale de Médecine* (Paris). 27: 157–159. *See also* Charpentier, 1883.

Jaggard, W. W. 1886. Two Recent Models of the Axis-Traction Forceps. *American Journal of Obstetrics.* 19: 421–425.

James, F. H. 1849. The Application of Atmospheric Pressure to Aid Delivery. *London Medical Gazette.* 8: 478–480.

James, Thomas C. *See* Harris, 1872a.

Janck (Ianckii), J. G. 1750. Commentatio de forcipe ac forfice ferramentis a Bingio chirurgo Hafniensi, inventis eorumque usus in partu difficili inventa describit. Lipsiae, apud I. C. Langenhemium.

Jardine, R. 1903. *Clinical Obstetrics.* London: Kimpton.

Jenks, E. W. 1879. Jenks's New Obstetric Forceps. *London Medical Record.* 7: 339.

Jewett, C. 1885. Notes on Hospital Obstetrics. *New York Medical Journal.* 42: 585—598.

———. 1895. The Axis Traction Forceps. *The American Gynecological Journal.* 6: 248.

———, Editor. 1899. *The Practice of Obstetrics by American Authors.* London: Kimpton.

Johnson, R. W. 1769. *A New System of Midwifery.* London: Wilson and Nicol.

Johnson, T. *See* Paré, 1665.

Johnstone, R. W. 1952. *William Smellie, the Master of British Midwifery.* Edinburgh: Livingstone.

Jonas, R. 1540. *Byrth of Mankynde.* English translation of Rösslin's *De partu hominis.* London: Raynolde.

Jones, E. W. P. 1960. Life and Works of Guillhemus Fabricius Hildanus. *Medical History.* 4: 112—134, 196–209.

Jones, G. R. 1972. David Daniel Davis, M.D., F.R.C.P. (1777–1841). *The Carmarthenshire Antiquary.* 8: 91–99.

Jörg, J. C. G. 1807. *Schriften zur Beförderung der Kenntniss des menschlichen Beckens.* Nuremberg and Leipzig: J. L. Schrooj.

Joulin, M. 1867. *Traité complet d'accouchements—diviseur céphalique.* Paris: Savy.

Kalindero, N. 1870. *Mémoire sur le céphalotripsie intra-cranienne par la méthode de M. le Dr F Guyon.* Paris: Coccoz.

Keiller, A. 1879. Axis Tractor. *Transactions of the Edinburgh Obstetrical Society.* 5: 54.

Kerr, J. M. 1908. *Operative Obstetrics.* London: Baillière, Tindall and Cox.

Kidd, G. H. 1867. Observations on the Construction of the Cephalotribe. *British Medical Journal.* 2: 335–337.

———. 1878–1879. New Midwifery Forceps. *Obstetrical Journal of Great Britain and Ireland.* 6: 720.

Kilian, H. F. 1835. *Geburtshüflicher Atlas.* Dusseldorf: Verlag von Arnz.

———. 1856. *Armamentarium Lucinae novum.* Bonn: E. Weber.

———. *See* Meadows, 1867.

Knight, S. T. 1860. A New Pattern for the Obstetrical Forceps. *Maryland and Virginia Medical Journal.* 14: 272–275. *See also* Braithwaite, J., and W. Braithwaite, Editors. 1860. *The Retrospect of Medicine.* 42: 299–301. London: Simpkin, Marshall. (Commonly called *Brathwaite's Retrospect.*)

Knox, J. S. *See* Parvin, 1890.

Kristeller, S. 1861. Dynamometrisch Vorrichtung an der Geburtszange. *Montschrift für Geburtskunde.* 17: 166–175.

Kuhn, W. and U. Tröhler. 1987. *Armamentarium obstetricium Gottingense.* Göttingen: Vandenhoeck and Ruprecht.

Kuntzsch. 1912. Über geburtshilfliche Extraktionen mit meinem Vakuumhelm. *Zentralblatt für Gynäkologie* 36: 893–895.

Küstner. *See* Witkowski, 1887.

La Motte, G. 1722. *Traité complet des accouchemens naturels, non naturels, et contre nature.* Paris: D'Houry.

———. 1746. *A General Treatise of Midwifery.* English translation of *Traité complet des accouchemens* by Thomas Tomkyns. London: Waugh.

Lanteneer. *See* Hubert, E., 1884.

Laroyenne, L. P. 1875. Des avantages réalisés par un perfectionnement facile à appliquer au forceps ordinaire destiné à permettre l'insertion des cordons de traction au centre des cuillers. *Lyon médical.* 19: 617–623.

Lazarewitch, J. 1868a. Induction of Premature Labour by Injection of the Fundus of the Uterus. *Transactions of the Obstetrical Society of London.* 9: 1–41.

———. 1868b. Instruments pour les opérations obstétricales. *Congrès Médical International de Paris (1867).* 1: 620–624.

———. 1869a. *Embryotome.* Kharkoff: Firenze.

———. 1869b. *Quelques opérations et instruments obstétricaux et gynécologiques.* Kharkoff: University Press.

———. 1877a. The Blunt Hook. *Transactions of the Obstetrical Society of London.* 28: 190—191.

———. 1877b. The Three Most Important Medical Instruments. T*ransactions of the International Medical Congress (1876).* Page 827.

———. 1881a. On the Curves of the Obstetric Forceps. *Transactions of the International Medical Congress, London.* 4: 243–271. London: J. W. Kolckmann.

———. 1881b. On the Curves of the Midwifery Forceps. *American Journal of Obstetrics.* 14: 914–917.

Leake, J. 1773. *The Description and Use of a New Pair of Forceps.* London: R. Baldwin.

———. 1781. *Practical Observations on the Child-bed Fever.* Fifth edition. London: Baldwin and Payne.

———. 1787. *Introduction to the Theory and Practice of Midwifery.* London: Baldwin and Murray.

Lee, R. G. 1844. *Lectures on the Theory and Practice of Midwifery, Delivered in the Theatre of St George's Hospital.* London: Longman.

———. 1848. *Clinical Midwifery.* Second Edition London: Churchill.

———. 1862. *Observations on the Discovery of the Original Obstetric Instruments of the Chamberlens.* London: Adlard.

———. 1875. Midwifery and Diseases of Women. Lecture IV. *St. George's Hospital Reports (1872–4).* 7: 42–43.

Leishman, W. 1880. *A System of Midwifery.* Third edition. Glasgow: James Maclehouse.

Le Page, J. F. 1883. On Axis Traction in Delivery with Obstetric Forceps. *British Medical Journal* 2: 768–769.

Levret, A. 1747. *Observations sur les causes et les accidens de plusieurs accouchemens laborieux.* Paris: Charles Osmont. Third edition: Paris: P. Alex Le Prieur, 1762.

———. 1751. *Suite des observations sur les causes et les accidens de plusieurs accouchemens laborieux, avec des remarques.* Paris: Delaguette.

———. 1753. *L'Art des accouchemens, demontré par des principes de physique et de mécanique.* Paris: Le Prieur. Second edition, 1761. Paris: Didot.

Long, M. 1872. A New Midwifery Forceps. *Lancet.* 1: 95.

Lowder, W. 1772. *Lectures on the Theory and Practice of Midwifery.* Unpublished manuscript of lecture notes.

Löwenthal, H. 1873. A New Forceps. *Medical Record (New York).* 8: 94–95. *See also* Braithwaite, J., and W. Braithwaite, Editors. 1874. *The Retrospect of Medicine.* London: Simpkin, Marshall. 49: 295–298. (Commonly called *Braithwaite's Retrospect.*)

Lucas, J. 1794. Hints on the Management of Women in Certain Cases of Pregnancy. *Memoirs of the Medical Society of London.* 2: 410–421.

Lusk, W. T. 1869. A New Cephalotribe. *New York Medical Journal.* 9: 525–526.

———. 1880a. The Forceps (with a Demonstration of the Tarnier Forceps), Version, and the Expectant Plan in Contracted Pelves. *Medical Record (N.Y.).* 17: 69–72.

———. 1880b. A Modification of the Tarnier Forceps. *American Journal of Obstetrics.* 13: 372–374.

———. 1882. *The Science and Art of Midwifery.* London: Lewis. Fourth edition, 1892.

Lyman, A. B. 1891. Lyman's Direct Axis Midwifery Tractor. *New York Medical Journal.* 54: 107–108.

Lyon, J. G. 1881. Removable Axis Traction Rods for Midwifery Forceps. *British Medical Journal.* 1: 425–426.

McCahey, P. 1890. Atmospheric Tractor: A New Instrument and Some New Theories in Obstetrics. *Medical and Surgical Reporter, Philadelphia.* 43: 619–623.

McClintock, A. H. 1876–1877. The Originator of the Double-curved Midwifery Forceps. *Obstetric Journal.* 4:330–334.

Macdonald, A. D. 1882. A New Indicating Axis Traction Forceps. *Lancet.* 2: 139–140.

McFerran, J. A. 1877. *The Obstetric Forceps. An Improvement in Their Construction.* Philadelphia.

———. 1884. Obstetric Forceps Jointed at the Junction of the Blades and Shanks. *Transactions of the Medical Society of Pennsylvania.* 16: 324–331.

McGillicuddy, T. J. 1889. A New Combined Axis-Traction Forceps to Be Used as an Alternative for Craniotomy. *American Journal of Obstetrics*. 22: 1247–1251.

Mackness, G. O. C. 1896. Some Modifications of Midwifery Forceps. *Transactions of the Edinburgh Obstetrical Society (1895-96)*. 21: 196–199. See also *Edinburgh Medical Journal*. 43: 237–240.

McLane, J. W. *See* Speert, 1963, and Baskett, 1996.

McLaurin, W. 1886. An Axis-Traction Midwifery Forceps with Sliding Blades. *Lancet*. 2: 402.

Madden, T. More. 1874a. On Certain Improvements in the Construction and Use of the Long and Short Midwifery Forceps. *British Medical Journal*. 1: 829–832.

———. 1874b. On Some Improvements in the Single and Double Curved Forceps and Their Use in Midwifery Practice. *Lancet*. 1: 865–867.

———. 1875. On the History and Use of the Short Straight Midwifery Forceps as a Tractor, and of the Long Double Curved Forceps as a Compressor and Lever. *Proceedings of the Dublin Obstetrical Society, Thirty-eighth Annual Session*. Pages 332–361.

———. 1888a. Recent Progress in Obstetrics and Gynaecology. *British Medical Journal*. 2: 343–346.

———. 1888b. Abridged Report of an Address on the Use of the Forceps and Its Improvement. *Lancet*. 2: 304–306.

Mann, M. D. and A. Hirst. 1889. *A System of Obstetrics and Gynecology by American Authors*. Volume 2, Part 1. Edinburgh and London: Pentland.

Mariaud. Circa 1875. Instrument catalogue. Paris.

Martin, A. E. 1873. Presentation to the Obstetrical Society of London (1872). *Transactions of the Obstetrical Society of London*. 14: 65–66.

Martin, E. 1862. *Hand-Atlas der Gynäkologie und Geburtshülfe*. Berlin: Hirschwald.

Mathew, G. Porter. 1898. An Improved Form of Axis-Traction Midwifery Forceps. *Lancet*. 2: 1484.

Mathieu, Maison. 1878. *Arsenal chirurgical*. Paris.

Mattei, A. 1855. *Essai sur l'accouchement physiologique*. Paris: Masson.

———. 1856. Nouveau Forceps. *Gazette des hôpitaux civils et militaires*. Paris. 75: 300.

———. 1859. A New Obstetric Forceps (Called Leniceps). *Gazette médicale de Paris*. 14: 52–53.

Maubray, J. 1724. *The Female Physician—to Which is Added the Whole Art of New Improv'd Midwifery*. London: Holland. Second edition, 1730.

Mauriceau, F. 1668. *Des Maladies des femmes grosses*. Paris: Henault, D'Houry, de Ninvelle, Coignara.

———. 1673. *The Accomplisht Midwife*. English translation of *Des Maladies des femmes grosses* by Hugh Chamberlen. London: Billingsley.

———. 1675. *Traité des maladies des femmes grosses*. Paris: D'Houry.

Maygrier, J. P. 1822. *Nouvelles Démonstrations d'accouchemens*. Paris: Béchet.

———. 1833. *Midwifery Illustrated*. English translation of *Nouvelles Démonstrations d'accouchemens* by A. Sidney Doane. New York: J. K. Moore.

Meadows, A., Editor. 1867. *Catalogue and Report of Obstetrical and Other Instruments Exhibited at the Conversazione of the Obstetrical Society of London*. London: Longmans, Green.

Meigs, C. D. 1849. *Obstetrics—The Science and the Art*. Philadelphia: Lea and Blanchard.

Mende, L. J. K. 1825. *Beobachtungen und Bemerkungen aus der Geburtshülfe und gerichtlichen Medizin*. Göttingen: Vandenhock und Ruprecht.

———. 1828. Beschreibung meine Kopfzange. *Gemeinsame Deutsche Zeitschrift für Geburtskunde*. 3: 274–291.

Mercurio, Scipione. 1601. *La Commare o riccoglitrice*. Venice: Ciotti.

Merriman, S. 1826. *A Synopsis of the Various Kinds of Difficult Parturition*. Fourth edition. London: Callow and Wilson.

Mesnard, J. 1753. *Le Guide des accoucheurs*. Second edition. Paris: De Bure.

Milne, A. 1868. Craniotomy and Cephalotripsy Contrasted; with Cases. *Edinburgh Medical Journal (1867–8)*. 23: 625–636.

Milne, J. S. 1907. *Surgical Instruments in Greek and Roman Times*. Oxford: Clarendon Press.

Mitchell, J. 1849. Who Invented the Air Tractor? Correspondence between Dr Simpson and Dr Mitchell. *London Medical Gazette*. 8: 519–521.

Mondotte. *See* Meadows, 1867.

Moore, N. 1918. *The History of St. Bartholomew's Hospital*. Volume 2. London: Pearson.

Moralès, J. 1871. Modification nouvelle au forceps. *Journal de médecine Bruxelles*. 52: 110–134.

Moreau, F. J. 1837. *Traité pratique des accouchemens*. Paris: Baillière.

———. 1844. *A Practical Treatise on Midwifery*. English translation of *Traité pratique des accouchemens* by T. F. Betton. Philadelphia: Carey and Hart.

Morgan, H. 1878. M. New Tractors for Midwifery Forceps. *British Medical Journal*. 1: 934.

Mulder, J. 1794. *Historia litteraria et critica forcipum et vectium obstetriciorium*. Leyden: Honkoop.

———. 1798. *Litterärische und kritische Geschichte der Zangen und Hebel in der Geburtshülfe*. German translation of *Historia litteraria et critica forcipum et vectium obstetriciorium* by Schlegel. Leipzig: Weidmann.

Mundé, P. 1873. The Cranioclast As Improved and Used by the Vienna School. *The American Journal of Obstetrics and Diseases of Women and Children*. 45: 1–38.

Murphy, E. W. 1852 *Lectures on the Principles and Practice of Midwifery*. London: Taylor, Walton and Maberly.

———. 1862. *Lectures on the Principles and Practice of Midwifery*. Second edition. London: Walton and Maberly.

Murray, J. J. 1859. Placenta Praevia—Air Pessary Used to Plug and Dilate the os uteri. *Medical Times and Gazette*. New series. 18: 596–597.

Murray, R. Milne. 1890–1891. The Axis-Traction Forceps; Their Mechanical Principles, Construction, and Scope. *Transactions of the Edinburgh Obstetrical Society*. 16: 58–89.

———. 1896. On Forceps with Adjustable Axis Traction; and on Forceps in Occipito-posterior positions of the Vertex. *Transactions of the Edinburgh Obstetrical Society (1895–96)*. 21: 171–181. See also *Edinburgh Medical Journal*. 1896–1897. 43: 228–237.

Mursinna, C. L. 1784–1786. *Abhandlung von den Krankheiten der Schwangeren*. Berlin: Himburg.

Naegele, F. C. 1829. *An Essay on the Mechanism of Parturition*. Translation of *Ueber den Mechanismus der Geburt* by Edward Rigby. London: Callow and Wilson.

———. 1830. *Lehrbuch der Geburtshülfe*. Heidelberg: J. C. B. Mohr.

Naegele, H. F. J., and W. L. Grenser. 1880. *Traité pratique de l'art des accouchments*. Paris: Baillière.

Neale, L. E. 1885. An Obstetrical Forceps. *American Journal of Obstetrics*. 18: 938–941, 1184.

Neville, W. C. 1886. Axis-Traction in Instrumental Delivery, with Description of a New and Simple Axis-Traction Forceps. *Dublin Journal of Medical Science*. 81: 97—109, 295–298.

Newham, S. 1865. Description of the "Guide-Hook", a New Obstetric Instrument. *Transactions of the Obstetrical Society of London*. 6: 7–9.

Nihell, E. 1760. *A Treatise on the Art of Midwifery*. London: Morley.

Oldham, H. 1855. On the Use of a Vertebral Hook in Some Cases of Difficult Delivery. *Lancet*. 1: 447.

Olivier, A. V. 1883. *De la conduite à tenir dans la présentation de l'extrémité pelvienne, mode des fesses, c'est à dire, avec relèvement des membres inférieurs sur le plan antérieur du foetus*. Paris: Delahaye et Lecrosnier.

Opie, T. 1888. Is the Frequent Use of Forceps Abusive?. *Transactions of the American Association of Obstetrics and Gynecology*. 1: 142–155.

Osborn, W. 1783. *An Essay on Laborious Parturition: In Which the Division of the symphysis pubis is Particularly Considered*. London: Cadell.

———. 1792. *Essays on the Practice of Midwifery*. London: Cadell.

Osiander, F. B. 1796. *Lehrbuch der Hebammenkunst*. Göttingen: J. G. Rosenbusch. *See also* Doran, 1913c.

Osiander, J. F. 1825. *Handbuch der Entbindungskunst*. Volume 3. Tubingen: Published by the author.

Ould, Fielding. 1742. *A Treatise in Midwifery in Three Parts*. Dublin: Oli Nelson and Charles Connor.

Pajot, Charles. 1863. De la céphalotripsie répétée sans tractions. *Gazette des hôpitaux civils et militaires*. 1: 513–532.

———. 1877. La séconde sur le forceps à aiguille. *Annals de gynécologie*. (Paris). 7: 321–362.

Paré, A. 1614. *Les oeuvres, corrigées et augmentées par luymesme, peu aupavant son décès*. Seventh edition. Paris: Buon.

———. 1665. *The Workes of That Famous Chirurgion Ambroise Parey. Translated out of Latine and Compared with the French by Tho. Johnson*. London: Clarke.

Parvin, T. 1890. *The Science and Art of Obstetrics*. Philadelphia: Lea Brothers.

Péan. *See* Baudelocque, J.-L., 1790 (English translation).

Pearse, T. F. 1887. Forceps with a Hinge. *British Gynaecological Journal*. 3: 182.

———. 1890. Note on Traction in the Use of Midwifery Forceps and on a New Instrument with a Perineal Curve. *British Medical Journal*. 2: 154.

Petit, A. 1798–1799. *Traité des maladies de femmes enceintes, des femmes en couche et des infants nouveaux nés rédigé sur les leçons d'Antoine Petit*. Paris: Baignères et Perral.

Petit, J. L. 1774. *Oeuvres complètes*. *See* Tarnier and Budin, 1901.

Piet, M. 1767. Observations sur l'usage du forceps courbé. *Journal de médicine, chirurgie et pharmacie etc.* Paris. 36: 264–268.

Pihan-Dufeillay. *See* Greenhalgh, 1866.

Pinard, A. 1879. Forceps (Instruments). In *Dictionnaire encyclopaedique des sciences médicales*. Edited by A. Dechambre. Fourth series; 3: 524–607. Paris: P. Asselin; G. Masson.

Playfair, W. S. *See* Greenhalgh, 1866 (discussion following paper).

———. 1869. Dr Barnes's Water Bags. *Medical Times and Gazette*. 2: 392–393.

Poullet, J. 1875a. Nouveau tracteur obstétrical. *Lyon médical*. 19: 90–101.

———. 1875b. Du sericeps et d'un nouveau tracteur obstétrical. *Archives de tocologie des maladies des femmes* (Paris). 2: 468–498.

———. 1881. Forceps souple à tractions indépendentes. *Gazette des hôpitaux civils et militaires*. Paris. 54: 1084. *See also Lyon médicale*. 1881. 38: 584–588.

———. 1883. *Des Diverses Espèces de forceps, leurs avantages et leurs inconvéniences*. Paris: Baillière.

———. 1884. Des principes sur lesquels doit reposer la construction d'un forceps; description d'un nouveau forceps. *Archives de tocologie des maladies des femmes* (Paris). 11: 569–603.

Power, D'A. 1927. "The Birth of Mankind or The Woman's Book." *The Library*. 8: 1–58.

Priestley, W. O. and H. R. Storer, Editors. 1855. *Obstetric Memoirs and Contributions of J. Y. Simpson*. Volume 1. Edinburgh: Black.

Pros, G. 1875. Réflexions sur l'importance de l'emploi des tractions mécaniques en obstétrique. *Gazette des hôpitaux civils et militaires*. Paris. 48: 707.

———. 1876. Sur l'application des tractions mécaniques aux accouchements à propos de nouveaux perfectionnements apportés à un appareil obstétrical. *Bulletin général de thérapeutique médicale et chirurgicale*. 91: 412–415, 450–453.

———. 1877. De la traction mécanique appliquée à l'art des accouchements. *Gazette obstétricale*. 6: 100–105, 113–116.

Pugh, B. 1754. *A Treatise of Midwifery*. London: Buckland.

Radcliffe, W. 1947. *The Secret Instrument*. London: Heinemann. Reprint with *Milestones in Midwifery* (Bristol: Wright, 1967). San Francisco: Norman Publishing, 1989.

Radford, T. 1839. On the Long Forceps. In *Essays on Various Subjects Connected with Midwifery*, 1–20. Manchester: Leech.

———. 1865. *Observations on the Caesarean Section and on Other Obstetric Operations*. Manchester.

———. 1867. *The Principles and Practice of Obstetric Medicine*. Fifth edition. London: Churchill.

———. 1869. Craniotomy and Caesarean Section. *Medical Times and Gazette*. 1: 61–62.

———. 1878. Remarks on the Use and Value of the Long Forceps. *British Medical Journal.* 2: 621–622.

Ramsbotham, F. H. 1834. Difficult Labour—Instruments. *London Medical Gazette.* 14: 337–344.

———. 1841. *Principles and Practice of Obstetric Medicine and Surgery.* First edition. London: Churchill. Fourth edition, 1856.

———. 1856. *Principles and Practice of Obstetric Medicine and Surgery.* Fourth edition. London: Churchill.

———. 1867. *Obstetric Medicine and Surgery.* Fifth edition. London: Churchill.

Ramsbotham, J. 1832. *Practical Observations in Midwifery.* London: Highley.

Rathlauw, J. P. 1747. *Het berugte geheim in de vroedkunde, van Rogier Roonhuysen ontdekt en uitgegeven op hooge order door Jan Pieter Rathlauw, vroedmeester.* Amsterdam: Zacharias Romberg.

Rawlins, R. 1817. Letter from Mr. Richard Rawlins, Surgeon, &c. Oxford, to One of the Editors, on His Invention of the Reflected Forceps. *The London Medical Repository.* 8: 212–213.

Raynolde, T. 1545. *The Byrth of Mankynde or the Woman's Book.* London.

Reid, W. L. 1878. On a New Form of Long Forceps. *Glasgow Medical Journal.* 10: 241–261.

———. 1889. Discussion. *British Medical Journal.* 1:231.

Reynolds, E. 1888. On Axis-Traction Forceps, the Principles of Their Construction and Their Value in Practice. *Boston Medical and Surgical Journal.* 118: 489–491.

Ribes, Champetier de. 1888. De l'accouchement provoqué. *Annales de gynécologie.* 30: 401–438.

Rigby, E. the Younger. 1841. *A System of Midwifery.* First edition. London: Whittaker.

Rist, Ignace. 1818. *Essai historique et critique sur le forceps.* Thesis, University of Strasbourg.

Ritchie, C. G. 1865. On the Operation of Cephalotripsy As Performed at Vienna by Professor Braun. *Transactions of the Obstetrical Society of London.* 6: 75–78.

Ritgen, F. F. 1829. Beschreibung einer Geburtszange mit Verlängerbaren und Verkürzbaren Löffeln. *Gemeinsame Deutsche Zeitschrift für Geburtskunde.* 4: 401–405.

Rizzoli, F. 1856. *Nuovi strumenti d'ostetricia.* Bologna: Tipo Governativa dalla Volpa e del Sassi.

Robertson, F. M. 1872. Modification of the Obstetrical Forceps, with Practical Remarks on Their Application. *American Journal of Obstetrics.* 5: 285–308.

Roler, E. O. F. 1874. A Modification of the Obstetric Forceps. *Medical Examiner (Chicago).* 15: 459.

Rolland, M. 1905. *Du Forceps lyonnais ou forceps à branches parallèles.* Lyon: A. Rey.

Rösslin, E. 1513. *Die swangern Frawen und hebammen Rosengarten.* Hagenau: H. Gran.

———. 1532. *De partu hominis.* Latin translation of *Die swangern Frawen und hebammen Rosengarten.* Frankfurt: Christianus Egenolphus.

———. 1540. *Byrth of Mankynde.* English translation of *Die swangern Frawen und hebammen Rosengarten* by R. Jonas. London: Raynolde.

Roussel. *See* Witkowski, 1892.

Rowland, B. 1981. *Medieval Woman's Guide to Health.* London: Croom Helm.

Roy, A. le. 1778. *Recherches historiques et pratiques sur la section de la symphyse de pubis, pratiquée pour suppléer, à l'opération césarienne, le 2 octobre 1777, sur la femme souchot.* Paris: Le Clerc.

Rueff, J. 1554. *Ein schön lustig Trostbüchle.* Zurich: C. Froschouer.

———. 1580. *De conceptu et generatione hominis.* Latin translation of *Ein schon lüstig Trostbüchle.* Frankfurt: Corvenus.

———. 1637. *The Expert Midwife, or An Excellent and Most Necessary Treatise of the Generation and Birth of Man.* English translation of *Ein schön lustig Trostbüchle.* London: E. Griffin.

Saleh, S. 1886. *Contribution à l'étude de la docimasie.* Number 205. Paris.

Sänger, M. 1881. Ueber Zangen mit Zugapparaten und axengemässe Zangenextraction. *Archiv für Gynaekologie.* 17: 382–443. *See also* Witkowski, 1887.

Sawyer, E. W. 1876. A New Obstetric Forceps. *Chicago Medical Journal and Examiner.* 33: 46–48.

———. 1885. The Continued Pelvic Curve in the Obstetric Forceps, with Remarks on the Forceps in General. *Chicago Medical Journal and Examiner.* 51: 15–22.

Saxtorph, J. S. and P. Scheel. 1804. *Matthias Saxtorphs gesammelte Schriften.* Copenhagen; Brummer.

Scanzoni, F. 1853. *Lehrbuch der Geburtshilfe.* Wien: L. W. Seidel. *See also* Meadows, 1867.

———. 1935. *Classical Contributions to Obstetrics and Gynaecology.* English translation of *Lehrbuch der Geburtshilfe* by H. Thoms. Springfield: Thomas.

Schlichting, J. D. 1747. *Embryulcia nova detecta; of, Eene heel nieuw en onbekende, dog nuttige behandelinge, in de meeste moeielyke baaringen op't spoedigste te helpen.* Amsterdam: Van Huen.

Schöller, J. V. 1842. *Kie küntsliche Frühgebert bewirkt durch den Tampon.* Berlin: W. Besser.

Schroeder, K. 1870. *Lehrbuch der Geburtshülfe.* Bonn: Cohen.

———. 1873. *Manual of Midwifery.* English translation of third edition of *Lehrbuch der Geburtshülfe* by C. H. Carter. London: Churchill.

Schuyler, W. D. 1884. A New Obstetric Forceps. *New York Medical Journal.* 39: 270–272.

Sermon, W. 1671. *The Ladies Companion or the English Midwife.* London: Thomas.

Sheraton, E. R. 1867. The Steel Fillet of E. R. Sheraton. *Transactions of the Obstetrical Society of London.* 8: 259–261.

Siebold, Adam Elias von. 1810–1812. *Lehrbuch der theoretisch-praktischen Entbindungskunde, zu seinen Vorlesungen für Aerzte, Wundärzte, und Geburtshelfer entworfen.* Nuremberg: J. L. Schrag.

Siebold, Eduard C. J. von. 1854. *Lehrbuch der Geburtshülfe.* Braunnschweig: Vieweg.

Siebold, Elias von. 1802. Wirceburgi dissertato inauguralis de forcipis obstetriciae requisitis. *Lucina.* Volume I. Part I. Pages 122–127. Leipzig: Jacobäer.

———. 1839–1845. *Versuch einer Geschichte der Geburtshülfe.* Berlin: Enslin.

Sigault, J. R. 1778. *Discours sur les avantages de la section de la symphise.* Paris: Quillau.

Simpson, A. R. 1880. Basilysis: A Suggestion for Comminuting the Fetal Head in Cases of Obstructed Labour. *Transactions of the Edinburgh Obstetrical Society.* 8: 427–439

———. 1880–1881. On Axis-Traction Forceps. *Edinburgh Medical Journal.* 26: 245—251, 289–300.

———. 1881. Axis-Traction Forceps. *British Medical Journal.* 1: 576–577.

———. 1882–1883. Again on Axis-Traction Forceps. *Transactions of the Edinburgh Obstetrical Society.* 8: 143–159. *See also Edinburgh Medical Journal.* 1884. 29: 289–303.

———. 1884a. The Latest Model of the Basilyst. *Edinburgh Medical Journal.* 29: 341–343.

———. 1884b. A Lecture on the History of Embryulcia. *British Medical Journal.* 2: 1178–1181, 1230–1233.

———. 1900. The Invention and Evolution of the Midwifery Forceps. *Scottish Medical and Surgical Journal.* 7: 465–495.

Simpson, J. Y. 1848. On the Mode of Application of the Long Forceps. *Edinburgh Monthly Journal of Medical Science.* 9: 193–196.

———. 1849a. On a Suction Tractor; or New Mechanical Power, as a Substitute for the Forceps in Tedious Labours. *Monthly Journal of Medical Science.* 9: 556–559.

———. 1849b. On the Air-Tractor, as a Substitute for the Midwifery Forceps. *Monthly Journal of Medical Science.* 9: 618–620.

———. 1867. On the Cephalotribe. *British Medical Journal.* 2: 337.

———. 1871. *Selected Obstetrical and Gynaecological Works.* Edited by J. Watts Black. Edinburgh: Clark.

———. 1872. On Cranioclasm: Modes of Delivery in Obstructed Labour. *Clinical Lectures on the Diseases of Women.* Edited by A. R. Simpson: Edinburgh: Adam and Charles Black.

Sloan, S. 1889. Antero-posterior Compression Forceps for Application at the Brim of Flat Pelves. *British Medical Journal.* 1: 229–233, 806.

Smellie, W. 1751. *Treatise on the Theory and Practice of Midwifery*. London: Wilson. Sixth edition, 1765. Dublin: Whitehouse.

———. 1754. *A Sett of Anatomical tables, with Explanations, and an Abridgement, of the Practice of Midwifery, with a View to Illustrate a Treatise on That Subject, and Collection of Cases*. London: Published by the Author.

———. 1876–1878. *Treatise on the Theory and Practice of Midwifery*. Edited and annotated by A. H. McClintock. London: New Sydenham Society.

Smith, A. H. 1879. The Pendulum Leverage of the Obstetric Forceps. *Transactions of the American Gynecological Society (1878)*. 3: 235–267.

———. 1882. Axis Traction with the Obstetric Forceps. *Transactions of the American Gynecological Society (1881)*. 6: 291–326.

Smith, J. 1884. A New Cephalotribe. *British Medical Journal*. 1: 1136.

Smith, W. Tyler. 1860. On the Abolition of Craniotomy from Obstetric Practice. *Transactions of the Obstetrical Society of London*. 1: 21–50.

Soranus. 1956. *Gynecology*. English translation of text from the first century A.D. by O. Temkin. Baltimore: Johns Hopkins

Speert, H. 1958. *Obstetric and Gynaecologic Milestones: Essays in Eponymy.* New York: Macmillan.

———. 1963. *The Sloane Hospital Chronicle*. Philadelphia: F. A. Davis.

———. 1973. *Iconographia Gyniatrica*. Philadelphia: F. E. Davis. Revised second edition, *Obstetrics and Gynecology: A History and Iconography*. San Francisco: Norman Publishing, 1994.

———. 1980. *Obstetrics and Gynecology in America: A History*. Chicago: American College of Obstetricians and Gynecologists.

Spiegelberg, O. 1878. *Lehrbuch der Geburtshülfe*. Lahr: Schauenberg.

———. 1887, *Textbook of Midwifery*. English translation of second edition of *Lehrbuch der Geburtshülfe* by J. B. Hurry. London: New Sydenham Society.

Spink, M. S. and G. L. Lewis. 1973. *Albucasis. On Surgery and Instruments. A Definitive Edition of the Arab Text with English Translation and Commentaries*. Berkeley: University of California Press.

Stanesco. *See* Charpentier, 1883.

Stark, J. C. 1794. *Archiv für die Geburtshülfe, Frauenzimmer und neugebohrner Kinder*. Jena: Euno.

Stearns, J. 1808. Account of the Pulvis Parturiens, a Remedy for Quickening Childbirth. *Medical Repository*. 11: 308–309.

———. 1822. Observations on the secale cornutum, or Ergot, with Directions for Its Use in Parturition. *Medical Record*. 32: 90.

Steele, A. B. 1875. The Vectis As an Obstetric Instrument. *Liverpool and Manchester Medical and Surgical Reports*. Pages 221–227.

Stein, G. G. 1804. *L'Art d'accoucher*. Paris: Croullebois.

Stein, G. W. 1782. *Kurze Beschreibung eines Labimeters*. Cassel: Schmiedt.

———. 1793. *Practische Anleitung zur Geburtshülfe*. Marburg: Neuen Akademischen Buchhandlung.

Stephenson, W. 1886. On the Principle of Traction Rods, with a Simple Suggestion Applicable to Any Forceps. *British Medical Journal*. 2: 411–412.

Sterne, L. 1847. *The Life and Opinions of Tristram Shandy, Gentleman*. London: Chidley.

Stewart, W. S. 1887. Improved Forceps. *Transactions of the International Medical Congress, Ninth Session*. Edited by J. B. Hamilton. 2: 328.

———. 1889. When Should the Obstetric Forceps Be Used, and What Form of Instrument Is Required? *Journal of the American Medical Association*. 13: 770–771.

Stillman, H. L. *See* Chalmers, 1971.

Stolz, J. A. *See* Naegele and Grenser, 1880.

Stuart, F. H. 1877. Obstetric Forceps with Short and Long Handles. *American Journal of Obstetrics and Diseases of Women and Children*. 10: 650–652.

Studley, W. H. 1882. Mechanism of Forceps, Labour, and the Principles of Forceps Construction. *American Journal of Medical Sciences*. 82: 87–103.

Swayne, J. G. 1876. On a New Form of Blunt Hook and Sling for Assisting Delivery in Cases of Breech Presentation. *Transactions of the Obstetrical Society of London*. 17: 313–317.

———. 1878. Effects of Forceps Delivery on the Infant. *British Medical Journal*. 2: 459–460.

Tarnier, E. S. 1877a. *Description de deux nouveaux forceps*. Paris: Lauwereyns.

———. 1877b. Un nouveau forceps. *Annales de gynécologie* (Paris). 7: 261–264.

———. 1881a. Perfectionnement dans la construction et dans l'application du forceps. *Transactions of the International Medical Congress, London*. 4: 239–243.

———. 1881b. Improvements in the Construction and Application of the Forceps. *American Journal of Obstetrics*. 14: 913.

———. 1883. *Nouveau Dictionnaire de médecine et de chirurgie pratiques*. Volume 12: *Embryotome*. Paris: Ballière et fils.

Tarnier, E. S. and P. Budin. 1901. *Traité de l'art des accouchements*. Volume 4. Paris: Steinheil.

Tarsitani, D. *See* Capuron, 1842–1843, 1843–1844.

Taylor, G. 1892. An Improved Aseptic Axis-Traction Forceps. *Lancet*. 2: 1449.

Taylor, I. E. 1876. Narrow Bladed Forceps. *American Journal of Obstetrics and Diseases of Women and Children*. 9: 495.

Thenance, J.-S. 1781. *Nouveau forceps non-croisé ou forceps du célèbre Levret perfectionné en 1781, avec la manière de s'en servir*. Lyon: Ballandre et Barret.

———. 1802. *Nouveau forceps non-croisé ou forceps du célèbre Levret perfectionné en 1781, avec la manière de s'en servir*. Lyon: Ballandre et Barret. Quoted in full in Rolland, 1905.

Thiery, M. 1992. Obstetric Forceps and Vectis: The Roots. *Acta belgicae historiae medicinae*. 5: 4–20.

Thirtle, J. H. 1910. A Sabbatarian Pioneer—Dr. Peter Chamberlain [sic]. *Transactions of the Baptist Historical Society*. 2: 9–30; 110–117.

Thomas, P. 1879. *Des méthodes, procédés, appareils et instruments dans les cas de présentation de l'epaule*. Paris: Delahaye.

Thomas, T. G. 1907. Symphyseotomy[sic] and hebotomy. In *The Practice of Obstetrics in Original Contributions by American Authors*. Edited by R. Peterson. London: Henry Kimpton.

Thoms, H. 1922. Outlining the Superior Strait of the Pelvis by Means of the X-ray. *American Journal of Obstetrics and Gynecology*. 4: 257–263.

———. 1933. *Chapters in American Obstetrics*. Springfield: Thomas. Second edition, 1961.

Tiemann, George. 1889. *American Armamentarium Chirurgicum*. New York: George Tiemann and Company. Reprint edition San Francisco: Norman Publishing, 1989.

Trefurt, J. H. C. 1844. *Ueber die Wendung des Kindes . . . Abhandlungen und Erfahrungen aus dem Gebiete der Geburtshülfe*. Göttingen: Vandenhoeck und Ruprecht.

Trelat, Ulysse, Jr. *See* Meadows, 1867.

Trotula. *De passionibus mulierum curandarum*. *See* Rowland, 1981, and Tuttle, 1976.

Tuttle, E. F. 1976. The Trotula and Old Dame Trot: A Note on the Lady of Salerno. *Bulletin of the History of Medicine*. 50: 61–72.

Uytterhoven, André. *See* Poullet, 1883, and Fry, 1889b.

Vacher, F. 1873. Remarks on a New Midwifery Forceps. *Liverpool and Manchester Medical and Surgical Reports*. 1: 77–84.

———. 1874. On Certain Improvements in the Hinged Short Forceps. *Liverpool and Manchester Medical and Surgical Reports*. 2: 99–100.

———. 1878. Note on an Improvement in the Short-Hinged Forceps. *Liverpool and Manchester Medical and Surgical Reports*. 6: 124–125.

Valette. 1857. Un forceps et un céphalotribe nouveau. *L'Union médicale de Paris*. 11: 347.

Vedder, M. R. 1878. An Improvement in the Obstetrical Forceps. *Medical Record (N.Y.)*. 13: 43–57, 224–225.

Vesalius, A. 1543. *De humani corporis fabrica libri septem*. Basel: Johannes Oporinus.

Voorhees, J. D. 1900. Dilatation of the Cervix by Means of a Modified Champetier de Ribes Balloon. *Medical Record*. 58: 361–366.

Wales. 1895. *See* Das, 1929.

Wallace, E. 1878. A New Cephalotribe. *Transactions of the American Medical Association*. 29: 487–489.

Wallace, W. *See* Harris, 1872b.

Waller, C. 1831. *Elements of Practical Midwifery; or, Companion to the Lying-in Room*. Second edition. London: Highley; Edinburgh: Oliver and Boyd.

Wasseige, A. 1876. Du crochet mousse articulé. *Annales de la Societé de Médecine-Chirugie de Liège*. 15: 81–105.

———. 1877. Lamineur céphalique. *Journal des sciences médicales*. 2: 265–266.

Weiss, J. 1831. *An Account of Inventions and Improvements of Surgical Instruments*. London: Longman, Rees, Orme, Brown and Green.

———. 1889. *Catalogue of Surgical Instruments, Apparatus and Appliances*. London.

Weissbrod, J. B. *See* Doran, 1913c.

Welchman, J. 1790. The Case of a Woman Who Underwent the Section of the symphysis pubis. *London Medical Journal*. 11: 46–56.

Wells, B. H. 1886. An Axis Traction Attachment Applicable to Any Variety of Forceps. *American Journal of Obstetrics*. 19: 487–488.

West, C. 1880. Annual Address. *Transactions of the Obstetrical Society of London*. 21: 1–19.

Westmacott, J. G. 1869. On the Use of the Whalebone Loop. *Transactions of the Obstetrical Society of London*. 11: 177–183.

White, J. P. *See* Barker, 1877.

Wiener, M. 1878. Cephalotribe, or Cranioclast (English translation). *American Journal of Obstetrics*. 11: 184–195.

Williams, J. W. 1903. *Obstetrics: A Textbook for the Use of Students and Practitioners*. New York: Appleton.

Wilson, A. 1985. William Hunter and the Varieties of Man-midwifery. In W*illiam Hunter and the Eighteenth Century Medical World*. Edited by W. F. Bynum and R. Porter. Cambridge: Cambridge University Press.

Wiltshire, A. 1877. Modifications of the Tarnier Forceps. *Transactions of the Obstetrical Society of London*. 19: 223–227.

Witkowski, G.-J. 1887. *Histoire des accouchements chez tous les peuples*. Paris: Steinheil.

———. 1892. *Anecdotes et curiosités historiques sur les accouchements*. Paris: Steinheil.

Wrigley, J. 1935. The Forceps Operation. *Lancet*. 3: 702–705.

Yonge, J. 1706–1707. An Account of Balls of Hair Taken from the Uterus and Ovaries of Several Women. *Philosophical Transactions of the Royal Society of London*. 25: 2387–2392.

Ziegler, A. 1848–1849. On a New Form of Craniotomy Forceps. *Monthly Journal of Medical Sciences*. 9: 770–777.

ILLUSTRATIONS

While every effort has been made to trace copyright holders, in some cases they could not be traced or may have been omitted inadvertently.

I gratefully acknowledge the facilities I have been given at the following museums and institutions and for access to photograph instruments in their possession:

Department of Obstetrics and Gynaecology, The Trinity Centre for Health Sciences, Dublin: Figures *18.17, 19.10, 19.16*.

Department of Obstetrics and Gynaecology, University College and Middlesex School of Medicine, London: Figures *5.4, 5.5, 6.9, 6.10, 8.24, 8.26, 18.24*.

Department of Obstetrics, University of Edinburgh: Figures *I.5, 3.8, 15.2, 15.3*.

Department of Obstetrics and Gynaecology, University of Liverpool: Figures *7.5, 7.12*.

First Department of Gynecology and Obstetrics, Charles University, Prague: Figure *18.16*.

The Royal College of Obstetricians and Gynaecologists: Figures *1.7, 2.6, 2.15, 3.2, 3.7, 3.12, 3.14, 3.15, 4.2, 4.3, 4.6, 4.7, 4.9, 4.11, 5.1, 5.2, 5.11, 5.22, 5.23, 5.24, 5.25, 6.1, 6.11, 6.17, 6.22, 6.26, 6.30, 6.31, 6.33, 6.34, 7.14, 7.15, 7.20, 8.3, 8.4, 8.9, 8.10, 8.11, 8.12, 8.27, 8.28, 8.29, 8.30, 9.11, 10.14, 10.21, 10.23, 12.1, 12.8, 12.10, 12.12, 13.7, 13.8, 13.9, 13.11, 13.12, 13.13, 13.16, 13.20, 13.21, 13.24, 14.4, 14.5, 14.22, 16.1, 16.7, 16.8, 16.10, 16.13, 16.16, 16.21, 16.22, 16.25, 16.26, 16.27, 16.28, 16.29, 16.30, 16.31, 17.1, 17.3, 17.7, 17.8, 17.9, 17.10, 18.2, 18.3, 18.5, 18.7, 18.8, 18.10, 18.12, 18.14, 18.15, 18.22, 18.23, 18.25, 18.26, 18.27, 19.2, 19.5, 19.28, 19.29, 19.30, 20.1, 20.2, 20.4, 20.5, 22.1, 22.6, 22.17, 22.18, 22.20, 22.21*.

The Royal College of Surgeons of England: Figures *19.9, 19.14, 19.18, 19.21, 22.22*.

The Science Museum, London: Figures *1.9, 1.11, 1.12, 2.8, 3.11, 3.13, 4.10, 5.7, 5.8, 5.12, 5.21, 6.12, 6.15, 8.15, 6.19, 6.20, 6.21, 6.23, 6.24, 6.25, 6.28, 6.29, 8.20, 8.23, 9.1, 9.3, 9.5, 9.8, 9.12, 9.13, 10.2, 10.3, 10.5, 10.7, 10.8, 10.16, 10.18, 10.25, 10.26, 12.5, 12.11, 12.14, 13.1, 13.4, 13.14, 14.7, 14.8, 14.17, 14.18, 16.5, 16.6, 16.9, 16.11, 16.14, 16.19, 16.20, 16.21, 16.23, 18.6, 18.9, 18.11, 18.35, 19.15, 19.17, 19.19, 19.31, 19.32, 19.34, 19.35, 19.38, 19.39, 22.4, 22.5, 22.7, 22.10, 22.11, 22.12, 22.19*.

York Medical Society: *Figure 3.9*.

I am indebted to the Librarians and staff of the following libraries for assistance in tracing references and for providing me with the material for the following illustrations:

The Royal College of Obstetricians and Gynaecologists: Figures *I.8, I.9, I.10, 1.1, 1.8, 2.1, 2.3, 2.4, 2.5, 2.7, 2.9, 2.10, 2.11, 2.12, 2.14, 3.1, 3.3, 3.4, 3.5, 3.6, 3.10, 4.1, 4.4, 4.5, 4.8, 5.6, 5.9, 5.10, 5.13, 5.14, 5.15, 5.19, 5.26, 5.28, 5.32, 6.14, 6.18, 6.27, 7.1, 7.2, 7.3, 7.4, 7.6, 7.8, 7.9, 7.10, 7.16, 8.2, 8.5, 8.13, 8.14, 8.16, 8.17, 9.4, 9.9, 9.10, 9.14, 9.16, 9.17, 9.18, 10.1, 10.17, 10.19, 10.20, 10.24, 11.1, 11.2, 11.4, 11.5, 11.6, 11.7, 11.8, 11.9, 11.10, 11.12, 11.13, 11.14, 11.19, 11.21, 12.2, 12.4, 12.7, 12.9, 12.15, 12.25, 13.2, 13.6, 13.10, 13.15, 13.17, 13.18, 13.19, 13.22, 13.23, 13.27, 13.28, 13.29, 14.1, 14.2, 14.3, 14.9, 14.10, 14.16, 14.20, 14.21, 14.23, 15.1, 15.5, 16.2, 16.3, 16.4, 16.12, 16.17, 16.18, 16.24, 16.32, 18.4, 18.18, 18.19, 18.20, 18.21, 18.31, 18.32, 18.33, 18.34, 19.20, 19.22, 19.24, 20.3, 20.8, 20.11, 20.12, 20.13, 20.14, 20.15, 21.1, 21.2, 21.5, 21.6, 22.2, 22.3, 22.8, 22.9, 22.13, 22.15, 22.16, 22.23, 23.24, 22.25, 22.26, 22.27*.

The Royal Society of Medicine: Figures 5.16, 5.17, 5.18, 5.20, 5.27, 5.30, 5.31, 6.16, 7.11, 7.13, 7.17, 7.18, 8.1, 8.6, 8.15, 8.19, 8.21, 9.6, 9.7, 10.6, 10.9, 10.10, 10.11, 10.12, 10.13, 10.15, 10.27, 11.3, 11.11, 11.15, 11.16, 11.17, 11.18, 11.20, 12.3, 12.6, 12.13, 12.16, 12.17, 12.18, 12.20, 12.21, 12.22, 12.23, 12.24, 13.3, 13.5, 13.26, 14.6, 14.11, 14.12, 14.13, 14.14, 14.15, 15.4, 17.4, 17.5, 17.6, 18.1, 18.13, 19.1, 19.3, 19.8, 19.11, 19.12, 19.13, 19.23, 19.25, 19.26, 19.27, 19.33, 19.36, 20.6, 20.7, 20.10, 21.3, 21.4.

The Wellcome Institute Library, London: Figures I.3, I.4, I.6, I.7, I.11, I.12, 1.10, 1.13, 1.14, 1.15, 1.16, 2.2, 2.13, 3.16, 5.3, 8.8, 8.18, 9.2, 10.4, 10.15.

The following illustrations are the subject of copyright and I acknowledge permission to reproduce them in this work:

Vandenhoeck and Ruprecht (*Armamentarium obstetricium Gottingense*. Kuhn and Tröhler, 1987.): Figure 5.29.

Edward Arnold and Company (*The Ventouse*. Chalmers JA, 1971): Figures 15.6, 15.7.

British Journal of Obstetrics and Gynaecology: Figures 6.32, 6.33, 6.34.

The Diplomate: Figures 1.3, 1.4, 1.5.

The Hunterian Society Transactions: Figures 3.17, 6.1.

Norman Publishing (*American Armamentarium Chirurgicum*. George Tiemann. Facsimile edition, 1989): Figures 7.7, 7.19, 8.22, 8.25, 9.15, 16.15, 19.4.

INDEX OF NAMES

References in *italics* indicate figures; those followed by "t" denote tables

Academy of Sciences of Paris, 239–240
Aitken, David William, 178, *179*
Aitken, John, 54, *55*, 72, 75, 147, *147*, 209, *209*–210, *226*, 227, 229, 263–264, *263*, *264*, *265*, *266*, 272, 275t
Albucasis, 1–2
Amand, Pierre, 22, *23*
Anderson, C. L., 96, *96–97*, 278t, 281t
Anderson, Tempest, 236, *238*, 257
Aquinas, St. Thomas, 214
Arnold, 267, *267*
Arnott, Neil, 195
Asdrubaldi, Francesco, 269
Assalini, Paolo, 141, *141–142*, 224, *225*, 238, *239*, 279t
Augusta, Princess Charlotte, 79
Auvard, Pierre Victor Alfred, 251–252, *253*
Aveling, J. H., 2, 11, 163, *163*
Avicenna, 1–2

Baglioni, S., 1
Ballantyne, J. W., 6
Barclay, John, 52, 125, *125*, 276t
Bar de Luc, Champion, 262
Bard, S., 98
Barker, Fordyce, 57, 173
Barnes, Fancourt, 246, *246*
Barnes, Robert, 86, 94–96, *95*, 129, 175, 185, 213, 214, 215, *215*, 242, 246, *250*, 250–251, 278t, 281t
Bartlett, J., 183
Barton, Lyman T., 280t
Baudelocque, A. C., 63
Baudelocque, J. L., 60, 62–63, *62–63*, 99–102, 199, 260, 262, 265, 266

Baudelocque, L.-A., 238–240, *239*
Baumers, M. R., 126, *128*
Beatty, John, 52, 57t, 123, *123–124*, 276t
Beatty, T. E., 88, *88*
Bedford, Gunning S., 103, *104–105*, 105
Benjamin, D., 189
Bernard, C., *142*, 143
Bethell, J. P., 102, *103*
Bing, Jens, 112, *113*
Bland, Robert, 20, 50–51, 57t
Blenkarne, W. L'Heureux, *116*, 116–117
Blond, Kasper, 255
Bloom, Regner, 19
Blot, Hippolyte, 223, *223*, 242, *242*
Blundell, James, 49–50, 90, 208, 225, 277t
Blunt, John, 45
Böehmer, A., 28
Boër, Lucas Johann, 57t, 74
Boivin, 57t
Bonney, Victor, 177, 281t
Bossi, L. M., 217, *217–218*
Boswell, J., 29
Bourgeois, Louise, 8
Boursier, Martin, 8
Bower, 147–149, *148*
Boyer, *271*
Braithwaite, James, 89–90, *90*, 121, 277t
Braun, Carl, 181, *181*, 214, 224, 225, *241*, 241–242, 251, *251*, 254, 255
Braun, G. A., 254
Bredin, John Noble, 109, *111*, 112
Breus, Carl, 181, *182*, 281t

Browne, O. D. T., 264
Brulatour, 118–119, *119*
Brunninghausen, Hermann Joseph, 71, *92*, *93*, 215
Bruyn, Johannes de, 207
Bullock, W. R., 65
Burge, John Henry Hobart, 120, *120*
Burns, John, 55, 213, 225
Burton, John, 37–38, *38*
Busch, D. W. H., 59, 68, 72, 267
Busch, John David, 68, 72, *73*, 75, *75*, 94
Butter, Alexander, 26, 29, 33

Cadran, *268*
Caldwell, William Edgar, 274
Cameron, Murdoch, 194, *194*, 281t
Campbell, C. J., 134, *135*
Campbell, W. M., 58
Cappie, James, *114*, 115
Carof, J., *115*, 115–116
Carus, C. G., 57t
Carwardine, H. H., 14
Cazeaux, P., 65, *65*, 126, 197
Cellier, Elizabeth, 37
Celsus, 1
Chailly-Honoré, Nicolas Charles, 240–241
Chalmers, J. A., 195
Chamberlen family, 9–16, *10*, *11*, *12*, *15*, 119, 200, 205, *205*
Chapman, Edmund, 25–26, *25–26*, 28, 275t
Charpentier, A., 119
Charrière, 272, *272*
Chassagny, M. 136–139, *136*, *139*, 140, 150, 154, 155
Christie, David, 164, *164*, 280t
Churchill, Fleetwood, 57t, 59, 87–88, *88*, 236t, 242, 273, 277t
Clark, John, 85, *86*, 276t
Clarke, Joseph, 45, 56t, 57t
Cleeman, R. A., 160, *161*
Cleveland, William Frederick, 221, *221*
Codd, William, 14
Collins, Robert, 54, *54*, 56t, 57t, 236t, 271, 272, 277t
Collyer, 267, *267*
Conquest, J. T., 113, *114*, 248, 249, 277t
Coutouly, P. V., 60, *61*, *62*, 117–118, *118*, 265, 266
Crainz, F., 1
Cullingworth, Charles, 175, 177

Das, Kedarnath, 14, 50, 53
Davan, 66
Davis, David, 80–85, *81–84*, 99, 102–103, 112–113, *113*, 208, 209, 229–230, *229*, *230*, 236, 237, 249, 257, *257*, 269, *269*, 279t

Davis, J. Hall, *250*, 251
Debenham, R. K., 204, *204*
De Bruin, Johannes, 19, 20
De Leurie, 93
Delore, Xavier, 151, 152, *153*
Demelin, L., 182, *182*
Denman, Thomas, 47–48, *48*, 51, 208, 221, *221*, 225, 275t
Depaul, John Anne Henri, 156
De Ribes, Champetier, 215–216, *215–216*
Dewees, W. B., 166, *167*, 193, *193*–194, 162–263
Dewees, William Potts, 63, 99–100, *100*
Dewhurst, J., 79
De Wind, Paulus, 17, 19, 29, 30
Dick, 130, *130*
Districtsloege, 212, *212*
Donald, Archibald, 238
Doran, A., 28, 38, 50, 67, 72, 112
Dorland, William Alexander Norman, 105
Douglas, James, 39
Douglas, William, 37
D'Outrepent, Joseph Servazius, 74
Draper, W., 121, *121*
Drinkwater, 24
Dubois, Antoine, 63–64, *64*, 279t
Dubois, Paul, 63–64, *64*, 279t
Dugès, Antoine Louis, 251, 267
Duke, Alexander, 150, *151*, 189
Duncan, J. Mathews, 94, *95*, 197, 223, *223*, 243, 244, 266, 267, 274, 278t
Duns, J., 195
Dupuy, John, 98
Dusée, 28–30, *31*, 32, 279t

Eardley-Wilmot, Robert, 202, 203–204
Earle, James I. Lumley, 268, 269
Eastlake, Henry Edward, 231–232, *232*
Edis, Arthur, 58
Elliot, G. T., *104–105*, 105, 280t
Evans, 54, 75

Felsenreich, T., 181, *182*
Ferguson, 268, 269
Ferguson, Haigh, 281t
Fisher, Robert W., 189, *190*
Flamant, R. P., 65
Forster, F. M. C., 96
Foulis, James, 185, *186*
Freke, John, 27, *27*, 109
Fries, *77*, 77
Froriep, Ludwig Friedrich von, *76–77*, 77

Fry, Henry D., 126, 128, *129*, 175, 194, *194*
Gaitskell, W., 208
Galabin, A. L., 129–130, 164, *164*, 280t
Gardner, W. S., 183
Gariel, M.-M., 214
Garrigues, Henry Jacques, 234–235, 261–262, *262*
Gayton, William, 86–87, *87*
Geijl, A., 18
Geminus, Thomas, 6
Germann, 272
Giffard, William, 27, *27*–28, 109
Gigli, Leonardo, 255, 262
Giordano, Scipione, 158, *158*
Glaister, J., 33
Godson, Clement, 223, *223*
Gordon, David, 115
Grattan, N., 191–193, *192*
Greenhalgh, Robert, 86, *86*–87, 220, 222, 223, 227, *268*, 269
Grégoire, 17, 28, *30*, 39
Greville, *187*, 281t
Grönning, 212, *212*
Guillemeau, Jacques, 5, 8, *226*, 227
Guillon, J. B., 78, *78*
Guyon, J. C. F., 245, *245*, 251

Haighton, John, 47, *47*, 90, 99, 275t
Hamilton, Alexander, 53, *53*–54, 112, *113*, 199, 214, 225, 227, 242–243, 276t
Hamilton, James, 54, 55, 90, 112, *113*
Hamon, L., *144*, 145, 155, *155*
Hardy, 56
Harper, Phillip H., 125
Harris, R. P., 98, 234, 260, 269, *269*
Hartmann, R., 169, *169*
Haslam, W. D., 116, *116*
Heidler, Hans, 255
Heister, Lorenz, 17, 22, *23*, 24
Hellier, J. B., 28
Hennig, Carl, 239, 240, *240*
Herbiniaux, G. M., 219, *220*
Herff, 165
Hermann, *167*, 167–168
Hewitt, Graily, 88, *88*, 242, 277t
Hicks, J. Braxton 173, 243, *243*, 247
Hildanus, Fabricius, 195
Hilliard, Robert Harvey, 185, *186*
Hippocrates, 3–4
Hirst, B. C., 117
Hodge, Hugh L., 101–102, *100*–*102*, 160
Hohl, A. F., 68, 69

Holland, Eardley, 79
Holland, Edmund, *163*, 163–164
Holmes, John Pocock, 222, 223, *248*, 249
Hopkins, J., 85–86, *86*, 214
Howitz, Frantz J. A. C., *270*, 271
Hubert, E., 168–169, *169*
Hubert, L. J., 168, *168*–*169*, 183, 201, *201*, 206, 207, 251, *252*
Huevel, Jean Baptiste van, 258–259, *259*, 271–272
Hunter, William, 38–39, 263
Huston, Robert M., 99, *99*
Hüter, 214

Jacquemier, Jean Marie, *256*, 257
Jaggard, William Wright, 170, 181
James, F. H., 196
James, Thomas C., 99, *100*
Janck, Johan Gottfried, 112
Jansen, 57t
Jardine, Robert, 251–252
Jenks, Edward W., *106*, 107
Jewett, Charles, *106*, 107, 183–184, *184*, 263
Johnson, Charles, 56t
Johnson, R. W., 3–4, 24, 52–53, *53*, 112, 160, *161*, 219, 231, *231*, 265, 276t
Johnston, George T., 56, 56t
Johnstone, R. W., 33
Jonas, R., 5
Jones, 222, 223
Jörg, Johan Christian Gottfried, *224*, 225
Joulin, M., 152, *152*–*153*, 257–258, *258*

Kalindero, N., 245
Keiller, Alexander, 115, 189
Kidd, George H., 243, *244*
Kielland, C. C. G., 281t
Kilian, H. F., 17, 57t, 63, 240, *240*
Kluge, 57t
Knight, S. T., *106*, 107
Knox, J. S., *167*, 167
Kristeller, Samuel, 151, *151*
Kuhn, W., 71–72, 207
Kuntzsch, 198
Küstner, 272, *273*

Labatt, Samuel, 56t
La Chapelle, 57t
La Motte, Guillaume, 16, 24
Laroyenne, Lucien Pierre, 162, *162*
Lazarewitch, J., 145, *145*, 199, 201, *201*, 214, 238, *256*, 257, 272, *272*, 279t

Leake, J., 126, *127*, 263
Le Doux, Gilles, 17
Lee, A. L., 49
Lee, Robert G., 213–214, *214*
Leishman, William, 243–244
Le Page, J. F., *188*, 189, 191–193, *193*
Le Roy, A., 260
Lever, 236t, *248*, 254, *254*
Levret, André, 39–44, *40–43*, 226, *228*, 229, 265, 279t
Levy, C. E. M., 109, *110*
Lewis, G. L., 2
Locarelli, 241, *241*
Lollini, 247, *247*, 251
Lowder, William, 47, *47*, 54, 275t
Löwenthal, H., 121–122, *122*
Luikart, Ralph Herbert, 108
Lusk, W. Thomas, 107, 173, 183, *183*, 204, 244, 246, *246*
Lyman, A. B., 189, *190*
Lyon, J. G., 177–178, *179*, 234, *235*

McCahey, Peter, 198, *198*
McClintock, A. H., 33, 56t
Macdonald, A. D., 191, *192*
McFerran, Joseph A., 191, *191*
McGillicuddy, Timothy J., 193, *193*
Mackness, George Owen Carr, 179, *179*
McLane, James W., *106*, 107–108
McLaurin, William, *188*, 189
Madden, T. More, 56, 88–89, *180*, 181
Maison Mathieu, 119
Mann, M. D., 117
Marginles, 196
Martin, A. E., 245, *245*
Martin, Eduard, 68, 70, *70*, 266, *267*
Mathew, George Porter 177, *178*, 278t, 281t
Mattei, A., 134, *134*, 142, 143, 152, *152*
Maubray, John, 22
Mauriceau, François, 4, 13, 22, *23*, 206, 226, 228–229, 231
May, 14
Mayer and Meltzer, *268*, 269
Maygrier, Jacques Pierre, 78
Meigs, Charles D., 99, 129
Mende, L. J. K., *76*, 77, 224, *225*, 241
Mercurio, Scipione, 2, *3*
Merriman, S., 57t, 220
Mesnard, Jacques, 136, *137*, 234, *235*
Miller, De Laskie, *111*, 112
Milliken, 267
Milne, A., 48

Milne, John Stewart, 1
Mitchell, James, 196
Moloy, Howard Carman, 274
Mondotte, *143*, 143–144
Moralès, J., 165, *165*
Moreau, F. J., 64, *65*
Morgan, Herbert, 150, *188*, 189
Moschner, 57t
Mulder, J., 24, 28, 32, 52–53
Mundé, Paul Fortunatus, 238–239, 251
Murphy, Edward, 57t, 89, *89*, 269, 277t
Murray, Jardine, 215
Murray, Robert Milne, 176, *177, 178*, 280t
Mursinna, C. L., 68, *68*

Naegele, Franz Carl, 57t, *71*, 71–72, 92, 223, *223*, 279t
Neale, L. E., 183, *184*
Neville, William, 185, *186–187*, 281t
Newham, Samuel, 232, *232*
Nihell, Elizabeth, 37

Oldham, H., 94, *95*, 221–223, *222*, 232–233, *233*
Olivier, A. V., 204, *205*
Opie, T., 175
Orme, David, 47, *47*, 275t
Osborn, William, *50–51*, 50–52, 55, 208, 225, 276t
Osiander, F. B., 67, *67*, 72, 160, *161*, 207
Osiander, J. F., 67
Ould, Fielding, 32, 226, *227*

Page, John, 28
Pajot, Charles, 119, *119–120*, 160, *161*, 167, 240, *240*
Palfyn, Johannes, 16–17, *16–17*, 32, 39
Paré, Ambroise, 4–5, 8, 22, 195, 196, 226, 227
Parvin, Theophilus, 128, 167, 204
Péan, 60, 64
Pearse, T. F., 109, *111*, 165, *165*
Petit, Antoine, 32
Petit, Jean Louis, 75, *75*
Piet, M., 60
Pinard, Adolphe, 72
Pineau, Severin, 260
Playfair, W. S., 205
Poullet, J. *135*, 139–141, *140, 141*, 156, *157*, 162, 165–167, *166*
Power, D'Arcy, 6
Preiss, 217, *218*
Priestley, W. H., 197
Pros, G., 155, *155*
Pugh, Benjamin, 28, *29*, 276t

Radcliffe, Walter, 9
Radford, Thomas, 90–91, *91*, 131, *131*, 211, 220, 277t, 278t
Ramsbotham, F. H., 57t, 91–93, *92*, 236t, 244, *248*, 249, 254, *254*, 273, *273*, 277t, 278t
Ramsbotham, J., 91
Rathlauw, Jan, *18*, 19, 136
Rawlins, R., 230
Raynolde, Thomas, 6–7
Reid, William, 128–129, *129*
Reynolds, E., 183
Ribes, Champetier de, 215–216, *215–216*
Riecke, 57t
Rigby, E., *92*, 93, 214
Rist, Ignace, 126
Ritchie, Charles George, 242
Ritgen, F. F., 132, *133*
Rizzoli, F., 212, *212*, 241, *241*, 272, *272*
Robertson, Francis Marion, 103, *103*, 210, *210*, 220
Rogers, N., 49
Roler, E. O. F., 105
Rolland, M., 136
Rösslin, Eucharius, 5, *7*
Roussel, 153, *153*, 158, *158*
Rueff, Jacob, 4, *7*, 7, 8

Saleh, Soubhy, 197, *197*
Sandborg and Vedler, 132, *132*
Sänger, Max, 162, *162–163*, 181
Sawyer, Edward Warren, 102, *103*
Saxtorph, Mathias, 109, *110*, 160
Scanzoni, Friedrich Wilhelm, 63, 197, *197*, 242, *242*, 256, 257
Schlichting, Daniel, *18*, 19–20, 136
Schroeder, K., 72
Schuyler, William David, 103, *104*
Scultetus, *226*
Sermon, William, 22
Shekleton, Robert, 56t
Sheraton, E. R., *202*, 203
Shippen, William Jr., 98
Siebold, 57t. See also Siebold, Elias von
Siebold, Adam Elias von, 71
Siebold, Eduard C. J. von, 70
Siebold, Elias von, 57t, *70*, 70–71, 99, 207
Sigault, J. R., 260
Simpson, A. R., 173, *174*, 175, *175*, 214, 225, 242, 251, *252*, 280t
Simpson, J. Y., 93–94, *93–94*, 110, 175, 195–197, *196*, 222, 223, 236t, 242–243, *243*, 249–250, *249*, 277t, 278t
Sloan, Samuel, *130*, 130–131

Smellie, William, 33–37, *35–37*, 161, 221, *221*, 226, 227–228, *228*, 265, 275t
Smith, Albert H., 117, *117*, 160, *161*, 173
Smith, James, 243, 245–246
Smith, W. Tyler, 236
Soranus of Ephesus, 4
Speert, H., 13, 214, 234
Spiegelberg, Otto von, 73–74, *74*, 279t
Spink, M. S., 2
Stanesco, *255*
Starke, J. C., 279t
Stearns, John, 98
Steele, A. B., 208, 209
Stein, G. W., 75, *76*, 270, 271
Stephenson, William, *188*, 189
Stewart, W. S., *148*, 149
Stillman, Herbert L., 197–198, *198*
Stolz, Joseph Alexis, 72–73, *73*, 279t
Storer, H. R., 197
Stuart, Francis H., 117, *117*
Studley, William Harrison, 185, *187*
Swayne, Joseph Griffiths, 131, 199, *201*

Targett, 254, *254*
Tarnier, Etienne Stéphane, 170–173, *171–172*, 216, 247, 258–259, *258*, *259*, 280t
Tarsitani, D., 66, *66*
Taylor, G., 165, *165*, 173
Taylor, Isaac E., 132, *133*, 134
Tennent, V. B., 98
Thenance, Jean-Simon, 66–67, 136, *138*
Thiery, M., 15
Thirtle, J. H., 11
Thomas, Pierre, 258, *258*
Thomas, T. G., 261
Thoms, Herbert, 98, 99, 274
Thynne, Andrew, 52, *52*, 276t
Tiemann, George, 102, 205, 235, 236, 244
Trelat, Ulysse Jr., *144*, 145
Tröhler, U., 71–72, 207
Trotula, 4
Tucker, Ervin A., *107*, 108, 280t
Tureau, 66
Tuttle, E. F., 4

Uytterhoven, André, 126, *128*

Vacher, Francis, 121, *121*
Valette, 136, *139*, 246, 247

Van der Ecken, *255*
Van Roonhuysen, 17–20, *20–21,* 206, *206*
Vedder, Maus R., 191, *191*
Vesalius, Andreas, 6–7
Voorhees, James Ditmar, *216,* 217

Wagstaff, *164,* 164–165, 280t
Walcher, Gustav Adolf, 217, *218*
Wales, 164–165
Walker, Dr. Chamberlen, 13, 28, *29,* 275t
Wallace, Ellerslie, 244
Wallace, William, 102, *103*
Waller, Charles, 90, *91*
Wasseige, *257,* 257–258
Weiss, John, 122, *146,* 147, 210, *210,* 223, *223*
Weissbrod, J. B., 68, *68*
Welchman, J. L., 263
Wells, Brooks H., 189–191, *190*
Wertt, 4
Westmacott, John G., *202,* 203
White, James Platt, 173
Wiener, M., 239
Williams, John Whitridge, 183, 263
Wiltshire, Alfred, 173
Winter, George, 251, *253*
Witkowski, G.-J., 59, 150, *151,* 158, 159
Woodham Mortimer Hall, 11, *11,* 14–15
Wrigley, J., 85, *97*

Yonge, James, 195
Young, Thomas, 52–53, *53,* 276t

Ziegler, Alexander, 52, 123, *124,* 234, *235,* 276t

INDEX OF SUBJECTS

References in *italics* indicate figures; those followed by "t" denote tables

air tractor, Simpson's. *See* vacuum extractors
antero-posterior forceps. *See also* asymmetric forceps
    craniotomy and, 130
    designs
        Baumers's, 126, *128*
        Cameron's, 194, *194*, 281t
        Dick's, 130, *130*
        Fry's, 128, *129*, 194, *194*
        McLaurin's, *188*, 189
        Reid's, 128–129, *129*
        Sandborg and Vedler's, 132, *132*
        Sloan's, *130*, 130–131
        Uytterhoven's, 126, *128*
    history of, 126
    indications for, 194
    purpose of, 126
    with axis traction. *See* axis traction, antero-posterior forceps with
apertorium, 7, *8*
Arabian medicine, 1
articulations
    in British practice, 66, *66*
    description of, 59
    in European practice, 59–60, 66, *66*
    modifications
        "block-lock," 67, *67*
        English lock, 34, *36*, *37*, 68–70
        French locks, 39–43, *40*, *41*, *42*, *43*, 59, 60
        lateral mortise, 70–71
        mortise, 59, 60
        pin-pivot, 71
        reversible lock, 66–67

artificial rupture of membranes, methods for, 213
    Lee's membrane perforator, 214, *214*
asymmetric forceps
    adjustable, for producing asymmetric blades, 132–135
    designs
        Baumers's, 126, *128*
        C. J. Campbell's, 134, *135*
        Dick's, 130, *130*
        Leake's, 126, *127*
        Mattei's, 134, *135*
        Poullet's, 134, *135*
        Radford's, 91, 131, *131*, 277t
        Reid's, 128–129, *129*
        Ritgen's, 132, *133*
        Sandborg and Vedler's, 132, *132*
        Sloan's, *130*, 130–131
        I. E. Taylor's, 132, *133*, 134
        Uytterhoven's, 126, *128*
    history of, 126
    indications for, 134
    summary overview of, 134–135
attachments for forceps. *See* dynamometers; tapes; tractors
axis traction. *See also* axis-traction forceps
    antero-posterior forceps with, 194
        Cameron's, 194, *194*, 281t
        Fry's, 194, *194*
        McLaurin's, *188*, 189
    criticisms of, 173
    definition of, 160
    developmental stages of, 160, *161*

axis traction (*continued*)
   geometric principles applied to
      description of, 167
      Hartmann's contributions, 169, *169*
      Hermann's contributions, 167, *167–168*
      L. J. Hubert's contributions, 168–169, *168–169*
      Murray's contributions, *176*, 177
      Neville's contributions, 185, *186*, 281t
      A. R. Simpson's contributions, 173, *174*, 175, *175*
      indications for, 194
axis-traction forceps
   adjustable, 177, *178*
      designs
         Mathew's, 177, *178*, 281t
         Murray's, 177, *178*, 280t
   American designs
      W. B. Dewees's, *193*, 193–194
      Jewett's, 183–184, *184*
      Lusk's, 183, *183*
      McFerran's, 191, *191*
      McGillicuddy's, 193, *193*
      Neale's, 183, *184*
      Studley's, 185, *187*
      Vedder's, 191, *191*
   in American practice, 183–184
   British designs
      D. W. Aitken's, 178, *179*
      Anderson-Neville's, 185, *187*, 281t
      Barnes-Neville's, 185, *187*, 281t
      Bonney's, 177, 281t
      Ferguson's, 281t
      Foulis's, 185, *186*
      Grattan's, 191–193, *192*
      Greville's, 281t
      Hilliard's, 185, *186*
      Le Page's, 191–193, *193*
      Macdonald's, 191, *192*
      Mackness's, 179, *179*
      Madden's, *180*, 181
      Neville's, 185, *186–187*
      A. R. Simpson's, 173, *174–175*, 175, 280t
         C. Braun's modifications, 181, *181*
         Breus's modifications, 181, *182*, 281t
         Cullingworth's modifications, 175–177
         Felsenreich's modifications, 181, *182*
   in British practice, 175–181, 185
   European designs
      C. Braun's, 181, *181*
      Breus's, 181, *182*, 281t
      Felsenreich's, 181, *182*
      Laroyenne's, 162, *162*
      Lyon's, 177–178, *179*
      Poullet's, 165–167, *166*
      Sänger's *162*, 162–163, 181
   with hinged shanks or handles, 191–194
      designs
         Le Page's, 191–193, *193*
         A. D. Macdonald's, 191, *192*
         McFerran's, 191, *191*
         McGillicuddy's, 193, *193*
         W. B. Dewees's, 193, *193*
         Vedder's, 191, *191*
   parallel, 182, *182*
   simplifying of, 185
   with stepped shanks. *See* stepped forceps
   Tarnier's contributions and designs. *See* Tarnier, Etienne Stéphane
   tractor attachments, 189–191
      designs
         Dukes's, 150, *151*, 189
         Fisher's, 189, *190*
         Le Page's, *188*, 189
         Lyman's, 189, *190*
         McLaurin's, *188*, 189
         Morgan's, *188*, 189
         Stephenson's, *188*, 189
         Wells's, 189–191, *190*

balloons, for inducing labor, 215–217
   designs
      R. Barnes's, 215, *215*
      De Ribe's, 215–216, *215–216*
      Tarnier's, 216
      Voorhees's, *216*, 217
baptism in utero
   effect on Caesarian section rate, 219
   Herbiniaux's device, 219, *220*
basilysts
   function of, 251
   L. J. Hubert's, 251, *252*
   A. R. Simpson's, 251, *252*
basilyst-tractor, 252
basiotribes
   Auvard's, 251–252, *253*
   Tarnier's, 251, *253*
blades, forceps. *See also* handles, detachable; hinged; interchangeable
   design variations
      asymmetric. *See* asymmetric forceps
      interchangeable

blades, forceps, interchangeable (*continued*)
    designs
        Brulatour's, 118–119, *119*
        Burge's, 120, *120*
        Cappie's, *114*, 115
        Carof's, 115–116, *115*
        Coutouly's, 117–118, *118*
        Pajot's, 119, *119–120*
    history of, 117
    interlocking male and female, 123–125
        designs
            Barclay's, 125, *125*, 276t
            J. Beatty's, 123, *123–124*, 276t
            Harper's, 125
            Ziegler's, 123, *124*, 276t
    rotating, 121–122
        Chassagny's design, 136, *139*
        Löwenthal's design, 121–122, *122*
"block-lock" modification, 67, *67*
Blond-Heidler saw, 255
blunt hooks, 211, *211*
    crotchets and, 211, *211*
bone pliers. *See* osteotomists
Brunninghausen lock, *92*, 93

Caesarian section
    baptism in utero and, 219
    in nineteenth-century practice, 219–220
        maternal mortality secondary to, 220, 244
    pelvic size considerations, 220
    prevalence of use, 220
    Raynolde's recommendations, 6–7
    seventeenth-century illustration of, *3*
calculus extractor, 5
cephalic version, 7
cephalometers, 147
    designs
        J. Aitken's, 54, *55*, 75, 147, *147*
        Evans's, 54, 75
cephalotomes, 254. *See also* embryotomes
    designs
        Tarnier's, 258, *258*, *259*
        Van Huevel's, 258–259, *259*
cephalotribes, 238–247
    in American practice, 244
        Lusk's, 244, 246, *246*
    in British practice, 242–244
        F. Barnes's, 246, *246*
        Duncan's, 243, *244*
        Hick's, 243, *243*, 247
        Kidd's, 243, *244*
        J. Y. Simpson's, 242, *243*
    combined instruments
        description of, 247
        designs
            Auvard's, 251–252, *253*
            Jardine's, 251–252
            Lollini's, 247, *247*
            Valette's, *246*, 247
            Winter's, 251–252, *253*
    in European practice, 238–242
        designs
            Assalini's *conquasator capitis*, 238, *239*
            L.-A. Baudelocque's, 238–240, *239*
            Blot's, 242, *242*
            C. Braun's, *241*, 241–242
            Hennig's *Kephalotryptor à crochets*, 240, *240*
            Kilian's, 240, *240*
            Locarelli's, 241, *241*
            Pajot's, 240, *240*
            Rizzoli's, 241, *241*
            Scanzoni's, 242, *242*
    fenestrated, 245–246
        designs
            F. Barnes's, 246, *246*
            Guyon's, 245, *245*, 251
            Lusk's, 244, 246, *246*
            Martin's, 245, *245*
            J. Smith's, *243*, 245–246
cephalotripsy. *See* cephalotribes
cervix
    dilation, sixteenth-century methods of, 7–8, *8*
    mechanical dilatation of, 215–218. *See also* balloons, for inducing labor
        Bossi's devices, 217, *217–218*
        Preiss's device, 217, *218*
        Walcher's device, 217, *218*
    slow-stretching of, for inducing labor, 214
chain saws, for fetal decapitation, 254–259
    designs
        Blond-Heidler's, 255
        Tarnier's *forceps-scie*, 259, *259*
        Van Huevel's *forceps-scie*, 258–259, *259*
        Joulin's *diviseur céphalique*, 257–258, *258*
Chamberlen family, 9–16
    education of, 11
    family tree of, *10*
    instruments

Chamberlen family, instruments (*continued*)
    fillets, *15*, 199, *200*
    forceps, 15, *15*
        commercial offering of, 13
        design of, 15
        development of, 14–15
        discovery of, 14
        secretive nature of, 13–14
        selling of design, 13, 15–16, 18–19
    levers, *15*, 205, *205*
  members of, 9–13, *10*
    Hugh Senior, 12–13
    Dr. Peter (third generation), 11–12
    Peter the Elder, 9, 11
    Peter the Younger, 9, 11
  public good schemes of, 11–12
  religious beliefs of, 11
  Woodham Mortimer Hall, 11, *11*, 12
Chassagny
  long forceps design, 136, *139*
  noncrossed forceps design, 136, *139*
  rotating forceps design
    description of, 139, *140*
    Trelat's forceps based on, *144*, 145
  sustained traction and
    advocacy of, 150, 155
    forceps à tractions soutenues, *154*, 155
  variety of designs, 136
cleidotomy
  cleidotomy scissors, 256, *257*
comminutors
  basilysts. *See* basilysts
  basiotribes. *See* basiotribes
  cephalotribes. *See* cephalotribes
  crainioclasts. *See* cranioclasts
  craniotomy forceps. *See* craniotomy forceps
  conquasator capitis, 238, *239*
  cranioclasts 247–251. *See also* craniotomy forceps in
    British practice
    designs
      R. Barnes's, *250*, 250–251
      Conquest's, *248*, 249
      D. Davis's, 249
      H. Davis's, *250*, 251
      Holmes's, *248*, 249
      Lever's, *248*
      F. H. Ramsbotham's, *248*, 249
      J. Y. Simpson's, *249*, 249–250
    cephalotribe and. *See* cephalotribes
    difficulties associated with, 242–243

    in European practice
      C. Braun's design, 251, *251*
    function of, 247, 249
    origins of, 247
    terminology, 249
craniometry, intrauterine, 274
craniotomes. *See* craniotomy forceps
craniotomy
  antero-posterior forceps as alternative to, 130
  attitudes to, 234–236
  frequency of, 56t, 236t, 238
  indications for, 238
  role of, 236–238
craniotomy forceps, 234–238. *See also* cranioclasts
  in Arabian medicine, 1–2
  crusher and tractor functions, 234
  designs
    Lyon's, 234, *235*
    nineteenth-century British, *235*
    Mesnard's, 234, *235*
    Ziegler's, 234, *235*
  frequency of use, 236t
  punch forceps for. *See* punch forceps
  traction use, 231
craniotractor, 251
crotchets. *See also* hooks
  birth canal trauma secondary to, 229
  blunt hook and, 211, *211*
  body, D. Davis's design, *229–230*, 230
  double, Smellie's design, *226*, 227, 228, *228*
  drill-crotchet, Eastlake's design, 231–232, *232*
  early eighteenth-century views of, 22, 24
  guarded, 228–230
    D. Davis's design, 229, *229–230*
    Levret's design, *226, 228*, 229
  simple, 227–228
    construction of, *227*, 227–228
    early types of, *226*, 227
    Guillemeau's design, *226*, 227
    operating principles, 227–228
  traction uses, 228
crushing forceps, 2, *2*. *See also* comminutors

Davis, David
  biographical information, 80
  crotchets designed by
    body, *229–230*, 230
    guarded, 229, *229–230*
  embryotomy knife designed by, 257, *257*
  embryulcia instruments designed by, *229–230*, 229–230

Davis, David (*continued*)
    forceps designed by
        American practice, use of, 99, 102–103
        common forceps, 80, *81*
        hinge modification, 80, *81*, 112–113, *113*
        illustration of complete set, *81*
        jointed blade, *83*, 83–84, 122
        measurements, 279t
        previously undescribed models, 84, *84*
        unequal breadth, *82*, 83
        unequal length, *82*, 83
    internal pelvimeter designed by, 269, *269*
    levers designed by, 208, *209*
decapitators. *See also* cephalotomes; embryotomes
    C. Braun's decollator, 254, *255*
    in British practice, 254, *254*
    crotchet, *255*, 256
    designs
        Lever's, 254, *254*
        F. H. Ramsbotham's, 254, *254*
        Scanzoni's *Auchenister*, 256, *257*
        Joulin's *diviseur céphalique*, 257–258, *258*
        Targett's, 254, *254*
    Greco-Roman hook, 1
    saws. *See* saws
detachable forceps handles. *See* handles, detachable
dynamometers
    forceps systems that incorporate
        Delore's pulley, 152, *153*
        Hamon's, 155, *155*
        Joulin's *aide-forceps*, 152, *152–153*
        Kristeller's forceps, 151, *151*
        Poullet's, 156, *156*, *157*
        Pro's, 155, *155*
    function of, 151
    origins of, 150
dystocia, 58t

embryotomes, 254–259. *See also* cephalotomes; decapitators
    designs
        D. Davis's embryotomy knife, 257, *257*
        Jacquemier's, 256, *257*
        Lazarewitch's, 256, *257*
        Stanesco's, *255*
        Tarnier's, 258, *258*
            forceps-scie, 259, *259*
        P. Thomas's, 258, *258*
        Van der Ecken's, *255*
        Van Huevel's *forceps-scie*, 258–259, *259*

embryulcia, 229
    comminutors for. *See* comminutors
    D. Davis's instruments for, 229–230, *229–230*, 257
    R. W. Johnson's instruments for, 231, *231*
ergot, for stimulating labor, 98, 131
extractors, 227–233
    crotchet. *See* crotchet
    designs
        Eastlake's drill-crotchet, 231–232, *232*
        Johnson's *embryulcus*, 231, *231*
        Mauriceau's *tire-tête*, 226, *227*
        Newham's Guide Hook, 232, *232*
        Oldham's vertebra hooks, 232–233, *233*
        Ould's *terebra occulta*, 226, *227*
    talons, 226, *227*
    vacuum. *See* vacuum extractors

falcetta, 262, *263*
fenestrated cephalotribes. *See* cephalotribes, fenestrated
fillets, 199–203
    abandonment of, 199, 205
    in American practice, 204–205
    in Arabian medicine, 1
    difficulties associated with, 199
    in European practice, 204
    flexible steel
        Sheraton's design, *202*, 203
    history of, 199
    introducers, or *porte-lacs*, 201, 204–205
        designs
            L. J. Hubert's, 201, *201*
            Lazarewitch's 201, *201*
            Olivier's, 204, *205*
            Swayne's, 199, *201*
    in Japanese practice, 199, *200*, 204, *205*
    materials for, 199
    in nineteenth-century practice, 203–205
    operating principles, 199, 201
    origins of, 25–26
    soft fillets
        designs
            Chamberlen's, 15, 199, *200*
            L. J. Hubert's, 201, *201*
            Swayne's, 199, *201*
        unidentified types of, 201–202
    whalebone
        designs
            Debenham's double interlocking, 204, *204*
            Eardley-Wilmot's, *202*, 203–204

fillets, whalebone, designs (*continued*)
    Olivier's, 204, *205*
    Westmacott's, *202*, 203
finger lugs. *See* finger rests
finger rests
  origins of, 72–74
  early forceps designs that integrated
    Brunninghausen's 71, *71*, 72
    J. D. Busch's, 72, *73*, 279t
    Levy's, 109, *110*
    Naegele's, 71, *71*, 72, 279t
    J. Y. Simpson's, *93*, 94, *94*, 278t
    Spiegelberg's, 73–74, *74*, 279t
    Stolz's, 72–73, *73*, 279t
foot forceps, 212, *212*
  designs
    Districtsloege's, 212, *212*
    Grönning's, 212, *212*
    Rizzoli's, 212, *212*
forceps, craniotomy. *See* craniotomy forceps
forceps, foot. *See* foot forceps
forceps, lithotomy, 22, *23*
forceps, obstetric
  in American practice
    Baudelocque's influence, 99–102
    Davis's influence, 99, 102–103
    designs
      Bartlett's, 183
      Barton's, 280t
      Bedford's, 103, *104*, 105
      Benjamin's, 189
      Bethell's, 102, *103*
      Burge's, 120, *120*
      Cleeman's, 160, *161*
      W. B. Dewees's, *166*, 167, 193, *193*
      W. P. Dewees's, 99–100, *100*
      Elliot's, *104*–105, *105*, 107, 280t
      Fry's, 126, 128, *129*, 194, *194*
      Gardner's, 183
      Hodge's, 100–102, *101*–*102*, 160
      Huston's, 99, *99*
      T. C. James's, 99, *100*
      Jenks's, *106*, 107
      Jewett's, *106*, 107, 183–184, *184*
      Knight's, *106*, 107
      Knox's, 167, *167*
      Löwenthal's, 121–122, *122*
      Luikart's, 108
      Lusk's, 107, 183, *183*
      McFerran's, 191, *191*
      McGillicuddy's, 193, *193*
      Miller's, *111*, 112
      McLane's, *106*, 107–108
      Neale's, 183, *184*
      Reynolds's, 183
      Robertson's, 103, *103*
      Roler's, 105
      Sawyer's, 102, *103*
      Schuyler's, 103, *104*
      A. H. Smith's, 117, *117*
      Stewart's, *148*, 149
      Studley's, 185, *187*
      I. E. Taylor's, 132–134, *133*
      Tucker-McLane's, *107*, 107–108, 280t
      Vedder's, 191, *191*
      W. Wallace's, 102, *103*
    during early nineteenth century, 99–102
    Meigs's views, 99, 129
    measurements, 280t
    during mid and late nineteenth century, 102–108
    Siebold's influence, *70*, 70–71, 99
  antero-posterior. *See* antero-posterior forceps
  articulation. *See* articulation
  asymmetric. *See* asymmetric forceps
  axis-traction. *See* axis-traction forceps
  in British practice
    barriers to use, 57
    designs
      D. W. Aitken's, 178, *179*
      J. Aitken's, 54, *55*, 72, 147, *147*, 275t
      Anderson's, 96, *96*, 97, 278t
      Aveling's, 163, *163*
      Barclay's, 125, *125*, 276t
      R. Barnes's, 94–96, *95*, 175, 278t
      J. Beatty's, 123, *123*, 276t
      T. E. Beatty's, 88, *88*, 277t
      Blenkarne's, 116–117, *116*
      Blundell's, 49–50, 277t
      Braithwaite's, 89–90, *90*, 277t
      Bredin's, 109, *111*, 112
      Bowers's, 147–149, *148*
      Burton's, 37–38, *38*
      Cameron's, 194, *194*, 281t
      C. J. Campbell's, 134, *135*
      Cappie's, *114*, 115
      Chamberlen's, 14–16, *15*
      Chapman's, 25–26, *25*–*26*, 28, 275t
      Christie's, 164, *164*
      Churchill's, 87–88, *88*, 277t
      Clark's, 85, *86*, 276t

forceps, in British practice, designs (*continued*)
    Collin's, 54, *54*, 277t
    Conquest's, 113–115, *114*, 277t
    Cullingworth's, 175–177
    Davis's, 80–84, *81–84*. *See also* Davis, David
    Denman's, 47–48, *48*, 275t
    Dick's, 130, *130*
    Draper's, 121, *121*
    Drinkwater's, 24
    Duncan's, 94, *95*, 278t
    Foulis's, 185, *186*
    Freke's, 27, *27*
    Galabin's, 129–130, 164, *164*, 280t
    Gayton's, 86–87, *87*
    Giffard's, 27, *27*–28
    Gordon's, 115
    Grattan's, 191–193, *192*
    Greenhalgh's, 86, *86*, 87
    Haighton's, 47, *47*, 275t
    A. Hamilton's, *53*, 53–54, 112, *113*, 276t
    Harper's, 125
    Haslam's, 116, *116*
    Hewitt's, 88, *88*
    Hilliard's, 185, *186*
    Holland's, 163–164, *163*
    Hopkin's, 85–86, *86*
    R. W. Johnson's, 52–53, *53*, 112, 160, *161*, 276t
    Leake's, 126, *127*
    Le Page's, 191–193, *193*
    Lowder's, 47, *47*, 275t
    Macdonald's, 191, *192*
    McLaurin's, *188*, 189
    Mackness's, 179, *179*
    Madden's, 88–89, *180*, 181
    Mathew's, 177, *178*, 281t
    Murphy's, 89, *89*
    Murray's, *176*, 177, 280t
    Neville's, 185, *186*, 187
    Oldham's, 94, *95*
    Orme's, 47, *47*, 275t
    Osborn's, *50–51*, 50–52, 276t
    Pearse's, 109, *111*, 165, *165*
    Pugh's, 28, *29*, 276t
    Radford's, 90–91, *91*, 278t
    F. H. Ramsbotham's, 91–93, *92*, 277t, 278t
    Reid's, 128–129, *129*
    Rigby's, 93
    A. R. Simpson's, *174*, 175, *175*, 280t
    J. Y. Simpson's, 93–94, *93–94*, 277t
    Sloan's, 130–131, *130*
    Smellie's, 34–37, *35–37*, 161, 275t. *See also* Smellie, William
    Swayne's, 131
    G. Taylor's, 165, *165*
    Thynne's, 52, *52*, 276t
    Vacher's, 121, *121*
    Wagstaff's, 164–165, *164*, 280t
    Walker's, 28, *29*, 275t
    Waller's, 90, *91*
    Weiss's, *146*, 147
    Wrigley's, *97*
    Young's, 52–53, *53*, 276t
    Ziegler's, 123, *124*, 276t
compression control. *See also* labimeters
    methods of, 74–78
conservative use, 56–58
Edinburgh School, 52–54, 276t
eighteenth century clinical applications of, 27–28
Evans of Oswestry's contributions, 54
history of, 24–28
    Hunter's contributions, 38–39
in European practice
    designs
        Assalini's, 141, *141–142*, 279t
        J. L. Baudelocque's, 60, 62–63, *62–63*, 99
        Baumers's, 126, *128*
        Bernard's, *142*, 143
        Bing's 112, *113*
        Boër's, 74
        C. Braun's, 181, *181*
        Breus's, 181, *182*, 281t
        Brulatour's, 118–119, *119*
        Brunninghausen's, 71, *71*
        D. W. H. Busch's, 72
        J. D. Busch's, 72, *73*, 279t
        Carof's, 115–116, *115*
        Cazeaux's, 65, *65*
        Chassagny's, 136, 139, *139*, *140*, 154, 155
        Coutouly's, 60, *61*, 117–118, *118*
        Delore's, 151, *152*, 153
        Demelin's, 182, *182*
        De Wind's, 30
        A. Dubois's, 63, *64*, 279t
        P. Dubois's, 63–64, *64*, 279t
        Dusée's, 28–30, *31*, 32, 279t
        Felsenreich's, 181, *182*
        Flamant's, 65
        Fries's, *77*, 77
        Froriep's, 76–77, *77*

forceps, in European practice, designs (*continued*)
    Grégoire's, 28, *30*, 39
    Guillon's, 78, *78*
    Hamon's, *144*, 145, 155, *155*
    Hartmann's, 169, *169*
    Hermann's, 167–168, *167*
    Hohl's, 68, *69*
    E. Hubert's, 168–169, *169*
    L. J. Hubert's, 168, *168*, *169*
    Kristeller's, 151, *151*
    Laroyenne's, 162, *162*
    Lazarewitch's, 145, *145*, 279t
    Levret's, 39–44, *40*–*43*, 279t. *See also* Levret, André
    Levy's, 109, *110*
    Lyon's, 177–178, *179*
    E. Martin's, 68, *70*, 70
    Mattei's, 134, *135*, 142, *143*
    Maygrier's, 78
    Mende's, 76, *77*
    Mesnard's, 136, *137*
    Mondotte's, 143–145, *143*
    Moralès's, 165, *165*
    Moreau's, 64, *65*
    Mursinna's, 68, *68*
    Naegele's, *71*, 71–72, 92, 279t
    Osiander's, 67, *67*
    Pajot's, 119, *119*–*120*
    Palfyn's, 16–17, *16*–*17*, 32, 39
    Péan's, 60, *64*
    J. L. Petit's, 75, *75*
    Piet's, 60
    Poullet's, 134, *135*, 139–141, *140*, *141*, 156, *157*, 165–167, *166*
    Prague school, 59, 60, 279t
    Rathlauw's, *18*, 19
    Ritgen's, 132, *133*
    Roussel's, *153*
    Sänger's, 162, *162*–*163*, 181
    Saxtorph's, 109, *110*
    Schlichting's, *18*, 19–20
    Siebold's, E. von, *70*, 70–71
    Spiegelberg's, 73–74, *74*, 279t
    Stein's, 75, *76*
    Stolz's, 72–73, *73*, 279t
    Tarnier's, 170–173, *171*, *172*, 280t
    Tarsitani's, 66, *66*
    Thenance's, 66–67, 136, *138*
    Trelat's, *144*, 145
    Uytterhoven's, 126, *128*
    Valette's, 136, *139*
    Weissbrod's, 67, *67*
  with folding blades. *See* blades, forceps
forceps delivery
  British conservatism regarding, 55–58, 56t
  in eighteenth- and nineteenth-century practice, 55–56
  in European practice, 56, 56t
  frequency of, 57t
  in Irish practice, 56, 56t
  Simpson's view of, 94
forceps-scie
  description of, 258
    Tarnier's design, 259, *259*
    Van Huevel's design, 258–259, *259*
with interchangeable blades. *See* blades, forceps
with interlocking male and female blades. *See* blades, forceps
with jointed blade. *See* blades, forceps
with labimeters. *See* labimeters
long. *See* long forceps
origins of
  Chamberlen family's role in. *See* Chamberlen family
  Johannes Palfyn's contributions, 16–17, *16*–*17*, 32, 39
  Van Roonhuysen family's role in, 17–21
parallel. *See* parallel forceps
with pelvic curve. *See* pelvic curve
with pressure-regulating devices. *See* pressure-regulating devices
rotating. *See* blades, rotating
short. *See* short forceps
with short and long handles. *See* handles, detachable
stepped. *See* stepped forceps
forceps longa et tersa, 8, *8*
forceps, punch. *See* punch forceps
fumigation
  for dead fetus extraction, 7
  for placenta extraction, 7

Greco-Roman surgical instruments, 1

handles
  curved
    in British practice, 163–165
    designs
      Aveling's forceps with, 163, *163*
      Christie's forceps with, 164, *164*
      Galabin's forceps with, 164, *164*, 280t
      Holland's forceps with, *163*, 163–164
      G. Taylor's forceps with, 165, *165*

handles, curved, designs (*continued*)
    Wagstaff's forceps with, *164*, 164–165, 280t
  development of, 163
  detachable. *See also* blades, interchangeable
    designs
      Bing's, 112, *113*
      Cappie's, *114*, 115
      Carof's, *115*, 115–116
      Conquest's, 113–115, *114*, 277t
      Coutouly's, 117–118, *118*
      A. H. Smith's, 117, *117*
      F. H. Stuart's, 117, *117*
      Valette's, 136, *139*
    for facilitating insertion of forceps, 112, *113*
  hinged
    description of, 109, *110–111*, 112
    designs
      Bing's, 112, *113*
      Blenkarne's, *116*, 116–117
      Braithwaite's, 89–90, *90*, 121, 277t
      Bredin's, 109, *111*, 112
      Cappie's, *114*, 115
      Carof's, *115*, 115–116
      Davis's, 112–113, *113*
      Draper's, 121, *121*
      Freke's, 27, *27*, 109
      A. Hamilton's, 112, *113*
      J. Hamilton's, 112, *113*
      Haslam's, *116*, 116
      Levy's, 109, *110*
      Miller's, *111*, 112
      Pearse's, 109, *111*
      Saxtorph's, 109, *110*
      Vacher's, 121, *121*
      Valette's, 136, *139*
    for facilitating insertion of forceps, 112, *113*
    origins of, 109
    transport and storage benefits, 109–112, *110–111*
  interchangeable
    history of, 117
    A. H. Smith's design, 117, *117*
    F. H. Stuart's design, 117, *117*
    short and long, 117, *117*
head crushers. *See* cephalotribes
hebotomy. *See* pubiotomy
herbal remedies, 22
hinged handles. *See* handles, hinged
hooks. *See also* crotchets
  blunt
    abandonment of, 211

    crotchets and, 211, *211*
    history of, 211
    in nineteenth-century practice, 211, *211*
    interchangeable, 211, *211*
  Greco-Roman, 1
  guide, Newham's, 232, *232*
  Paré's, *226*, 227
  traction. *See* axis traction, tractor attachments
  vertebra, Oldham's, 232–233, *233*
hydrostatic bags, for inducing labor
  designs
    R. Barnes's, 215, *215*
    De Ribe's, 215–216, *215–216*
    Tarnier's *ballon*, 216
    Voorhees's, 216, *217*

induction and stimulation of labor
  in American practice, 216–217
  in British practice, 213–214
  disagreements regarding, 213
  ergot for, 98
  in European practice, 213
  indications, 213
  methods for
    artificial rupture of membranes, 214, *214*
      Lee's perforator, 213–214, *214*
    intracervical rubber balloons. *See* hydrostatic bags
    laminaria tents, 214
    mechanical dilatation of cervix. *See* cervix, mechanical dilatation of
    medical methods, 214
  premature, 48, 213
instruments. *See also specific instrument*
  herbal remedies *versus*, 22
interchangeable blades. *See* blades, forceps, interchangeable
intracervical rubber balloons, for inducing labor. *See* hydrostatic bags

Kephalotryptor, Martin's, *70*
Kephalotryptor à crochets, Hennig's, 240, *240*

labimeters. *See also* pressure-regulating devices
  designs
    J. D. Busch's, *75*, 75
    Guillon's, 78, *78*
    Maygrier's, 78
    Mende's, *76*, 77
    Stein's, 75, *76*

labimeters (*continued*)
    introduction of, 75
lamineur céphalique, 257, 257–258
lateral mortise articulation, 70–72
leniceps
    Mattei's design, *142*, 143
    Mondotte's modifications, *143*, 143, 145
levers
    application, guidelines for, 208
    in British practice, 207–208
        designs
            Chamberlen's, *15*, 205, *205*
            D. Davis's, 208, *209*
            Gaitskell's, 208
            Radford's interchangeable set, *211*
    in European practice, 207
        designs
            Herbiniaux's, 219, *220*
            L. J. Hubert's, *206*, 207
            Mauriceau's, 206
            Van Roonhuysen family's, 20, *20–21*, 205, *206*
    fenestrated blade use, 207–208
    flexible
        J. Aitken's, *209*, 209–210, 226, *227*
        Robertson's, 210, *210*
        Weiss's, 210, *210*
    folding, *207*, 207–208
    geographical differences in designs, 206–207
    history of, 205
    methods of use, 206
    origins of, 20
Levret, André
    biographical information, 39
    childbirth recommendations, 43–44
    forceps of, 39–44, *40–43*
        French modifications from, 59–66
        pelvic curve, 39, 43, *43*
        recommendations regarding use of, 43–44
        Smellie's design and, comparisons between, 43, *43*
        measurements, 279t
    guarded crotchet, *228*, 229
    instruments designed by, 39
    pelvimetry contributions, 265
    tire-tête, 39, *40*, *41*
lithotomy forceps, 22, *23*
locks. *See* articulations
long forceps. *See also* individual types and designs and appendix of measurements
    in American practice, 98–107
        measurements, 280t

    designs. *See* forceps designs
    with diverging shanks. *See* shanks, diverging
    in European practice
        measurements, 279t, 280t, 281t
        origins. *See* Levret
    with hinged shanks. *See* shanks, hinged
    limitations of, 93, 170
    in nineteenth-century British practice, 90–97
        axis traction. *See* axis traction
        changing designs, 90
        characteristics of, 90
        definitions, 90, 93–94
        long curved, 90–96, *91–97*, 278t
        long straight, 90, *91*, 277t
        measurements, 93–94, 277t–278t
            Rigby's criteria, 92, 93
    with parallel shanks. *See* shanks, parallel

man-midwives
    in American practice, 98
    in British practice, 47–52
    cartoon images of, 45, *46*
    criticisms of, 37, 45
    educational courses for, 98
    evolution of, 32
    factors influencing the development of, 33
    midwives opposition to, 36–37, 45
    in seventeenth-century France, 13, 22
metreurynters. *See* hydrostatic bags
midwifery
    ancient teaching regarding, 3–4
    Catholicism effects on, 4
    in early nineteenth-century practice, 45
    early texts regarding, 3–8, *6*, *7–8*
    in fourteenth-century practice, 4
    male involvement in, 5, 22. *See also* man-midwives
    in Middle Ages, 3–8
    in seventeenth-century practice, 4
    in sixteenth-century practice, 4, 6–8
midwives
    ancient functions of, 5
    education of, 5, 45
    male. *See* man-midwives
    opposition to man-midwives, 36–37, 45
    in sixteenth-century practice, 5
    textbooks for, 5–8
Midwives Act of 1902, 9

noncrossed forceps. *See* parallel forceps

operative delivery
  British conservatism regarding, 55–58, 56t
  in eighteenth- and nineteenth-century practice, 55–56
  in European practice, 56, 56t, 59
  frequency of, 57t, 58
  in Irish practice, 56, 56t
Osiander, maneuver devised by, 160, *161*, 173
osteotomists
  Davis's designs
    cutting force of, 236
    indications for, 236
    longitudinal, *237*
    oval, *237*

Pajot's maneuver, 160, *161*, 167
parallel forceps, 136–149
  in American practice, 149
    Stewart's design, *148*, 149
  in British practice, 147–148
    designs
      J. Aitken's, 147, *147*, 275t
      Bowers's, 147–149, *148*
      McLaurin's, *188*, 189
      Weiss's, *146*, 147
  in European practice, 136–146
    designs
      Assalini's, 141, *141*–*142*, 279t
      Bernard's, *142*, 143
      Chassagny's, 136, *139*, *140*, 141
      Hamon's, *144*, 145
      Lazarewitch's, 145, *145*, 279t
      Mattei's, *134*, *135*, *142*, 143
      Mesnard's, 136, *137*
      Mondotte's, *143*, 143, 145
      Poullet's, 139–141, *140*
      Thenance's, 66–67, 136, *138*
      Trelat's, *144*, 145
      Valette's 136, *139*
parallel shanks. *See* shanks, parallel
pelvic curve of forceps blades
  description of, 28, *33*
  limitations of, 93
  origins of
    Levret's contribution, 39, *40*, *41*, 43, *43*
    Pugh's contribution, 28
    Smellie's contribution, 36, *36*
  in trephine perforators, 225, *225*
pelvimeters. *See also* pelvimetry
  combined external and internal
    designs
      J. Aitken's, 265, *266*
      Boyer's, *271*
      Charrière's, 272, *272*
      Collin's, 272, *272*
      Germann's, 272
      Küstner's, 272, *273*
      Lazarewitch's, 272, *272*
      Rizzoli's, 272, *272*
      Van Huevel's, 271–272
  external
    designs
      Arnold's, 267, *267*
      J. L. Baudelocque's, 265, *266*
      Collyer's, 267, *267*
      Dugès's, 267
      Duncan's, 266, *267*
      Martin's, 266, *267*
      Milliken's, *267*
      Stein's *grand pelvimètre*, 270, *271*
  internal
    designs
      Asdrubaldi's, 269
      Cadran's, *268*
      Coutouly's, 265, *266*
      Davis's, 269, *269*
      Earle's, *268*, 269
      Ferguson's, *268*, 269
      Greenhalgh's, *268*, 269
      Harris's, 269, *269*
      Howitz's, *270*, 271
      Mayer and Meltzer's, *268*, 269
      Stein's *petit pelvimètre*, 270, *271*
pelvimetry. *See also* pelvimeters
  acceptance of, 273–274
  in British practice, 265–267, 268–269, *269*
  in European practice, 265, *266*, 270, *271*
  history of, 265
  in nineteenth-century practice, 265–274
  intrauterine craniometry and, 274
  radiological, 274
  rudimentary methods of, 273
pelviotomy. *See* pubiotomy
perce-crâne, Mauriceau's, 22
perforators, 219–225
  double crossover
    designs
      Greenhalgh's, *222*, 223
      Holmes's, *222*, 223
      Oldham's, 221–223, *222*

perforators (*continued*)
   membrane. *See* artificial rupture of membranes
   method of use, 225
   screw-operated
      Weiss's design, 223, *223*
   spear
      description of, 220–221
      designs
         R. W. Johnson's, 231, *231*
         Mauriceau's, 226, *227*
         Ould's, 226, *227*
         Robertson's, *220*
   spring-loaded
      designs
         Blot's, 223, *223*
         Duncan's, 223, *223*
         Godson's, 223, *223*
         Jones's, 222, *223*
         Naegele's, 223, *223*
         J. Y. Simpson's, 222, *223*
   trephine
      description of, 225
      designs
         Assalini's, *224*, 225
         Braun's, *224*, 225
         Jörg's, *224*, 225
         Mende's, *224*, 225
      operating principles of, 225
   wedge-scissor, 221
      description of, 221
      designs
         Cleveland's, 221, *221*
         Denman's, *220*, 221
         Smellie's, *220*, 221
perineal steps, in shank. *See* stepped forceps
placenta expulsion, ancient methods, 7
podalic version, 4–5, 22, 49, 219
Poullet, J.
   axis-traction forceps design, 165–167, *166*
   forceps général, 134, *135*
   forceps souple à tractions indépendantes, 156, *157*
   mechanical tractor design, 156, *157*
   noncrossed forceps design, 139–141, *140*
   sericeps design, 156, *156*
pressure-regulating devices. *See also* labimeters
   designs
      J. Aitken's, 54, *55*, 75
      Elliot's, *104*, 105, 107
      Evans's, 75
      Fries's, 77, *77*

      Froriep's, 76, 77, *77*
      Mende's, 76, 77
      Petit's, 75, *75*
   function of, 74–75
pubiotomy (hebiotomy), 262
   J. Aitken's saw for, 262, *264*
   definition of, 262
   Gigli's saw for, 262
   origins of, 262
pulvis parturiens, 98
punch forceps
   C. L. Anderson's design, 236, *238*
   Davis's osteotomists, 236, *237*

rotating blades. *See* blades, rotating
rostrum anatis, 8

saws, for fetal decapitation
   Blond-Heidler's, 255
   Gigli's, 255
   Tarnier's *forceps-scie*, 259, *259*
   Van Huevel's *forceps-scie*, 258–259, *259*
   Jacquemier's, 256, *257*
   Joulin's *diviseur céphalique*, 257–258, *258*
shanks
   diverging, in Irish practice, 87–89
      description of, 87
      designs
         T. E. Beatty's, 88, *88*, 277t
         Churchill's, 87–88, *88*, 277t
         Hewitt's, 88, *88*, 277t
         Madden's, 88–89
   hinged, in axis-traction forceps, 191–194. *See also*
      blades, hinged; handles, hinged
      description of, 191
      designs
         Grattan's, 191–193, *192*
         Macdonald's, 191, *192*
         McFerran's, 191, *191*
         McGillicuddy's, 193, *193*
         Vedder's, 191, *191*
      purpose of, 191
   parallel
      introduction in Britain, 90
      introduction in America, 105–107
short forceps. *See also individual types and designs and appendix of measurements*
   in American practice, 99
   in British practice, 47–54

short forceps (*continued*)
    introduction by Smellie, 34
    introduction of pelvic curve, 36
    methods of use, 86–87, 89
    during late eighteenth, early nineteenth century
        in Dublin, 54
        in Edinburgh, 52–54
        in London, 47–52
    during mid nineteenth century, 85–87
    compressive force of, 89
    measurements, 129, 276t
    methods of use, 89
Simpson, A. R.
    axis-traction forceps, *174–175*, 175, 280t
        Cullingworth's modifications, 175–177
        Felsenreich's modifications, 181, *182*
    basilyst designed by, 251, *252*
    classification of destructive instruments, 234
Simpson, J. Y.
    air tractor design, 195–197, *196*. *See also* vacuum extractors
    destructive instruments designed by
        cephalotribe, 242–243, *243*
        cranioclasts, 249–250, *249*
        perforators, 222, *223*
    long forceps designed by, 93–94, *93–94*
        C. L. Anderson's modifications, 96, *96*, *97*, 278t
        R. Barnes's modifications, 94, *95*, 278t
        Duncan's modifications, 94, *95*, 278t
        Oldham's modifications, 94, *95*
        measurements, *93*, *94*, 278t
    short straight forceps designed by, 93, *93*, 277t
skull base, crushing of
    instruments for. *See* basilysts; cranioclasts
Smellie, William
    advertisements regarding courses offered by, 34, *34*
    biographical information, 33–34
    criticisms of, 36–38, 45
    double crotchet designed by, 226, 228, *228*
    forceps designed by, 34–37, *35–37*
        curved forceps, 36, *37*
        "English lock," 34
        history of, 33–34
        Levret's design and, comparisons between, 43, *43*
        measurements, 35–36, 275t
        modifications, 35–36
        pelvic curve modification, 36, *37*
        recommendations regarding use of, 34–35
        straight forceps, 35
        wooden design, 34, *35*

    pelvimetry contributions, 265
    self-assessments of work, 34
    Treatise on the Theory and Practice of Midwifery, 34
spear perforators. *See* perforators, spear
speculum matricis, 7, 8
sphenotresia. *See* basilysts
stepped forceps. *See also* handles, curved
    in American practice
        W. B. Dewees's design, *166*, 167, 193
        Knox's design, 167, *167*
    in British practice
        designs
            Aveling's, 163, *163*
            Christie's, 164, *164*
            Galabin's, 164, *164*, 280t
            Pearse's, 165, *165*
            G. Taylor's, 165, *165*
            Wagstaff's, 164, *164*–165, 280t
            Wales's, 164–165
    development of, 163
    in European practice
        designs
            Hermann's, 167–168, *167*
            E. Hubert's, 168–169, *169*
            Moralès's *forceps à trois courbures*, 165, *165*
            Poullet's, 165, *166*
stone forceps, 22, *23*
suction tractor, for vacuum extraction of fetus. *See* vacuum extractors
symphysiotomy. *See also* pubiotomy
    Aitken's saw for, 263–264, *264*
    in American practice, 262–263
    Bar de Luc's saw for, 262
    Baudelocque's analysis of, 260
    in British practice, 263–264
    in European practice, 260–262
    history of, 260–261
    indications for, 264
    maternal mortality from, 260–261
    origins of, 260
    problems associated with, 260
    techniques for
        J. Aitken's, 263–264, *264*
        French, 261, *261*
        Garrigues's, 261–262, *262*
        Italian, 261
        Neapolitan, 261–262, *262*
        Sigault's, 260
    versus Caesarian section, 260, 264

talons, *226, 227*
tapes (lacs), 160, *162*–163
Tarnier, Etienne Stéphane,
    axis-traction forceps designed by, 170–173, *171–172*, 280t
        early designs, 170, *171*
        forceps à branches croisées et à manches immobiles, *171*
        later designs, *172*, 173
        American response to, 173, 175
        British response to, 173
        European response to, 173
        modifications based on. *See also individual types and designs and appendix of measurements*
            American, 183–184, *183–184*
            British, *174*, 175–181, *175–176, 178–180*
            European, 181–182, *181–182*
    forceps-scie, 259, *259*
terebra occulta, *226, 227*
tire-tête
    designs
        Amand's, 22, *23*
        Levret's, 39, *40–41*
        Mauriceau's, 22, *23*, *226, 227*
    traction uses, 231
traction
    aids for. *See also* axis traction; tapes; tractors
    auto-traction
        description of, 158
        Giordano's *forcipe a staffe briglie*, 158, *158*
        Roussel's report of, 158, *158*
    craniotomy forceps for, 231
    force
        devices for measuring. *See* dynamometers
        Pajot's maneuver for improving, 160, *161*, 167
        pulley system for, 152, *153*
        tapes effect on, 160, *162*
    sustained (*tractions soutenues*)
        Chassagny's advocacy of, 150, 155
        Chassagny's *forceps à tractions soutenues*, *154*, 155
        Delores's system, 152–155, *153*
        Hamon's device for, 155–156, *155*
        Joulin's *aide-forceps* for, 152, *152–153*
        Mattei's device for, 152, *152*
        Poullet's *forceps souple à tractions independantes*, 156, *157*
        Poullet's *sericeps*, 156, *156*
        Pro's portable tractor, 155, *155*
        Roussel's *aide-forceps*, *153*

tractors. *See also* axis-traction forceps, traction attachments; traction
    basilyst-tractor, *252*
    mechanical. *See* traction, sustained
transforator, 251, *252*
trephine perforators. *See* perforators, trephine
turning rods, *202, 203*

United Company of Barber-Surgeons, 5, 9

vacuum extractors, 195–198
    designs
        Kuntzsch's *Vakuumhelm*, 198
        McCahey's, 198, *198*
        Saleh's, 197, *197*
        J. Y. Simpson's air tractor, 195–197
            abandonment of, 197
            clinical uses, 196
            criticism of, 196
            operating principles of, 195
            specifications, 195
        Stillman's, 197–198, *198*
    evolution of, 195
    Mitchell's claim, 196
    principle of, 195
    Yonge's cupping glass, 195
Van Roonhuysen family, 17–21
    lever design, 20, *20*, 206, *206*
    possible link with Chamberlen family, 18–19
    Rathlauw's association with, 19
    Schlichting's claim, 19
vectis. *See* levers
vertebra hooks
    Oldham's design, 232–233, *233*

whalebone fillets. *See* fillets, whalebone
wire écraseurs, 254–255. *See also* forceps-scie

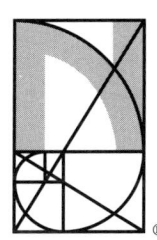

THE OBSTETRICIAN'S ARMAMENTARIUM was printed by Braun Brumfield, Inc., of Ann Arbor, Michigan, on acid-free 70-pound paper. The text was set in Pagemaker 6.5 by Paul Benkman of Tiki Bob Publishing & Design, San Francisco, using Minion and Syntax typefaces from Adobe Systems.

Members of the staff at Norman Publishing who participated in this project were Justin E. Aff, Editorial Assistant; Natalie J. Coleman, Editorial Assistant; Jeremy M. Norman, Publisher; and Martha Nicholson Steele, Managing Editor. The edition was completed in April 2000.